Biochemical Actions of Hormones

Volume XII

Contributors

SALVATORE M. ALOJ

MICHAEL ANTONIOU

CARTER BANCROFT

MIHIR R. BANERJEE

ELMUS G. BEALE

PETER F. BLACKMORE

SUZANNE BOURGEOIS

MARTIN L. BROCK

STEPHEN E. BUXSER

OLIVIER CIVELLI

J. H. CLARK

DANIELA CORDA

PRISCILLA S. DANNIES

JAMES DOUGLASS

RONALD M. EVANS

JOHN H. EXTON

JUDITH C. GASSON

GREGORY G. GICK

DARYL K. GRANNER

EVELYN F. GROLLMAN

EDWARD HERBERT

GARY L. JOHNSON

MARCIA E. JOHNSON

LEONARD D. KOHN

CLAUDIO MARCOCCI

B. M. MARKAVERICH

GERARD MARTENS

DIANA MARVER

KELLY E. MAYO

GEOFFREY H. MURDOCH

RICHARD D. PALMITER

PATRICIA PUMA

HAIM ROSEN

MICHAEL G. ROSENFELD

CARLO M. ROTELLA

DAVID J. SHAPIRO

ROBERTO TOCCAFONDI

DONATELLA TOMBACCINI

BRUCE A. WHITE

R. C. WINNEKER

Biochemical Actions of Hormones

Edited by GERALD LITWACK

Fels Research Institute
Health Sciences Center
School of Medicine
Temple University
Philadelphia, Pennsylvania

VOLUME XII

1985

ACADEMIC PRESS, INC.
(Harcourt Brace Jovanovich, Publishers)

Orlando   San Diego   New York   London

Toronto   Montreal   Sydney   Tokyo

ACADEMIC PRESS, INC.
Orlando, Florida 32887

United Kingdom Edition published by
ACADEMIC PRESS INC. (LONDON) LTD.
24–28 Oval Road, London NW1 7DX

Library of Congress Cataloging in Publication Data
(Revised for vol. 12)
Main entry under title:

Biochemical actions of hormones.

    Includes bibliographies and indexes.
    1. Hormones––Collected works. I. Litwack, Gerald.
II. Axelrod, Julius. Date.   [DNLM: 1. Hormones.
2. Physiology. WK 102 B615]
QP571.B56   574.19'27   70–107567
ISBN 0–12–452812–0 (v. 12)

PRINTED IN THE UNITED STATES OF AMERICA

85 86 87 88   9 8 7 6 5 4 3 2 1

Contents

1.   Generation of Diversity of Opioid Peptides

Edward Herbert, Olivier Civelli, James Douglass,
Gerard Martens, and Haim Rosen

2.   Polypeptide Hormone Regulation of Prolactin Gene Transcription

Geoffrey H. Murdoch, Ronald M. Evans, and
Michael G. Rosenfeld

7. Mechanisms Involved in the Actions of Calcium-Dependent Hormones

Peter F. Blackmore and John H. Exton

8. Steroid and Polypeptide Hormone Interaction in Milk-Protein Gene Expression

Mihir R. Banerjee and Michael Antoniou

9. Control of Prolactin Production by Estrogen

Priscilla S. Dannies

10. Genetic and Epigenetic Bases of Glucocorticoid Resistance in Lymphoid Cell Lines

Suzanne Bourgeois and Judith C. Gasson

Contents

Contributors

Numbers in parentheses indicate the pages on which the authors' contributions begin.

Salvatore M. Aloj (457), Section on the Biochemistry of Cell Regulation, Laboratory of Biochemical Pharmacology, National Institute of Arthritis, Diabetes, Digestive and Kidney Diseases, National Institutes of Health, Bethesda, Maryland 20205

Michael Antoniou (237), Tumor Biology Laboratory, School of Biological Sciences, University of Nebraska-Lincoln, Lincoln, Nebraska 68588

Carter Bancroft (173), Molecular Biology and Virology Department, Sloan Kettering Institute, New York, New York 10021

Mihir R. Banerjee (237), Tumor Biology Laboratory, School of Biological Sciences, University of Nebraska-Lincoln, Lincoln, Nebraska 68588

Elmus G. Beale* (89), Diabetes and Endocrinology Research Center, Departments of Internal Medicine and Biochemistry, Veterans Administration Medical Center, The University of Iowa College of Medicine, Iowa City, Iowa 52240

Peter F. Blackmore (215), Howard Hughes Medical Institute and Department of Physiology, Vanderbilt University School of Medicine, Nashville, Tennessee 37232

Suzanne Bourgeois (311), Regulatory Biology Laboratory, The Salk Institute for Biological Studies, San Diego, California 92138

Martin L. Brock† (139), Department of Biochemistry, University of Illinois, Urbana, Illinois 61801

*Present address: Department of Anatomy, Texas Tech University Health Science Center, School of Medicine, Lubbock, Texas 79430.
†Present address: Imperial Cancer Research Fund Laboratories, P.O. Box 123, Lincoln Inn Fields, London WC2A 3PX, England.

Stephen E. Buxser* (433), Department of Biochemistry, University of Massachusetts Medical Center, Worcester, Massachusetts 01605

Olivier Civelli (1), Department of Chemistry, University of Oregon, Eugene, Oregon 97403

J. H. Clark (353), Department of Cell Biology, Baylor College of Medicine, Houston, Texas 77030

Daniela Corda (457), Section on the Biochemistry of Cell Regulation, Laboratory of Biochemical Pharmacology, National Institute of Arthritis, Diabetes, Digestive and Kidney Diseases, National Institutes of Health, Bethesda, Maryland 20205

Priscilla S. Dannies (289), Department of Pharmacology, Yale University School of Medicine, New Haven, Connecticut 06510

James Douglass (1), Department of Chemistry, University of Oregon, Eugene, Oregon 97403

Ronald M. Evans (37), Molecular Biology and Virology Laboratory, The Salk Institute for Biological Studies, San Diego, California 92138

John H. Exton (215), Howard Hughes Medical Institute and Department of Physiology, Vanderbilt University School of Medicine, Nashville, Tennessee 37232

Judith C. Gasson (311), Division of Hematology-Oncology, Department of Medicine, UCLA School of Medicine, Los Angeles, California 90024

Gregory G. Gick (173), Molecular Biology and Virology Department, Sloan Kettering Institute, New York, New York 10021

Daryl K. Granner† (89), Diabetes and Endocrinology Research Center, Departments of Internal Medicine and Biochemistry, Veterans Administration Medical Center, The University of Iowa College of Medicine, Iowa City, Iowa 52240

*Present address: Pharmaceutical Research and Development, Cell Biology Research Group, The Upjohn Company, Kalamazoo, Michigan 49001.

†Present address: Department of Physiology, Vanderbilt University, Nashville, Tennessee 37232.

Evelyn F. Grollman (457), Section on the Biochemistry of Cell Regulation, Laboratory of Biochemical Pharmacology, National Institute of Arthritis, Diabetes, Digestive and Kidney Diseases, National Institutes of Health, Bethesda, Maryland 20205

Edward Herbert (1), Department of Chemistry, University of Oregon, Eugene, Oregon 97403

Gary L. Johnson (433), Department of Biochemistry, University of Massachusetts Medical Center, Worcester, Massachusetts 01605

Marcia E. Johnson (173), Molecular Biology and Virology Department, Sloan Kettering Institute, New York, New York 10021

Leonard D. Kohn (457), Section on the Biochemistry of Cell Regulation, Laboratory of Biochemical Pharmacology, National Institute of Arthritis, Diabetes, Digestive and Kidney Diseases, National Institutes of Health, Bethesda, Maryland 20205

Claudio Marcocci* (457), Section on the Biochemistry of Cell Regulation, Laboratory of Biochemical Pharmacology, National Institute of Arthritis, Diabetes, Digestive and Kidney Diseases, National Institutes of Health, Bethesda, Maryland 20205

B. M. Markaverich (353), Department of Cell Biology, Baylor College of Medicine, Houston, Texas 77030

Gerard Martens (1), Department of Chemistry, University of Oregon, Eugene, Oregon 97403

Diana Marver (385), Departments of Internal Medicine and Biochemistry, University of Texas Health Science Center, Southwestern Medical School, Dallas, Texas 75235

Kelly E. Mayo† (69), Howard Hughes Medical Institute and Department of Biochemistry, University of Washington, Seattle, Washington 98195

Geoffrey H. Murdoch (37), Eukaryotic Regulatory Biology Program,

*Present address: Cattedra di Endocrinologia e Medicina Costituzionale, Universitá di Pisa, Via Roma 67, 56100 Pisa, Italy.
†Present address: Molecular Biology and Virology Laboratory, The Salk Institute for Biological Studies, San Diego, California 92138.

School of Medicine, University of California, San Diego, La Jolla, California 92037

Richard D. Palmiter (69), Howard Hughes Medical Institute and Department of Biochemistry, University of Washington, Seattle, Washington 98195

Patricia Puma* (433), Department of Biochemistry, University of Massachusetts Medical Center, Worcester, Massachusetts 01605

Haim Rosen (1), Department of Chemistry, University of Oregon, Eugene, Oregon 97403

Michael G. Rosenfeld (37), Eukaryotic Regulatory Biology Program, School of Medicine, University of California, San Diego, La Jolla, California 92037

Carlo M. Rotella (457), Section on the Biochemistry of Cell Regulation, Laboratory of Biochemical Pharmacology, National Institute of Arthritis, Diabetes, Digestive and Kidney Diseases, National Institutes of Health, Bethesda, Maryland 20205

David J. Shapiro (139), Department of Biochemistry, University of Illinois, Urbana, Illinois 61801

Roberto Toccafondi (457), Section on the Biochemistry of Cell Regulation, Laboratory of Biochemical Pharmacology, National Institute of Arthritis, Diabetes, Digestive and Kidney Diseases, National Institutes of Health, Bethesda, Maryland 20205

Donatella Tombaccini (457), Section on the Biochemistry of Cell Regulation, Laboratory of Biochemical Pharmacology, National Institute of Arthritis, Diabetes, Digestive and Kidney Diseases, National Institutes of Health, Bethesda, Maryland 20205

Bruce A. White† (173), Molecular Biology and Virology Department, Sloan Kettering Institute, New York, New York 10021

R. C. Winneker (353), Department of Cell Biology, Baylor College of Medicine, Houston, Texas 77030

*Present address: Collaborative Research, Inc., 128 Spring Street, Lexington, Massachusetts 02173.

†Present address: Department of Anatomy, University of Connecticut Health Center, Farmington, Connecticut 06032.

Preface

This volume emphasizes aspects of molecular biology with respect to hormone action. The first part of the book contains a number of chapters dealing with gene expression, transcription, RNA stabilization, and protein synthesis. E. Herbert and collaborators describe the opioid peptides. Prolactin gene expression is a system described from the point of view of gene regulation by G. H. Murdoch, R. M. Evans, and M. G. Rosenfeld, and also by C. Bancroft *et al.* The control by estrogen is detailed in a chapter by P. S. Dannies. Gene regulation by glucocorticoids is the subject of work by K. E. Mayo and R. D. Palmiter with the metallothionein gene and by D. K. Granner and E. G. Beale with tyrosine aminotransferase and phosphoenolpyruvate carboxykinase expression. D. J. Shapiro and M. L. Brock report on the roles of estrogen in the transcription and stabilization of vitellogenin mRNA. P. F. Blackmore and J. H. Exton describe mechanisms involved in the actions of calcium-dependent hormones. M. R. Banerjee and M. Antoniou narrate the multiple hormonal controls of milk-protein gene expression. S. Bourgeois and J. C. Gasson describe the genetic basis of glucocorticoid resistance in cell cultures. The remainder of the volume is dedicated to the description of various receptors: J. H. Clark's laboratory reports on estrogen and antiestrogen binding sites; D. Marver describes the mineralocorticoid receptor; G. L. Johnson's laboratory summarizes its findings regarding the nerve growth factor receptor; and L. D. Kohn's laboratory describes the thyrotropin receptor. This volume, then, stresses modern molecular biology as it pertains to hormone action as well as basic work with hormone receptors. Consequently, it should appeal both to endocrinologists and to workers in the field of molecular biology.

Gerald Litwack

CHAPTER 1

Generation of Diversity of Opioid Peptides

Edward Herbert, Olivier Civelli, James Douglass,
Gerard Martens, and Haim Rosen

Department of Chemistry
University of Oregon
Eugene, Oregon

BIOCHEMICAL ACTIONS OF HORMONES, VOL. XII

I. INTRODUCTION

During the past two decades, a great variety of small peptides that mediate specific physiological responses in animals have been discovered. These peptides, called *neuroendocrine peptides,* are the messenger molecules that convert neural signals into physiological responses and may serve both as neurotransmitters or neuromodulators in the nervous system and as hormones in the circulatory system. It is, therefore, not surprising to find them in a side variety of tissues. For example, the adrenocorticotropin (ACTH) endorphin family of peptides is found in the anterior and neurointermediate lobes of the pituitary, in several sites in the brain, and in the intestine, the placenta, and the immune system.

The structures of neuroendocrine peptides have been determined largely by classic amino acid sequencing techniques. However, their mode of synthesis could not be studied in detail until recombinant DNA techniques were developed. As a result, it was shown that the small neuroendocrine peptides are synthesized in the form of large polypeptide precursors. Determination of amino acid sequences of these precursors culminated in the discovery of an important new class of proteins, called polyproteins (or polyfunctional proteins) because they serve as precursors to more than one biologically active peptide. Indeed, one of these precursors, proenkephalin, is the source of as many as eight different bioactive peptides that must be excised from the precursors to become active. These peptides then may act in concert to coordinate complex behavioral responses.

The domains of the biologically active peptides in the precursors are usually flanked by pairs of basic amino acid residues, indicating that trypsinlike enzymes and carboxypeptidases are involved in producing bioactive peptides from precursors, as in the case of conversion of proinsulin to insulin (Steiner *et al.*, 1980). The proteolytic cleavages are often not the only events necessary to obtain a bioactive peptide from a precursor; specific amino acid residue modifications are also involved. For example, the precursors contain sequences that can specify attachment of oligosaccharides. Other forms of modification may include phosphorylation, amidation, acetylation, sulfation, and methylation of particular amino acids.

Hence, polyproteins can give rise to the variety of peptides necessary to mediate complex behavioral responses. However, this is not the only mechanism used to create diversity in the production of bioactive peptides. All steps that mediate the expression of a gene coding for a polyprotein can be involved in generating this type of diversity. Expression of a polyprotein gene can be regulated differently in different tissues. For example, glucocorticoids affect pro-opiomelanocortin (POMC) gene expression in the anterior but not in the neurointermediate lobe of the pituitary. Tissue-specific expression of neuroendocrine peptide genes can result from alternate modes of splicing of a pre-mRNA copied from a single gene. This diversity-generating mechanism leads to the formation of different mRNAs and, therefore, of different precursors in different tissues, as in the case of expression of the calcitonin gene (Amara *et al.*, 1982). Also, regulation of a complex behavior can be controlled by a family of genes producing related sets of bioactive peptides. These genes may be expressed selectively in different cells involved in the behavior pattern such as occurs in egg-laying behavior in the marine invertebrate *Aplysia californica* (Scheller *et al.*, 1983). In some instances it is the polypeptide precursor itself that is processed to different bioactive products in different tissues. This type of tissue-specific processing appears to be related to different sets of processing enzymes in each tissue. Finally, diversity of expression also occurs during the last step in the production of bioactive peptides, their secretion into the extracellular space. The secretion of bioactive peptides may be controlled by neural signals in one tissue and by hormones in another tissue, as in the secretion of POMC peptides from the anterior and neurointermediate lobes of the pituitary. Thus, diversity in the production of neuroendocrine peptides can occur at almost all levels of gene expression.

Diversification of neuroendocrine peptides is perhaps best illustrated by the opioid peptide family. More than 16 different endogenous peptides have been identified that exhibit opioid ativity in various bioassays. The first of these peptides to be isolated were the pentapeptides Met- and Leu-enkephalin (Hughes *et al.*, 1975). The other opioid peptides are C-terminal extensions of either Met- or Leu-enkephalin as shown in Fig. 1. β-Endorphin, for example, is a C-terminal extension of Met-enkaphalin, whereas dynorphin and the neo-endorphin are C-terminal extensions of Leu-enkephalin.

During the past 4 years it has been shown through the use of recombinant DNA technology and protein chemistry that all of the known opioid peptides are derived from three different precursor proteins (Fig. 2). The first opioid precursor protein to be characterized was pro-opiomelanocortin (POMC), which gives rise to the opioid, β-endorphin, and a variety of other peptides

β-endorphin (31 amino acids)	Tyr·Gly·Gly·Phe·Met·Thr·Ser·Glu·Lys·Ser·Gln·Thr·Pro·Leu·Val·Thr·Leu·Phe·Lys·Asn·Ala·Ile·Ile·Lys·Asn·Ala·Tyr·Lys·Lys·Gly·Glu^{31}
Peptide E	Tyr·Gly·Gly·Phe·Met·Arg·Arg·Val·Gly·Arg·Pro·Glu·Trp·Trp·Met·Asp·Tyr·Gln·Lys·Arg·Tyr·Gly·Gly·Phe·Leu^{25}
Met-enk·Arg·Phe	Tyr·Gly·Gly·Phe·Met·Arg·Phe^{7}
Met-enk·Arg·Gly·Leu	Tyr·Gly·Gly·Phe·Met·Arg·Gly·Leu^{8}
Met-enkephalin	Tyr·Gly·Gly·Phe·Met
Leu-enkephalin	Tyr·Gly·Gly·Phe·Leu
Dynorphin 1–17	Tyr·Gly·Gly·Phe·Leu·Arg·Arg·Ile·Arg·Pro·Lys·Leu·Lys·Trp·Asp·Asn·Gln^{17}
Dynorphin 1–8	Tyr·Gly·Gly·Phe·Leu·Arg·Arg·Ile^{8}
α-Neo-endorphin	Tyr·Gly·Gly·Phe·Leu·Arg·Lys·Tyr·Pro·Lys^{10}
β-Neo-endorphin	Tyr·Gly·Gly·Phe·Leu·Arg·Lys·Tyr·Pro^{9}
Dynorphin B or Rimorphin	Tyr·Gly·Gly·Phe·Leu·Arg·Arg·Gln·Phe·Lys·Val·Val·Thr^{13}

FIG. 1. Structure of some opioid peptides. The sequences of Met-enkephalin and Leu-enkephalin are in boxes.

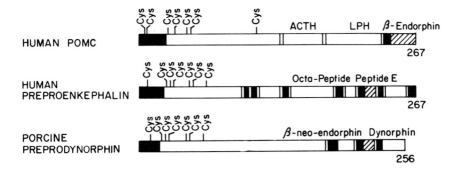

FIG. 2. Schematic representation of the three opioid polypeptide precursors. The black box at the N terminus represents the signal sequence. Cys indicates the presence of a cysteine residue in the precursor. Some of the bioactive peptides are indicated. The black boxes in the precursors indicate the presence of an enkephalin sequence. Pairs of basic amino acid residues are indicated by a bar.

including adrenocorticotropin (ACTH) and α-, β-, and γ-melanocyte–stimulating hormones (MSH) (Nakanishi *et al.*, 1979). The second precursor protein to be characterized was proenkephalin, which contains six copies of Met-enkephalin and one copy of Leu-enkephalin (Comb *et al.*, 1982; Gubler *et al.*, 1982; Noda *et al.*, 1982a). In the adrenal medulla this precursor gives rise to a number of different opioid peptides including Met- and Leu-enkephalin, peptide E, which contains one copy of Met-enkephalin and one copy of Leu-enkephalin, peptide F, which contains two copies of Met-enkephalin, and Met-enkephalin-Arg-Gly-Leu (Kilpatrick *et al.*, 1981a). The third precursor is prodynorphin, which contains three copies of Leu-enkephalin and gives rise to the opioids dynorphin and β-neo-endorphin (Kakidani *et al.*, 1982) (Figs. 1 and 2). The integrity of the enkephalin sequence is essential for the morphinomimetic activity of all of these peptides. Some remarkable similarities in the structure of the opioid peptide precursors are revealed in Fig. 2. First, the precursors are almost all the same length and the sequences of the biologically active peptides are confined almost exclusively to the C-terminal half of the precursors. The N-terminal region of each precursor is rich in cysteine residues, and the distribution of these residues is similar in each case, indicating that formation of disulfide bridges may be essential for stabilizing the protein in conformations required for correct processing. Finally, the biologically active domains in each precursor are flanked on both sides by pairs of basic amino acid residues, creating potential cleavage sites for trypsinlike enzymes (Fig. 2).

II. APPROACHES AND STRATEGIES USED IN CHARACTERIZING THE OPIOID PEPTIDE PRECURSOR PROTEINS

A. The Peptide Chemistry Approach

The first step in analyzing a precursor molecule by the peptide chemistry approach is to prepare antibodies that will specifically recognize the corresponding bioactive peptide. For example, POMC was first identified by the use of antibodies directed against ACTH and β-endorphin (Mains *et al.*, 1977; Roberts and Herbert, 1977). Since most of the bioactive peptides are of small size, they have often been coupled to carriers in order to increase their immunogenicity. Sometimes the antibodies are directed against a terminal amino acid of the peptide fragment. This type of antibody would have a reduced affinity for the precursor molecule, however. Because of this problem, the peptide precursors must be proteolytically cleaved before the immunoassay step. Following this treatment, the intermediate forms of the bioactive peptides can be detected by the antibody. The latter approach has been used to identify enkephalin-containing precursor peptides in the adrenal medulla and brain.

When trying to identify polyprotein precursors, the choice of the starting tissue is critical. One must take into account whether the bioactive peptide is synthesized in a tissue or transported to that tissue, the number of different cell types that make up the tissue, and the ability of that tissue to be maintained in primary culture if radiolabeling (pulse-chase) techniques are to be employed to characterize the precursor molecule.

Once the choice of tissue has been made, the material is homogenized and total cellular protein is extracted under denaturing conditions in the presence of protease inhibitors. At this point, the precursor protein is either directly immunoprecipitated from the total polypeptide extract, as in the case of POMC, or the extract is fractionated in order to isolate the precursor in relatively pure form. High-performance liquid chromatography (HPLC) is proving to be a very powerful technique for the isolation of relatively pure proteolytic cleavage fragments of specific polyproteins. This technique, which has been used for the identification of dynorphin- and enkephalin-containing peptides (Udenfriend and Kilpatrick, 1983; Goldstein *et al.*, 1979), is rapid and allows one to analyze large volumes of tissue extract with extremely high resolution. Further characterization of the precursor may involve gel chromatography (to determine the size of the precursor) and peptide mapping or partial sequencing (to determine the structure of the precursor).

The peptide and immunochemical approaches allow the characterization not only of the intact precursors, but also of the naturally occurring intermediates of processing. Although these techniques permit one to follow the fate of the primary translation product from its synthesis to the final maturation of the bioactive peptide(s), they do not provide any means of studying other levels of gene expression. The nucleic acid approach has been adopted by a number of laboratories to study gene structure, transcription, and RNA processing and to quantitate levels of mRNA.

B. The Nucleic Acid Approach

1. Cell-Free mRNA Translation

The general procedure in cell-free mRNA translation includes purification of the poly(A) mRNA population, translation in a cell-free protein-synthesizing system, immunological purification of the precursor, and analysis of the precursor by gel electrophoresis. A complete discussion of the application of this approach is contained in a recent review (Douglass *et al.*, 1984).

2. Recombinant DNA Approach

The recombinant DNA approach has been used to determine the complete amino acid sequence of numerous bioactive peptide precursors. The general complementary DNA (cDNA) cloning procedure is outlined as follows. A total population of poly(A) mRNAs (or a partially enriched fraction) is enzymatically transcribed into cDNA by the action of reverse transcriptase. This reaction is primed by the hybridization of oligo(dT) to the poly(A) region of the mRNA. The single-stranded cDNA molecules are converted to their double-stranded form by incubation with DNA polymerase and inserted into a bacterial vector. These chimeric molecules are introduced into bacterial cells to generate a "library" of cDNA clones. The clones containing the peptide precursor cDNA of interest are then isolated from the cDNA "library," and the cDNA inserts are sequenced in order to obtain the sequence of the precursor protein.

The isolation of cDNA clones for many neuropeptide mRNA species has proven to be very difficult because of the low levels of these species of mRNA. For example, prodynorphin mRNA makes up less than 0.01% of the total poly(A) mRNA population in the hypothalamus. Hence, the isolation of cDNA clones for prodynorphin requires the construction of extremely large cDNA libraries and demands the use of highly efficient cloning techniques (Okayama and Berg, 1982).

Various screening methods have been developed for the identification of specific cDNA clones. The choice of method is usually dependent on the concentration of peptide precursor mRNA in the total poly(A) mRNA population. If the level of precursor mRNA is high, as in the case of POMC mRNA in the pituitary, total enzymatically radiolabeled mRNA (Nakanishi *et al.*, 1978) can be used as a screening probe. Because of the high level of these specific sequences, one can be relatively sure that at least one of the cDNA clones that hybridizes with the total radiolabeled mRNA will contain the sequence corresponding to the desired polyprotein precursor. For detecting less abundant or rare cDNA clones like proenkephalin or prodynorphin, a screening strategy involves the use of synthetic oligodeoxynucleotide probes. Oligomers complementary to sequences in the opioid precursor mRNA molecule are synthesized chemically. In general, the oligomers are complementary to the mRNA sequences that code for the opioid peptides themselves. The oligomers are labeled with radioactive phosphate at their 5' end and applied to nitrocellulose filters containing lysed clones that represent the entire cDNA library. When hybridization is carried out under the proper conditions, the oligonucleotide probe will bind selectively to the complementary nucleotide sequence and the location of the hybridizing cDNA clone can be detected by autoradiography. This approach has an advantage over other approaches in that it can be used to detect virtually any cDNA clone of interest, provided that peptide sequence information is available.

Several factors must be taken into account when the sequence of an oligonucleotide probe is designed. First, because of the degeneracy of the genetic code it is usually necessary to synthesize pools of oligomers corresponding to all possible codons in the mRNA sequence. While the synthesis of oligomer pools ensures a perfect match with the specific mRNA sequence, it also reduces selectivity in the screening by increasing the possibility of hybridization of oligomers with different clones sequentially related to the clone of interest, referred to as "false positive" clones. This problem is particularly vexing in screening cDNA clones transcribed from complex mRNA populations such as those that exist in the brain. Second, the size of the oligomer is also important. Generally, oligomers 14 to 17 bases in length are adequate to ensure selectivity in screening complex cDNA libraries. When using probes of this size, relatively stringent hybridization conditions can be employed, thus reducing the number of positive cDNA clones with only partially correct hybridizing sequences (Wallace *et al.*, 1979; Agarwal *et al.*, 1981).

Oligonucleotide probe pools have been used to detect cDNA clones that code for full-length bovine and human preproenkephalin (Noda *et al.*, 1982a; Gubler *et al.*, 1982; Comb *et al.*, 1982). In both species cDNA was transcribed from mRNA that contained less than 0.1% preproenkephalin mRNA. Oligomers, 14 or 15 nucleotides in length, served as hybridization probes for the isolation of partial (Gubler *et al.*, 1982) or full-length (Comb *et al.*, 1982) preproenkephalin cDNA clones.

Brain tissue is believed to contain as many as 100,000 species of mRNA, compared to roughly 10,000 species for most other tissues. The high complexity of brain tissue mRNA increases the chances of detecting false positive cDNA clones in cDNA libraries, particularly when one screens with pools of oligomers instead of single oligomers. Detection of false positives with mismatched sequences occurs during screening because the hybridization conditions cannot be made selective enough to prevent oligomers with slightly different AT/GC ratios from forming stable complexes with the DNA.

We have encountered this problem during the isolation of a porcine prodynorphin cDNA clone. One hundred thirty thousand hypothalamic cDNA clones were screened with a pool of eight different tetradecamers complementary to the sequence that codes for the C-terminal portion of dynorphin (1–17). The AT/GC ratio of these oligomers varied between 1 and 2.5. Hybridizations carried out at 35 or 42°C in a buffer containing 0.6 M NaCl/ 0.06 M Na citrate led to the detection of 10 different cDNA clones, which were subjected to sequencing. The region of homology between the oligomer probes used and the sequences of the clones detected is shown in Fig. 3 (the mismatched bases are underlined). One can see that in all but one clone, the core of the oligomer matched perfectly, whereas the 5' and 3' ends did not. All of these clones, therefore, could be classified as false positives since none of them codes for an entire dynorphin (1–17) sequence. (The sequences adjacent to the oligomer regions were totally different from the published prodynorphin cDNA sequence.) It is also noteworthy that no clones were isolated with more than two mismatches. This is a measure of the stringency of the hybridization conditions used. The generation of the false positive clones is principally due to the complexity of the mRNA population used, as evidenced by the difficulty in obtaining specific brain cDNAs (Furutani *et al.*, 1983) compared to other organs.

To avoid the isolation of false positive clones, a different strategy for the use of synthetic oligonucleotides has been devised: the generation of specifically primed cDNA libraries. In this approach, oligonucleotides are designed to hybridize to a specific sequence in the 3' region of the mRNA of interest. When cDNA synthesis is primed with these oligonucleotides the resulting cDNA library is enriched for the cDNA clone of interest. A second oligonucleotide pool, designed to recognize a sequence 5' to the one recognized by the primer, is used as a hybridization probe to detect the correct cDNA clone.

This methodology introduces another level of specificity in the charac-

Edward Herbert et al.

terization of a particular cDNA clone by allowing the synthesis of only a restricted number of cDNA species specific for a particular sequence. However, we have found in practice that this approach does not abolish the synthesis of false positive clones, but only reduces their numbers. Indeed, we applied this approach to the isolation of the prodynorphin cDNA using a 17-base oligomer as primer for the cDNA reaction. This primer hybridizes 460 bases 5' to a tetradecamer used for screening. We were able to obtain 15,000 specifically primed clones. Three positive clones were identified by screening with the tetradecamer. The sequence of two of these clones showed that they fall into the class of the false positive clones (Fig. 3), the

```
Tetradecamer:    5'  T G  G   T T  G   T C C C A  T   T T   3'
                          A         A              C

A
   H 20-1:             - - T G A T T G T C C C A C A G - -
                                                    ___
   H 27-2:             - - T G T T T G T C C C A T T T - -
                               _
   H 35  :             - - T A G T T G T C C C A T T T - -
                              _
   S 87  :             - - T A G T T A T C C C A C T T - -
                              _
   S 93  :             - - A G G T T G T C C C A C T G - -
                                                      _
   S 99  :             - - - - - - - - - C C C A C C T - -
                                                  _
   S 205 :             - - A T G T T A T C C C A T T T - -
                           _ _
   S 206 :             - - T T G T T G T C C C A T T G - -
                                                      _
   S 208 :             - - T G A T T A T C C C A C C T - -
                                                  _
                                            G
                                            ↙
   S 22  :             - - T G A T T A T C C C A T T T - -

_____

B
   ssp 2-3  :          - - A A G T T G T C C C A C T T - -
                           _ _
   ssp 1-11 :          - - C G T T T G T C C C A C T T - -
                           _ _ _
```

FIG. 3. Partial sequences of the dynorphin "false positive" clones. Sequences of the synthetic tetradecamers complementary to the mRNA sequence of dynorphin (13–17) are shown on top of the figure. These tetradecamers, enzymatically labeled with ^{32}P, were used as probes for the detection of clones related to the dynorphin sequence. (A) Partial sequences of the clones isolated from hypothalamic cDNA library primed by oligo(dT). (B) Partial sequences of the clones isolated from a hypothalamic specifically primed cDNA library. In this case, the cDNA synthesis was initiated by hybridization of a synthetic oligomer 17 bases long, complementary to the bases situated 360 bases downstream of the stop codon on the prodynorphin mRNA. Only part of the sequences is shown; the rest of the sequences did not correspond to the known prodynorphin precursor sequence. The bases that form a mismatch with the oligomers are underlined.

third being the desired prodynorphin clone. Therefore, specific priming proved to be critical in overcoming the problem posed by the complexity of the brain mRNAs. The partial prodynorphin cDNA clone obtained by this specific-priming procedure can then serve as a highly specific probe in the screening of oligo(dT)-primed cDNA library. One can also use this technique to obtain the sequence of the 5' end of mRNAs, a task often difficult to reach for long mRNAs. This powerful approach has been used for the detection of the full-length sequence of two opioid precursors: procnkephalin (Noda *et al.*, 1982a) and prodynorphin (Kakidani *et al.*, 1982).

To summarize, then, various approaches have been used to determine the amino acid sequence and structural organization of polyprotein precursors. Over the past few years, the recombinant DNA approach has proven to be the most powerful. cDNA clones can be used not only to determine the sequence of protein precursors, but to determine the structure of the polyprotein genes as well.

III. STRUCTURE OF OPIOID PEPTIDE GENES

A. ISOLATION OF GENOMIC CLONES

Some of the cDNA clones mentioned above have been used as hybridization probes to isolate genomic DNA fragments coding for the respective peptide precursor mRNA molecule. These genomic DNA fragments are, in general, isolated from λ genomic libraries. λ genomic libraries consist of large genomic DNA fragments, usually 10,000–20,000 base pairs (bp) in length, which have been randomly inserted into specially constructed λ phage vectors (Lawn *et al.*, 1978). These chimeric molecules are packaged into viable λ phage particles and are used to infect a lawn of bacteria. The resulting plaques are transferred to nitrocellulose filters and screened by plaque hybridization using the cDNA clone as a hybridization probe (Benton and Davis, 1977). DNA fragments from the resulting genomic clones are subcloned into a plasmid vector or the double-stranded replicative form DNA of the phage M13 for sequence analysis (Messing *et al.*, 1977; Sanger *et al.*, 1977). In some cases, the entire gene for a given polyprotein is quite large, so multiple positively hybridizing λ clones must be isolated.

Many eukaryotic genes contain coding regions (exons) that are separated by noncoding intervening sequences (introns). Intronic regions may be quite large (>10,000 bp). Hence, Southern blotting (Southern, 1975) is usually employed to determine which regions of DNA isolated from a λ genomic clone actually contain exonic sequences, thus facilitating a rapid sequence analysis of the coding regions. The same type of analysis can also yield information concerning the copy number of a gene in a particular genome.

The occurrence of split genes in eukaryotic genomes has led to a hypothesis that introns separate functional domains in the gene coding regions, thus allowing for rapid evolution of novel peptides (Doolittle, 1978; Gilbert, 1978). Indeed, several polyprotein genes are organized such that exonic regions code for unique functional regions of the precursor polypeptide (Bell *et al.*, 1983; Schmale *et al.*, 1983). However, the opioid peptide genes do not have intronic regions separating exonic regions that code for individual bioactive peptides.

B. Opioid Peptide Gene Structure

The pro-opiomelanocortin gene structure has been determined for human (Whitfeld *et al.*, 1982; Chang *et al.*, 1980; Cochet *et al.*, 1982), bovine (Nakanishi *et al.*, 1980; 1981), rat (Drouin and Goodman, 1980), and mouse (Notake *et al.*, 1983; Uhler *et al.*, 1983) species. The overall structure of the POMC gene is highly conserved among these different species. The human and rat proenkephalin and prodynorphin genes have also been isolated (Noda *et al.*, 1982b; Comb *et al.*, 1983; Horikawa *et al.*, 1983). The general organization of the proenkephalin and prodynorphin genes is remarkably similar to that of the human POMC gene and is schematically diagrammed in Fig. 4. All three genes have large 3′ exons that contain the nucleotides coding for all of the biologically active peptides and the majority of the N-terminal portions of the precursors. Note that the 3′ untranslated region of the prodynorphin gene is much larger than that of the other two genes. Some 3 kilobases (kb) upstream (5′) is a smaller exon that contains sequences coding for the remainder of the amino-terminal portion of the precursor molecule, the initiator methionine, and a few bases of the 5′ untranslated region of the mRNA. The remaining sequences coding for the 5′ untranslated region of the mRNA are found farther upstream on either one (POMC) or two (proenkephalin and prodynorphin) exons. The prodynorphin gene differs from the other two genes in that its first exon is large.

The structural similarities between these three genes in humans suggest that they may have arisen via a common evolutionary mechanism. The human POMC and proenkephalin genes are not, however, closely linked in the genome. POMC has been localized to chromosome 2 (Owerbach *et al.*, 1981), while the proenkephalin gene is located on chromosome 12 (M. Comb, personal communication). The location of the prodynorphin gene is not known.

The 3′ exons of all the opioid genes contain regions of intrasequence

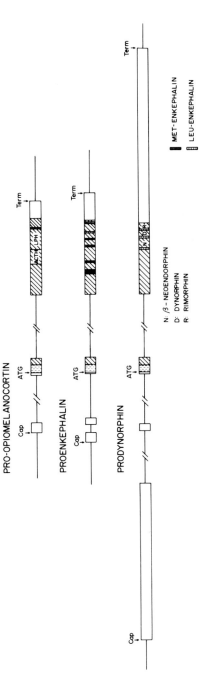

FIG. 4. Structural comparison of the human POMC, proenkephalin, and prodynorphin genes. Lines indicate introns; boxes indicate exons. ATG indicates the initiator methionine; Term indicates the mRNA 3′ end. Cap shows the start of transcription. Dashed boxes indicate the signal peptide; hatched boxes, the extent of the coding region. The different enkephalin sequences are indicated.

homology. In POMC, three repetitive nucleotide regions are present (approximately 50 nucleotides in length) that code for α, β, and γ-melanocyte–stimulating hormone. In human proenkephalin there are seven regions of internal nucleotide sequence homology (approximately 25 bp in length) that code for the biologically active enkephalin moieties. This observation has led to the suggestion that the POMC and proenkephalin genes have evolved via a series of duplication and rearrangement events of ancestral MSH-like sequences and enkephalinlike sequences, respectively (Nakanishi *et al.*, 1980; Noda *et al.*, 1982b).

Southern blotting experiments and the isolation of genomic clones from λ genomic libraries have implied that only one proenkephalin and one POMC gene are present in the human genome. The same holds true for the number of POMC genes in the bovine and rat genome. In contrast, two groups (Notake *et al.*, 1983; Uhler *et al.*, 1983) have reported the presence of two POMC genes in the mouse genome, one of which is a pseudogene. The pseudogene exhibits 92% homology with 533 base pairs of the functional POMC gene, including the coding regions for ACTH and β-lipotropin (β-LPH). However, the presence of a premature translation termination codon and a mutation in a codon for a dibasic amino acid cleavage site within the protein predicts that β-endorphin would not be present in the translation product, and ACTH would not be cleaved from the precursor by a trypsinlike cleavage enzyme. Thus, the POMC pseudogene in the mouse cannot encode a functional precursor protein similar to the POMC precursor. Finally, the mouse POMC pseudogene sequence is flanked on both sides by direct repeats 10 bp in length. This observation raises the interesting possibility that the pseudogene may have arisen via the formation of an aberrant transcript of the functional gene followed by the insertion of its cDNA copy into the mouse genome (Notake *et al.*, 1983).

C. COMPARATIVE ASPECTS OF PROENKEPHALIN GENES IN THE HUMAN, RAT, AND AMPHIBIAN

Analysis of protein sequences in different species in order to determine conserved regions constitutes an approach to understanding which sequences may be functionally significant. The proenkephalin amino acid sequences are known in the human (Comb *et al.*, 1982) and bovine species (Noda *et al.*, 1982a; Gubler *et al.*, 1982), and the nucleotide sequence of the proenkephalin gene has been reported in humans (Comb *et al.*, 1983; Noda *et al.*, 1982b). We have examined the rat proenkephalin gene and found that its overall structural organization is very similar to that of the human; the sizes and positions of the corresponding introns and exons are almost identical in these two species. In addition, we have cloned and sequenced the main exons of two different proenkephalin genes in the South African clawed toad, *Xenopus laevis*, which diverged from the main line of vertebrate evolution some 350 million years ago. The sizes of the two main exons of the toad genes are identical, and their organization is remarkably similar to that of the main exons of the rat and human genes (Martens and Herbert, 1984). The main exon in *Xenopus* codes for 216 amino acids, which is slightly less than the number coded for in the human (221 amino acids) (Comb *et al.*, 1983). Each of the toad proenkephalins contains five copies of Met-enkephalin and one copy of Met-enkephalin-Arg-Gly-Tyr and one Met-enkephalin-Arg-Phe (Martens and Herbert, 1984). Met-enkephalin-Arg-Gly-Leu and Leu-enkephalin, two enkephalin sequences present in human, bovine, and rat proenkephalin, are not found in the *Xenopus* sequence. Thus, amphibian proenkephalin contains no Leu-enkephalin sequences, suggesting that a switch from a Met-enkephalin to a Leu-enkephalin sequence in the mammalian proenkephalins occurred less than 350 million years ago.

The distribution of enkephalin sequences appears to be very similar among human, bovine, rat, and *Xenopus* proenkephalin. Some of the spacer regions between the enkephalin sequences have a high degree of amino acid homology, while others have diverged to a considerable extent. It is interesting to note that the highly conserved regions between enkephalin units 2 and 3, 5 and 6, and 6 and 7 correspond to enkephalin-containing peptides (ECPs) isolated from bovine adrenal medulla (peptides F, E, and B, respectively). The high degree of conservation of these peptides (especially of the highly potent opioid peptide E) might point to an important physiological role for them, both in mammals and in lower vertebrates. The enkephalin sequences in both mammalian and amphibian precursors are flanked by pairs of basic amino acids, suggesting that similar processing mechanisms are used in both mammals and amphibians. In mammals, the cysteine residues in three opioid precursor proteins are located in almost identical positions in the N-terminal region. It has been suggested that this region is important for proper folding of the precursor molecule in order to ensure correct processing. The conservation of the cysteine residues in the proenkephalin sequences of the four species reinforces this concept. Thus, the high conservation of proenkephalin sequences in mammals and amphibians suggests that the enkephalins and ECPs have an important physiological function(s) in a wide range of vertebrates (Martens and Herbert, 1984).

The two nonallelic *Xenopus* proenkephalin genes likely result from a genomic duplication in *X. laevis*, which was previously postulated on the basis of the chromosome number and DNA content per cell in different *Xenopus* species (Bisbee *et al.*, 1977). Finally, a polymorphism has been revealed in one of the toad proenkephalin genes. With restriction mapping and sequence analysis it was established that the allelic variation is due to an insertion/deletion of a 1-kb DNA fragment, approximately 1.5 kb 5′ from the main exon (Martens and Herbert, 1984). The inserted DNA had the characteristics of a transposable element and appeared to belong to a family of repetitive sequences that are transcribed during embryonic development of *X. laevis.*

IV. TRANSCRIPTIONAL AND POSTTRANSCRIPTIONAL REGULATION OF OPIOID PEPTIDE GENE EXPRESSION

The tissue levels of numerous bioactive peptides derived from polyproteins can be altered by a variety of synthetic and naturally occurring substances. In this section we will document some examples in which various regulators are altering opioid peptide levels as the result of changes in the level of mRNA that codes for these peptides. The following questions will be addressed: (1) Which tissues are actively transcribing polyprotein genes? (2) What are some of the characteristics of these genes that make them transcriptionally active? (3) How are transcriptionally active polyprotein genes regulated *in vivo?*

A. DETECTION OF mRNA CODING FOR VARIOUS POLYPROTEINS

A polyprotein cDNA clone or λ genomic clone can be used as a hybridization probe for detecting and quantifying the corresponding mRNA. The following examples illustrate how the Northern blot procedure (Alwine *et al.*, 1977; Thomas, 1980) has been used to determine the tissue-specific distribution of mRNA coding for various opioid peptides.

Study of the distribution of POMC mRNA in various rat brain tissues shows that the hypothalamus, amygdala, and cerebral cortex contain POMC transcripts (mRNA), while the cerebellum and midbrain do not (Civelli *et al.*, 1982). In addition, POMC transcripts in the amygdala and cortex appear to be slightly smaller in size than POMC transcripts isolated from the hypothalamus. The distribution of proenkephalin mRNA in these same tissues has been measured (Tang *et al.*, 1983) and proenkephalin transcripts are detected (in order of abundance) in the striatum, hypothalamus, cerebellum, midbrain, hippocampus, and cortex.

These data provide two important pieces of information. First, the distribution of POMC mRNA in the rat brain is different from that of proenkephalin mRNA. For example, the rat cerebellum contains relatively high levels of proenkephalin transcripts but no detectable POMC mRNA. Since opioid peptides are derived from both precursor molecules, proenkephalin-derived peptides may play an important role in this region of the brain, while β-endorphin (from POMC) does not. Second, the levels of mRNA can be correlated with the levels of the bioactive peptides derived from POMC or proenkephalin. In most cases a direct correlation is observed, confirming that the bioactive peptides previously detected in these tissues by radioimmunoassay are present as a result of direct synthesis in those tissues, and not of transport to those tissues from a secondary site of synthesis.

Several groups (Hudson *et al.*, 1981; Gee and Roberts, 1982) have used POMC cDNA as a hybridization probe to study the differential expression of the POMC gene in the various lobes of the rat pituitary. Using these probes, approximately 3–5% of anterior lobe cells appear to contain POMC transcripts, while greater than 90% of the intermediate lobe cells show cytoplasmic localization of POMC mRNA. By combining immunohistochemical methods with *in situ* hybridization histochemistry it has also been shown that the same cells contain both POMC peptides and POMC mRNA (Gee and Roberts, 1982). These data suggest that the presence of the POMC peptides in these cells is due to their local synthesis and is not the result of uptake from the plasma.

Unquestionably, *in situ* hybridization histochemistry is a valuable tool, which will enable us in the future to localize the cellular sites of expression of polyproteins.

B. Characteristics of Transcriptionally Active Polyprotein Genes

Gene expression in eukaryotic cells is influenced by a wide variety of factors. The TATA box (or Hogness/Goldberg) (Goldberg, 1979) is involved in fixing the start point of transcription and also affects the transcriptional efficiency *in vivo* (Breathnach and Chambon, 1981; Grosschedl and Birnsteil, 1980). The level of methylation in the neighborhood of a gene can also affect the transcriptional activity of that gene (Felsenfeld and McGhee, 1982). In addition, the structure of the chromatin of actively transcribing genes may differ from that of nontranscribing genes (Weisbrod, 1982). The following studies will serve to illustrate how various strategies are being used to determine the factors that are involved in the transcriptional activation of polyprotein genes.

A cloned human POMC gene has been ligated to SV40 DNA, introduced into COS monkey cells, and transcribed from its own promoter (Mishina *et al.*, 1982). Deletion mutants in the 5' region of the gene were generated to determine the effects of these sequences on transcription of the gene *in vivo*. If nucleotide +1 is the first base of the primary transcript, deletion of sequences from −20 to −40 (containing the TATA box) completely abolishes accurate transcription from the POMC promoter. This result suggests that the TATA box region is a distinct promoter element of the human POMC gene.

A unique feature of the human POMC promoter region is that the deletion of sequences from −53 to −59 results in a threefold enhancement of the transcriptional efficiency. This region overlaps with a continuous stretch of GC pairs present −48 to −56 bp upstream from the cap site. The GC stretch itself or its specific pattern of methylation may depress transcription of the gene, and its partial removal may, therefore, increase the transcriptional efficiency of the human POMC gene.

C. Regulation of Expression of Transcriptionally Active Polyprotein Genes

Many compounds alter the levels of bioactive paptides. Some of these substances change the rate of processing of the precursor molecules. Others regulate the rate of transport or secretion of the bioactive peptides following their release from the precursor molecule. In this section we will discuss how transcriptionally active polyprotein genes are regulated *in vivo* by various substances and by other unique control mechanisms.

V. REGULATION OF POMC GENE EXPRESSION

A. Factors Affecting Secretion of POMC Peptides from the Pituitary

The secretion of POMC-derived peptides is regulated differently in the anterior (AL) and neurointermediate (NIL) lobes of the rat pituitary. In the anterior lobe, the secretion of POMC-derived peptides is positively regulated by corticotropin-releasing factor (CRF) (Vale *et al.*, 1981) and negatively regulated by endogenous glucocorticoids released from the adrenal cortex (Watanabe *et al.*, 1973a; Fleischer and Rawls, 1970). Glucocorticoids also inhibit POMC production in AL corticiotrophs but have no effect on NIL cells that produce POMC (Yates and Maran, 1974).

In the NIL, dopaminergic neurons from the hypothalamus impinge on

POMC-containing cells and inhibit the release of POMC-derived peptides (Vermes *et al.*, 1980; Farah *et al.*, 1982). As expected, the administration of dopamine antagonists such as haloperidol stimulates the release of POMC peptides from the NIL (Höllt and Bergmann, 1982), and increases the levels of POMC peptides within the NIL (Höllt *et al.*, 1982; Lepine and Dupont, 1981). These agents have no effect on the release of POMC peptides from anterior lobe corticotrophs.

The experiments that follow demonstrate that the same factors that affect secretion of POMC peptides from the pituitary also affect the levels of POMC mRNA in a tissue-specific fashion.

B. POMC Gene Regulation in the Anterior Lobe

Cell-free protein translation assays indicate that the level of POMC mRNA activity in whole rat pituitary is increased two- to fivefold by adrenalectomy (Nakanishi *et al.*, 1979). Administration of dexamethasone (DEX) to adrenalectomized rats resulted in a marked suppression of POMC mRNA activity. The lobes of the pituitary were not separated from one another in this study. Hence, the contribution of each lobe to the POMC mRNA response could not be accurately evaluated.

Cell-free translation assays were also used to determine the effects of steroid hormones on POMC mRNA activity in the mouse anterior pituitary tumor cell line (AtT-20-D$_{16v}$) that secretes ACTH and endorphin (Nakamura *et al.*, 1978; Roberts *et al.*, 1979). The addition of DEX to culture medium reduced the level of POMC mRNA activity to 30–40% of that in untreated cells. This translational activity of POMC occurs without affecting the rate of processing of POMC to ACTH and β-endorphin (Roberts *et al.*, 1979).

More recently, mouse and rat POMC cDNA clones have been used as hybridization probes to accurately determine the effects of adrenalectomy and subsequent DEX administration on POMC mRNA levels in the rat anterior lobe (Herbert *et al.*, 1981; Schachter *et al.*, 1983; Birnberg *et al.*, 1983). Eight hours after adrenalectomy the levels of POMC mRNA increased markedly, reaching 15- to 20-fold the control level at 18 days postoperation. When DEX was administered to rats 8 days after adrenalectomy, these events were reversed (Birnberg *et al.*, 1983), and after five daily injections of DEX, POMC mRNA had returned to control levels (Fig. 5).

The large changes in POMC mRNA levels in the anterior pituitary after adrenalectomy raised the question of whether glucocorticoids regulate POMC gene expression at the level of transcription. To test this possibility, POMC transcription rates were assayed by the nuclear transcription method, which measures the number of RNA polymerase molecules transcribing

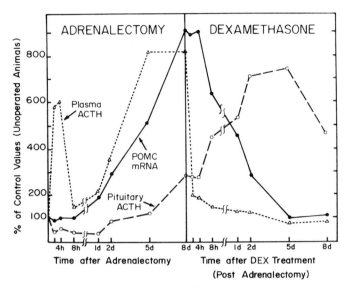

Fɪɢ. 5. Effects of adrenalectomy and dexamethasone treatment on the level of POMC mRNA and peptides in the anterior lobe of the rat pituitary. Plasma and pituitary ACTH peptide levels were determined by radioimmunoassay; POMC mRNA levels, by solution hybridization (Birnberg *et al.*, 1983). Adrenalectomy was performed at time 0. Eight days after adrenalectomy, some of the rats were given dexamethasone by subcutaneous injection.

POMC genes in a given time period (1 and 4 hours after adrenalectomy). The results show that the rate of transcription increases by 20-fold in the anterior pituitary within 1 hour of adrenalectomy. The observed increase in transcription rate was completely suppressed by administration of DEX to animals immediately after adrenalectomy.

Within 2 hours of adrenalectomy, plasma ACTH levels (Fig. 5) increased more than sixfold and were accompanied by a dramatic drop in pituitary ACTH (endorphin levels that are not shown followed ACTH levels closely). This is compatible with rapid enhancement of release of ACTH from the anterior pituitary following adrenalectomy, leading to a depletion of anterior pituitary ACTH. As POMC mRNA levels increase, there is a gradual increase in pituitary ACTH, which returns to control levels 5 days after adrenalectomy. Note that within 2 hours of initiation of dexamethasone treatment a sharp decrease in plasma ACTH levels occurs, indicating a rapid inhibition of ACTH release from the anterior pituitary. These results suggest that glucocorticoids have two separate actions on POMC gene expression in the anterior pituitary. The first action is an inhibition of secretion of ACTH/ endorphin peptide, and the second is an inhibition of transcription of the POMC gene. Both of these effects occur very rapidly (within 1 hour of administration of DEX). If transcription of the POMC gene increases within an hour of treatment, then why does it take 8–24 hours to observe a change in POMC mRNA levels after adrenalectomy or dexamethasone treatment? One likely explanation is that the pool of POMC mRNA is so large in the anterior pituitary that changes in the rates of transcription take a long time to be reflected in the size of the mRNA pool. The preceding effects are specific to POMC gene expression in the anterior lobe; POMC mRNA levels and the rate of transcription of the POMC gene in the NIL are not altered by adrenalectomy or by DEX administration (Schachter *et al.*, 1983; Birnberg *et al.*, 1983).

In situ hybridization has been used to determine that the increase in POMC mRNA levels in the anterior lobe following adrenalectomy is due to a number of factors, including enlarged cell volume and an increase in the numbers of POMC-producing cells (Gee and Roberts, 1982). This technique clearly allows for a more refined analysis of the factors involved when a heterogeneous tissue is being studied.

How are glucocorticoids affecting the levels of POMC transcripts in the anterior lobe? The model that has the most support is that a soluble glucocorticoid-receptor complex translocates to the nucleus in anterior lobe corticotrophs, binds to a specific region near the POMC gene, and exerts a primary effect at the level of transcription (Watanabe *et al.*, 1973b). This possibility is supported by studies that show sequence similarities in the 5'-flanking region between the bovine POMC gene and the mouse α-globin and β-globin genes, all of which are negatively regulated by glucocorticoids (Nakanishi *et al.*, 1981). Also, a 21-bp segment in the 5'-flanking region of the human POMC gene (distinct from the sequences mentioned previously) has been identified that shares homology with a DNA sequence in the 5'-flanking regions of two other glucocorticoid-regulated genes (rat growth hormone and the mouse mammary tumor virus long-terminal-repeat). Clearly, more studies remain to be done before this particular regulatory mechanism is understood.

C. POMC Gene Regulation in the Neurointermediate Lobe

Cell-free translation studies (Höllt *et al.*, 1982) and RNA dot blotting (Chen *et al.*, 1983) have been used to study the effects of dopamine agonists and antagonists on POMC mRNA levels in the rat NIL. Administration of the dopamine antagonist, haloperidol, results in a four- to six-fold (time-and-dose-dependent) increase in the level in NIL POMC mRNA. This stimulatory effect is observed as early as 6 hours after administration. In contrast, ergocryptine, a dopamine agonist, decreases two- to three-fold the level of POMC mRNA in the rat NIL (Chen *et al.*, 1983). The time-dependent changes in POMC mRNA levels and the magnitude of these changes suggest that dopaminergic compounds modulate POMC mRNA levels in the NIL in the same fashion as they regulate POMC peptide secretion. The mechanisms underlying dopaminergic modulation of POMC mRNA levels in the NIL remain to be elucidated.

It is also worthwhile to note that dopaminergic compound have no effect on POMC mRNA levels in the anterior lobe (Chen *et al.*, 1983).

D. Differential Regulation of the POMC Gene

Glucocorticoids alter the level of POMC mRNA in the AL, but have no effect on POMC mRNA levels in the NIL. Autoradiographic studies with labeled steroids have shown that there is no uptake of glucocorticoids in the nuclei of POMC-producing cells in the NIL (Warembourg, 1975; Rees *et al.*, 1977). Thus, NIL cells do not appear to contain functional glucocorticoid receptors.

The experiments described above also revealed that changes in the rate of secretion of POMC-derived peptides from the AL following adrenalectomy or DEX treatment were much more rapid than the change observed in the level of POMC mRNA. These data suggest that secretion of POMC peptides and transcription of the POMC gene are differentially regulated by glucocorticoids in the AL (Birnberg *et al.*, 1983).

POMC mRNA levels in the NIL are affected by dopaminergic compounds, while no effect is observed on the maintenance of POMC mRNA levels in the AL. This tissue-specific regulation could be due to the fact that dopamine receptors are present on NIL cells but are not associated with AL corticotrophs (Gudelsky *et al.*, 1980; Nansel *et al.*, 1979).

VI. PROENKEPHALIN GENE REGULATION

Daily injections in rats for 2–3 weeks with haloperidol, a dopamine receptor antagonist, increases twofold the level of Met-enkephalin in the striatum (Hong *et al.*, 1978; 1979). These data suggest that the prolonged blockage of dopamine receptors by haloperidol accelerates the synthesis of the enkephalin precursor molecule.

To investigate the possibility that haloperidol was modulating the level of proenkephalin mRNA in the striatum, cell-free translation and immunoprecipitation (Sabol *et al.*, 1983) as well as Northern blotting techniques

(Tang *et al.*, 1983) were employed. Following chronic haloperidol treatment for 3 weeks, the levels of proenkephalin mRNA in the striatum were increased two- (Sabol *et al.*, 1983) to fourfold (Tang *et al.*, 1983), consistent with the concomitant elevation of striatal Met-enkephalin content. Thus, haloperidol elevates the Met-enkephalin content in the striatum primarily by increasing the proenkephalin mRNA content in that tissue. This effect was specific to the striatum since haloperidol had no effect on maintaining proenkephalin mRNA levels in the rat hypothalamus, cortex, or hippocampus (Tang *et al.*, 1983).

VII. TRANSLATIONAL AND POSTTRANSLATIONAL CONTROL OF PRODUCTION OF OPIOID PEPTIDES

A. INTRODUCTION

Opioid peptides become active only after they are cleaved out of their precursor molecules. In some cases other modifications such as glycosylation, phosphorylation, amidation, or acetylation must also occur in order to activate these peptides. Amino acid sequences specify the enzymatic processes that lead to activation of the neuroendocrine peptides. These processes usually occur in a well-defined order as the proteins and peptides move through compartments in the secretion pathway.

Most of the domains of the opioid peptides in the precursors are flanked by pairs of basic amino acid residues (either Lys-Arg, Lys-Lys, or Arg-Arg), suggesting that trypsinlike enzymes are involved in the cleavage reaction. A carboxypeptidase-like enzyme is thought to remove the C-terminal basic amino acid to produce the bioactive peptide. However, other types of cleavage recognition sites are also used, including a single Arg site in proenkephalin and prodynorphin (to be discussed later).

Carboxy-terminal amidation has been observed in the formation of α-MSH from POMC (Eipper *et al.*, 1983; Bradbury *et al.*, 1982; Scott *et al.*, 1973, 1976) and a Met-enkephalin octapeptide from proenkephalin (Weber *et al.*, 1983; Matsuo *et al.*, 1983). The C-terminal amino acid of peptides that undergo amidation is followed by a glycine residue in the precursors, which is involved in transfer of the amino group and is cleaved from the peptide during the amidation reaction (Eipper *et al.*, 1983; Bradbury *et al.*, 1982).

Glycosylation of a protein at asparagine residues requires the sequence Asp-x-Thr or -x-Ser (Marshall, 1974; Hubbard and Ivatt, 1981). Glycosylation can also occur at serine or threonine residues (Marshall, 1974; Hubbard and Ivatt, 1981). POMC is known to be glycosylated. Human and bovine proenkephalin also have Asp-x-Thr sequences. However, since not all such sequences are glycosylated in a protein, it is not possible to predict which precursors will contain these oligosaccharides. In order to demonstrate the existence of oligosaccharides, one must isolate the protein and analyze its carbohydrate content or carry out pulse-label studies with radioactive sugars.

Other posttranslational modifications have been detected in the processing of POMC, including phosphorylation (Raese *et al.*, 1980; Bennett *et al.*, 1981a,b; Eipper and Mains, 1982), acetylation (Zakarian and Smyth, 1980; Smyth *et al.*, 1979; Eipper and Mains, 1981; Liotta *et al.*, 1981; Seizinger and Höllt, 1980; Akil *et al.*, 1981), sulfation (Hosphina *et al.*, 1982), and methylation (D. Chelsky, personal communication).

B. APPROACHES TO THE STUDY OF PROCESSING OF OPIOID PEPTIDE PRECURSORS

In order to determine the events involved in the processing of a protein precursor, it is necessary to have a system in which one can perform pulse-label and pulse-chase experiments. Most of the tissues that synthesize neuroendocrine precursors consist of mixed populations of cells in which the cells of interest comprise only a small proportion of the total population of cells. Tumor tissues and cell lines derived from precursor peptide-producing cells have been used as simplified model systems for the study of biosynthesis and the processing of neuroendocrine peptides because the cell population is relatively homogeneous. For example, detailed information about the processing of POMC has been obtained by the use of a mouse anterior pituitary cell line designated AtT-20-D$_{16V}$ (Yasamura, 1968). Pulse-label and pulse-chase studies with radioactive amino acids and sugars have helped define the steps involved in the processing of POMC in AtT-20 cells (Mains and Eipper, 1976; Roberts *et al.*, 1978; Eipper *et al.*, 1976; Phillips *et al.*, 1981). A complete review of the processing of POMC in AtT-20 cells is presented by Eipper and Mains (1980) and Herbert *et al.* (1980).

C. TISSUE-SPECIFIC PROCESSING OF POMC, PROENKEPHALIN, AND GASTRIN

1. Processing of POMC in Anterior and Neurointermediate Lobes of the Rodent Pituitary

Cultures of anterior and neurointermediate lobes of the rat pituitary provide viable and convenient systems for studying expression of POMC-derived peptides. In addition to the tissue-specific differences in regulation of hormone release described earlier, there are marked differences in the types of peptides derived from the ACTH-β-LPH portion of the precursor in the two lobes of the pituitary. The anterior lobe contains predominantly the steroidogenic hormone $ACTH_{1-39}$, while the intermediate lobe of the pituitary contains high levels of α-MSH ($ACTH_{1-13}$ with an acetylated N terminus and an amidated C terminus) and corticotropin-like intermediate lobe peptide (CLIP) ($ACTH_{18-39}$), as shown in Fig. 6 (Scott *et al.*, 1974, 1976; Roberts *et al.*, 1978; Mains and Eipper, 1975, 1979; Eipper and Mains, 1978; Kraicer, 1977; Gianoulakis *et al.*, 1979). Thus, $ACTH_{1-39}$ is further processed in the neurointermediate lobe to yield α-MSH and CLIP (Scott *et al.*, 1973). The lobes of the rodent pituitary also differ in the amounts of β-LPH, β-endorphin, and acetylated derivatives of β-endorphin that they contain. While the anterior lobe contains mainly β-LPH, the neurointermediate lobe has predominantly β-endorphin and derivatives of β-endorphin (Zakarian and Smyth, 1980; Smyth *et al.*, 1979; Eipper and Mains, 1981; Liotta *et al.*, 1981; Seizinger and Höllt, 1980; Akil *et al.*, 1981; Baizman *et al.*, 1979; Baizman and Cox, 1978; Loeber *et al.*, 1979; Lissitzky *et al.*, 1978) (see Fig. 6). Despite the differences in the ACTH/endorphin peptides in the two lobes of the pituitary, the forms of POMC they contain are very similar (Roberts *et al.*, 1978; Rosa *et al.*, 1980).

Pulse-label and pulse-chase studies with rodent pituitary cells show that the initial cleavages and glycosylation steps in the processing of POMC are the same in the two lobes of the pituitary (Roberts *et al.*, 1978; Eipper and Mains, 1978; Rosa *et al.*, 1980; Hinman and Herbert, 1980). As shown in Fig. 6, glycosylation of the N-terminal portion of POMC occurs first in the γ-MSH region of the molecule. About half of the POMC molecules are also glycosylated at Asn residue 29 in the ACTH portion of the molecule. The latter site is not present in bovine (Li *et al.*, 1958), human (Lee *et al.*, 1961), or porcine ACTH (Shepherd *et al.*, 1956). After glycosylation is complete, cleavage occurs between ACTH and β-LPH, resulting in the formation of glycosylated ACTH intermediates and β-LPH, as in $AtT-20-D_{16V}$ cells. Another cleavage then occurs to release glycosylated and unglycosylated forms of ACTH (Roberts *et al.*, 1978; Mains and Eipper, 1979; Eipper and Mains, 1978; Rosa *et al.*, 1980; Hinman and Herbert, 1980) and an N-terminal fragment. In the rodent anterior pituitary, processing essentially ceases at this point, but in the neurointermediate lobe ACTH is processed to α-MSH and CLIP by cleavage in the middle of the molecule. The N-terminal fragment of ACTH is then trimmed back to 13 residues ($ACTH_{1-13}$), presumably by carboxypeptidases, amidated at the C terminus and acetylated at the N terminus (Scott *et al.*, 1973, 1974; Jackson and Lowry, 1980). The β-LPH portion of POMC is cleaved in the NIL to form γ-LPH and β-endorphin. β-Endorphin is then acetylated at its N terminus and shortened by removal of four C-terminal amino acids (Zakarian and Smyth, 1980; Smyth *et al.*, 1979;

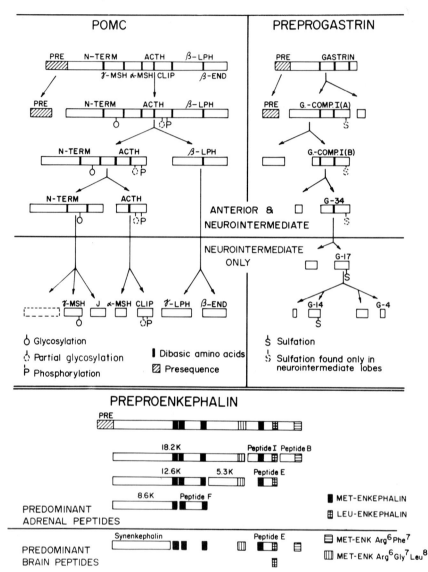

FIG. 6. Tissue-specific processing pathways of opioid peptide precursors. Processing of POMC in the anterior and the neurointermediate lobe of the pituitary is shown at the upper left. This tissue-specific processing is compared to the preprogastrin processing taking place in the same cells as POMC at the upper right. Predominant preproenkephalin-derived peptides found in the bovine adrenal gland and brain, are depicted at the bottom. Abbreviations: PRE, presequence; N-TERM, N-terminal peptide; J, joining peptide; CLIP, corticotropin-like intermediate lobe peptide; β-END, β-endorphin; β- and γ-LPH, β- and γ-lipotropin; α- and γ-MSH, α- and γ-melanocyte stimulating hormones; G-comp I(A) and I(B), gastrin component I(A) and I(B); G-34, -17, -14, -4, gastrin-34, -17, -14, -4.

Eipper and Mains, 1981). Acetylation of β-endorphin at its N terminus destroys its analgesic activity. Hence, this modification might be a way of regulating the amount of active endorphin available in the NIL.

Recent evidence suggests that the N-terminal portion of POMC is also cleaved extensively in the pituitary. Cleavage at Arg^{49}-Lys^{50} (Fig. 7), the first pair of basic amino acids in POMC, would be expected to give rise to a cysteine-rich N-terminal fragment. Although this peptide fragment has not yet been purified, immunoassays suggest it is present in the pituitary (Eleman et al., 1982). Proteolytic cleavage at the next pair of basic amino acid residues in rodent POMC (Fig. 7) would be expected to give rise to a 24–amino acid peptide, γ_3-MSH, which has a glycosylation site at Asn^{65} in all species shown. A glycosylated form of Lys-γ_3-MSH has been shown to be present in the intermediate lobe of bovine and rat pituitaries (Hammond et al., 1982; Esch et al., 1981; Browne et al., 1981). Bovine, human, and porcine POMC have an additional pair of basic amino acids (Arg^{62}-Arg^{63}) which, if cleaved, would give rise to γ_2-MSH, a dodecapeptide. Since a glycine is present at the C terminus of this peptide, amidation might be expected to occur, forming a peptide ending in Phe-NH_2. This peptide has been detected in the NIL of bovine pituitary (Browne et al., 1981; Shibasaki et al., 1980) but not in the anterior pituitary (Tanaka et al., 1983; Shibasaki et al., 1981). Hence, the N terminus of POMC is more completely processed in the NIL of the pituitary than in the anterior pituitary (Eleman et al., 1981; Hope and Lowry, 1981; Esch et al., 1981; Pederson et al., 1982; Tanaka et al., 1981), as already demonstrated for the ACTH and β-LPH domains.

Cleavage of the N-terminal fragment of POMC also occurs at the Lys-Arg site just preceding ACTH (Fig. 7), forming an acidic peptide called joining, or J, peptide (Seidah et al., 1981; Noe, 1981), which varies in length from 19 amino acids (mouse and rat) to 31 amino acids (human) (Seidah et al., 1981; Browne et al., 1982; Umagat et al., 1982). In mouse, rat, and human, Lys-

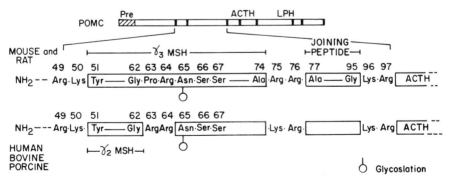

FIG. 7. Structure and processing of the amino-terminal portion of POMC in various species.

Arg is preceded by a Gly residue, raising the possibility of amidation of the Glu residue in this peptide. The amidated form of this peptide has been reported to be present in human pituitary (Browne *et al.*, 1982).

These results show that cleavage occurs at all of the pairs of basic amino acid residues contained in POMC (Figs. 6 and 7). POMC has also been shown to be phosphorylated in the AL and NIL of rat pituitary (Bennett *et al.*, 1981a,b). Because of the importance of phosphorylation in modulating cellular activities, an attempt was made to determine whether physiological factors might control the extent of phosphorylation *in vivo* and in cultured rat pituitary cells. No correlation could be found between the extent of phosphorylation and stimulation of ACTH release by CRF or cAMP (Mains and Eipper, 1983). Also, no major differences were found between the degree of phosphorylation of ACTH peptides in anterior and neurointermediate lobes of the pituitary (Eipper and Mains, 1982).

Almost all of the POMC-derived products shown in Fig. 6 arise by proteolytic cleavages at Lys-Arg sites. It appears that in mammals this sequence is preferred as a cleavage site over Arg-Arg or Lys-Lys (as in the case of conversion of proinsulin to insulin).

Noteworthy in relation to the tissue-specific processing of POMC, immunostaining studies with gastrin-specific antibodies (Larsson and Rehfeld, 1981) have revealed that these peptides are present in the same cells that contain POMC in the AL and NIL of the porcine pituitary. The precursor to gastrin is also present in this tissue. An exciting finding is that the gastrin precursor is processed differently in the two lobes of the pituitary. In the anterior pituitary, higher molecular weight forms of unsulfated gastrin predominate, including component I and gastrin-34 (Rehfeld and Larsson, 1981), whereas in the neurointermediate lobe, a sulfated lower molecular weight form of gastrin (gastrin-17) is a major product. Therefore, the results show that the processing of the gastrin precursor in the AL and NIL of the pituitary parallels that of POMC in these cells. A very interesting question is whether production and release of gastrin peptides are regulated in the same manner as POMC peptides in the two lobes of the pituitary.

2. Processing of Proenkephalin

Detection of immunoreactive enkephalin peptides in the bovine adrenal medulla provided impetus for using this tissue to study biosynthesis of enkephalins (Schultzberg *et al.*, 1978a,b). Since these subjects have been reviewed in depth recently (Udenfriend and Kilpatrick, 1983; Lewis and Stern, 1983), we will present only a brief summary emphasizing tissue-specific differences in processing of proenkephalin.

A variety of enkephalin-containing peptides (ECPs) are present in adrenal medulla (Yang *et al.*, 1979; Viveros *et al.*, 1979; Lewis *et al.*, 1979) and brain (Rossier *et al.*, 1980; Boarder *et al.*, 1982), in addition to the pentapeptides, Met- and Leu-enkephalin. Figure 6 shows the biosynthetic relationship of these peptides in the adrenal medulla and brain. The arrangement of the six Met-enkephalin and one Leu-enkephalin units in preproenkephalin is presented first. Met-enkephalin-Arg[6]-Phe[7] is present at the C-terminal part of the precursor, and the octapeptide product, Met-enkephalin-Arg[6]-Gly[7]-Leu[8], comprises the amino acid sequence 186–193 in the precursor (Rossier *et al.*, 1980; Boarder *et al.*, 1982; Stern *et al.*, 1979, 1980a; Kilpatrick *et al.*, 1981a). Larger ECPs containing more than one enkephalin sequence are also observed, including peptide E, which has a Met-enkephalin at its N terminus and a Leu-enkephalin at its C terminus, and peptide F, which has a Met-enkephalin sequence at each end (Jones *et al.*, 1978; Kilpatrick *et al.*, 1981c; Stern *et al.*, 1980b). These smaller ECPs are derived from larger peptides. For example, peptide E arises from peptide I by cleavage at a Lys-Arg site, and peptide F comes from still larger fragments, which have also been characterized (Jones *et al.*, 1982a,b) (Fig. 6). It is still not clear which of these peptides are end products of processing and which are intermediates. Bioassays indicate that peptide E (Kilpatrick *et al.*, 1981c), Met-enkephalin-Arg[6]-Phe[7], and Met-enkephalin-Arg[6]-Gly[7]-Leu[8] (Inturrisi *et al.*, 1980; Audiger *et al.*, 1980) are very potent opioids. However, peptide F and larger ECPs are not very active in assays of opioid activity (Kilpatrick *et al.*, 1981c). The bioactivity assays suggest that peptide E and the smaller ECPs are the true end products of biosynthesis, whereas the larger fragments are intermediates in processing.

The proenkephalin peptide sequences flanked by Lys-Arg or Lys-Lys sites are cleaved out of the precursor, whereas the Met-enkephalin sequence in peptide E that has an Arg-Arg on its C terminus is not released from the precursor.

An amidated octapeptide ECP has recently been isolated from bovine brain and human pheochromocytoma (a tumor of the adrenal medulla). This peptide, which results from cleavage at a single Arg residue in peptide E (Weber *et al.*, 1983; Matsuo *et al.*, 1983), is the first amidated opioid peptide that has been isolated. Cleavage at a single Arg residue also occurs in the processing of several other precursors, including proAVP (producing a glycopeptide) (Land *et al.*, 1982), prodynorphin (Weber *et al.*, 1982; Minamino *et al.*, 1980; Seizinger *et al.*, 1981; Fischli *et al.*, 1982; Kilpatrick *et al.*, 1982a; Cone *et al.*, 1983), procholecystokinin (Rehfeld, 1980), and progrowth-hormone-releasing-factor (Gubler *et al.*, (1983).

As in the case of POMC, the processing of proenkephalin is tissue specific. The major products of processing in the adrenal medulla are the higher molecular weight ECPs, whereas in the brain one finds mainly the enkephalins and other small ECPs (Udenfriend and Kilpatrick, 1983; Weber *et al.*, 1983; Liston *et al.*, 1983).

Little is known about the function of enkephalin peptides produced by the adrenal medulla. These peptides are released into the circulation (Kilpatrick *et al.*, 1981b; Viveros *et al.*, 1982), and denervation of the gland has been shown to increase the level of ECPs in the adrenal medulla (Lewis *et al.*, 1980). However, the target organs for these peptides are unknown.

The processing of ECPs is particularly interesting because these peptides are present in the same secretory vesicles as epinephrine (Viveros *et al.*, 1979), another major secretory product of the chromaffin cells. The production and release of enkephalins and epinephrins are coordinately regulated (Viveros *et al.*, 1979). It would be very important to know the level of gene expression at which this regulation occurs.

Several mechanisms can be proposed to explain tissue-specific processing of neuroendocrine peptide precursors. One is the existence of a different set of processing enzymes in different tissues. The environment at the sites of processing could also differ in different tissues. Another possibility is a difference in the structures of the precursor molecules in different tissues. In the latter case, a sequence difference in the precursor molecule would dictate how the precursor is processed in each tissue. Different translational modifications of the precursor might also account for tissue differences in processing. Different precursors could arise by selective expression of one or more of a family of genes in each tissue or from a single gene by alternate modes of splicing, as in the case of the calcitonin/calcitonin gene related peptide (CGRP) gene. Most of the evidence to date suggests that differential processing of POMC occurs at the level of processing enzymes in the pituitary. First, there is only one POMC gene in the mouse (Uhler *et al.*, 1983) and rat (J. Drouin, personal communication) species; second, an extensive search for different forms of mRNA that might code for different POMC forms in the two lobes of the pituitary has been negative (Herbert *et al.*, 1983); and third, posttranslational modifications of POMC appear to be the same in the two lobes of the pituitary.

Differential processing of proenkephalin in the adrenal modulla and brain also appears to be determined by differences in processing enzymes because only one proenkephalin gene can be detected in these species (Comb *et al.*, 1983).

Thus, different sets of processing enzymes appear to be responsible for tissue-specific expression of neuroendocrine peptides. Posttranslational processing makes up the last steps in the cascade of events leading to expression of the polyprotein genes and appears to be a major mechanism for generating diverse sets of peptides in the neuroendocrine system.

The question finally arises as to why nature has made large proteins for the generation of small peptides. Neuroendocrine peptides become active only after they have been liberated from the precursor molecule and properly modified. Other portions of the amino acid sequence of the precursor may, therefore, be necessary for specifying interactions involved in compartmentalization and activation of the proteins during secretion.

Polyproteins contain either multiple copies of a single type of bioactive peptide or a set of functionally distinct bioactive peptides. Thus, a single mRNA transcript that codes for diverse bioactive peptides can be generated. The production of precursors containing multiple copies of the same bioactive peptide may be a way of more efficiently producing a neuroendocrine peptide. On the other hand, the production of different bioactive peptides from a single precursor provides a means of coordinating the synthesis of functionally related peptides that may act together to mediate a distinct behavioral response. The evolution of this type of precursor may well have paralleled the evolution of the diffuse neuroendocrine system in higher organisms.

REFERENCES

Agarwal, K. L., Brunstedt, J., and Noyes, B. E. (1981). *J. Biol. Chem.* **256**, 1023–1028.

Akil, H., Veda, Y., Lin, H. L., and Watson, S. J. (1981). *Neuropeptides* **1**, 429–446.

Alwine, J. C., Kemp, D. J., and Stark, G. R. (1977). *Proc. Natl. Acad. Sci. U.S.A.* **74**, 5350–5354.

Amara, S. G., Jonas, V., Rosenfeld, M. G., Ong, E. S., and Evans, R. M. (1982). *Nature (London)* **298**, 240–244.

Audiger, Y., Mazarguil, H., Rossier, J., and Cros, J. (1980). *Eur. J. Pharmacol.* **68**, 237–238.

Baizman, E. R., and Cox, B. M. (1978). *Life Sci.* **22**, 519–524.

Baizman, E. R., Cox, B. M., Osman, O. H., and Goldstein, A. (1979). *Neuroendocrinology* **28**, 402–409.

Bell, G. I., Santerre, R. F., and Mullenbach, G. T. (1983). *Nature (London)* **302**, 716–718.

Bennett, H. P. J., Brown, C. A., and Solomon, S. (1981a). *Biochemistry* **20**, 4530–4538.

Bennett, H. P. J., Brown, C. A., and Solomon, S. (1981b). *Proc. Natl. Acad. Sci. U.S.A.* **78**, 4713–4717.

Benton, W. D., and Davis, R. W. (1977). *Science* **196**, 180–182.

Birnberg, N., Lissitzky, J.-C., Hinman, M., and Herbert, E. (1983). *Proc. Natl. Acad. Sci. U.S.A.* **80**, 6982–6986.

Bisbee, C. A., Baker, M. A., Wilson, A. C., Hadji-Azimi, I., and Fischberg, M. (1977). *Science* **195**, 785–787.

Boarder, M. R., Lockfield, A. J., and Barchas, J. D. (1982). *J. Neurochem.* **38**, 299–304.

Bradbury, A. F., Finnie, M. D. A., and Smyth, D. G. (1982). *Nature (London)* **298**, 686–689.

Breathnach, R., and Chambon, P. (1981). *Annu. Rev. Biochem.* **50**, 349–383.

Browne, C. A., Bennett, H. P. J., and Solomon, S. (1981). *Biochem. Biophys. Res. Commun.* **100**, 336–343.

Browne, C. A., Bennett, H. P. J., and Solomon, S. (1982). *Anal. Biochem.* **123**, 201–208.

Chang, A. C. Y., Cochet, M., and Cohen, S. (1980). *Proc. Natl. Acad. Sci. U.S.A.* **77**, 4890–4894.

Chen, C. L. C., Dionne, F. T., and Roberts, J. L. (1983). *Proc. Natl. Acad. Sci. U.S.A.* **80**, 2211–2215.

Civelli, O., Birnberg, N., and Herbert, E. (1982). *J. Biol. Chem.* **257**, 6783–6787.

Cochet, M., Chang, A. C. Y., and Cohen, S. N. (1982). *Nature (London)* **297**, 335–339.

Comb, M., Seeburg, P. H., Adelman, J., Eiden, L., and Herbert, E. (1982). *Nature (London)* **295**, 663–666.

Comb, M., Rosen, H., Seeburg, P., Adelman, J., and Herbert, E. (1983). *DNA* **2**, 213–229.

Cone, R., Weber, E., Barchas, J. D., and Goldstein, A. (1983). *J. Neurosci.* **3**, 2146–2152.

Doolittle, R. (1978). *Nature (London)* **272**, 581–582.

Douglass, J., Civelli, O., and Herbert, E. (1984). *Annu. Rev. Biochem.* **53**, 665–715.

Drouin, J., and Goodman, H. M. (1980). *Nature (London)* **288**, 610–613.

Eipper, B. A., and Mains, R. E. (1978). *J. Supramol. Struct.* **8**, 247–256.

Eipper, B. A., and Mains, R. E. (1980). *Endocr. Rev.* **1**, 1–27.

Eipper, B. A., and Mains, R. E. (1981). *J. Biol. Chem.* **256**, 5689–5695.

Eipper, B. A., and Mains, R. E. (1982). *J. Biol. Chem.* **257**, 4907–4915.

Eipper, B. A., Mains, R. E., and Guenzi, D. (1976). *J. Biol. Chem.* **251**, 4121–4126.

Eipper, B. A., Glembotski, C. C., and Mains, R. E. (1983). *J. Biol. Chem.* **258**, 7292–7298.

Eleman, R., Hakanson, R., Larsson, I., Sundler, F., and Thorell, J. I. (1982). *Endocrinology (Baltimore)* **111**, 578–583.

Esch, F. S., Shibasaki, T., Bohlen, P., Wehrenberg, W. B., and Ling, N. (1981). *Peptides (N.Y.)* **2**, 485–488.

Farah, J. M., Malcolm, D. S., and Mueller, G. P. (1982). *Endocrinology (Baltimore)* **110**, 657–659.

Felsenfeld, G., and McGhee, J. (1982). *Nature (London)* **296**, 602–603.

Fischli, W., Goldstein, A., Hunkapiller, M., and Hood, L. (1982). *Proc. Natl. Acad. Sci. U.S.A.* **79**, 5435–5437.

Fleischer, N., and Rawls, W. E. (1970). *Am. J. Physiol.* **4**, 367–404.

Furutani, Y., Morimoto, Y., Shibahara, S., Noda, M., Takahashi, H., Hirose, T., Asai, M., Inayama, S., Hayashida, H., Miyata, T., and Numa, S. (1983). *Nature (London)* **301**, 537–540.

Gee, C. E., and Roberts, J. L. (1982). *DNA* **2**, 157–163.

Gianoulakis, C., Seidah, N. G., Routhier, R., and Chrétien, M. (1979). *J. Biol. Chem.* **254**, 11902–11906.

Gilbert, W. (1978). *Nature (London)* **271**, 501.

Goldberg, M. L. (1979). Ph.D. Thesis, Stanford University, Stanford, California.

Goldstein, A., Tachibana, S., Lowney, L. I., Hunkapiller, M., and Hood, L. E. (1979). *Proc. Natl. Acad. Sci. U.S.A.* **76**, 6666–6670.

Grosschedl, R., and Birnsteil, M. L. (1980). *Proc. Natl. Acad. Sci. U.S.A.* **77**, 1432–1436.

Gubler, U., Seeburg, P. H., Gage, L. P., and Udenfriend, S. (1982). *Nature (London)* **295**, 206–209.

Gubler, U., Monahan, J. J., Lomedico, P. T., Bhatt, R. S., Collier, K. J., Hoffman, B. J., Bohlen, P., Esch, F., Ling, N., Zeytin, F., Brazeau, P., Poonian, M. S., and Gage, L. P. (1983). *Proc. Natl. Acad. Sci. U.S.A.* **80**, 4311–4314.

Gudelsky, G. A., Nansel, D. D., and Porter, J. C. (1980). *Endocrinology (Baltimore)* **107**, 30–34.

Hammond, G. L., Chung, D., and Li, C. H. (1982). *Biochem. Biophys. Res. Commun.* **108**, 118–123.

Herbert, E., Roberts, J. L., Phillips, M., Allen, R., Hinman, M., Budarf, M., Policastro, P., and Rosa, P. (1980). *Front. Neuroendocrinol.* **6**, 67–101.

Herbert, E., Birnberg, N., Lissitzky, J.-C., Civelli, O., and Uhler, M. (1981). *Neurosci. Newsl.* **12**, 16–27.

Herbert, E., Oates, E., Martens, G., Comb, M., Rosen, H., and Uhler, M. (1983). *Cold Spring Harbor Symp. Quant. Biol.* **48**, 375–384.

Hinman, M., and Herbert, E. (1980). *Biochemistry* **19**, 5395–5402.

Höllt, V., and Bergmann, M. (1982). *Neuropharmacology* **21**, 147–154.

Höllt, V., Haarmann, I., Seizinger, B. R., and Hertz, A. (1982). *Endocrinology (Baltimore)* **110**, 1885–1891.

Hong, J. S., Yang, H. Y. T., Fratta, W., and Costa, E. (1978). *J. Pharmacol. Exp. Ther.* **205**, 141–147.

Hong, J. S., Yang, H. Y. T., Gillin, J. C., Di Giulio, A. M., Fratta, W., and Costa, E. (1979). *Brain Res.* **160**, 192–195.

Hope, J., and Lowry, P. J. (1981). *Front. Horm. Res.* **8**, 44–61.

Horikawa, S., Takai, T., Toyosato, M., Takahashi, H., Noda, M., Kakidani, H., Kubo, T., Hirose, T., Inayama, S., Hayashida, H., Miyata, T., and Numa, S. (1983). *Nature (London)* **306**, 611–614.

Hoshina, H., Hortin, G., and Boime, I. (1982) *Science* **217**, 63–64.

Hubbard, S. C., and Ivatt, R. J. (1981). *Annu. Rev. Biochem.* **50**, 555–584.

Hudson, P., Penschow, J., Shine, J., Ryan, G., Niall, H., and Coghlan, J. (1981). *Endocrinology (Baltimore)* **108**, 353–356.

Hughes, J., Smith, T. W., Kosterlitz, H. W., Fothergill, L. A., Morgan, B. A., and Morris, H. R. (1975). *Nature (London)* **258**, 577–579.

Inturrisi, C. E., Umans, J. G., Wolff, D., Stern, A. S., Lewis, R. V., Stein, S., and Udenfriend, S. (1980). *Proc. Natl. Acad. Sci. U.S.A.* **77**, 5512–5514.

Jackson, S., and Lowry, P. J. (1980). *Ann. N.Y. Acad. Sci.* **86**, 205–219.

Jones, B. N., Stern, A. S., Lewis, R. V., Kimura, S., Stein, S., Udenfriend, S., and Shively, J. E. (1978). *Arch. Biochem. Biophys.* **204**, 392–395.

Jones, B. N., Shively, J. E., Kikpatrick, D. L., Kojima, K., and Udenfriend, S. (1982a). *Proc. Natl. Acad. Sci. U.S.A.* **79**, 1313–1315.

Jones, B. N., Shively, J. E., Kilpatrick, D. L., Stern, A. S., Lewis, R. V., Kojima, K., and Udenfriend, S. (1982b). *Proc. Natl. Acad. Sci. U.S.A.* **79**, 2096–2100.

Kakidani, H., Furutani, Y., Takahashi, H., Noda, M., Morimoto, Y., Hirose, T., Asai, M., Inayama, S., Nakanishi, S., and Numa, S. (1982). *Nature (London)* **298**, 245–249.

Kilpatrick, D. L., Jones, B. N., Kojima, K., and Udenfriend, S. (1981a). *Biochem. Biophys. Res. Commun.* **103**, 698–705.

Kilpatrick, D. L., Lewis, R. V., Stein, S., and Udenfriend, S. (1981b). *Proc. Natl. Acad. Sci. U.S.A.* **77**, 7473–7475.

Kilpatrick, D. L., Taniguchi, T., Jones, B. N., Stern, A. S., Shively, J. E., Hulliman, J., Kimura, S., Stein, S., and Udenfriend, S. (1981c). *Proc. Natl. Acad. Sci. U.S.A.* **78**, 3265–3268.

Kilpatrick, D. L., Wahlström, A., Lahm, H. W., Blacher, R., and Udenfriend, S. (1982a). *Proc. Natl. Acad. Sci. U.S.A.* **79**, 6480–6483.

Kilpatrick, D. L., Wahlström, A., Lahm, H. W., Blacher, R., and Udenfriend, S. (1982b). *Proc. Natl. Acad. Sci. U.S.A.* **79**, 6680–6683.

Kraicer, J. (1977). *Front. Horm. Res.* **4**, 200–222.

Land, H., Schutz, G., Schmale, H., and Richter, D. (1982). *Nature (London)* **295**, 299–303.

Larsson, L. I., and Rehfeld, J. F. (1981). *Science* **213**, 768–770.

Lawn, R. M., Fritsch, E. F., Parker, R. C., Lake, G. B., and Maniatis, T. (1978). *Cell* **15**, 1157–1163.

Lee, T. H., Lerner, A. B., and Buettner-Janusch, V. (1961). *J. Biol. Chem.* **236**, 2970–2974.

Lepine, J., and Dupont, A. (1981). *Endocr. Soc.* **108**, 385 (abstr.).

Lewis, R. V., and Stern, A. S. (1983). *Annu. Rev. Pharmacol. Toxicol.* **23**, 353–372.

Lewis, R. V., Stern, A. S., Rossier, J., Stein, S., and Udenfriend, S. (1979). *Biochem. Biophys. Res. Commun.* **89**, 822–829.

Lewis, R. V., Stern, A. S., Kilpatrick, D. L., Gerber, L. D., and Rossier, J. (1980). *J. Neurosci.* **1**, 80–82.

Li, C. H., Dixon, J. S., and Chung, D. (1958). *J. Am. Chem. Soc.* **80**, 2587–2588.

Liotta, A. S., Yamaguchi, H., and Krieger, D. T. (1981). *J. Neurosci.* **1**, 585–595.

Lissitzky, J.-C., Morin, O., Dupont, A., Labrie, F., Seidah, N. G., Chrétien, M., Lis, M., and Coy, D. H. (1978). *Life Sci.* **11**, 1715–1726.

Liston, D. R., Vanderhaeghen, J.-J., and Rossier, J. (1983). *Nature (London)* **302**, 62–65.

Loeber, J. G., Verhoef, J., Burbach, J. P. H., and Wilter, A. (1979). *Biochem. Biophys. Res. Commun.* **86**, 1288–1295.

Mains, R. E., and Eipper, B. A. (1975). *Proc. Natl. Acad. Sci. U.S.A.* **72**, 3565–3569.

Mains, R. E., and Eipper, B. A. (1976). *J. Biol. Chem.* **251**, 4115–4120.

Mains, R. E., and Eipper, B. A. (1979). *J. Biol. Chem.* **254**, 7885–7894.

Mains, R. E., and Cipper, B. A. (1983). *Endocrinology (Baltimore)* **112**, 1986–1995.

Mains, R. E., Eipper, B. A., and Ling, N. (1977). *Proc. Natl. Acad. Sci. U.S.A.* **74**, 3014–3018.

Marshall, R. D. (1974). *Biochem. Soc. Symp.* **40**, 17–26.

Martens, G., and Herbert, E. (1984). *Nature (London)* **310**, 251–254.

Matsuo, H., Miyata, A., and Mizuma, K. (1983). *Nature (London)* **305**, 721–723.

Messing, J., Gronenborn, B., Muller-Hill, B., and Hofschneider, P. H. (1977). *Proc. Natl. Acad. Sci. U.S.A.* **74**, 3642–3646.

Minamino, N., Kangawa, K., Fukada, A., and Matsuo, H. (1980). *Biochem. Biophys. Res. Commun.* **95**, 1475–1481.

Mishina, M., Kurosaki, T., Yamamoto, T., Notake, M., Masu, M., and Numa, S. (1982). *EMBO J.* **1**, 1533–1538.

Nakamura, M., Nakanishi, S., Sueoka, S., Imura, H., and Numa, S. (1978). *Eur. J. Biochem.* **86**, 61–66.

Nakanishi, S., Inoue, E. A., Kita, T., Numa, S., Chang, A. C. Y., Cohen, S. N., Nunberg, J., and Schimke, R. T. (1978). *Proc. Natl. Acad. Sci. U.S.A.* **75**, 6021–6025.

Nakanishi, S., Inoue, A., Kita, T., Nakamura, M., Chang, A. C. Y., Cohen, S. N., and Numa, S. (1979). *Nature (London)* **278**, 423–427.

Nakanishi, S., Terahashi, Y., Noda, M., Notake, M., Watanabe, Y., and Numa, S. (1980). *Nature (London)* **287**, 752–755.

Nakanishi, S., Teranishi, Y., Watanabe, Y., Notake, M., Noda, M., Kakidani, H., Jingami, H., and Numa, S. (1981). *Eur. J. Biochem.* **115**, 429–438.

Nansel, D. D., Gudelsky, G. A., and Porter, J. C. (1979). *Endocrinology (Baltimore)* **105**, 1073–1077.

Noda, M., Furutani, Y., Takahashi, H., Toyosato, M., Hirose, T., Inayama, S., Nakanishi, S., and Numa, S. (1982a). *Nature (London)* **295**, 202–206.

Noda, M., Teranishi, Y., Takahashi, H., Toyosato, M., Notake, M., Nakanishi, S., and Numa, S. (1982b). *Nature (London)* **297**, 431–434.

Noe, B. D. (1981). *J. Biol. Chem.* **256**, 4940–4946.

Notake, M., Tobimatsu, T., Watanabe, Y., Takahashi, H., Mishina, M., and Numa, S. (1983). *FEBS Lett.* **156**, 67–71.

Okayama, H., and Berg, P. (1982). *Mol. Cell. Biol.* **2**, 161–170.

Owerbach, D., Rutter, W. J., Roberts, J. L., Whitfeld, P. L., Shine, J., Seeburg, P. H., and Shows, T. B. (1981). *Somatic Cell Genet.* **7**, 359–369.

Pederson, R. C., Ling, N., and Brownie, A. C. (1982). *Endocrinology (Baltimore)* **110**, 825–834.

Phillips, M. A., Budarf, M. L., and Herbert, E. (1981). *Biochemistry* **20**, 1666–1675.

Raese, J. D., Boarder, M. R., Makk, G., and Barchas, J. D. (1980). *Adv. Biochem. Pyschopharmacol.* **22**, 377–383.

Rees, H., Stumpf, W., Sar, M., and Petrusz, P. (1977). *Cell Tissue Res.* **182**, 347–356.

Rehfeld, J. F. (1980). *In* "Gastrointestinal Hormones" (G. B. J. Glass, ed.), pp. 433–449. Raven Press, New York.

Rehfeld, J. F., and Larsson, L.-I. (1981). *J. Biol. Chem.* **256**, 10426–10429.

Roberts, J. L., and Herbert, E. (1977). *Proc. Natl. Acad. Sci. U.S.A.* **74**, 4826.

Roberts, J. L., Phillips, M., Rosa, P. A., and Herbert, E. (1978). *Biochemistry* 17, 3609–3618.

Roberts, J. L., Budarf, M. L., Baxter, J. D., and Herbert, E. (1979). *Biochemistry* 18, 4907–4915.

Rosa, P., Policastro, P., and Herbert, E. (1980). *J. Exp. Biol.* **89**, 215–237.

Rossier, J., Audigier, Y., Ling, N., Cros, J., and Udenfriend, S. (1980). *Nature (London)* **288**, 88–90.

Sabol, S. L., Yoshikawa, K., and Hong, J. S. (1983). *Biochem. Biophys. Res. Commun.* **113**, 391–399.

Sanger, F., Nicklen, S., and Coulson, A. R. (1977). *Proc. Natl. Acad. Sci. U.S.A.* **74**, 5463–5467.

Schachter, B. S., Johnson, L. K., Baxter, J. D., and Roberts, J. L. (1983). *Endocrinology (Baltimore)* **110**, 1442–1444.

Scheller, R. H., Jackson, J. F., McAllister, L. B., Rothman, B. S., Mayeri, E., and Axel, R. (1983). *Cell* **32**, 7–22.

Schmale, H., Heinsohn, S., and Richter, D. (1983). *EMBO J.* **2**, 763–767.

Schultzberg, M., Hokfelt, T., Lundberg, J. M., Terenius, L., Elfin, L. G., and Elde, R. D. (1978a). *Acta Physiol. Scand.* **103**, 475–477.

Schultzberg, M., Lundberg, J. M., Hokfelt, T., Terenius, L., Brand, J., Elde, R. D., and Goldstein, M. (1978b). *Neuroscience* **3**, 1169–1186.

Scott, A. P., Ratcliff, J. G., Rees, L. H., Bennett, H. P. J., Lowry, P. J., and McMartin, C. (1973). *Nature (London), New Biol.* **244**, 65–67.

Scott, A. P., Lowry, P. L., Ratcliff, J. G., Rees, L. H., and Landon, J. (1974). *J. Endocrinol.* **61**, 355–364.

Scott, A. P., Lowry, P. J., and van Wimersma Greidanus, T. B. (1976). *J. Endocrinol.* **70**, 197–205.

Seidah, N. G., Rochemont, J., Hamelin, J., Benjannet, S., and Chrétien, M. (1981). *Biochem. Biophys. Res. Commun.* **102**, 710–716.

Seizinger, B. R., and Höllt, V. (1980). *Biochem. Biophys. Res. Commun.* **96**, 535–543.

Seizinger, B. R., Höllt, V., and Hertz, A. (1981). *Biochem. Biophys. Res. Commun.* **102**, 197–205.

Shepherd, R. G., Willson, S. D., Howard, K. S., Bell, P. H., Davis, S. B., Eigner, E. A., and Shakespeare, N. E. (1956). *J. Am. Chem. Soc.* **78**, 5067–5076.

Shibasaki, T., Ling, N., and Guillemin, R. (1980). *Biochem. Biophys. Res. Commun.* **96**, 1393–1399.

Shibasaki, T., Ling, N., Guillemin, R., Silver, M., and Bloom, F. (1981). *Regul. Pept.* **2**, 43,–52.

Smyth, D. G., Massey, D. E., Zakarian, S., and Finnie, M. D. A. (1979). *Nature (London)* **279**, 251–254.

Southern, E. M. (1975). *J. Mol. Biol.* **98**, 503–517.

Steiner, D. F., Quinn, P. S., Shu, J. C., March, J., and Tager, H. S. (1980). *Ann. N.Y. Acad. Sci.* **343**, 1–16.

Stern, A. S., Lewis, R. V., Kimura, S., Rossier, J., Gerber, L. D., Brink, L., Stein, S., and Udenfriend, S. (1979). *Proc. Natl. Acad. Sci. U.S.A.* **76**, 6680–6683.

Stern, A. S., Lewis, R. V., Kimura, S., Rossier, J., Stein, S., and Udenfriend, S. (1980a). *Arch. Biochem. Biophys.* **205**, 606–613.

Stern, A. S., Jones, B. M., Shively, J. E., Stein, S., and Udenfriend, S. (1980b). *Proc. Natl. Acad. Sci. U.S.A.* **78**, 1962–1966.

Tanaka, I., Nakai, Y., Nakao, K., Oki, S., Fukata, J., and Imura, H. (1981). *Clin. Endocrinol.* **15**, 353–361.

Tanaka, I., Nakai, Y., Nakao, K., Oki, S., Yoshimasa, T., and Imura, H. (1983). *J. Clin. Endocrinol. Metab.* **56**, 1080–1083.

Tang, F., Costa, E., and Schwartz, J. P. (1983). *Proc. Natl. Acad. Sci. U.S.A.* **80**, 3841–3844.

Thomas, P. S. (1980). *Proc. Natl. Acad. Sci. U.S.A.* **77**, 5201–5205.

Udenfriend, S., and Kilpatrick, D. L. (1983). *Arch. Biochem. Biophys.* **221**, 309–323.

Uhler, M., Herbert, E., D'Eustachio, P., and Ruddle, F. D. (1983). *J. Biol. Chem.* **258**, 9444–9453.

Umagat, H., Kucera, P., and Wen, L. F. (1982). *J. Chromatogr.* **239**, 463–474.

Vale, W., Speiss, J., Rivier, C., and Rivier, J. (1981). *Science* **213**, 1394–1397.

Vermes, I., Mulder, G. H., Smelik, P. G., and Tilders, F. J. H. (1980). *Life Sci.* **27**, 1761–1768.

Viveros, O. H., Diliberto, E. V., Hazum, E., and Chang, K. J. (1979). *Mol. Pharmacol.* **16**, 1101–1108.

Viveros, O. H., Wilson, S. P., and Chang, K.-J. (1982). *In* "Regulatory Peptides" (E. Costa and M. Trabucchi, eds.), pp. 217–224. Raven Press, New York.

Wallace, R. B., Shaffer, J., Murphy, R. F., Bonner, J., and Hirose, T. (1979). *Nucleic Acids Res.* **6**, 3543–3557.

Warembourg, M. (1975). *Cell Tissue Res.* **161**, 183–191.

Watanabe, H., Nicholson, W. E., and Orth, D. N. (1973a). *Endocrinology (Baltimore)* **93**, 411–416.

Watanabe, H., Orth, D. N., and Taft, D. O. (1973b). *J. Biol. Chem.* **248**, 7625–7679.

Weber, E., Evans, C. J., and Barchas, J. D. (1982). *Nature (London)* **299**, 77–79.

Weber, E., Esch, F. S., Bohlen, P., Paterson, S., Corbett, A. D., McKnight, A. T., Kosterlitz, H. W., Barchas, J. D., and Evans, C. J. (1983). *Proc. Natl. Acad. Sci. U.S.A.* **80**, 7372–7366.

Weisbrod, S. (1982). *Nature (London)* **297**, 289–295.

Whitfeld, P. L., Seeburg, P. H., and Shine, J. (1982). *DNA* **1**, 133–143.

Yang, H.-Y. T., Costa, E., Diguilio, A., Fratta, W., and Hong, J. S. (1979). *Fed. Proc., Fed. Am. Soc. Exp. Biol.* **38**, 364–366.

Yasamura, T. (1968). *Am. Zool.* **8**, 285–305.

Yates, F. E., and Maran, J. W. (1974). *In* "Handbook of Physiology" (E. Knobil and W. H. Sawyer, eds.), Sect. 7, Vol. IV, Part 1, pp. 367–404.

Zakarian, S., and Smyth, D. G. (1980). *Nature (London)* **288**, 613–615.

CHAPTER 2

Polypeptide Hormone Regulation of Prolactin Gene Transcription

Geoffrey H. Murdoch

Eukaryotic Regulatory Biology Program
School of Medicine
University of California, San Diego
La Jolla, California

Ronald M. Evans

Molecular Biology and Virology Laboratory
The Salk Institute for Biological Studies
San Diego, California

Michael G. Rosenfeld

Eukaryotic Regulatory Biology Program
School of Medicine
University of California, San Diego
La Jolla, California

BIOCHEMICAL ACTIONS OF HORMONES, VOL. XII

I. INTRODUCTION

The interaction of peptide hormones with specific plasma membrane re-ceptors can generate a diversity of intracellular signals, which regulate a variety of molecular events. Because these signals have the potential to independently regulate discrete domains of biological effects, it is critical to identify the precise site(s) at which control of each complex cellular process occurs in order to elucidate the underlying molecular mechanisms. In this review we describe the regulation of prolactin biosynthesis by peptide hor-mones as a model for peptidergic regulation of gene expression. Because the regulation of specific eukaryotic gene expression can occur at multiple levels (Darnell, 1982), the initial issue is to define which components of the biosyn-thetic machinery are regulated by polypeptide hormones. A clonal rat pitui-tary cell line (GH) was utilized for these investigations, because these cells produce growth hormone and prolactin and express receptors for several peptide hormones (for reviews, see Martin and Tashjian, 1977; Bancroft, 1981). Peptide hormones such as thyrotropin releasing hormone (TRH) and epidermal growth factor (EGF) were established to rapidly increase prolac-tin gene expression acting exclusively at the level of transcription. The tran-scriptional responsivity of the prolactin gene to peptide hormones is confer-red by specific genomic sequences located in the 5′ region of the prolactin gene. It is proposed that these sequences interact with specific protein factors that are modified as a consequence of the hormone–receptor interac-tion; one potential peptide enhancer protein is described. Each polypeptide hormone exerts rapid transcriptional effects over an unexpectedly large ge-nomic domain encompassing 5–10% of active polymerase II–catalyzed tran-scription units. These data are consistent with the notion that peptide hor-mones, in a fashion analogous to the effects of steroid hormones, can rapidly alter the transcription of a large subset of genes and thereby alter cellular phenotype by synthetic events as well as via protein modification.

II. REGULATION OF PROLACTIN SYNTHESIS BY PEPTIDE HORMONES

A. TRANSCRIPTIONAL STIMULATION OF THE PROLACTIN GENE BY TRH AND EGF

Following binding to specific high-affinity plasma membrane receptors, polypeptide hormones modulate cellular function by regulating a variety of molecular events. Some of these events, such as the polarization of the plasma membrane, the alterations in activities of cytoplasmic enzymes, and the release of storage granules, are rapid, exhibiting kinetics nearly identical to the occupancy of the plasma membrane receptors by the peptide regulator. Only since the introduction of recombinant DNA technology have the means been available to study the initial hormonal effects on specific protein biosynthesis. Prior measurements of the accumulation of the induced protein product had suggested that hormonal effects on gene expression were late, perhaps indirect, consequences of plasma membrane events. Recent advances in molecular biology and the cloning of specific mRNAs allow a clear delineation of the initial mechanisms by which peptide hormones modulate gene expression because they permit quantitation of cytoplasmic levels of specific mRNAs and of gene-specific transcription rates. The structural organization of the rat prolactin gene is diagrammed in Fig. 1. As shown in Fig. 2, the polypeptide hormones TRH and EGF rapidly stimulate transcription of the prolactin gene approximately tenfold (Murdoch *et al.*, 1982a, 1983), with corresponding increases in nuclear RNA precursors

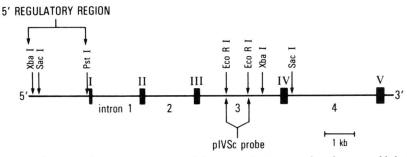

FIG. 1. The rat prolactin gene. A map of the rat prolactin gene, based upon published sequence data (Gubbins *et al.*, 1980; Chien and Thompson, 1980; Cooke and Baxter, 1982) is presented to diagram the position of a 1 kb intervening sequence subclone that was used to quantitate prolactin gene transcription in the studies reviewed in this chapter.

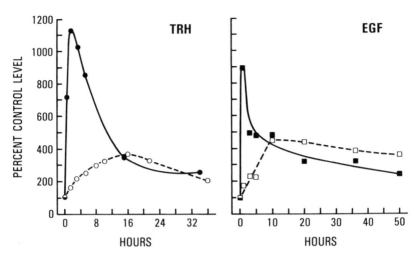

FIG. 2. Transcriptional regulation of the prolactin gene expression by TRH ($3 \times 10^{-7}\ M$) and EGF ($5 \times 10^{-8}\ M$). Closed symbols represent the kinetics of stimulation of prolactin gene transcription, and open symbols represent prolactin mRNA. The basal prolactin gene transcription rate was approximately 2 ppm/kb probe size.

(Potter *et al.*, 1981). While the maximal transcriptional effects are typically observed 30–60 minutes after addition of either hormone, a significant stimulation occurs by 2 minutes. Figure 2 also shows the time course of accumulation of cytoplasmic prolactin mRNA that results from this transcriptional stimulation. The initial burst of prolactin gene transcription produces a doubling of prolactin mRNA within hours, although cytoplasmic prolactin mRNA levels do not reach their maximum levels until 16–20 hours following the addition of hormone. Analysis of cytoplasmic RNA prepared 2 hours after hormone addition reveals that the newly synthesized prolactin mRNA is ~150 nucleotides longer than that already present in the cytoplasm. Removal of the polyA tracts by hybridization to oligo(dT) followed by ribonuclease H digestion altered the size of both species of prolactin mRNA to a single 830 nucleotide species, documenting that the appearance of a new species of prolactin mRNA following hormone treatment reflected the longer mean poly(A) tract of newly synthesized mRNA transcripts. These data suggest that the stimulation of prolactin mRNA accumulation after addition of TRH or EGF is the direct consequence of very rapid modulations of transcriptional events.

A second characteristic feature of the effects of peptide hormones on prolactin gene expression is a rapid attenuation of the transcriptional stimulation and the subsequent lack of response to re-addition of hormone (Murdoch *et al.*, 1982a, 1983). We refer to this effect of peptide hormones on prolactin gene expression, the rapid stimulation followed by desensitization, as a "burst-attenuation" transcriptional response. The TRH stimulation begins to attenuate within 1 hour and decays with a half-time of approximately 7 hours. This decay rate is nearly identical to the half-time of TRH receptor down-regulation (Hinkle and Tashjian, 1975). EGF-stimulated prolactin gene transcription also desensitizes with kinetics similar to EGF-receptor down-regulation described in other systems (Haigler *et al.*, 1980). There are clearly several potential mechanisms for this attenuation; however, the similarity of the kinetics of down-regulation and attenuation suggests that the desensitization is occurring at the plasma membrane. This hypothesis is supported by the observation that TRH produces a nearly maximal transcriptional stimulation in cultures of GH cells in which prolactin transcription has attenuated to the prior addition of EGF. Similar results were obtained with EGF in cells desensitized to TRH. Although there is marked desensitization in the magnitude of the transcriptional stimulation, there does not appear to be any time-dependent alteration in the efficacy of these hormones. Thus, dose response curves of prolactin mRNA accumulation after 8, 20, and 30 hours of treatment with TRH, corresponding to early, maximal, and desensitized levels of message, show no significant time-dependent shift in the hormone concentration producing half-maximal stimulation (ED-50s) (Fig. 3).

The stimulation of prolactin gene transcription produced by each hormone appears sufficient to account completely for the subsequent accumulation of cytoplasmic mRNA. In other model systems of polypeptide hormone action, such as the stimulation by prolactin of casein mRNA accumulation in breast tissue, it has been suggested that the accumulation of a specific mRNA is the result of a modest stimulation in gene transcription accompanied by a substantial increase in the stability of the cytoplasmic mRNA (Guyette *et al.*, 1979). The kinetics of the prolactin mRNA accumulation argue against analogous hormonal effects of prolactin mRNA stability in the GH cell system. Prolactin mRNA accumulation in response to treatment with TRH or EGF ceases concomitant with attaining parity with the level of the transcriptional stimulation. This occurs approximately 16 hours after addition of TRH and 10 hours after addition of EGF. The half-life of prolactin mRNA has not been measured directly; however, the decay of cytoplasmic prolactin mRNA levels following removal of hormone and the half-time of accumulation in the presence of a constant transcriptional stimulation (see Section III,C) suggest a half-life of prolactin mRNA in GH cells of approximately 8 hours. This estimate of half-life is compatible with the kinetics of prolactin mRNA accumulation following the burst-attenuation transcriptional response to either EGF or TRH.

In some systems, such as the stimulation of insulin synthesis by glucose, there appears to be regulation at the level of mRNA translation (Itoh and

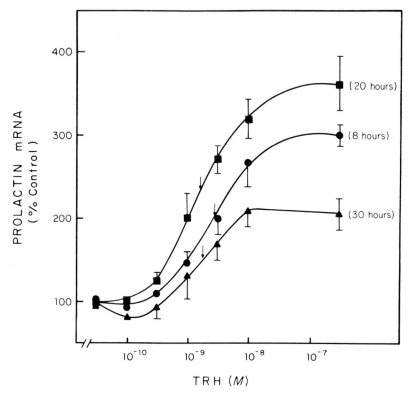

FIG. 3. Dose–response curves of the induction of prolactin mRNA levels by TRH. GH cell cultures were treated with various concentrations of TRH for 8 (●), 20 (■), or 30 (▲) hours. Prolactin mRNA was quantitated as described in Potter *et al.* (1981).

Okamoto, 1980; Cordell *et al.*, 1982). In contrast, TRH appears to increase prolactin production only at the level of mRNA synthesis. Thus, dose–response curves of the stimulation of prolactin mRNA levels by a series of TRH analogs (Fig. 4), reveal an ED-50 exactly the same as that reported for the stimulation of prolactin production measured by media accumulation (Hinkle *et al.*, 1974). In normal pituitary cells, dopamine agonists increase the intracellular prolactin degradation rate (Dannies and Rudnick, 1980) as well as inhibiting prolactin transcription and decreasing mRNA levels (Maurer, 1980, 1981). Although GH cells do not have functional dopamine receptors (Malarkey *et al.*, 1977), there is evidence that the stability of newly synthesized prolactin in GH cells is regulable (Kiino and Dannies, 1981). However, the time course of TRH-stimulated prolactin synthesis, measured by pulse labeling and immunoprecipitation, exactly parallels the kinetics of message accumulation (Murdoch *et al.*, 1983). Therefore, although specific protein biosynthesis is potentially regulable at multiple levels, TRH appears to modulate prolactin synthesis in GH cells via effects solely at the level of prolactin gene transcription.

B. The 5' Portion of the Prolactin Gene Transfers Hormonal Regulation to Unregulated Gene Products

The ability of peptide hormones to regulate transcription of the prolactin gene as a consequence of binding to plasma membrane receptors suggests that there must be a biochemical mechanism to transfer the signal to the nucleus. In prokaryotic organisms, the interaction of DNA-binding proteins with specific nucleotide sequences present in the promoter region of regulated genes suggests a general mechanism for regulating transcription (de Crombrugghe *et al.*, 1971; Zubay *et al.*, 1970; for review, see Peterkofsky, 1976). The role of specific DNA sequences in the acceptor mechanism of steroid hormones was intentionally explored because of the similarity be-

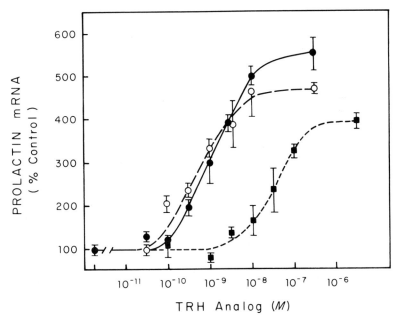

Fig. 4. Dose–response curves of the induction of prolactin mRNA by TRH analogs. GH cell cultures were treated for 24 hours with various concentrations of TRH (○), *t*-methyl-His TRH (●), or *N*-methyl-prolylamide TRH (■).

tween their receptor system and bacterial regulatory mechanisms. The resultant studies have suggested that this type of regulation continues to be utilized by eukaryotic organisms. Several types of data support this conclusion. First, recent studies of the transcriptional regulation of mouse mammary tumor virus by glucocorticoids have suggested that the steroid–receptor complex does bind to specific DNA sequences present within the integrated viral genome (Payvar *et al.*, 1981; Govinden *et al.*, 1982; Phahl, 1982; Chandler *et al.*, 1983). Similar data has been reported with respect to endogenous genes (Mulvihill *et al.*, 1982; Compton *et al.*, 1983). Second, analysis of the regulation of fusion genes containing specific genomic sequences following introduction into heterologous cell types reveals that the transcriptional regulation of a series of genes, including α_2-globulin, mouse mammary tumor virus, ovalbumin, and both rat and human growth hormone by glucocorticoids or other steroid hormones, or thyroid hormone, is determined solely by 5′-flanking DNA sequences present within the gene, provided that the recipient cell has the appropriate receptors (e.g., Lee *et al.*, 1981; Kurtz, 1981; Robins *et al.*, 1982; Doehmer *et al.*, 1982; Huang *et al.*, 1982; Page and Parker, 1983; Dean *et al.*, 1983). Recent studies have placed such regulatory sequences within regions of 50–60 nucleotides. Although the precise sequence of the acceptor site is not unequivocally identified, these studies do suggest that specific DNA sequences, rather than the packaging of a gene or its position in a region of a chromosome, are the critical determinants of its ability to be transcriptionally regulated by steroid hormones.

To investigate the possibility that the ability of a gene to be transcriptionally regulated by peptide hormones is also encoded in specific DNA sequences, a hybrid gene was constructed using the 5′ region of the prolactin gene (including the noncoding promoter region, the TATA box, and portions of the first prolactin coding exon) and the 3′ coding region of the growth hormone gene [including the noncoding growth hormone introns, the poly(A) addition signal, and the presumed terminator region]. Figure 5 is a diagram of the recombinant vector used to transfect this gene into heterologous cells. It also contains portions of the bacterial plasmid pBR322 to allow its replication in *Escherichia coli* and a selectable marker, the bacterial gene conferring resistance to the neomycin family of antibiotics (Southern and Berg, 1982). This vector was transfected, using the technique of calcium phosphate coprecipitation, into a cell line with well-characterized EGF receptors, A431 cells (Haigler *et al.*, 1978; Carpenter *et al.*, 1979). Several clonal lines were isolated by selection with the neomycin analog G418 and found to contain either single or multiple integrated copies of the vector (Supowit *et al.*, 1983). Those that contain the hybrid gene in a nonrearranged form produce an mRNA that utilizes the expected cap site and that is

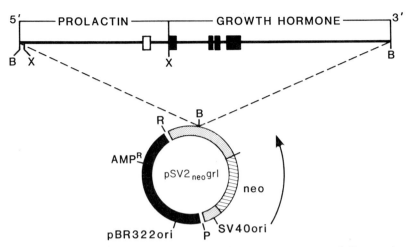

Fig. 5. Construction of a plasmid containing a fusion gene consisting of 5' rat prolactin genomic and coding information of the rat growth hormone gene. This plasmid (pSV2$_{neo}$grl) was used for DNA-mediated gene transfer experiments; a series of clonal transfected human A431 cell lines were analyzed.

polyadenylated and spliced to generate the predicted 1 kb mature transcript. Figure 6 shows the effect of addition of EGF to cultures of one such clonal line containing a single integrated copy of the transfected gene. There is a marked (fourfold) increase in the cellular content of the hybrid mRNA. The time course of accumulation and the maximum amount of stimulation are nearly identical to that produced by EGF in GH cells. However, the absolute levels of the hybrid mRNA are nearly 40 times less than prolactin mRNA in GH cells. This difference is the consequence of a greatly reduced basal transcription rate. While EGF typically stimulates prolactin gene transcription in GH cells from a basal rate of 2 ppm (parts per million) to nearly 20 ppm, the basal transcription rate of the hybrid gene in A431 cells is unmeasurable and increases to ~0.3 ppm in cells treated with EGF for 50 minutes. These data indicate that EGF acts to increase the transcription rate of the transfected hybrid gene and that the ability of EGF to stimulate the transcription of the prolactin gene is conferred by DNA sequences present in the 5' portion of the prolactin gene. Therefore, the basic principles dictating regulation of gene expression are analogous for peptide and steroid hormones. Recent data have localized the sequences conferring transcriptional regulation of the prolactin gene by EGF, TRH, phorbol esters, and cAMP to 170 base pairs of 5' flanking and noncoding genomic information (unpublished).

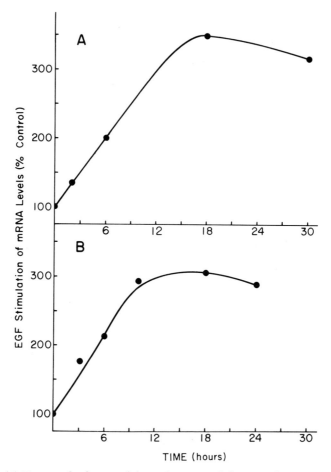

FIG. 6. (A) Kinetics of induction of the prolactin growth hormone fusion gene product by EGF in a clonal transfected A431 cell line (grl-i clone in this experiment). (B) The kinetics of prolactin mRNA induction in GH cells are shown for comparison.

C. Hormone-Induced Phosphorylations of Nuclear Proteins

While specific DNA sequences adjacent to the 5′ promoter region of the prolactin gene confer responsivity to peptide hormones, the nature of the signal generated by the peptide hormone–receptor interaction that interacts with this regulatory sequence is unknown. In GH cells, a portion of internalized EGF-receptor complexes have been reported to bind directly to the nucleus, leading to the suggestion that peptide hormones might interact directly with chromatin (Johnson *et al.*, 1980). Although the kinetic argument is not definitive, the relative rapidity of the time course of EGF-stimulated transcription compared to that of receptor accumulation at the nucleus makes it tempting to speculate that occupancy of plasma membrane receptors results in the generation of a second messenger, which transports the signal to the nucleus. In GH cells, both TRH and EGF stimulate the phosphorylation of a modest number of uncharacterized cytoplasmic proteins (Sobel and Tashjian, 1983; Drust *et al.*, 1982), and the phosphorylation of a specific nuclear protein is one plausible mechanism by which peptide hormones could affect transmission of their signal to the 5′-regulatory DNA

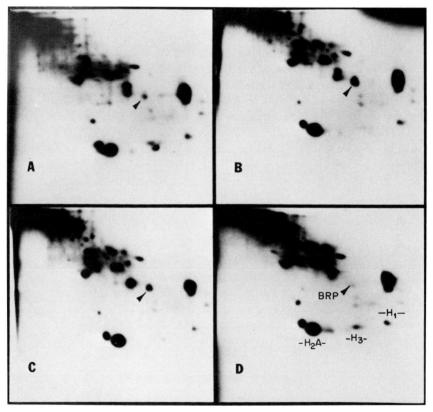

FIG. 7. Phosphorylation of a novel basic nuclear protein (BRP). Each panel is an autoradiograph of a two-dimensional gel of acid-soluble nuclear proteins using acid–urea–triton in the first dimension and SDS–PAGE in the second dimension. (A) Control GH cells. (B) GH cells treated for 45 minutes with 8 BrcAMP (2.5 mM). (C) Cells treated for 45 minutes with TRH (3×10^{-7} M). (D) GH cells treated for 45 minutes with the calcium ionophore A23187 (1.5 μM).

sequences. Figure 7 demonstrates the hormone-regulated phosphorylation of one candidate acid-soluble nuclear chromatin-associated protein. The phosphorylation of this basic regulated phosphoprotein (BRP) is stimulated up to tenfold by both TRH and EGF (Murdoch *et al.*, 1983, 1984). The phosphorylation of BRP by TRH parallels both kinetically and pharmacologically the stimulation of prolactin gene transcription. Increased phosphorylation can be detected 2 minutes after addition of TRH, is maximal between 30 and 60 minutes, and returns to nearly control levels within 36 hours.

The physical properties of BRP distinguish it from all known histone and HMG proteins. BRP is found almost exclusively bound to chromatin, from which it can be extracted by 0.4 M sulfuric acid or 0.35 M NaCl. However, unlike histone, H_1, or HMG proteins, it precipitates in 5% perchloric acid. As shown in Fig. 7, BRP migrates in SDS polyacrylamide gels with the same apparent molecular weight as the major H-1 histone isotypes. However, because it migrates more slowly in the acid–urea–triton dimension, it must differ in either charge or hydrohobicity (Franklin and Zweidler, 1977). BRP is present in the adrenal cortex and in the liver and medullary thyroid carcinoma cell lines, as well as in A431 cells. A protein in the superior cervical ganglia whose phosphorylation is regulated by NGF (Yu *et al.*, 1980) could be similar to BRP. TRH and EGF stimulate phosphorylation of 3–5 distinct sites on BRP, all of which are on serine residues (Waterman *et al.*, 1983). BRP phosphorylation thus provides an additional useful marker of the nuclear events induced by TRH and EGF, and its phosphorylation consistently parallels the regulation of prolactin gene transcription.

D. Peptide Hormones Exert Transcriptional Effects over Large Genomic Domains

BRP is approximately as abundant as HMG-14 or HMG-17 based on Coomasie blue staining; therefore, it is likely to have a wide chromatin distribution. If BRP phosphorylation were critical for the mediation of the transcriptional effects of TRH and EGF, it would be predicted that the prolactin gene would be one of a fairly large domain of hormonally regulated genes. An estimate of the size of this genomic domain was obtained by measuring the total number of RNA polymerase II complexes actively transcribing before ane after hormonal treatment. As illustrated in Fig. 8, TRH and EGF each stimulate the amount of α-amanitin–sensitive transcription up to twofold. This transcriptional response cannot be attributed to a nonspecific stimulation in the efficiency of polymerase II activity, because the

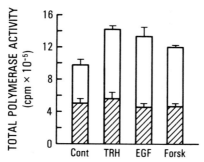

FIG. 8. Effects of TRH and EGF on total transcription. Purified nuclei from control GH cells or cells incubated for 30 minutes in the presence of TRH ($3 \times 10^{-7} M$), EGF ($3 \times 10^{-8} M$), or forskolin ($10^{-6} M$), were allowed to run off nascent transcripts in the presence (notched bars) or absence (total bars) of α-amanitin (0.8 μM). The height of the open bars reflects total RNA polymerase II template activity as described in Murdoch *et al.* (1983).

transcription rate of the growth hormone gene and eight constitutively expressed genes was not affected (Murdoch *et al.*, 1983). TRH appears to stimulate the transcription of each gene in its domain rapidly, with the maximal increase in total transcription occurring within 30 minutes, followed by a rapid attenuation (Murdoch *et al.*, 1983). In addition, this responsive domain is as sensitive to TRH regulation as the prolactin gene because both events are half-maximally stimulated at 3 nM TRH.

E. The Transcriptional Effects of TRH and EGF Are Additive

Prolactin gene transcription appears to be stimulated by TRH, EGF, bombesin, and elevated cAMP levels. However, it remains to be determined whether each peptide hormone exerts independent direct effects on the prolactin gene, implying the potential existence of multiple peptide responsive regulatory sequences within a single transcription unit. Alternatively, there may simply be multiple specific receptors that interact with the same signal transduction system. Traditionally, the distinction between independent and convergent regulatory systems is suggested by determining whether the effects of individual hormones are additive. The combined effects of TRH and EGF were studied because each initially interacts with a discrete plasma membrane receptor and because it has been documented that the stimulation of prolactin synthesis and prolactin mRNA levels by these hormones is additive (Murdoch *et al.*, 1984). Because each hormone has been shown to induce a transcriptional response that rapidly desensitizes, the observed additivity could be the result of either additive initial transcriptional effects or a summation of late submaximal transcriptional stimulations. To definitively address the question of additivity, the combined transcriptional effects of maximal concentrations of TRH and EGF were measured 30 minutes after hormone addition. As shown in Fig. 9, the rapid maximal transcriptional effects of each hormone are clearly additive in moderately dense cultures of rapidly growing cells.

The additivity of the transcriptional stimulations by TRH and EGF in appropriate culture conditions is compatible with the existence of separable independent effects directly on the prolactin gene. However, the additivity could also be occurring at a point of convergence of separate rate-limiting transduction systems. This latter possibility is supported by the observation that, under conditions of additive transcriptional effects, the phosphorylation of BRP by TRH and EGF is also additive. The description of other systems, e.g., cases in which a single enzyme is regulated by phosphorylations at multiple specific sites by independent kinase systems suggested that BRP itself might represent such a point of convergence. Because tryptic

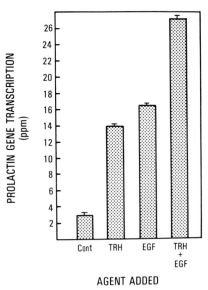

AGENT ADDED

FIG. 9. Additive effects of TRH and EGF on prolactin gene expression. Nascent transcripts were quantitated by *in vitro* run-off and DNA excess hybridization following 45 minutes of hormonal treatment. TRH was added at 3×10^{-7} *M*; EGF, at 5×10^{-8}.

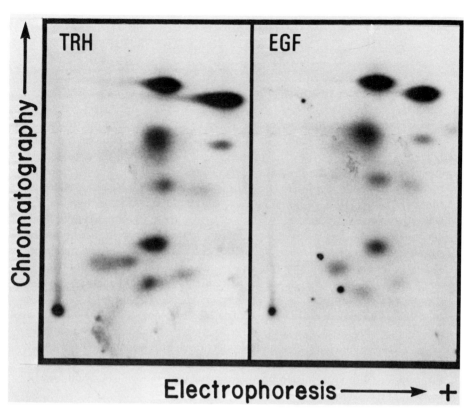

FIG. 10. Tryptic phosphopeptide map of BRP, labeled in the intact cells following hormonal treatment for 30 minutes in GH cells. The five major phosphopeptides are consistently observed, and they are identical in both TRH- and EGF-treated cells. Since adjacent basic residues often generate two tryptic peptides, the minimum number of phosphoaminoacid residues is three.

phosphopeptide maps of BRP (Fig. 10) suggest that EGF and TRH stimulate the phosphorylation of the same tryptic fragments, the additivity reflects either a greater percentage of BRP protein phosphorylated or the use of different residues within identical tryptic fragments. Detailed analysis of the 5′ genomic sequences of the prolactin gene conferring TRH and EGF regulation to hybrid fusion genes will determine whether the hormonal regulation is determined by common or discrete DNA sequences. Preliminary studies of the transcriptional domain stimulated by these hormones suggest that TRH and EGF affect overlapping, but not identical, domains.

III. TRANSDUCTION MECHANISMS OF TRH-STIMULATED PROLACTIN GENE TRANSCRIPTION

A. SUMMARY OF THE INITIAL EFFECTS OF TRH IN GH CELLS

While hormonal regulation of specific enzyme activity via modification can often be reconstructed *in vitro*, hormonal control of complex processes such as transcription or secretion have not yet proved tractable to such a direct biochemical approach. The crucial facts required to understand hormonal regulation of gene expression are the precise genomic sequences which confer TRH- and EGF-dependent transcriptional regulation on the prolactin gene, the protein(s) associated with those sequences, and the potential modification of these factors by hormones. A parallel issue is to define which signaling mechanism(s) generated by receptor–hormone interaction is responsible for mediating the transcriptional response to the hormone. To investigate this latter issue, we have applied kinetic and pharmacological approaches, in combination with genetic analyses, to gain insight into the relationship between prolactin gene transcription and several cellular processes suggested by other investigators to mediate the intracellular effects of TRH. These include an elevation in cytosolic calcium, a stimulation of cAMP levels, and an activation of the phosphatidylinositol cycle. A brief review of the evidence supporting each postulate is presented as a background to the experimental data.

Appreciation of the importance of calcium ions in the transduction of hormonal signals has evolved significantly since Douglas's description of stimulus-secretion coupling (Taraskevich and Douglas, 1977). That calcium is involved in the mechanism of action of TRH was initially suggested by studies that demonstrated that EGTA and cobalt ions were able to inhibit the stimulation of prolactin release and production (Gautvik and Tashjian, 1973; Tashjian *et al.*, 1978). Electrophysiologic studies provided evidence compatible with the possibility that calcium ions might be a second messenger of TRH. TRH greatly enhances the frequency of calcium spike potentials in both GH cells and a subpopulation of pituicytes (Kidokoro, 1975; Taraskevich and Douglas, 1977; Ozawa and Kimura, 1979). Although this channel is not well characterized, it is probably distinct from the voltage-dependent channel present in neural and cardiac tissue (Gershenogorn, 1980; Geras *et al.*, 1983). TRH induces both an influx and efflux of cellular calcium ions, but produces a transient net increase in cytoplasmic free calcium concentrations measurable by Quin 2 fluorescence (Gershengorn and Thaw, 1983). In the absence of extracellular calcium, TRH produces a similar elevation in cytoplasmic calcium by mobilizing calcium from intracellular compartments. The site of these intracellular stores probably includes both mitochondrial and endoplasmic reticulum and, potentially, the plasma membrane (Ronning *et al.*, 1982; Thaw *et al.*, 1982). The resultant elevation of cytoplasmic calcium levels could mediate the intracellular effects of TRH. It is possible that a portion of the TRH-dependent cytoplasmic phosphorylations could be mediated by a calcium-dependent kinase because they are reproduced by addition of calcium to cytosolic preparations (Drust and Martin, 1982).

Although recent studies of the mechanism of action of TRH have emphasized the role of calcium or phosphatidylinositol turnover (see Sections III,A and III,C), the first mechanism of action suggested for TRH in GH cells was a stimulation of cAMP levels (Labrie *et al.*, 1975). It has recently been reported that there is a strong calcium dependence of the stimulation of adenylyl cyclase by TRH (Broström *et al.*, 1983; Gautvik *et al.*, 1983). Although the net elevation of cAMP levels is modest in comparison with that produced by the peptide hormone VIP, TRH has been reported to stimulate a cytoplasmic cAMP-dependent protein kinase (Gautvik *et al.*, 1977). A subset of the cytoplasmic phosphorylations induced by TRH can be mimicked by agents known to stimulate cAMP (Drust *et al.*, 1982). Cholera toxin and cAMP analogs have been previously documented to reproduce many of the effects of TRH in GH cells, including the stimulation of prolactin synthesis and release (Martin and Tashjian, 1977).

An alternative second messenger system postulated to be activated in response to TRH is the activation of the phosphatidylinositol cycle. In this enzymatic cycle, which is activated by a variety of hormones in many different tissues, phosphatidylinositol is sequentially cleaved to diacylglycerol and phosphoinositol, then converted first to phosphatidic acid and finally back to phosphatidylinositol (for review, see Berridge, 1981; Farese, 1983). The intermediates that are transiently produced by the cycling of the pathway are believed to initiate a cascade of cellular effects. For example, phosphatidic acid is suggested to act as a calcium ionophore, phosphoinositol may signal release of cellular calcium stores, and diacylglycerol can be a source of arachidonic acid for prostaglandin synthesis. A recently elucidated consequence of stimulating the phosphatidylinositol cycle is the activation of a novel cytoplasmic protein kinase referred to as C-kinase (Takai *et al.*, 1979a,b; Kishimoto *et al.*, 1980; Niedel *et al.*, 1983; for review, see Nishizuka, 1983). This kinase is maximally activated in the presence of phospholipid by a combination of calcium and diacylglycerol, also called diolein. The requirement for diolein can also be met by the various tumor-promoting phorbol esters (Castagna *et al.*, 1982). Because these agents bind and activate C-kinase with the same rank order as their effects on the growth or differentiated function of a variety of cell types, it has been suggested that C-kinase may be the critical cellular receptor for phorbol esters. These compounds may, therefore, allow investigations of the cellular consequences of C-kinase activation independent of other potential effects of phosphatidylinositol cycle stimulation. The role of each of these potential mediators in hormone-induced modification of prolactin gene transcription is considered in the subsequent sections.

B. THE ROLE OF CALCIUM

In specific serum-free media, decreasing extracellular calcium concentrations is reported to exert a dramatic effect on both basal prolactin mRNA levels and the ability of TRH and EGF to stimulate message accumulation (White and Bancroft, 1983). We have attempted to determine whether there is a specific calcium-dependent step in TRH regulation of prolactin gene expression. Agents that disrupt cellular calcium homeostasis do inhibit the ability of TRH to increase prolactin gene transcription; i.e., cobalt ions completely block prolactin gene transcriptional stimulation (Fig. 11) and BRP phosphorylation (Fig. 12) by TRH. The specificity of this effect is demonstrated by the lack of effect on growth hormone gene transcription. The documentation of this specific effect of cobalt on prolactin biosynthesis is possible because the rapid transcriptional effects are quantitated long before

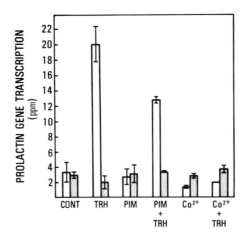

FIG. 11. Effects of calcium-modulating agents on TRH-stimulated prolactin gene transcription. The transcription of the prolactin gene (open bars) and growth hormone (stippled bars) were quantitated by nuclear run-off assay in unstimulated GH cells or cells treated for 45 minutes with TRH ($3 \times 10^{-7} M$) in the presence or absence of either pimozide (1 μM) or cobalt chloride (1 mM). Results are the mean of duplicate experiment determinations.

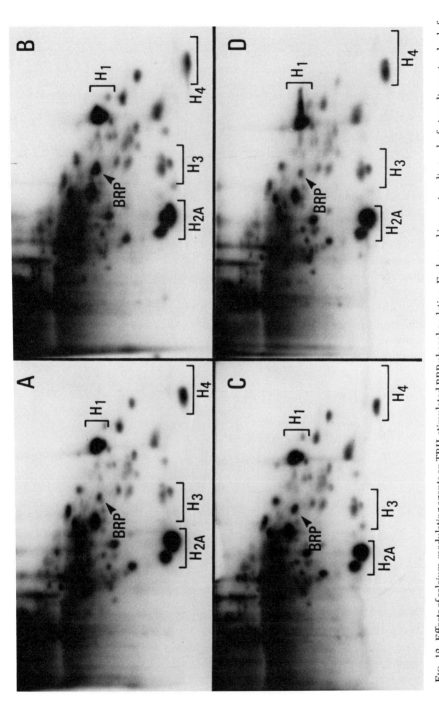

FIG. 12. Effects of calcium-modulating agents on TRH-stimulated BRP phosphorylation. Each panel is an autoradiograph of a two-dimensional gel of phosphorylated nuclear basic proteins isolated from cells after a 30-minute treatment with agents. (A) Unstimulated cells. (B) Cells incubated with TRH (3×10^{-7} M). (C) Cells incubated with TRH in the presence of pimozide (1 μM). (D) Cells incubated with TRH in the presence of cobalt chloride (1 mM).

any toxic effects of cobalt on the cell are manifest. The ability of antipsychotic drugs, which bind to calmodulin in a calcium-dependent manner (Levin and Weiss, 1979) and which interfere with other calcium-dependent processes (Kuo *et al.*, 1980; Thaw *et al.*, 1982), to antagonize hormonal stimulation, is often cited as evidence that a calmodulin-dependent process mediates the hormonal effect (Conn *et al.*, 1981). These agents inhibit TRH-stimulated prolactin mRNA accumulation and prolactin gene transcription (Fig. 8) with the same rank order as their affinity for calmodulin (pimozide/chlorprothixene/trifluperazine). One micromolar pimozide produces inhibitions of prolactin mRNA accumulation and TRH-stimulated prolactin gene transcription by 50 and 45%, respectively, and comparably inhibits the ability of TRH to stimulate BRP phosphorylation (Fig. 12). The fact that cobalt and pimozide inhibit both nuclear effects of TRH suggests that they interfere with TRH's second messenger system rather than directly inhibiting prolactin gene transcription. If the transient elevation in cytoplasmic calcium concentration produced by TRH itself mediates the transcriptional effects of TRH, pharmacologic alteration of cytoplasmic calcium should mimic the response. As shown in Fig. 13, neither calcium ionophores, A23187 and ionomycin, nor membrane depolarizing agents, 50 mM potassium and 4-aminopyridine, stimulate prolactin gene transcription. These agents also exert no effect on

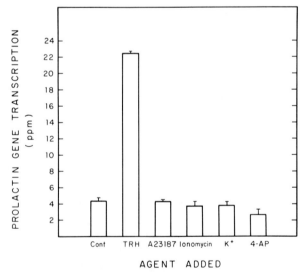

AGENT ADDED

FIG. 13. Effects of agents inducing prolactin secretion on prolactin gene transcription in GH cell cultures. The effects of 50 minutes of incubation with TRH (3×10^{-7} M), the calcium ionophores A23187 (1.5 μM) or ionomycin (3 μM), K$^+$ (50 mM), or 4-amino purine (0.3 mM) are shown.

BRP phosphorylation (Fig. 7). However, all of these agents have been shown to stimulate release of prolactin from GH cells, presumably by raising cytoplasmic calcium. Therefore, the nuclear events that lead to the increase in prolactin synthesis are clearly separable from prolactin release. These data suggest that the release of storage vesicles from the cytoplasm does not exert a pull on the transcriptional apparatus and that the two processes are probably independently regulated events. The inability of secretagogues to elicit nuclear effects cannot be ascribed to a simultaneous independent toxic process because they do not inhibit the ability of TRH to stimulate prolactin gene transcription.

These pharmacological studies suggest that, although calcium ions play a role in the effects of TRH on gene expression, elevation of cytoplasmic calcium is either not required or insufficient to mediate the transcriptional effects. One possible explanation is that the critical nuclear phosphorylation is the product of a calcium-dependent protein kinase that has additional regulatory cofactors. This possibility can be evaluated by examining the calcium dependence of BRP phosphorylation in homogenates of control and TRH-treated GH cells. As shown in Fig. 14, BRP kinase remains active in homogenates of TRH-treated cells. Addition of calcium to control homogenates does not reproduce this phosphorylation, although calcium-dependent phosphorylations are clearly observed. The phosphorylation of BRP in homogenates of TRH-treated cells is not decreased by chelation of free calcium with EGTA, although the modest stimulations of the calcium-dependent phosphorylations in the TRH-treated homogenates are abolished. Therefore, it is likely that TRH does stimulate calcium-dependent kinase(s), but that the nuclear events, for which BRP phosphorylation is a marker, are not directly mediated by a calcium-dependent kinase.

C. The Role of Cyclic AMP

Addition of cAMP to dopamine-treated pituitary cells increases prolactin mRNA by reversing the inhibition of prolactin transcription produced by dopamine (Maurer, 1981), which could indicate either that cAMP acts in the pituitary by interfering with the dopamine receptor mechanism or that it directly effects prolactin gene transcription. Therefore, the effects of cAMP on prolactin gene expression were studied in GH cells, where cholera toxin and derivatives of cAMP clearly stimulate prolactin synthesis (Dannies *et al.*, 1976). As shown in Fig. 15, cAMP analogs or forskolin, a diterpene which directly activates adenylyl cyclase, produce a fourfold stimulation in prolactin gene transcription and prolactin mRNA accumulation in GH cells (Murdoch *et al.*, 1982b). The rapid transcriptional response leads to a commensu-

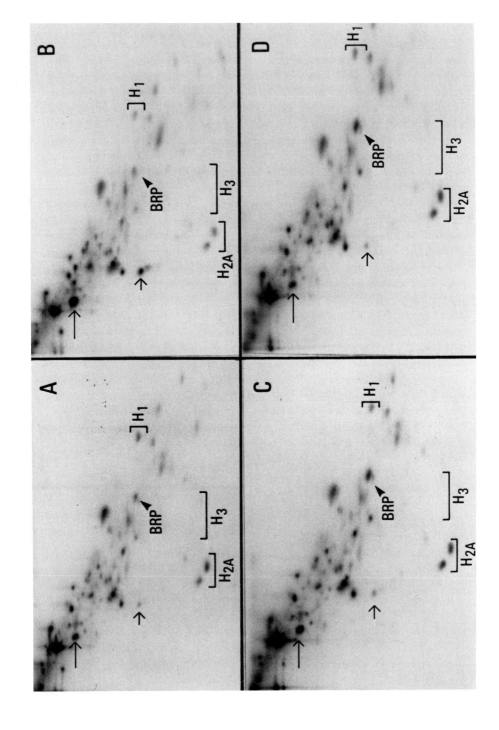

rate accumulation of prolactin mRNA. In contrast to the stimulation produced by peptide hormones, there is no attenuation of the transcriptional response. Therefore, the half-time of prolactin mRNA accumulation provides a reasonable estimate of the mRNA half-life. In addition to increasing prolactin gene transcription, foreskolin treatment also stimulates BRP phosphorylation (Murdoch *et al.*, 1982b). Although forskolin and TRH exert similar nuclear effects, a more detailed analysis demonstrates that cAMP does not mediate the transcriptional effects of TRH. First, the stimulation of prolactin gene transcription by cAMP is reproducibly no more than half that produced by the peptide hormones TRH or EGF. The simultaneous elevation of cytoplasmic calcium with the calcium ionophore A23187 does not further increase prolactin gene transcription stimulated by cAMP. Although purified BRP protein can act as a substrate of the cAMP-dependent protein kinase, TRH does not increase the activity of this kinase in the nucleus. Figure 16 shows phosphopeptide maps of histone, H1. Addition of forskolin to GH cell cultures leads to the phosphorylation of the H_1 peptide containing the serine residue Ser 37, which is the specific site of the cAMP-dependent protein kinase (Langan, 1969). TRH does not induce phosphorylation of this site. Finally, cobalt chloride blocks both the stimulation of prolactin gene transcription (Fig. 17) and phosphorylation of BRP induced by forskolin, but does not inhibit the phosphorylation of histone H_1 (Waterman *et al.*, 1984). The most likely explanation of the effect of cAMP on prolactin gene transcription is that the stimulation of cAMP-dependent protein kinase leads to a secondary activation of that messenger system activated by TRH. An example of this type of secondary effect of cAMP is the enhancement of calcium spike potentials in pancreatic islet cells (Henquin *et al.*, 1983).

D. The Role of C-Kinase

Treatment of GH cells with 12-O-tetradecanoyl-phorbol-13-acetate (TPA), one of the more potent phorbol esters, produces many of the same effects as TRH and EGF, including shape change, growth inhibition, and stimulation

---

FIG. 14. Effects of calcium ions on *in vitro* BRP phosphorylation in homogenates of (A, B) unstimulated or (C, D) TRH-treated GH cell cultures. After a 30-minute incubation with TRH ($3 \times 10^{-7} M$), control and treated cells were homogenized and labeled *in vitro* with [^{32}P]ATP for 90 seconds prior to preparation of acid-soluble nuclear proteins. In (B) 0.6 mM calcium chloride was included in the *in vitro* phosphorylation reaction. In (D) 0.5 mM EGTA was included in the *in vitro* reaction. Autoradiographs of two-dimensional gels are shown; arrows point to two phosphoproteins which show increased phosphorylation in the presence of calcium.

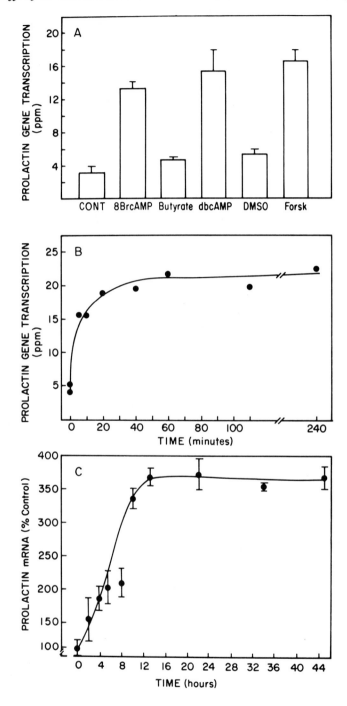

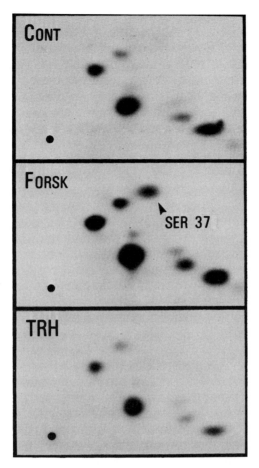

FIG. 16. Tryptic phosphopeptide maps of histone H_1 isolated from untreated GH4 cells (control) or cultures incubated with 10^{-6} M forskolin, or 3×10^{-7} M TRH for 30 minutes. The arrow indicates the phosphopeptide containing Ser 37, the site of cAMP-dependent phosphorylation.

FIG. 15. Stimulation of prolactin gene expression by cAMP. (A) The effects of addition of 8 BrcAMP (2.5 mM), dibutyryl cAMP (1mM), or forskolin (10^{-6} M) to GH cells on prolactin gene transcription. (B) The kinetics of forskolin stimulation of prolactin gene transcription in GH cells. (C) The kinetics of prolactin mRNA accumulation in response to forskolin. [Data from Murdoch *et al.* (1982b).]

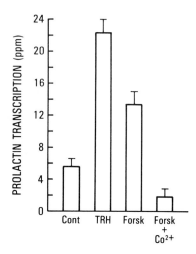

Fig. 17. Effect of cobalt ions on cAMP-stimulated prolactin gene transcription. Prolactin gene transcription was quantitated by measurement of nascent transcripts in isolated nuclei from GH4 cells that have been treated for 50 minutes with forskolin (10^{-6} M) in the presence and absence of 1 mM cobalt chloride. The parallel stimulation produced by TRH (3×10^{-7} M) is shown for comparison. Results are the mean ±SEM of triplicate determinations.

of prolactin production (Osborne and Tashjian, 1981). The effect of TPA on prolactin gene transcription is illustrated in Fig. 18. TPA typically stimulates prolactin gene transcription almost to the same extent that TRH does. However, in those experiments where it produces a slightly smaller stimulation, simultaneous addition of calcium ionophore restores the full effect. Additionally, TPA induces a phosphorylation of BRP nearly equal to that produced by TRH, and the simultaneous addition of A23187 generates a full response. One possible explanation of this data is that, while the elevation in cytosolic calcium produced by TRH allows full activation of C-kinase, TPA fulfills only the diolein requirement (Nishizuka, 1983; Grosveld *et al.*, 1982; Shenk, 1981), and the extent of kinase activation by TPA depends on the level of cytosolic calcium at the time of experiment. Finally, TPA regulation of prolactin gene expression is conferred by 5' genomic sequences, and documented by DNA-mediated gene transfer experiments (Supowit *et al.*, 1983).

Although these effects of phorbol esters suggest that C-kinase could itself mediate the stimulation of prolactin gene transcription by TRH, it is unlikely that C-kinase is acting directly in the nucleus. C-kinase is an amphipathic molecule, and it becomes associated with cell membranes during the process of activation. Subcellular fractionations suggest that little, if any, becomes associated with the nucleus. These studies provide the basis for designing

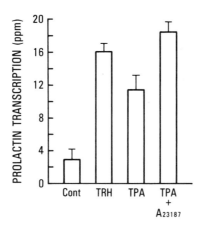

Fig. 18. The effect of tumor promoters on prolactin gene expression. The effect of treating GH cultures for 30 minutes with TRH ($3 \times 10^{-7} M$), with the phorbol ester TPA ($2 \times 10^{-7} M$), or with TPA ($2 \times 10^{-7} M$) in the presence of the calcium ionophore A23187 (1.5 μM). Results are the average $\pm$ SEM of triplicate determinations. The effects of calcium ionophore alone are shown in Fig. 13.

future experiments utilizing DNA-mediated gene transfer to elucidate the potential mechanisms of TRH-regulated nuclear effects.

IV. THE POTENTIAL SIGNIFICANCE OF TRANSCRIPTIONAL REGULATION BY PEPTIDE HORMONES

Understanding the mechanisms by which regulatory substances modify gene expression and thereby alter cellular phenotype represents a fundamental question for understanding developmental processes and physiological homeostasis in higher eukaryotes. In the case of regulatory agents that bind to receptors within the cell, such as steroid hormones, the initial predictions that the receptor–ligand complex would bind to specific genomic sequences and modify gene transcription have received substantial experimental support. However, for polypeptide hormones, there has been no unifying conceptual framework by which to explain their effects on gene expression. Studies of TRH effects on specific gene expression in a well-characterized model system, as reviewed in this chapter, have provided insight into the mechanisms by which polypeptide hormones exert their effects on protein synthesis. First, it is now clear that these hormones can rapidly (within 1–2 minutes) alter the transcription of specific genes. Because it has been reported that specific nuclear proteins widely distributed in chromatin can be modified in response to polypeptide hormones (Langan, 1969; Murdoch *et al.*, 1982b), models that predict either general alterations in chromatin structure or that involve binding of modified proteins to specific genomic sequences are consistent with available data. Analysis of determinants of hormonal regulation of the prolactin gene by polypeptide hormones establishes the principle that the structural requirement for transcriptional regulation is similar for both peptide and steroid hormones, because regulation is conferred by recognition of specific genomic DNA sequences by proteins or other factors. While in the case of steroid hormones it is probable that the regulatory factor binding to specific genomic sequences and modulating transcription is the steroid–receptor complex, the mediator for peptide hormone effects is likely to differ fundamentally in that it is discrete from the receptor and instead modified by hormone–receptor interactions. The corollary of this putative modification event is the necessity of a mechanism by which binding of hormone to a plasma membrane receptor generates a signal that reaches the nucleus. TPA mimics the actions of TRH on both prolactin gene transcription and BRP phosphorylation; in addition, the 5′-flanking region of the prolactin gene contains determinants for the transcriptional response to TPA. Because TPA appears to activate C-kinase, activation of C-kinase may provide the basis of the modifications necessary for initiation of nuclear events; however, the protein kinase actually mediating nuclear phosphorylation events is apparently not calcium-dependent, and, therefore, is activated consequent to C-kinase activation.

The ability of a series of peptide hormones to transcriptionally regulate a single prolactin transcription unit raises a fundamental question regarding the number of regulatory sites present in the 5′ region flanking the gene. It is tempting to speculate that there exists a series of discrete regulatory sites in close structural proximity because EGF and TRH appear to modulate overlapping but distinct genomic domains. We have proven by S1 mapping procedures that the identical 5′ CAP site is utilized, irrespective of which inductive agent is used, indicating that the discrete regulatory sites all dictate use of the same initiation site. While peptide and steroidal regulatory substances share a requirement for specific genomic sequences to confer their effects, there are distinct physiologic regulatory differences between the two classes of hormones. For example, modulation of gene expression in response to alterations in homeostasis can be regulated more acutely by peptide than by steroid hormones. This is not a consequence of the transduction system, but rather because of the more rapid fluctuations in the circulating concentrations of peptide hormones, as exemplified by the extremely rapid and dramatic alterations in the concentrations of hypophysiotropic regulators in the hypothalamic–pituitary portal circulation. The half-life of neuropeptides in synaptic clefts may be even shorter. In addition, many cells have receptors dictating responsivity to a large number of peptide regulators; these receptors themselves are under complex regulation. For example, in GH cells, estrogens are known to increase the number of TRH receptors (Gershengorn *et al.*, 1979), while glucocorticoids and vitamin D inhibit the TRH receptor down-regulation. If receptor down-regulation were the mechanism of the rapid attenuation of the transcriptional response, it would not be surprising that vitamin D potentiates the stimulation of prolactin biosynthesis by TRH (Murdoch and Rosenfeld, 1981). Under certain conditions, the transcriptional attenuation for some genes may be so rapid that the resultant mRNA accumulates significantly only in the presence of a steroid hormone inhibiting the attenuation process. In situations where the attenuation of transcriptional stimulation was decreased or minimal, dramatic alterations in the cellular phenotype might be the predicted result; such a phenomenon may be critical in cells in which peptide hormones induce pleiotropic effects such as differentiation or growth events. Conversely, pathological expression of genes during transformation events may reflect activation of the transcriptional domain characteristic of a particular polypeptide regulator. The very complexity of transcriptional control by polypeptide hormones generates a series of unanswered questions, all the more tantalizing because their solution promises to yield unexpected and fundamental insights into homeostatic regulatory mechanisms utilized by higher eukaryotes.

ACKNOWLEDGMENTS

The data of Scott Supowit and Ellen Potter regarding the regulation of the transfected "grolactin" gene, and of Marian Waterman regarding multifactorial regulation of prolactin gene transcription and of sites of hormone-stimulated BRP phosphorylation are presented in this chapter and will be independently reported in reviewed manuscripts. This chapter and the studies described therein benefited from discussions with Rodrigo Franco and Marcia Barinaga.

REFERENCES

Bancroft, F. C. (1981). *In* "Functionally Differentiated Cell Lines" (G. Sato, ed.) pp. 47–59. Alan Liss, Inc., New York.

Berridge, M. J. (1981). *Mol. Cell. Endocrinol.* **24,** 115–140.

Broström, M. A., Broström, C. O., Brotman, L. A., and Green, S. S. (1983). *Mol. Pharmacol.* **23,** 399–408.

Cachelin, A. B., de Peyer, J. E., Kokubun, S., and Reuter, H. (1983). *Nature (London)* **304,** 462–464.

Carpenter, G., King, L., and Cohen, S. (1979). *J. Biol. Chem.* **254,** 4884–4891.

Castagna, M., Takai, Y., Kaibuchi, K., Sauo, K., Kikkana, U., and Nishizuka, Y. (1982). *J. Biol. Chem.* **257,** 7847–7851.

Chandler, V. L., Maler, B. A., and Yamamoto, K. R. (1983). *Cell* **33**, 489–499.
Chien, Y. H., and Thompson, E. B. (1980). *Proc. Natl. Acad. Sci. U.S.A.* **77**, 4583–4587.
Compton, J. G., Schrader, W. T., and O'Malley, B. (1983). *Proc. Natl. Acad. Sci. U.S.A.* **80**, 16–20.
Conn, P. M., Rogers, D. C., and Sheffield, T. (1981). *Endocrinology (Baltimore)* **109**, 1122–1126.
Cooke, N. E., and Baxter, J. D. (1982). *Nature (London)* **297**, 603–606.
Cordell, B., Diamond, D., Smith, S., Punter, J., Schone, H. H., and Goodman, H. M. (1982). *Cell* **31**, 531–5442.
Dannies, P. S., and Rudnick, M. S. (1980). *J. Biol. Chem.* **255**, 2776–2781.
Dannies, P. S., Gautvik, K. M., and Tashjian, A. H. (1976). *Endocrinology (Baltimore)* **98**, 1147–1159.
Darnell, J. E. (1982). *Nature (London)* **297**, 365–371.
Dean, D. C., Knoll, B. J., Risen, M. E., and O'Malley, B. W. (1983). *Nature (London)* **305**, 551–554.
de Crombrugghe, B., Chen, B., Anderson, W. C., Nissley, P., Gottesman, M., Pastan, I., and Perlman, R. L. (1971). *Nature (London)* **231**, 139.
Doehmer, J., Barinaga, M., Vale, W., Rosenfeld, M. G., Verma, I. M., and Evans, R. M. (1982). *Proc. Natl. Acad. Sci. U.S.A.* **79**, 2268–2271.
Douglas, W. W. (1968). *Br. J. Pharmacol.* **34**, 451–463.
Drust, D. S., and Martin, T. F. J. (1982). *J. Biol. Chem.* **257**, 7566–7573.
Drust, D. S., Sutton, C. A., and Martin, T. F. J. (1982). *J. Biol. Chem.* **257**, 3306–3312.
Farese, R. V. (1983). *Endocr. Rev.* **41**, 78–95.
Franklin, S. G., and Zweidler, A. (1977). *Nature (London)* **266**, 273–274.
Gautvik, K. M., and Tashjian, A. H. (1973). *Endocrinology (Baltimore)* **92**, 573–583.
Gautvik, K. M., Walaas, E., and Walaas, O. (1977). *Biochem. J.* **162**, 379–386.
Gautvik, K. M., Gordeladze, J. O., Jahnsen, T., Haug, E., Hansson, V., and Lystad, E. (1983). *J. Biol. Chem.* **258**, 10304–10311.
Geras, E., Rebecchi, M. J., and Gershengorn, M. C. (1983). *Endocrinology (Baltimore)* **110**, 901–906.
Gershengorn, M. C. (1980). *J. Biol. Chem.* **255**, 1801–1803.
Gershengorn, M. C., and Thaw, C. (1983). *Endocrinology (Baltimore)* **113**, 1522–1524.
Gershengorn, M. C., Marcus-Samuels, B. E., and Geras, E. (1979) *Endocrinology (Baltimore)* **105**, 171–178.
Govinden, M. B., Spiess, E., and Majors, J. (1982). *Proc. Natl. Acad. Sci. U.S.A.* **79**, 5157–5161.
Grosveld, G. C., de Buer, E., Shewmaker, C. K., and Flowell, R. A. (1982). *Nature (London)* **295**, 120–126.
Gubbins, E. J., Maurer, R. A., Lagrimmi, M., Erwin, C. R., and Donelson, J. C. (1980). *J. Biol. Chem.* **255**, 8655–8662.
Guyette, W. A., Matuski, R. J., and Rosen, J. M. (1979). *Cell* **17**, 1013–1023.
Haigler, H., Ash, J. F., Singer, S. J., and Cohen, S. (1978). *Proc. Natl. Acad. Sci. U.S.A.* **75**, 3317–3321.
Haigler, H. T., Maxfield, F. R., Willingham, M. C., and Pastan, I. (1980). *J. Biol. Chem.* **255**, 1239–1241.
Henquin, J.-C., Schmeer, W., and Meissner, H. P. (1983). *Endocrinology (Baltimore)* **112**, 2218–2223.
Hinkle, P. M., and Tashjian, A. H. (1975). *Biochemistry* **14**, 3845–3851.
Hinkle, P. M., Woroch, E. L., and Tashjian, A. H. (1974). *J. Biol. Chem.* **249**, 3085–3090.
Huang, A. L., Ostrowski, M. C., Bernard, D., and Hager, G. L. (1982). *Cell* **27**, 245–255.

Itoh, N., and Okamoto, H. (1980). *Nature (London)* **283**, 100–102.

Johnson, L. K., Vlodavsky, I., Baxter, J. D., and Gospodarowicz, D. (1980). *Nature (London)* **287**, 340–343.

Kidokoro, Y. (1975) *Nature (London)* **258**, 741–742.

Kiino, D. R., and Dannies, P. S. (1981). *Endocrinology (Baltimore)* **109**, 1264–1269.

Kishimoto, A., Takai, Y., Mori, T., Kikkawa, U., and Nishizuka, Y. (1980). *J. Biol. Chem.* **255**, 2273–2276.

Kuo, J. F., Andersson, R. G. G., Wise, B. C., Mackerlova, L., Salomonsson, I., Brackett, N. L., Katoh, N., Shoji, M., and Wrenn, R. W. (1980). *Proc. Natl. Acad. Sci. U.S.A.* **77**, 7039–7043.

Kurtz, D. T. (1981). *Nature (London)* **291**, 629–631.

Labrie, F., Borgeat, P., Lemay, A., Lemaire, S., Barden, N., Drouin, J., Lemaire, I., Jolicoeur, P., and Bélanger, A. (1975). *Adv. Cyclic Nucleotide Res.* **5**, 787–801.

Langan, T. (1969). *Biochemistry* **64**, 1276–1283.

Lee, F., Mulligan, R., Berg, P., and Ringold, G. (1981). *Nature (London)* **294**, 228.

Levin, R. M., and Weiss, B. (1979). *J. Pharmacol. Exp. Ther.* **208**, 454–459.

Malarkey, W. B., Groshong, J. C., and Milo, G. E. (1977). *Nature (London)* **266**, 640–641.

Martin, T. F. J., and Tashjian, A. H. (1977). *In* "Biochemical Actions of Hormones" (G. Litwack, ed.), Vol. 4, pp. 270–317. Academic Press, New York.

Maurer, R. A. (1980). *J. Biol. Chem.* **255**, 8092–8097.

Maurer, R. A. (1981). *Nature (London)* **294**, 94–97.

Mulvihill, E. R., Le Pennec, J. P., and Chambon, P. (1982). *Cell* **24**, 621–632.

Murdoch, G. H., and Rosenfeld, M. G. (1981). *J. Biol. Chem.* **256**, 4050–4055.

Murdoch, G. H., Potter, E., Nicholaisen, A. K., Evans, R. M., and Rosenfeld, M. G. (1982a). *Nature (London)* **300**, 192–194.

Murdoch, G. H., Rosenfeld, M. G., and Evans, R. M. (1982b). *Science* **218**, 1315–1317.

Murdoch, G. H., Franco, R., Evans, R. M., and Rosenfeld, M. G. (1983). *J. Biol. Chem.* **258**, 15329–15335.

Murdoch, G. H., Waterman, M., Evans, R. M., and Rosenfeld, M. G. (1984). Submitted for publication.

Niedel, J. E., Kuhn, L., and Vandenbark, G. R. (1983). *Proc. Natl. Acad. Sci. U.S.A.* **80**, 36.

Nishizuka, Y. (1983). *Trends Biochem. Sci.* **8**, 13–16.

Osborne, R., and Tashjian, A. H. (1981). *Endocrinology (Baltimore)* **108**, 1164–1170.

Ozawa, S., and Kimura, N. (1979). *Proc. Natl. Acad. Sci. U.S.A.* **76**, 6017–6020.

Page, M. J., and Parker, M. G. (1983). *Cell* **32**, 495.

Payvar, F., Wrange, O., Carlstedt-Duke, J., Okret, S., Gustafsson, J. A., and Yamamoto, K. (1981). *Proc. Natl. Acad. Sci. U.S.A.* **78**, 6628–6632.

Peterkofsky, A. (1976). *Adv. Cyclic Nucleotide Res.* **7**, 1.

Phahl, M. (1982). *Cell* **31**, 475–482.

Potter, E., Nicholaisen, A. K., Ong, E. S., Evans, R. M., and Rosenfeld, M. G. (1981). *Proc. Natl. Acad. Sci. U.S.A.* **78**, 6662–6666.

Robins, D. M., Park, I., Seeburg, P. W., and Axel, R. (1982). *Cell* **29**, 623.

Ronning, S. A., Heathey, G. A., and Martin, T. F. J. (1982). *Proc. Natl. Acad. Sci. U.S.A.* **79**, 6294–6298.

Schonbrunn, A., Krasnoff, M., Westendorf, J. M., and Tashjian, A. H. (1980). *J. Cell Biol.* **85**, 786–797.

Shenk, T. (1981). *Curr. Top. Microbiol. Immunol.* **93**, 25–40.

Sobel, A., and Tashjian, A. H. (1983). *J. Biol. Chem.* **258**, 10312–10324.

Southern, P. J., and Berg, P. (1982). *J. Mol. Appl. Genet.* **1**, 327.

Supowit, S. E., Potter, E., Evans, R. M., and Rosenfeld, M. G. (1983). *Proc. Natl. Acad. Sci. U.S.A.* **81**, 2975–2979.

Takai, Y., Kishimoto, A., Iwasa, Y., Kawahasa, Y., Mori, T., and Nishizuka, Y. (1979a). *J. Biol. Chem.* **254**, 3692–3695.

Takai, Y., Kishimoto, A., Kikkawa, U., Mori, T., and Nishizuka, Y. (1979b). *Biochem. Biophys. Res. Commun.* **91**, 1218–1224.

Taraskevich, P. S., and Douglas, W. W. (1977). *Proc. Natl. Acad. Sci. U.S.A.* **74**, 4064–4067.

Tashjian, A. H., Lomedico, M. E., and Maina, D. (1978). *Biochem. Biophys. Res. Commun.* **81**, 798–806.

Thaw, C., Wittlin, S. D., and Gershengorn, M. C. (1982). *Endocrinology (Baltimore)* **111**, 2138–2140.

Waterman, M., Murdoch, G. H., Evans, R. M., and Rosenfeld, M. G. (1984). Submitted for publication.

White, B. A., and Bancroft, F. C. (1983). *J. Biol. Chem.* **258**, 4618–4622.

Yu, M. W., Tolson, N. W., and Guroff, G. (1980). *J. Biol. Chem.* **255**, 10481–10492.

Zubay, G., Schwartz, D., and Beckwith, J. (1970). *Proc. Natl. Acad. Sci. U.S.A.* **66**, 104.

CHAPTER 3

Glucocorticoid Regulation of Metallothionein Gene Expression

Kelly E. Mayo* and Richard D. Palmiter

Howard Hughes Medical Institute and Department of Biochemistry
University of Washington
Seattle, Washington

*Present address: Molecular Biology and Virology Laboratory, The Salk Institute for Biological Studies, San Diego, California 92138.

BIOCHEMICAL ACTIONS OF HORMONES, VOL. XII

I. INTRODUCTION

A. METALLOTHIONEINS

The metallothioneins (MTs) are a group of small cysteine-rich proteins that have a high capacity to bind certain heavy metals. These proteins are thought to function in the detoxification of harmful metals, such as cadmium and mercury, and in the metabolism of essential metals, such as zinc and copper (Kojima and Kägi, 1978; Brady, 1982). Most vertebrates have two polymorphic forms of metallothionein that differ in amino acid sequence; these are designated MT-I and MT-II. The 61–amino acid protein contains 20 cysteine residues that are involved in coordination of heavy metals. The positioning of these cysteines is absolutely conserved between species and between metallothioneins I and II. Structural studies indicate that the protein consists of two metal-binding domains: an amino-terminal domain in which 3 metal atoms are bound by 9 cysteines, and a carboxy-terminal domain in which 4 metal atoms are bound by 11 cysteines (Otvos and Armitage, 1980; Winge and Miklossy, 1982). Synthesis of the metallothioneins can be induced by heavy metals, an observation compatible with their proposed role in metal metabolism and detoxification (Kägi and Nordberg, 1979). In addition, metallothionein levels can be raised in animals by a variety of stresses (Oh *et al.*, 1978). This is due, at least in part, to a direct effect of glucocorticoid hormones on metallothionein synthesis (Karin and Herschman, 1979). This chapter will review some of the recent advances in the molecular biology of the metallothioneins. Although emphasis will be placed upon glucocorticoid regulation of metallothionein genes, it will be useful to compare and contrast results obtained for heavy metal regulation of these genes.

B. METALLOTHIONEIN GENES

We use the mouse as a model system for studying metallothionein gene regulation, and have described previously the generation of cDNA and genomic clones corresponding to the mouse *MT-I* gene (Durnam *et al.*, 1980). The structure of this gene is depicted in Fig. 1. More recently, both mouse (Searle *et al.*, 1984) and human (Karin and Richards, 1982) MT-II genes have been isolated. The size and exon/intron boundaries of these genes conform to the basic structure shown for the mouse *MT-I* gene (Fig. 1). Although there appears to be a single *MT-I* and *MT-II* gene in mice, the human *MT* genes comprise a family of about 11 closely related members (Karin and

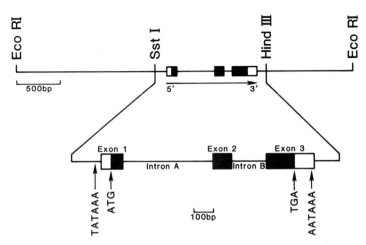

Fɪɢ. 1. Structure of the mouse metallothionein-I gene. The exons are indicated as boxes and the introns as lines. Coding regions are shaded. Consensus sequences thought to be involved in the initiation of transcription, the initiation and termination of translation, and polyadenylation are indicated. Intron A interrupts between amino acids 9 and 10; intron B, between amino acids 31 and 32 of the 61–amino acid metallothionein protein. The arrow indicates the direction of transcription. The *Sst* I to *Hind* III fragment was used as a hybridization probe for most of the experiments described.

Richards, 1982), and there are multiple monkey *MT* genes (Schmidt and Hamer, 1983).

II. REGULATION OF THE MOUSE *MT-I* GENE BY GLUCOCORTICOIDS

A. Assays for Regulation

It is becoming clear from results in a variety of prokaryotic and eukaryotic systems that there are multiple control steps at which the level of a specific gene product can be regulated (Darnell, 1982). Thus, in interpreting the results of gene regulation experiments, it is important to consider the assay being used. We utilize four basic assay systems for measuring *MT* gene expression. To measure MT protein, we label cells or tissues with [^{35}S]cysteine and separate and identify the labeled MT by a variety of chromatographic or electrophoretic techniques. We measure MT-I mRNA amounts by solution hybridization with ^{32}P-labeled MT-I cDNA (Durnam and Palmiter, 1983). To directly measure *MT-I* gene transcription, we perform RNA polymerase "run-on" experiments using nuclei isolated from control or induced cells, a technique that essentially measures the number of RNA polymerase molecules transcribing the gene at the time the nuclei are isolated (McKnight and Palmiter, 1979). Lastly, to easily assay MT promoter activity, we use a fusion gene containing the regulatory/promoter regions of the *MT-I* gene linked to a *Herpesvirus simplex*-1 thymidine kinase *(TK)* structural gene (Brinster *et al.*, 1982). This allows us to assay *MT-I* gene promoter activity enzymatically.

B. Regulation in Mice

The observation that a variety of physical and chemical stresses increase the synthesis of MTs in rat liver (Oh *et al.*, 1978), led Karin and Herschman (1979) to examine the effect of glucocorticoid hormones on metallothionein synthesis. Using cultured HeLa cells, they were able to demonstrate a direct effect of the synthetic glucocorticoid, dexamethasone, on MT synthesis. With the availability of recombinant DNA probes for the mouse *MT-I* gene, it became possible to analyze the mechanisms by which glucocorticoids regulate metallothionein synthesis. Using these probes, Hager and Palmiter (1981) showed that administration of dexamethasone to mice dramatically increased the rate of transcription of the *MT-I* gene in liver. Lesser inductions were measured in other tissues, the extent of induction apparently being regulated, at least in part, by the number of glucocorticoid receptors in various target tissues. Thus, glucocorticoids seem to be important regulators of metallothionein gene expression *in vivo*. Although the exact physiological role of MT induction by glucocorticoids is unknown, possible roles include a hormonal modulation of zinc homeostasis and a general protective involvement of MT in the stress response. Glucocorticoids also appear to be physiological mediators of MT induction in the fetal liver during embryonic development (Quaife *et al.*, 1985).

C. Regulation in Mouse Cell Lines

Because of the difficulty in controlling the localization and concentration of glucocorticoids administered to mice, we turned to cultured mouse cell lines to study glucocorticoid regulation of the mouse *MT-I* gene in more detail. For most of these experiments we used the mouse sarcoma-180 cell line (S180), in which the synthesis of the metallothioneins is substantially

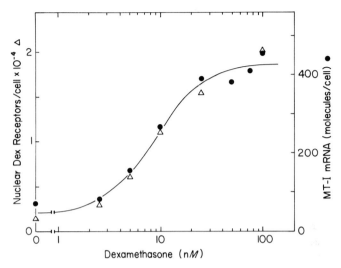

FIG. 2. Dose–response relationship for glucocorticoid induction of the mouse metallothio-nein-I gene. MT-I mRNA amounts (●———●) were measured by solution hybridization to MT-I cDNA 8 hours after treatment of mouse S180 cells with the indicated amount of dex-amethasone. Nuclear glucocorticoid receptors (△———△) were determined as described (Mayo and Palmiter, 1981a) 1 hour after addition of dexamethasone.

induced by both heavy metals and glucocorticoids (Mayo and Palmiter, 1981a). Figure 2 shows the dose–response relationship obtained when MT-I mRNA was measured in these cells following treatment with the synthetic glucocorticoid, dexamethasone. MT-I mRNA levels were induced ninefold with a maximal dose of the hormone (100 nM); the induction was half-maximal at 8 nM dexamethasone. Figure 2 also shows that the induction of MT-I mRNA was directly proportional to an increase in the number of glucocorticoid receptors associated with nuclear binding sites following dex-amethasone addition. While we utilized only the synthetic glucocorticoid dexamethasone for our experiments, Karin and Herschman (1980) demon-strated that naturally occurring glucocorticoids are also effective inducers of MT synthesis and that other classes of steroid hormones do not induce MT synthesis.

The kinetics of several parameters associated with glucocorticoid-induced MT synthesis are shown in Fig. 3. Figure 3B indicates that the rate of MT synthesis and the amount of MT-I mRNA began to increase within 30 min-utes of addition of dexamethasone to S180 cells. Both reached maximal levels after about 8 hours and remained high as long as the hormone was present.

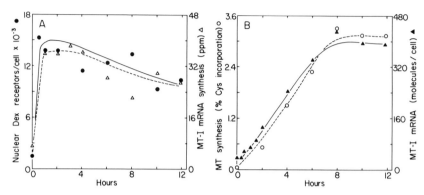

FIG. 3. Kinetics of glucocorticoid-induced mouse metallothionein-I gene expression. In all cases, 100 n*M* dexamethasone was added to mouse S180 cells at time zero. (A) Nuclear glucocorticoid receptors (●———●) measured as described in Mayo and Palmiter (1981a). MT-I mRNA synthesis (△---△) in parts per million of pulse-labeled ³H-RNA that is MT-I specific as determined by filter hybridization. (B) MT-I mRNA accumulation (▲———▲) determined by solution hybridization to MT-I cDNA. MT synthesis (○---○) measured by [³⁵S]cysteine incorporation and gel filtration.

These kinetics do not suggest a role for translational control in the regulation of MT synthesis. To determine whether increased MT synthesis and MT-I mRNA accumulation in response to glucocorticoids are due to increased *MT-I* gene transcription, MT-I mRNA synthesis was measured by pulse labeling S180 cells with [³H]uridine at various times following dexamethasone addition. Fig. 3A shows that MT-I mRNA synthesis was maximal within 1 hour of hormone addition and that the kinetics of nuclear localization of the glucocorticoid receptor closely paralleled those for MT-I mRNA synthesis. Because the half-life of MT-I mRNA is only about 2–4 hours, the pulse-labeling technique used for measuring MT-I mRNA synthesis in Fig. 3 might not be an accurate reflection of actual *MT-I* gene transcription. Therefore, we also used the nuclear "run-on" technique described in Section IIA to measure *MT-I* gene transcription following glucocorticoid administration to S180 cells. These results indicate that glucocorticoids directly increase *MT-I* gene transcription (Mayo and Palmiter, 1982; Beach *et al.*, 1981). Analysis of multiple experiments in which we have measured induction of MT-I mRNA and *MT-I* gene transcription in mouse S180 cells treated with glucocorticoids indicates that MT-I mRNA levels increase about tenfold, but that *MT-I* gene transcription increases only about five- to eightfold. This suggests that glucocorticoids might also increase slightly the stability of MT-I mRNA; however, it is clear that glucocorticoid-induced MT synthesis is largely due to increased *MT-I* gene transcription.

III. COMPARISONS TO HEAVY METAL REGULATION

A. DIFFERENTIAL RESPONSIVENESS TO METALS AND GLUCOCORTICOIDS

In several ways, the characteristics of MT induction by metals or glucocorticoids are very similar. Like glucocorticoids, metals exert their effect by directly increasing *MT-I* gene transcription (Durnam and Palmiter, 1981). The kinetics of the metal induction are also very similar to those seen for glucocorticoid induction of the *MT-I* gene (Durnam and Palmiter, 1981). However, an examination of the extent of the induction by these two agents in a variety of mouse tissues and cell lines reveals substantial differences. *In vivo*, these differences are somewhat difficult to analyze because the inductions are influenced by a variety of factors. For example, there is a generally good correlation between the amount of Cd taken up by various organs and their ability to induce MT-I mRNA in response to Cd; the best inductions are observed in tissues such as liver, kidney, and intestine, all of which absorb large amounts of Cd (Durnam and Palmiter, 1981). Also, as mentioned previously, the ability of various organs to induce MT-I mRNA in response to glucocorticoids appears to be at least partially determined by the number of glucocorticoid receptors present in these organs. For example, glucocorticoids are much more effective inducers in liver, which has a large number of glucocorticoid receptors, than in kidney, which has far fewer glucocorticoid receptors (Hager and Palmiter, 1981). Lastly, it is difficult to estimate what proportion of the cells in any given tissue is able to respond to either metals or glucocorticoids. Despite these complications, some general conclusions can be drawn from considering the induction in an organ such as the liver, which responds well to both metals and glucocorticoids. Analysis of either MT-I mRNA levels or *MT-I* gene transcription in liver reveals that Cd can elicit a response that is twice as large as that obtained with dexamethasone (Durnam and Palmiter, 1981; Hager and Palmiter, 1981). Thus, metals seem to be somewhat more effective inducers of MT-I than glucocorticoids.

When the inductions of MT-I mRNA by Cd or glucocorticoids in mouse cell lines are compared, a similar result is obtained; in general, metals are better inducers than glucocorticoids (Mayo and Palmiter, 1981a). In addition, it is clear that most cultured mouse cell lines respond to metals in a very similar manner, wheras the response to glucocorticoids is much more variable. Following maximal induction of a variety of mouse cell lines derived from diverse tissues with Cd, MT-I mRNA levels are about 1000 to 1500 molecules/cell in all of the lines (Mayo and Palmiter, 1981a). In contrast, maximal dexamethasone-induced MT-I mRNA levels in these same cell lines range from 150 to 850 molecules/cell. Only in mouse L cells was the induction by glucocorticoids similar to that with cadmium. Furthermore, this variability in responsiveness to glucocorticoids cannot be adequately explained by variations in the number of glucocorticoid receptors. This can be demonstrated by considering the induction in two cell lines, the sarcoma line S180, and the hepatoma line hepa 1A. Both have similar basal levels of MT-I mRNA and, in both, this level is increased 20- to 25-fold following Cd addition. However, MT-I mRNA is induced about tenfold by dexamethasone in the S180 cells, but only about twofold in the hepa 1A cells (Mayo and Palmiter, 1981a). Direct measurements of *MT-I* gene transcription indicate an eightfold dexamethasone-induced increase in S180 cells and essentially no increase in hepa 1A cells (Beach *et al.*, 1981). Both of these cell lines have approximately the same number of glucocorticoid receptors (K. Mayo, unpublished results). Thus, the hepatoma line seems to be deficient in some factor other than the glucocorticoid receptor necessary for glucocorticoid-induced *MT-I* gene transcription.

B. Independent Regulation by Metals and Glucocorticoids

Responses to steroid hormones have been broadly divided into two classes: primary responses, which are very rapid and independent of ongoing protein synthesis, and secondary responses, which often begin after some lag period and appear to require prior synthesis of intermediary proteins (Yamamoto and Alberts, 1976). Because glucocorticoids are known to stimulate zinc uptake by mammalian cells (Cox, 1968), it is conceivable that glucocorticoids exert their effect by increasing the cellular content of this inducing metal and are, therefore, indirect inducers of the *MT-I* gene. To test this idea, we examined the relationship between dexamethasone-induced zinc uptake and *MT-I* gene expression in mouse S180 cells (Mayo and Palmiter, 1981a). These experiments indicated that (1) growth of S180 cells in a chemically defined medium depleted of zinc did not inhibit MT-I mRNA accumulation in response to dexamethasone, (2) the glucocorticoid-induced increase in zinc uptake was not measurable until about 4 hours after hormone addition, whereas MT-I mRNA began to increase within 30 minutes, and (3) dexamethasone induced MT-I mRNA in the presence of the protein synthesis inhibitor cyclohexamide, a drug that blocks dexamethasone-induced zinc uptake. These results argue that the induction of MT-I mRNA by glucocorticoids is a primary response. Similar results have been obtained for glucocorticoid induction of human metallothioneins (Karin *et al.*, 1980).

Metals also appear to be primary inducers of *MT-I* gene transcription in that the response is very rapid, independent of protein synthesis, and occurs in chemically defined media lacking any hormones (K. Mayo, unpublished results). Thus, metals and glucocorticoids represent two distinct classes of inducers that work via direct but independent mechanisms.

C. METAL–GLUCOCORTICOID INTERACTIONS

Because metals and glucocorticoids act independently to induce *MT-I* gene transcription, they might potentially also act additively or synergistically. We first examined this possibility by inducing S180 cells with optimal doses of either Cd or dexamethasone, or both, and found that the induction with the combination of inducers was always limited to that seen with Cd alone. Because glucocorticoid receptors are reported to contain sensitive sulfhydryl groups that might interact with Cd (Granberg and Ballard, 1977), we examined the effect of Cd on the number of nuclear glucocorticoid receptors in S180 cells and found this number was decreased tenfold (Mayo and Palmiter, 1982). We have, therefore, used zinc, a metal normally present in growing cells, to address the question of whether metals and glucocorticoids together can induce more MT-I mRNA than either agent alone. Table I shows results from two independent experiments that suggest that zinc and dexamethasone are able to act nearly additively to induce MT-I mRNA in mouse S180 cells. Interestingly, the MT-I mRNA levels achieved with this combination of inducers is higher than that seen in these cells with optimal doses of any single inducer, including Cd; this implies that metal-induced transcription of the *MT-I* gene must be limited by factors other than the maximal rate at which the gene can be transcribed. These results suggest

TABLE I

INTERACTION OF METALS AND GLUCOCORTICOIDS TO INDUCE
METALLOTHIONEIN-I mRNA IN MOUSE S180 CELLS

Treatment	MT-I mRNA (molecules/cell)	
	Experiment 1	Experiment 2
Control	55	50
Dexamethasone[a]	660	665
Zinc[b]	950	1100
Dexamethasone + zinc	1610	1750

[a]S180 cells were treated for 8 hours with 100 nM dexamethasone.
[b]S180 cells were treated for 8 hours with 60 μM ZnSO$_4$.

that *in vivo* the combined effects of glucocorticoids, physiological metals such as zinc, and perhaps other inducers will determine the ultimate level of *MT-I* gene expression.

IV. REGULATION OF THE MOUSE *MT-I* GENE IN NEW ENVIRONMENTS

A. Cadmium-Resistant Cell Lines

The metallothioneins are believed to play a major role in the sequestration and detoxification of some harmful metals. Consistent with this role is the observation that cultured cell lines selected for resistance to cytotoxic metals overproduce metallothioneins (Rugstad and Norseth, 1978). It is now clear that in mouse cell lines a major mechanism for overproducing metallothioneins is amplification of *MT* genes (Beach and Palmiter, 1981; Beach *et al.*, 1981). We selected in a stepwise manner a derivative of the previously described S180 cell line resistant to normally toxic amounts of Cd (Cd^R S180), and found that in these cells the *MT-I* gene is amplified about tenfold (Mayo and Palmiter, 1982). We then used this cell line to study the effect of gene amplification on the hormonal regulation of the mouse *MT-I* gene.

As mentioned in Section III,C, cadmium inactivates the glucocorticoid receptor. It was therefore necessary to completely remove Cd from the Cd^R cells prior to performing experiments on the regulation of amplified *MT-I* genes. This was accomplished by growing Cd^R cells in nonselective medium for 8 days. At the end of this withdrawal period, these cells (Cd^R-WD) do not contain detectable amounts of Cd, have decreased amounts of MT-I mRNA and MT protein, and retain the majority of the amplified *MT-I* gene copies (Mayo and Palmiter, 1982). Figure 4 shows the effect of Cd or dexamethasone addition on MT-I mRNA levels and *MT-I* gene transcription in both normal (Cd^S) S180 cells and the cadmium-resistant- withdrawn variant (Cd^R-WD). The results are expressed on a per gene copy basis so that identical regulation in the two cell types can be indicated by equivalent height of the two sets of histograms. Figure 4 shows that regulation of the *MT-I* gene by Cd is directly proportional to gene dosage; this suggests that the amplified *MT-I* gene copies in Cd^R cells are regulated by Cd in a manner identical to that observed for the original unamplified *MT-I* gene in Cd^S S180 cells. Figure 4 also shows that dexamethasone-induced MT-I mRNA accumulation and *MT-I* gene transcription in Cd^R-WD cells are only about one-sixth of the values expected considering gene dosage; this suggests that the amplified *MT-I* gene copies in Cd^R cells are essentially nonresponsive to glucocor-

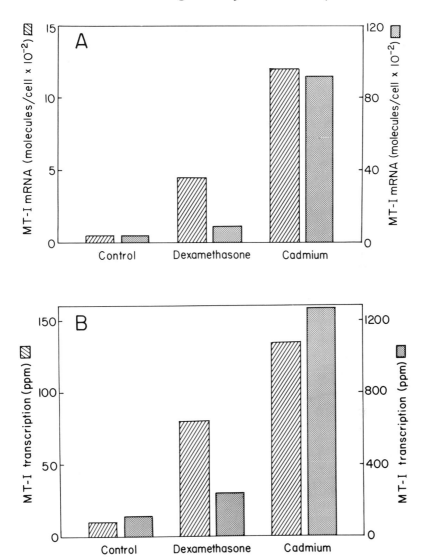

FIG. 4. Regulation of the mouse metallothionein-I gene in normal and cadmium-resistant mouse S180 cells. Cross-hatched histograms represent Cd^S S180 cells, and stippled histograms represent Cd^R-WD S180 cells as described in the text. The scale for Cd^R-WD cells is eightfold greater than that for Cd^S cells; this corresponds to the difference in *MT-I* gene number in these two cell lines. Both cell lines were induced with 100 nM dexamethasone; Cd^S cells, with 20 μM CdSO$_4$; and Cd^R-WD cells, with 120 μM CdSO$_4$. (A) MT-I mRNA levels determined 8 hours after induction; (B) *MT-I* gene transcription measured 1 hour after induction.

ticoids. A more detailed clonal analysis of Cd^R cells indicated that all of the cells within the population are deficient in their response to dexamethasone (Mayo and Palmiter, 1982).

The selective loss of glucocorticoid-regulated *MT-I* gene expression following amplification of the gene is not a unique property of the S180 cell line. Cadmium-resistant variants of hepatoma 1A and Friend erythroleukemia cells also have amplified *MT-I* genes that are regulated normally by Cd but are nonresponsive to glucocorticoids although, as noted previously, the *MT-I* gene in hepa 1A cells is essentially nonresponsive to glucocorticoids even prior to amplification (Beach *et al.*, 1981). We have considered two types of explanations for this loss of hormone responsiveness. Because steroid hormone receptors are generally believed to bind to specific high-affinity sites near those genes that they regulate (Yamamoto and Alberts, 1976; Gorski and Gannon, 1976), it is possible that such a binding site might not be coordinately amplified with the *MT-I* structural gene in Cd^R cells. However, recent experiments with other steroid hormone–responsive genes suggest that cloned genes generally containing a few kilobases or less of DNA flanking the gene retain hormonal regulation following transfer into mammalian cells (Buetti and Diggelman, 1981; Kurtz, 1981; Robins *et al.*, 1982) and contain specific binding sites for steroid receptor proteins (Payvar *et al.*, 1981; Mulvihill *et al.*, 1982; Govindan *et al.*, 1982). We know that at least 25 kb of DNA flanking the *MT-I* gene are coamplified in the Cd^R S180 cells (Mayo and Palmiter, 1982). We therefore consider it to be unlikely that important regulatory sites remain unamplified. An alternate explanation is that during development glucocorticoid responsiveness is established by appropriate modifications of DNA or chromatin constituents (for example, methylation or nucleosome phasing) and that such an epigenetic chromatin structure is neither selected for nor appropriately maintained during the process of gene amplification. Consistent with this notion is the observation that several characteristics of nuclease hypersensitivity at the 5' end of the *MT-I* gene become altered when the gene is amplified, suggesting that the chromatin structure in this region has been altered in some manner (Senear and Palmiter, 1983).

B. Transfected Cell Lines

We have used DNA-mediated transfection of mammalian cells as a functional test to define DNA sequences necessary for expression and regulation of the mouse *MT-I* gene. Two vectors containing selectable marker genes were constructed for these experiments. The first vector, pMT-TK, includes a 4 kb *Eco* R1 fragment of mouse DNA including the *MT-I* gene and both 5'-

and 3'-flanking sequences (see map in Fig. 1) as well as the *Herpesvirus simplex*-1 TK gene. This vector was used for transfection of homologous mouse L_{TK}^- cells. The second vector, pMT-GPT, includes the same 4 kb genomic fragment containing the *MT-I* gene and the *Escherichia coli* xanthine–guanine phosphoribosyl transferase (*GPT*) gene. This vector was used for transfection of heterologous human HeLa$_{HGPRT}^-$ cells.

Because human *MT* gene sequences do not hybridize to mouse *MT-I* gene probes when appropriate hybridization conditions are used, it is possible to specifically measure the expression of the transfected genes when the pMT-GPT vector is used to transfect human cells. We isolated a number of cell clones containing pMT-GPT after transfection with CaPO$_4$–DNA precipitates (Graham and Van der Eb, 1973) and selection in HAT medium (Szybalski *et al.*, 1962). Table II shows the results of experiments in which the regulation of these transfected *MT-I* genes by Cd and glucocorticoids was examined. Results obtained with two different pMT-GPT transformants are presented. pMT-GPT-23 contained about two copies of the transfected gene, wheras pMT-GPT-5 contained about ten copies; in both cases the transfected genes were integrated at a single site into high-molecular-weight DNA, presumably a human chromosome (Mayo *et al.*, 1982). Both of these clones expressed the transfected mouse *MT-I* gene at a level corresponding to the relative *MT-I* gene copy number (Table II). In each clone, MT-I mRNA was induced about twofold by dexamethasone and about sixfold by Cd. When *MT-I* gene transcription rates were measured, only Cd increased transcription of the transfected genes (Table II). This same result was ob-

TABLE II

REGULATION OF THE MOUSE METALLOTHIONEIN-I GENE FOLLOWING TRANSFECTION INTO HUMAN CELLS

Cell line	MT-I gene copy number[a]	MT-I mRNA[b] (molecules/cell)			MT-I Gene transcription[c] (ppm)		
		Control	Dex[d]	Cd[e]	Control	Dex	Cd
HeLa$_{HGPRT-}$	0	0	0	0	6	6	6
pMT-GPT-23	2	100	205	610	20	20	90
pMT-GPT-5	10	840	1400	4645	100	100	400

[a]Copy number was estimated using Southern blotting techniques (Mayo and Palmiter, 1982).
[b]Determined by solution hybridization to MT-I cDNA.
[c]Transcription reactions were as described (McKnight and Palmiter, 1979), and values are corrected for 50% efficiency.
[d]Induction was for 1 hour with 100 nM dexamethasone.
[e]Induction was for 1 hour with 40 μM CdSO$_4$.

tained for four additional pMT-GPT transformants (Mayo *et al.*, 1982). Because glucocorticoids do not induce transcription of the transfected genes, we presume that the twofold dexamethasone-induced increase in MT-I mRNA is a consequence of a small effect on MT-I mRNA stability, consistent with previous results (Section II,C).

A possible explanation for the inability of glucocorticoids to appropriately regulate the mouse *MT-I* gene in transfected human cells is that the human glucocorticoid receptor or other human regulatory proteins might not productively recognize and interact with mouse DNA regulatory regions. To test this possibility, homologous mouse cells were transfected with the vector pMT-TK, and transformed clones were isolated. Although analysis of these clones is complicated by the background contributed by the endogenous mouse *MT-I* gene, the results clearly indicate that in eight clones examined the transfected *MT-I* genes were transcriptionally regulated by Cd but not by glucocorticoids (Mayo and Palmiter, 1981b; Mayo *et al.*, 1982). In contrast, the endogenous mouse *MT-I* gene in these same cells was transcriptionally regulated by both agents. It is possible that the fragment of mouse DNA used for these experiments, which contains 1.7 kb of DNA flanking the 5' side of the *MT-I* gene, does not contain those sequences necessary for glucocorticoid inducibility. However, we again favor the interpretation proposed previously for the loss of glucocorticoid responsiveness by amplified *MT-I* genes (Section IV,A), that hormonal regulation is dependent upon a developmentally controlled gene commitment process that cannot be appropriately reproduced following either gene amplification or transfection.

Mouse cells have also been transfected with a cloned fusion gene including the mouse *MT-I* gene promoter/regulatory region and the human growth hormone structural gene on a bovine papilloma virus vector (Pavlakis and Hamer, 1983). In this case, the transfected genes are present in 10–100 copies/cell and remain episomal rather than integrated into a host chromosome. The hybrid mRNA made by this fusion gene was inducible by Cd, but not by dexamethasone, consistent with our results. In contrast, Karin and co-workers (1984a) found that when the human *MT-II* gene was transfected into rat cells it was appropriately regulated by Cd and glucocorticoids in some transformants, although only Cd was effective in others. The finding that only some of the transformants were glucocorticoid inducible (Karin *et al.*, 1984a) is consistent with the notion that chromatin environment plays an important role in determining glucocorticoid responsiveness. The explanation for the different results obtained for the mouse *MT-I* and human *MT-II* genes is unclear. It seems unlikely to be due to differences between the *MT-I* and *MT-II* genes, because we have recently found that the mouse *MT-II* gene is regulated by Cd but not by glucocorticoids following transfection

(Searle *et al.*, 1984). There may be inherent differences in the *MT* genes from these two species.

C. SOMATIC CELL HYBRIDS

Our results with amplified and transfected *MT-I* genes indicate that the chromosomal environment of the gene might play a role in its regulation by glucocorticoids. We therefore wondered whether the *MT-I* gene would remain glucocorticoid inducible if an entire mouse chromosome containing this gene were placed in a new environment, such as a heterologous mammalian cell. In collaboration with Dr. David Cox (University of California, San Francisco), we tested this idea by examining mouse *MT-I* gene expression in hamster/mouse somatic cell hybrids that retain only a few mouse chromosomes. The mouse *MT-I* gene has been mapped to mouse chromosome 8 (Cox and Palmiter, 1983). We therefore examined six different hamster/mouse hybrid clones that contain mouse chromosome 8, as well as several other mouse chromosomes. By choosing appropriate hybridization conditions, expression of the mouse *MT-I* gene can be monitored without a substantial contribution from the endogenous hamster *MT* genes. Table III shows results obtained when these six clones, as well as several controls not

TABLE III

REGULATION OF THE MOUSE METALLOTHIONEIN-I GENE IN HAMSTER/MOUSE SOMATIC CELL HYBRIDS

		MT-I mRNA (molecules/cell)[a]		
Clone number	Mouse chromosome 8[b]	Control	Dexamethasone[c]	Cd[d]
12 (parental)	−	5	30	110
2	−	30	30	160
8	−	5	10	100
3	+	80	90	775
5	+	115	230	500
11	+	130	180	650
1	+	140	180	875
9	+	195	650	995
10	+	130	680	1150

[a]Determined by solution hybridization to MT-I cDNA using conditions that eliminate most hybridization to hamster MT mRNAs.

[b]Markers for various mouse chromosomes are described in detail by Cox and Palmiter (1983).

[c]Induction was for 24 hours with 100 nM dexamethasone.

[d]Induction was for 8 hours with 30 μM CdSO$_4$. The small Cd induction seen in clones without mouse chromosome 8 is induction of hamster MT mRNA.

containing mouse chromosome 8, were induced with Cd or dexamethasone. All of the six clones containing mouse chromosome 8 express the *MT-I* gene and, in all six, MT-I mRNA was inducible by Cd. In two of these six clones, MT-I mRNA was also induced by glucocorticoids (Table III). Thus, in at least some cases, the *MT-I* gene can be regulated by glucocorticoids when it is present in its normal chromosomal environment within a heterologous cell type.

We are not certain why all of the clones containing mouse chromosome 8 do not respond to glucocorticoids. However, because these cell lines generally carry several mouse chromosomes, it is possible that the presence or absence of mouse chromosomes other than 8 affect glucocorticoid regulation of the *MT-I* gene. In this respect, it is interesting to note that two of the three clones that include mouse chromosome 18 (clones 1, 9, and 10 in Table III) respond to glucocorticoids, whereas each of three clones that do not include mouse chromosome 18 (clones 3, 5, and 11) are nonresponsive to glucocorticoids. The mouse glucocorticoid receptor gene has been mapped to mouse chromosome 18 (Francke and Gehring, 1980); perhaps the presence of the mouse receptor protein is required for glucocorticoid-regulated mouse *MT-I* gene expression. Because we have not yet unambiguously determined which mouse chromosomes are present in each of the hybrid clones described in Table III, it remains possible that other chromosomes are common to the glucocorticoid-responsive clones.

D. Activated Lymphoid Cells

Genetic approaches to studying the mechanisms by which glucocorticoids regulate specific genes have led to the isolation of several variant classes of the mouse lymphoid cell lines S49 and W7 that are nonresponsive to glucocorticoids (Sibley and Tomkins, 1974; Bourgeois and Newby, 1977). Because we were interested in using these variant cell lines to study glucocorticoid regulation of the *MT-I* gene, we first tested the normal parental S49 and W7 cell lines to determine whether the *MT-I* gene was inducible by metals and glucocorticoids. To our surprise, we found that these cell lines do not express the *MT-I* gene at detectable levels (Mayo and Palmiter, 1981a). We have since found that the *MT-I* gene can be activated in these lymphoid cell lines in at least three different ways. First, treatment with the DNA methylation inhibitor 5-azacytidine results in *MT-I* gene expression (Compere and Palmiter, 1981). Second, lymphoid cell lines resistant to normally toxic amounts of Cd can be selected in a stepwise manner, and these cells eventually begin to express the *MT-I* gene (K. Mayo, unpublished results). Third, cells that express the *MT-I* gene can be isolated following UV mutagenesis and single-step selection in Cd (Lieberman *et al.*, 1983).

We analyzed lymphoid cell lines in which the *MT-I* gene was activated by these various schemes to determine whether the gene was rendered inducible by metals and glucocorticoids. These results are summarized in Table IV. We found that in each of the three cases the *MT-I* gene could be induced by Cd, but not by glucocorticoids. In the case of 5-azacytidine–activated cells, a small (twofold) induction of MT-I mRNA by glucocorticoids was observed (Compere and Palmiter, 1981). However, based upon our results with transfected *MT-I* genes (Section IV,B), we surmise that this is due to MT-I mRNA stabilization, not to increased *MT-I* gene transcription. In each of the three activated lymphoid cell lines described, there was a loss of methylated cytosine residues from all of the *Hpa* II sites in the vicinity of the *MT-I* gene. Thus, in each case, demethylation of many sites in and around the *MT-I* gene is correlated with expression and metal regulation of the gene. These results with activated lymphoid cell lines are similar to those obtained for the hepatoma 1A cell line (Section III,A); in each case, the endogenous *MT-I* gene can be regulated by metals, the *MT-I* genes have normal flanking sequences, and the cells contain high levels of the glucocorticoid receptor, yet it appears that the *MT-I* gene remains altered in some manner such that it is not regulated by glucocorticoids.

TABLE IV

REGULATION OF THE MOUSE METALLOTHIONEIN-I GENE
IN ACTIVATED LYMPHOID CELL LINES

	MT-I mRNA (molecules/cell)[a]		
Treatment of cells	Control	Dexamethasone	Cd
None	0	0	0
Stepwise selection for Cd resistance[b]	165	165	490
5-Azacytidine[c]	20	40	500
UV mutagenesis/Cd selection[d]	10	10	120

[a]MT-I mRNA was determined by solution hybridization to MT-I cDNA. Inductions were with 100 n*M* dexamethasone for 8 hours, or with $CdSO_4$ as indicated.

[b]Cells were selected for growth in 50 μ*M* Cd and were withdrawn from selective media for 8 days. Reinduction was with 50 μ*M* $CdSO_4$.

[c]See Compere and Palmiter (1981) for details of 5-azacytidine activation. Induction was with 10 μ*M* $CdSO_4$.

[d]See Lieberman *et al.* (1983) for selection scheme. Cells were selected for growth in 5 μ*M* Cd and were withdrawn from selective media for 8 days. Reinduction was with 5 μ*M* $CdSO_4$.

E. TRANSGENIC MICE

Because many of our results argue that chromatin structure or gene commitment might play a role in glucocorticoid-regulated *MT-I* gene expression, we also examined the influence of development on eventual regulation of the *MT-I* gene. Transgenic mice that develop from fertilized eggs microinjected with a metallothionein–thymidine kinase fusion gene (Section II,A) were used for this purpose. These mice contain multiple copies of the fusion gene integrated at a single chromosomal site. Because integration into the mouse genome is an early event following microinjection, these fusion genes progress through development as part of an otherwise normal mouse chromosome (Brinster *et al.*, 1981). Four mice that showed good metal regulation of metallothionein–thymidine kinase fusion genes were tested with glucocorticoids; in all cases the fusion gene was nonresponsive (Palmiter *et al.*, 1982). Thus, progression through development alone does not seem to be sufficient to generate a glucocorticoid-responsive state. In all transgenic mice examined, integration did not occur via homologous recombination with the endogenous mouse *MT-I* gene; the microinjected *MT-I* gene sequences are, therefore, not present in their normal chromosomal position. Perhaps position effects are also a determining factor in generating glucocorticoid responsiveness.

V. SUMMARY

Glucocorticoid hormones have been shown to play a major role in regulating the synthesis of the metallothioneins. They act via specific hormone receptors to increase transcription of the *MT-I* gene in mouse cells and tissues. This induction is rapid, does not require ongoing protein synthesis, and is independent of other inducers of metallothionein synthesis. Metals act in a similar manner to independently regulate synthesis of the metallothioneins. More recently, we have discovered that inflammation, mimicked by injection of bacterial endotoxin (lipopolysaccharide), also induces MT-I mRNA independently of the other inducers (Durnam *et al.*, 1984). The metallothionein genes, therefore, provide an excellent model system for studying eukaryotic gene regulation.

We found that, when the mouse *MT-I* gene is activated in lymphoid cells, amplified, or transferred to other cells, it invariably retains information necessary for its metal-regulated expression, but loses the ability to be regulated by glucocorticoids. Based upon this evidence, we have proposed that hormonal regulation of the *MT-I* gene depends upon gene commitment, a process that normally occurs at a critical point in development and results in a replicable *cis* acting change in DNA or chromatin structure that allows subsequent productive interaction with glucocorticoid receptors. Further work to test this idea and to identify critical aspects of *MT-I* gene chromatin structure is necessary. It is encouraging that a human *MT-II* gene retains hormonal regulation following gene transfer (Karin *et al.*, 1984a). Karin *et al.* (1984b) have recently defined two stretches of DNA near the human *MT-II* gene promoter that seperately mediate induction of the gene by either heavy metals or glucocorticoid hormones. The glucocorticoid-responsive element is coincident with the DNA-binding site for the glucocorticoid hormone receptor.

The physiological implications and consequences of glucocorticoid-regulated metallothionein synthesis remain poorly understood. Certainly, some cells that are not glucocorticoid inducible, or that fail to make MTs at all, are able to survive and divide, indicating that metallothioneins are not essential for survival. Nevertheless, the fact that they are present in most tissues and regulated by a variety of stimuli suggests that they must play an important role in times of stress and inflammation. The induction by MTs by glucocorticoids or inflammation results in sequestration of available metals such as zinc and copper. In some situations, this results in decreased serum concentrations of these metals. How the relocation of these essential metals helps protect an organism in times of stress and inflammation is not clear. During normal development of the mouse, MTs are induced to high levels in the fetal liver, apparently in response to a surge in maternal glucocorticoid production during the last few days of gestation (Quaife *et al.*, 1985). In this case, the sequestration of zinc and copper by MTs may provide a storage function for later development. Clearly, at both the molecular and cellular level, much remains to be understood about the regulation of the metallothionein genes by glucocorticoids.

REFERENCES

Beach, L. R., and Palmiter, R. D. (1981). *Proc. Natl. Acad. Sci. U.S.A.* **78**, 2110–2114.
Beach, L. R., Mayo, K. E., Durnam, D. M., and Palmiter, R. D. (1981). *ICN-UCLA Symp. Mol. Cell. Biol.* **23**, 239–248.
Bourgeois, S., and Newby, R. F. (1977). *Cell* **11**, 423–430.
Brady, F. O. (1982). *Trends Biochem. Sci.* 7(4), 143–145.
Brinster, R. L., Chen, H. Y., Trumbauer, M., Senear, A. W., Warren, R., and Palmiter, R. D. (1981). *Cell* **27**, 223–231.
Brinster, R. L., Chen, H. Y., Warren, R., Sarthy, A., and Palmiter, R. D. (1982). *Nature (London)* **296**, 39–42.
Buetti, E., and Diggelman, H. (1981). *Cell* **23**, 335–345.
Compere, S. J., and Palmiter, R. D. (1981). *Cell* **25**, 233–240.
Cox, D., and Palmiter, R. D. (1983). *Hum. Genet.* **64**, 61–64.
Cox, R. P. (1968). *Mol. Pharmacol.* **4**, 510–521.
Darnell, J. E., Jr. (1982). *Nature (London)* **297**, 365–371.
Durnam, D. M., and Palmiter, R. D. (1981). *J. Biol. Chem.* **256**, 5712–5716.

Durnam, D. M., and Palmiter, R. D. (1983). *Anal. Biochem.* **131**, 385–393.
Durnam, D. M., Perrin, F., Gannon, F., and Palmiter, R. D. (1980). *Proc. Natl. Acad. Sci. U.S.A.* **77**, 6511–6515.
Durnam, D. M., Hoffman, J. S., Quaife, C. J., Benditt, E. P., Chen, H. Y., Brinster, R. L., and Palmiter, R. D. (1984). *Proc. Natl. Acad. Sci. U.S.A.* **81**, 1053–1056.
Francke, U., and Gehring, U. (1980). *Cell* **22**, 657–664.
Gorski, J., and Gannon, F. (1976). *Annu. Rev. Physiol.* **38**, 425–450.
Govindan, M. V., Spiess, E., and Majors, J. (1982). *Proc. Natl. Acad. Sci. U.S.A.* **79**, 5157–5161.
Graham, F. L., and Van der Eb, A. J. (1973). *Virology* **52**, 456–467.
Granberg, J. P., and Ballard, P. L. (1977). *Endocrinology (Baltimore)* **100**, 1160–1168.
Hager, L. J., and Palmiter, R. D. (1981). *Nature (London)* **291**, 340–342.
Kägi, J. H. R., and Nordberg, M., eds. (1979). "Metallothionein." Birkhaeuser, Basel.
Karin, M., and Herschman, H. R. (1979). *Science* **204**, 176–177.
Karin, M., and Herschman, H. R. (1980). *J. Cell. Physiol.* **103**, 35–40.
Karin, M., and Richards, R. I. (1982). *Nature (London)* **299**, 797–802.
Karin, M., Anderson, R. D., Slater, E., Smith, K., and Herschman, H. R. (1980). *Nature (London)* **286**, 295–297.
Karin, M., Haslinger, A., Holtgreve, H., Cathala, G., Slater, E., and Baxter, J. D. (1984a). *Cell* **36**, 371–379.
Karin, M., Haslinger, A., Holtgreve, H., Richards, R. I., Krauter, P., Westpal, H. M., and Beato, M. (1984b). *Nature* **308**, 513–519.
Kojima, Y., and Kägi, J. H. R. (1978). *Trends Biochem. Sci* **3**, 90–93.
Kurtz, D. T. (1981). *Nature (London)* **291**, 629–631.
Lieberman, M., Beach, L. R., and Palmiter, R. D. (1983). *Cell* **35**, 207–214.
McKnight, G. S., and Palmiter, R. D. (1979). *J. Biol. Chem.* **254**, 9050–9058.
Mayo, K. E., and Palmiter, R. D. (1981a). *J. Biol. Chem.* **256**, 2621–2624.
Mayo, K. E., and Palmiter, R. D. (1981b). *In* "Gene Amplification" (R. T. Schimke, ed.), pp. 67–73. Cold Spring Harbor Lab. Cold Spring Harbor, New York.
Mayo, K. E., and Palmiter, R. D. (1982). *J. Biol. Chem.* **257**, 3061–3067.
Mayo, K. E., Warren, R., and Palmiter, R. D. (1982). *Cell* **29**, 99–108.
Mulvihill, E., Lepennec, J.-P., and Chambon, P. (1982). *Cell* **28**, 621–632.
Oh, S. H., Deagen, J. T., Whanger, D. D., and Weswig, P. H. (1978). *Am. J. Physiol.* **234**, E282–E285.
Otvos, J. D., and Armitage, I. M. (1980). *Proc. Natl. Acad. Sci. U.S.A.* **77**, 7094–7098.
Palmiter, R. D., Chen, H. Y., and Brinster, R. L. (1982). *Cell* **29**, 701–710.
Pavlakis, G. N., and Hamer, D. H. (1983). *Proc. Natl. Acad. Sci. U.S.A.* **80**, 397–401.
Payvar, F., Wrange, O., Carlstedt-Duke, J., Okret, S., Gustafsson, J. A., and Yamamoto, K. R. (1981). *Proc. Natl. Acad. Sci. U.S.A.* **78**, 6628–6632.
Quaife, C., Mottet, N. K., and Palmiter, R. D. (1985). Submitted for publication.
Robins, D. M., Paek, I., Seeburg, P. H., and Axel, R. (1982). *Cell* **29**, 623–631.
Rugstad, H. E., and Norseth, T. (1978). *Biochem. Pharmacol.* **27**, 647–650.
Schmidt, C. J., and Hamer, D. H. (1983). *Gene* **24**, 137–146.
Searle, P. F., Davison, B. L., Stuart, G. W., Wilke, T. M., Norstedt, G., and Palmiter, R. D. (1984). *Mol. Cell. Biol.* **4**(7), 1221–1230.
Senear, A. W., and Palmiter, R. D. (1983). *Cold Spring Harbor Symp. Quant. Biol.* **47**, 539–547.
Sibley, C. H., and Tomkins, G. M. (1974). *Cell* **2**, 221–227.
Szybalski, W., Szybalski, E. H., and Ragni, G. (1962). *Natl. Cancer Inst. Monogr.* **7**, 75–89.
Winge, D. R., and Miklossy, K. A. (1982). *J. Biol. Chem.* **257**, 3471–3476.
Yamamoto, K. R., and Alberts, B. M. (1976). *Annu. Rev. Biochem.* **45**, 721–746.

CHAPTER 4

Regulation of the Synthesis of Tyrosine Aminotransferase and Phosphoenolpyruvate Carboxykinase by Glucocorticoid Hormones

Daryl K. Granner* and Elmus G. Beale †

Diabetes and Endocrinology Research Center
Departments of Internal Medicine and Biochemistry
Veterans Administration Medical Center
The University of Iowa College of Medicine
Iowa City, Iowa

*Present address: Department of Physiology, Vanderbilt University, Nashville, Tennessee 37232.

†Present address: Department of Anatomy, Texas Tech University Health Science Center, School of Medicine, Lubbock, Texas 79430.

BIOCHEMICAL ACTIONS OF HORMONES, VOL. XII

I. INTRODUCTION AND HISTORICAL PERSPECTIVE

Mechanisms that provide for the differentiation, replication, and growth of cells, repairing and replacing cells and their components, responding to an altered environment, and supplying a constant source of energy, are essential to the survival of multicellular organisms. It is likely that all of these processes, some more clearly adaptive than others, are regulated by a variety of different classes of molecules. One of these classes is the steroid hormones, which are in many ways the prototypical mammalian regulatory molecule. Their structure, although relatively simple in design and variation compared to proteins, allows them to participate in diverse regulatory processes of cell growth and differentiation (estrogens, androgens, progestins, and glucocorticoids), ion balance (mineralocorticoids), and a variety of metabolic pathways (glucocorticoids). Steroid hormones generally act by regulating the transcription of specific genes (see Anderson, 1984, for review), although there are enough well-documented exceptions to prevent this from being a rule (Wasserman and Smith, 1978). The purpose of this chapter is to review how glucocorticoid hormones enhance the synthesis of the hepatic enzymes tyrosine aminotransferase (TAT) and phosphoenolpyruvate carboxykinase (PEPCK).

A. DEVELOPMENT OF THE BASIC PRINCIPLES OF REGULATION

The spectacular advances in experimental molecular biology, which have taken studies of gene regulation to a level unimagined a few years ago, tend to obscure the major achievements that provided the foundation for these very studies. The importance of the fundamental concepts derived from these earlier studies merits a short review, and this also provides some perspective on the accelerating rate with which new advances are being made in this area (see Fig. 1).

The concept that the conversion of foodstuffs into cellular constituents or into energy involved an orderly progression of discrete biochemical reactions, each catalyzed by an enzyme, first began to be developed around the turn of this century. It took some time for this notion to gain general acceptance, but by the 1950s the basic metabolic pathways had been defined. Subsequent experiments in this area focused on the coordination of these complex pathways. An important event in this regard was the formulation by a number of investigators, including the Coris, Soskin, Notkins, and Levine, of the hypothesis that hormones might provide the means of metabolic coordination (Levine, 1981).

Another extremely important concept began to emerge in the early 1940s. Prior to that time, a cell was thought to consist of a membrane that separated a fixed set of enzymatically catalyzed reactions from the environment. Since the cell was capable of self-replication, this implied a constancy of these

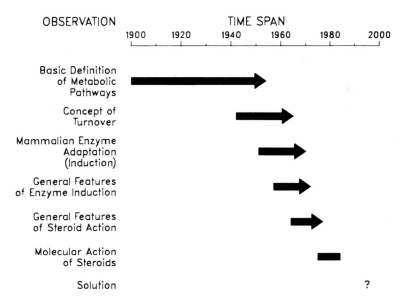

FIG. 1. Evolution of studies of enzyme induction. This figure represents the major developments that have contributed to the current understanding of hormonal regulation of enzyme synthesis. The length of the arrow approximates the time span required for the development of these concepts and coincides with the dates discussed in the text. "Molecular Action of Steroids" is shown without a point since this has not been resolved yet.

reactions from generation to generation. Hence, it was inferred that a cell's endowment of enzymes did not change. This arrangement, although conservative, lacks the key ingredient now recognized as one of the fundamental features of biological systems—flexibility. Schoenheimer, in some of the first experiments to use isotopes, showed in 1942 that cellular constituents were actually in a dynamic state. Schoenheimer (1942) accomplished this by feeding rats water composed of heavy hydrogen (D_2O) and measuring its rate of incorporation into fat. Subsequently, using a single injection of an amino acid containing the heavy isotope of nitrogen (^{15}N), other investigators showed that the half-time ($t_{1/2}$) of liver protein nitrogen was 7 days (Shemin and Rittenberg, 1946). Several years later, using a more sensitive assay in which tritium-labeled water was administered for 125 days as the tracer, a much more comprehensive study of the turnover of many body constituents was performed (Thompson and Ballou, 1956). Of particular interest to the subject of this review was the observation that liver proteins could be separated into two classes according to relative rates of turnover. One group, comprising about 3% of total protein, had a very slow $t_{1/2}$, about 140 days. The major group consisted of two subclasses that turn over much more rapidly, one with a $t_{1/2}$ of 4.5 days and another with a $t_{1/2}$ of 12 days. These observations led to the development of concepts about turnover that play a role in designing enzyme induction experiments to this day. The net result of turnover can be static or dynamic. In a static state, the pool of molecules is replenished by synthesis, transport from an inactive compartment of the cell, or transformation of inactive form, to active forms of the molecules at the same rate at which the molecules are being degraded, inactivated, or transported out of an active compartment of the cell. In a dynamic state, the pool increases or decreases because of altered rates of these processes, primarily synthesis or degradation in the case of enzyme induction or deinduction. Turnover provides the mechanism for flexibility. More rapid and accurate changes in response to the internal or external environment can be accomplished by making subtle adjustments to an ongoing synthesis–degradation process than by employing an "all or none" mechanism that would involve starting from scratch.

Thus, the basic observations that resulted in the definition of the metabolic pathways, the concept that the enzymatic reactions that govern these pathways are regulated and the demonstration that proteins turn over, certainly were prerequisites for studies of enzyme regulation by hormones.

B. Development of the Concept of Enzyme Induction

Enzyme induction, the adaptive increase in the number of molecules of a specific enzyme, is a relatively new biological concept that is scarcely older than the era of "molecular biology." The observation that cellular components turn over (Schoenheimer, 1942; Shemin and Rittenberg, 1946; Thompson and Ballou, 1956) led to the emergence of the concept that complex organisms could show adaptive responses to their environment. In the 1940s, it was shown that remarkable changes in the amount of enzymes in microorganisms occur, generally in response to alterations of substrate concentration (Dubos, 1940; Monod, 1947; Spiegelman, 1946), but a similar phenomenon was not demonstrated in mammalian cells until 1951. In that year, two papers provided the first demonstration of enzyme "adaptation," or induction as it is now known, in a mammalian tissue. Knox and Mehler (1951) showed that tryptophan, whether given by oral, subcutaneous, or intraperitoneal routes to rabbits, rats, and guinea pigs, resulted in a six- to eightfold increase in the activity of the enzyme now known as tryptophan oxygenase (TO). This was a rapid response. The increase occurred within several hours, and enzyme activity returned to the basal value within 15–20 hours. Although unprecedented in mammalian tissues, this substrate-induced "adaptive increase" was very similar to that noted in microorganisms. Even more novel was the observation that a variety of other compounds, such as tyrosine, kynurenine, phenylalanine, and histidine, which were not substrates of TO, were also effective inducers. In a subsequent paper, Knox showed that these substances only induced TO when the animals had an intact pituitary–adrenal axis (Knox, 1951). This axis was known to be involved in adaptation to stress (Selye, 1946), and Knox noted that several of the animals injected with the nonsubstrate compounds were irritable and became agitated. When adrenalectomized rats failed to respond to these compounds and to adrenaline (epinephrine), Knox hypothesized that adrenal cortical hormones were involved. Purified preparations of glucocorticoids had just become available and, when tested, were found to induce TO in adrenalectomized rats (Thompson and Mikuta, 1954). Thus, the hypothesis was confirmed.

By 1956, many examples of changes of enzyme activity in response to adrenalectomy, thyroidectomy, hypophysectomy, and diabetes could be cited (Knox *et al.*, 1956). Shortly thereafter, glucocorticoids were found to induce TAT (Lin and Knox, 1957), and the era of research on the hormonal regulation of enzyme induction was under way. This topic has been the subject of several excellent review articles (Kenney, 1970; Pitot and Yatvin, 1973; Schimke, 1973; Gelehrter, 1976).

C. MECHANISM OF ENZYME INDUCTION

In addition to demonstrating an adaptive response of a mammalian enzyme, the original observations by Knox and Mehler (1951) were important in another way; these investigators proposed that the change in TO activity was due to an increased *amount* of the enzyme. Their statement, "The production of a potential increase in metabolism by increasing the amount of enzyme, but without affecting the catalytic activity of a given amount of enzyme may therefore be a general means of metabolic regulation," although self-evident today, was written at a time when efforts to define the action of hormones were largely confined to cell-free systems. Steroid hormones were thought to act as co-factors; hence the mind-set was that hormones altered catalytic activity. Not surprisingly, the few effects obtained were usually inhibitory (Dorfman, 1952) and were not related to the effect expected from endocrine organ ablation (Knox *et al.*, 1956). Until the paper by Knox (1951), and to a considerable extent for at least another decade, the fact that steroid hormone action required an intact cell that was capable of protein synthesis was not given serious consideration.

Proof that increased activity of an enzyme was due to an increased amount of the protein required a purified protein, a specific antibody, and a specific immunoprecipitation assay. Such evidence was obtained for TAT (Kenney, 1962a) and for TO (Feigelson and Greengard, 1962). The concept of turnover implied that an increased amount of protein could result from an increased rate of synthesis, from a decreased rate of degradation, or from some combination of these processes. The theoretical basis for such experiments was defined by Schimke and co-workers, who showed that tryptophan slowed hepatic TO degradation while hydrocortisone enhanced TO synthesis (Schimke *et al.*, 1965; Berlin and Schimke, 1965). Kenney (1962b) had shown that rat liver TAT synthesis was also enhanced by hydrocortisone and that this effect was sufficient to account for the increase of enzyme activity.

The next major advance came when Jacob and Monod (1961) proposed that specific mRNAs direct the synthesis of each protein, a concept that was quickly adapted to studies of hormonal regulation of proteins in eukaryotic cells. Unfortunately, many of the enzymes of interest exist in very small amount, so it took several years before specific assays of mRNA activity or amount, measured by various cell-free translation systems or by hybridization to specific cDNA probes, were established. In the meantime, results obtained from experiments using various inhibitors of RNA synthesis were used to make inferences about the mediating role of mRNA. Since many of these compounds, most notably actinomycin D, inhibited glucocorticoid induction of TAT (Greengard and Acs, 1962; Thompson *et al.*, 1966), TO (Greengard and Acs, 1962), and PEPCK (Shrago *et al.*, 1963), it was assumed that ongoing mRNA synthesis was necessary for the response. This assumption required considerable faith and more than a few leaps of logic but, as we will discuss, in these instances the prediction was confirmed by the more direct mRNA assays. Table I illustrates the sequence in which studies of

TABLE I
GLUCOCORTICOID INDUCTION OF HEPATIC ENZYMES

| | Enzyme | | |
Process	TAT	TO	PEPCK
Increased enzyme activity	1957	1954	1963
Increased enzyme amount	1962	1962	—
Increased enzyme synthesis	1962	1965	1975
Increased mRNA activity	1976	1973	1977
Increased mRNA amount	1983	1982	1983
Increased mRNA transcription	—	1983	1983

enzyme induction generally proceed and provides a comparison of the years in which such studies were published for three hepatic proteins.

D. MECHANISMS OF STEROID HORMONE ACTION

The original discovery of hormone-binding "receptors" came from the work of Talwar *et al.* (1964), who showed that estradiol was tightly bound to a high-molecular-weight component in uterine cytosol. The definition, localization, characterization, and function of steroid receptors has received a great deal of attention in recent years, and several excellent reviews of the role of glucocorticoid receptors in the action of this class of hormones have been published (King and Mainwaring, 1974; Rousseau, 1975; Leung and Munck, 1975; Munck and Leung, 1976; Cake and Litwack, 1975; Baxter, 1976; Baxter and Ivarie, 1978; Rousseau and Baxter, 1979). The general scheme is as follows. The glucocorticoid enters the target cell and binds to a specific cytoplasmic receptor. An "activation" process, which requires heat and salt *in vitro*, then occurs, and this enables the steroid–receptor complex to enter the nucleus, where it binds to selected regions of the DNA and/or chromatin. This interaction results in altered transcription of selected genes and an altered cellular phenotype. Although there are several thousand steroid–receptor binding sites in the nucleus of a target cell, the cellular phenotype, as defined by the different proteins synthesized, is not changed very much. Fewer than 1% of the hepatic cell proteins constitute the glucocorticoid domain, as judged by the studies of Ivarie and O'Farrell (1978) and O'Farrell and Ivarie (1979). One interpretation of their observation is that this class of steroid hormone, although it binds to many nuclear sites, influences the expression of very few genes. Since the hormone could affect the size and charge of proteins through *in vivo* posttranslational modification, a more direct assessment of the gene domain influenced by glucocorticoids can be made by looking at the products synthesized by poly(A)$^+$ RNA in a cell-free system (see below).

There is considerable biochemical (King and Mainwaring, 1974; Rousseau, 1975; Leung and Munck, 1975; Munck and Leung, 1976; Cake and Litwack, 1975; Baxter, 1976; Baxter and Ivarie, 1978; Rousseau and Baxter, 1979) and genetic (Yamamoto *et al.*, 1976) evidence that glucocorticoid receptors bind to DNA, but selective binding, in a region likely to affect gene transcription, was only demonstrated recently (Payvar *et al.*, 1981; Govindan *et al.*, 1982; Geisse *et al.*, 1982; Pfahl, 1982). It was also recently demonstrated that steroid–receptor binding to specific DNA sequences actually affected transcription of a specific gene. This observation required that a putative regulatory region of DNA, which contained specific glucocorticoid–receptor binding sites, could confer regulation to a gene ordinarily unresponsive to glucocorticoids. Portions of two different genes were used to effect this result. The production of mammary tumor virus (MTV) RNA in infected HTC cells is increased severalfold by glucocorticoid hormones (Ringold *et al.*, 1975). This increase is due to enhanced transcription of the MTV genome (Ringold *et al.*, 1977; Ucker *et al.*, 1981), and several studies show that this virus contains all the information required for glucocorticoid action (Huang *et al.*, 1981; Yamamoto *et al.*, 1981; Groner *et al.*, 1982). All retroviruses contain long-terminal-repeat (LTR) DNA segments of varying length and DNA sequence. The mammary tumor virus LTR contains glucocorticoid–receptor binding sites (Payvar *et al.*, 1981; Govindan *et al.*, 1982; Geisse *et al.*, 1982; Pfahl, 1982) and the initiation site for transcription of the MTV genome. To test whether these two sites are functionally linked, Lee *et al.* (1981) fused the MTV long-terminal-repeat segment to the dihydrofolate reductase (DHFR) gene, which is ordinarily not responsive to glucocorticoid hormones. The resultant fusion gene, put into a cell that was unable to produce DHFR itself, produced enhanced amounts of DHFR in response to dexamethasone. Therefore, the enhanced expression of DHFR in this fusion gene construction must have been conferred by the LTR segment isolated from the *MTV* gene. A more precise localization of the glucocorticoid–receptor sites that are coupled to transcription initiation was provided by the experiments of Chandler *et al.* (1983), who fused specific fragments of the LTR segment to the herpes simplex thymidine kinase gene, which also is not normally influenced by glucocorticoids. These experiments, by no means the only ones of this type, serve to illustrate how the model of glucocorticoid action has been extended over the past few years.

The general features of steroid hormone action and enzyme induction have been outlined. The rest of this chapter will deal with how these principles have been applied to the regulation of the synthesis of the hepatic enzymes TAT and PEPCK by glucocorticoid hormones.

II. REGULATION OF TYROSINE AMINOTRANSFERASE BY GLUCOCORTICOID HORMONES

A. GENERAL FEATURES OF TYROSINE AMINOTRANSFERASE

Tyrosine aminotransferase (L-tyrosine:2-oxoglutarate aminotransferase; EC.2.6.1.5; TAT) is an enzyme that catalyzes the first and rate-limiting step of tyrosine degradation. The end result of this is the formation of fumarate and acetoacetate. The precise metabolic purpose of TAT is unclear, but it may be to prevent the accumulation of toxic levels of tyrosine. TAT is absent in hereditary hypertyrosinemia, a condition that is associated with multiple abnormalities in humans (Goldsmith *et al.*, 1973) and that is indirectly lethal to mink since it results in poor pelts (Goldsmith *et al.*, 1981). A secondary purpose of TAT may be to provide ketogenic and gluconeogenic substrates. TAT is found only in liver or liver-derived cell lines and is a dimeric molecule consisting of two identical 53,000 M_r subunits. Earlier reports of multiple forms, some of which were allegedly subject to differential regulation by various hormones, has recently been explained. A protease that selectively cleaves a 4000 M_r piece from the carboxy terminus of TAT causes much of the heterogeneity, as does the presence of mitochondrial aspartate aminotransferase, which can transaminate tyrosine. The metabolic role of TAT and the intracellular processing of this enzyme have been discussed in detail in an earlier review article (Hargrove and Granner, 1984).

Tyrosine aminotransferase is subject to regulation by a number of compounds, including several hormones (Granner and Hargrove, 1983). Current evidence indicates that all changes in TAT activity are due to changes in its rate of synthesis and/or degradation. Although TAT undergoes a number of posttranslational modifications, there is no evidence that these contribute to alterations in catalytic activity (Hargrove and Granner, 1984).

B. INDUCTION OF TYROSINE AMINOTRANSFERASE IN RAT LIVER

The induction of TAT by glucocorticoid hormones represents one of the earliest examples of hormonal induction of a mammalian enzyme. In the late 1950s, Lin and Knox (1957, 1958) injected intact or adrenalectomized rats with hydrocortisone and noted a fivefold increase in hepatic TAT activity 5 hours later. The rapidity and extent of the response, coupled with the relative ease of performing the enzymatic assay, made this a very attractive system, and it quickly became a favored model for studying the mechanism of action of glucocorticoid hormones. This phenomenon has subsequently been documented in perfused rat liver (Barnabei and Sereni, 1960; Goldstein *et al.*, 1962; Hager and Kenney, 1968), fetal liver organ culture (Wicks, 1969), and at least four different tissue culture lines (Pitot *et al.*, 1964; Thompson *et al.*, 1966; Gerschenson *et al.*, 1970; Richardson *et al.*, 1969). Consequently, the induction of TAT by glucocorticoids is regarded as being a fundamental characteristic of the hepatic parenchymal cell.

The question raised by Knox and Mehler (1951) a decade earlier anticipated the strategy employed in the early 1960s and subsequent years, to define this effect of glucocorticoid hormones. The first objective in defining an induction phenomenon, whether at the level of protein or mRNA, is to determine whether the alteration is due to a change in the activity or the amount of the molecule in question. If the amount of a protein (or mRNA) is increased, the next step is to determine whether this is due to increased synthesis or decreased degradation. The approach to these questions is epitomized in several studies by Kenney, who used partially purified TAT (Kenney, 1959) to prepare an antiserum that was then used to show that the induction of rat liver TAT catalytic activity by hydrocortisone was associated with a commensurate increase in the amount of TAT protein (Kenney, 1962a). Using this antiserum to immunoprecipitate TAT from pulse-labeled hepatic proteins, he then demonstrated that the increase of TAT protein was due to increased synthesis and not to stabilization of the protein against degradation (Kenney, 1962b). This series of studies certainly helped provide the conceptual framework of induction phenomena in mammalian tissues, and a number of interesting biological questions have subsequently been addressed using TAT regulation as the model and the general approach outlined above. These include (a) the actions of a number of hormones, (b) the "permissive" action of glucocorticoids, (c) the neonatal development and differentiation of proteins, (d) the association between malignant transformation and dedifferentiation, (e) the diurnal variation of proteins, and (f) the role cytoplasmic factors and chromatin modification play in the regulation of the synthesis of specific proteins (see Granner and Hargrove, 1983, for a review).

C. TAT INDUCTION IN CULTURED HEPATOMA CELLS

The intact animal systems imposed several experimental limitations; hence, the development of simpler, more defined systems for studying these questions in mammalian cells represent another major advance. One of the most effective solutions to this problem is to study cells in culture. Efforts to grow mammalian cells in culture began shortly after the turn of the century, but met with little consistent success until the 1950s. For the next several years, most attention was given to establishing lines of cells in culture and then defining the nutritional requirements for their growth. Once this was accomplished, a cell line was generally not used for any other purpose. There was, in fact, considerable skepticism that such cells could be used to study regulatory phenomena.

The induction of TAT in the H4IIE cells, a line derived from the chemically induced Reuber H35 rat hepatoma, was the first demonstration of enzyme induction in a cultured cell of hepatic origin (Pitot *et al.*, 1964). These investigators added 10^{-6} *M* cortisone acetate to the culture medium and noted a rapid increase of TAT activity, comparable to that noted in rat liver (Lin and Knox, 1957, 1958; Kenney, 1962a). Soon thereafter, Thompson *et al.* (1966) showed that TAT could be induced in HTC cells, a different cell line derived from the chemically induced Morris rat hepatoma 7288c. The general features of TAT induction in HTC cells were the same as in rat liver with respect to the kinetics and magnitude of the induction, the necessity for ongoing protein and RNA synthesis, and the observation that only steroids with glucocorticoid activity, as opposed to other types of steroids, were effective (Thompson *et al.*, 1966). During the next few years, many details of TAT induction were defined in HTC cells, and it is reasonable to say that several of these would have been difficult, if not imposible, to obtain from studies using rats. Many of the key features of TAT induction in HTC cells are illustrated diagrammatically in Fig. 2. When a maximally effective concentration of the synthetic glucocorticoid dexamethasone is added at time zero (case A), there is a 2-hour lag before TAT activity begins to increase. After 2 hours, the enzyme activity steadily increases until it reaches a plateau (after approximately 12 hours) at levels eight- to tenfold higher than in untreated control cells (case B) (Thompson *et al.*, 1966). This new steady state is maintained as long as the cells are exposed to the inducer (Granner *et al.*, 1970). Removal of the dexamethasone by washing the cells (case C) results in a prompt *deinduction* of enzyme activity, and the rate of decline is comparable to the turnover time of the protein (Granner *et al.*, 1970). This induction requires ongoing RNA and protein synthesis, since it is prevented when either actinomycin D (case D) or cycloheximide (case E) are added at the same time as the dexamethasone (Thompson *et al.*, 1966).

A number of critical biological processes, including gluconeogenesis, glycogenolysis, and lipolysis, achieve maximal rates only when glucocorticoid hormones are present (Granner, 1979). This important function of glucocorticoids, which has been termed the permissive effect, is poorly understood in molecular terms, but the phenomenon can be studied in HTC cells. Whereas cAMP analogs result in a four- to fivefold induction of hepatic TAT (Wicks *et al.*, 1974), the same compounds are much less effective when

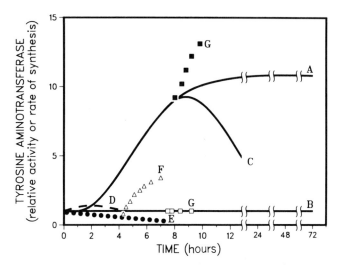

Fɪɢ. 2. Tyrosine aminotransferase induction in HTC cells. This figure depicts several events in the induction of TAT by dexamethasone in HTC cells. The time after addition of dexamethasone and other substances is shown on the abscissa, and the relative amount of TAT catalytic activity or TAT synthesis is shown on the ordinate. The various treatment conditions (A–G) are described in detail in the text. In cases B and G, no dexamethasone was added to the HTC cells. Case A represents the induction seen when maximally effective concentrations of the inducer are added. Case C represents the deinduction that results when the inducer is removed. Cases D and E show that induction is prevented if either actinomycin D or cycloheximide is added with the inducer. If the latter is removed (Case F), there is a rapid induction of TAT. Case G illustrates the fact that Bt₂cAMP is ineffective in control cells but is an excellent inducer in cells first treated with dexamethasone.

added to HTC cells (Case G, open squares; Granner *et al.*, 1968a; Granner, 1976). But, if the HTC cells are first exposed to dexamethasone and then to dibutyryl cAMP, a rapid additional increase of TAT activity is seen (case G, closed squares; Granner, 1976). This *reinduction*, the restoration of responsiveness to cAMP, exceeds the TAT level that can be achieved by any treatment with the steroid alone, but absolutely depends on the presence of the glucocorticoid. Therefore, it is an excellent example of a permissive effect. A more detailed analysis of this problem should be forthcoming, given the availability of this cultured cell system, assays for mRNA^{TAT}, and the imminent elucidation of details about the structure of the gene and associated regulatory regions.

Thompson *et al.* (1966) showed that cycloheximide prevented the induction of HTC cell TAT by dexamethasone. This likely meant that the increase of catalytic activity resulted from *de novo* synthesis of the enzyme, but a direct assessment of this was necessary. In studies analogous to those described above, TAT was purified from rat liver, and an antiserum that showed perfect cross-reactivity between rat and HTC cell TAT was developed (Granner *et al.*, 1968b). This antiserum was then used to show that induction involved *de novo* synthesis of TAT and not conversion from an inactive to an active enzyme (Granner *et al.*, 1970). In all of the instances illustrated in Fig. 2 or described above, there was an excellent correlation between enzyme catalytic activity and the rate of TAT synthesis (Granner *et al.*, 1968b, 1970; Hayashi *et al.*, 1967; Tomkins *et al.*, 1966). As we will discuss, there is also a good correlation of these processes with mRNA[TAT] levels.

Other examples of the special manner in which cultured cells have contributed to our understanding of TAT induction and glucocorticoid action merit further consideration. A number of investigators helped establish the central role of the glucocorticoid receptor in TAT induction and, in so doing, elucidated many general features of this receptor that relate to its association with many other biological events. This topic is reviewed in detail in a book dedicated to Gordon Tomkins, in whose laboratory and with whose inspired direction many of these studies were conducted (Baxter and Rousseau, 1979).

Regulatory mutants, which are instrumental in elucidating control mechanisms in bacteria, are difficult to obtain in mammalian cells. However, valuable information has been obtained by studying TAT induction in various phases of the generation cycle of hepatoma cells. The mammalian cell cycle consists of an ordered series of events demarcated by the periods of DNA synthesis (S phase) and mitosis (M). These discrete events are separated by two "gaps," G_1 and G_2. It was known for some time that rates of protein and RNA synthesis varied markedly in the cell cycle; thus, it was possible that specific cycle-dependent regulatory mechanisms might be occurring. This prediction proved to be correct, as illustrated by the series of studies of TAT regulation in HTC cells by Martin and co-workers (1969a,b; Martin and Tomkins, 1970) and studies of TAT regulation in HTC and RLC cells (Sellers and Granner, 1974). The basic observation is that the generation cycle in HTC and RLC cells can be divided into steroid-sensitive (last two-thirds of G_1 and S) and steroid-insensitive (G_2, M, and early G_1) phases. Since this approach should prove useful in elucidating the mechanisms that control steroid responsiveness at the gene level, a brief review of some of the experiments follows.

Fig. 3A illustrates the response of randomly growing cultures of HTC and RLC cells to 10^{-5} M dexamethasone. In each case, TAT activity begins to increase after the customary short lag period, and within 3 hours, the values are always greater than those noted in uninduced cells. The new steady state, some five times greater than noted in control cells in this experiment,

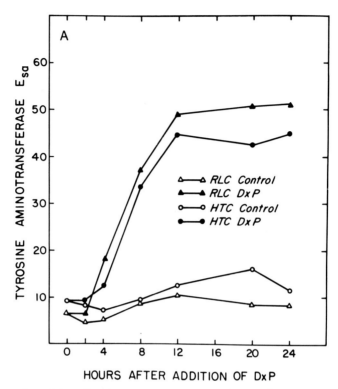

FIG. 3A. Effect of the cell cycle on tyrosine aminotransferase induction. Experiment was performed using randomly growing HTC or RLC cells suspended at a concentration of 400,000 cells/ml. The cultures were divided, and 10^{-5} M dexamethasone phosphate (DxP) was added to one half. Aliquots were taken at the times indicated for the determination of TAT catalytic activity. [Adapted from Sellers and Granner (1974).]

was reached in about 12 hours (Sellers and Granner, 1974). We then compared TAT induction in randomly growing cells to that obtained in synchronized cells that were blocked in mitosis with colcemid and then released into G_1. Dexamethasone was added at the beginning of G_1, and, while both random and "early G_1" cells eventually showed a four- to sixfold induction of TAT (Fig. 3B), the lag period before the enzyme increased was several hours longer in HTC or RLC cells synchronized at the onset of G_1 than in the randomly growing cells. This suggested that the cells were resistant to dexamethasone in early G_1 but that, at some point, this was a readily reversible phenomenon.

This delayed response to dexamethasone in cells synchronized in G_1 led to a more complete analysis, as shown in Fig. 4. The results of these experiments, with HTC cells shown in panel A and RLC cells shown in panel B,

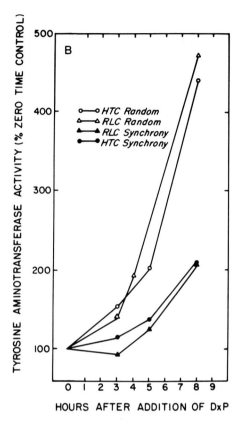

Fɪɢ. 3B. Effect of the cell cycle on tyrosine aminotransferase induction. Experiment was conceptually similar to that of Fig. 3A except that some HTC and RLC cells were synchronized in mitosis with colcemid and then allowed to enter G_1 by removal of the colcemid at time zero. DxP was added at this time. [Adapted from Sellers and Granner (1974).]

can be summarized as follows: (a) In both cell lines, basal TAT activity is higher in M and early G_1 than later in G_1 or in S, and a distinct decline begins about 2–3 hours into G_1; (b) RLC and HTC cells show no response to dexamethasone in M phase; (c) there is a period of 2–3 hours in early G_1 when both cell lines are refractory to dexamethasone, since TAT activity 5 hours into G_1 is the same when the hormone is added at time zero (onset of G_1) or at 2 hours into G_1; and (d) addition of dexamethasone later in G_1 or in S results in a rapid induction of TAT activity in both cell lines. It is noteworthy that, while the maximal rate of synthesis of TAT in randomly growing cells depends on the constant presence of the steroid (see Example A in Fig. 1), HTC or RLC cells induced before synchronization and then released into G_1 maintain a predetermined rate of TAT synthesis whether or not the

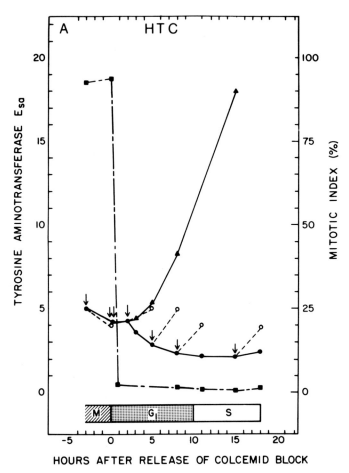

Fig. 4. Effect of the cell cycle on tyrosine aminotransferase induction. HTC cells (A) and RLC cells (B) were synchronized by colcemid block. Cells were divided into two flasks after removal of the mitotic block. The mitotic index is represented by (■—·— — · —■). One flask served as a control and as a stock for aliquots that were exposed to DxP at 2, 5, 8, and 14 hours into the cell cycle as indicated by the single arrow (↓). DxP was added to the other flask at the beginning of G_1, as indicated by the double arrow (↓↓). Inductibility during mitosis was examined by exposure to DxP in the continued presence of colcemid. The various test conditions are represented as follows: control (●———●); DxP added at beginning of G_1 (▲———▲); DxP added at each time indicated in the cell cycle (○- - -○). [Adapted from Sellers and Granner (1974).]

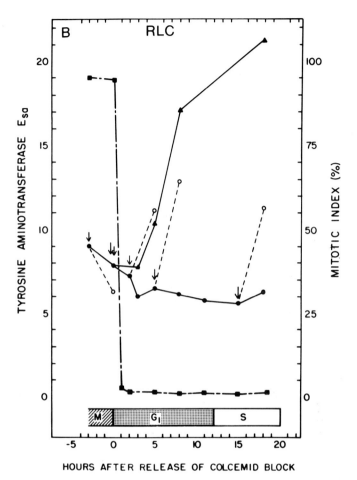

Fig. 4. (*continued*)

steroid is present. Thus, although TAT synthesis occurs throughout the cell cycle, it is enhanced by glucocorticoids only during finite periods. This internal regulation, which is likely exerted at the gene level, appears to offer a unique opportunity to study glucocorticoid action. Contemporary techniques of molecular biology have not been applied to this problem as yet.

D. REGULATION OF mRNA^{TAT} ACTIVITY

The inference that ongoing RNA synthesis was required for the induction of TAT by glucocorticoids arose from two observations. First, actinomycin D inhibited TAT induction in both liver (Greengard and Acs, 1962) and HTC cells (Thompson *et al.*, 1966). Second, a specific RNA that allowed for TAT synthesis accumulated during the 2-hour lag period between the addition of steroid and the first appearance of an increase in TAT activity (Peterkofsky and Tomkins, 1967, 1968; Steinberg *et al.*, 1975). This second conclusion, reached through a series of experiments illustrated as case F in Fig. 2, was obtained as follows. Dexamethasone and the protein synthesis inhibitor cycloheximide were added simultaneously to HTC cells. No TAT induction occurs in this circumstance. Several hours later the inhibitor was removed, whereupon TAT activity immediately increased, without the usual lag. This suggested that a substance, presumed then to be mRNA^{TAT}, accumulated in the absence of protein synthesis, and upon removal of the cycloheximide it was translated into TAT (Peterkofsky and Tomkins, 1967). Subsequent experiments, some using actinomycin D to inhibit RNA synthesis, helped pinpoint the appearance of this substance to a time about 30 minutes after the addition of the steroid (Peterkofsky and Tomkins, 1968; Steinberg *et al.*, 1975). The next step was to directly measure the mRNA that codes for TAT.

The difficulties encountered in establishing an assay that could be used to reliably quantitate the activity or amount of mRNA^{TAT} in liver or HTC cells have been discussed (Granner and Hargrove, 1983). Several groups used protein-synthesizing systems derived from oocytes, wheat germ extracts, or nuclease-treated rabbit reticulocyte lysates to quantitate mRNA^{TAT} activity (Nickol *et al.*, 1976; Roewekamp *et al.*, 1976; Diesterhaft *et al.*, 1977). The latter proved to be the most reliable. Figure 5A illustrates an experiment in which the reticulocyte lysate assay was used to quantitate the effect of glucocorticoid hormones on TAT catalytic activity and mRNA^{TAT} activity in rat liver. The problems involved in measuring mRNA^{TAT} arose from its relative scarceness; Fig. 5A shows that mRNA^{TAT} constitutes about 0.03% of total poly(A)$^+$ RNA in liver. The intraperitoneal injection of hydrocortisone results in a six- to sevenfold increase in mRNA^{TAT}, with the peak level occurring about 5 hours after the injection. The mRNA^{TAT} then declines, probably because of metabolism and excretion of the inducer. The kinetics and magnitude of this response are very similar to those of TAT catalytic activity, and proportional increases of both were noted after the intraperitoneal injection of hydrocortisone. This increase of mRNA^{TAT} was prevented when the rats were also injected with cordycepin and actinomycin D (Fig. 5B), hence the unsurprising conclusion that ongoing RNA synthesis was required (Diesterhaft *et al.*, 1980).

The relationship of mRNA^{TAT} to TAT synthesis and catalytic activity has been studied in more detail in HTC cells. The results of several of these experiments are summarized in Fig. 6. This depiction represents the average values of three separate experiments in which dexamethasone was added

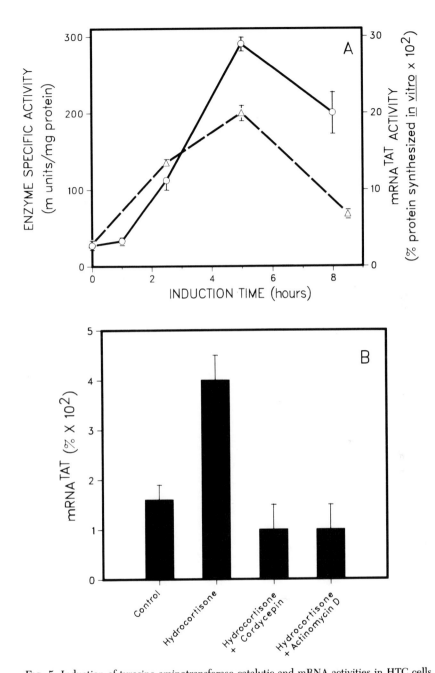

FIG. 5. Induction of tyrosine aminotransferase catalytic and mRNA activities in HTC cells. (A) The kinetics of induction of rat liver TAT activity (O————O) and mRNA^{TAT} activity (△--△) were compared at various times after the intraperitoneal injection of hydrocortisone. (B) Adrenalectomized rats were treated for 1 hour; then the livers were isolated and mRNA^{TAT} activity was determined. Rats were treated with saline, hydrocortisone, hydrocortisone plus cordycepin, or hydrocortisone plus actinomycin D. [Adapted from Diesterhaft *et al.* (1977).]

to HTC cells at time zero. The first thing to note is that these cells have approximately the same relative amount of mRNA^{TAT} as liver. An increase of mRNA^{TAT} from the basal value of 0.03% of total poly (A)$^+$ RNA was noted within 30 minutes of the addition of the steroid to the culture medium (Fig. 6). This effect preceded the increase of TAT synthesis, which in turn occurred before the increase of TAT catalytic activity. The dexamethasone-induced steady-state level of all three processes was 8–10 times greater than in control HTC cells. Given this, and the observation that the increase of mRNA^{TAT} anticipates the increase of TAT synthesis, we suggested that mRNA^{TAT} was rate limiting (Olson *et al.*, 1980). This conclusion was strengthened by the observation that there is a direct relationship between mRNA^{TAT}, TAT synthesis, and TAT catalytic activity throughout the range of effective dexamethasone concentrations (Fig. 7). The same relationship was obtained when steroids such as 11,β-hydroxyprogesterone or deoxycorticosterone, which are known to be suboptimal inducers, were employed. We also applied this comparison to variant HTC cells that were selected because of their inability to increase TAT activity in response to dexamethasone (Thompson *et al.*, 1977). These cells have a lower basal level of both TAT and mRNA^{TAT} [about 0.01% of total poly(A)$^+$ RNA] than wild-

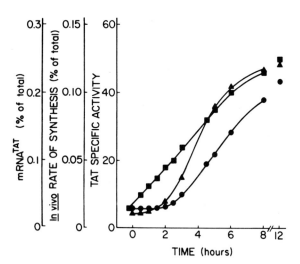

Fig. 6. Kinetics of tyrosine aminotransferase induction in HTC cells. Dexamethasone was added to HTC cells at time zero and aliquots were removed at various times thereafter for determination of mRNA^{TAT} activity (■———■), the *in vivo* rate of synthesis of TAT (▲———▲), and TAT catalytic activity (●———●). The values represent the mean of three separate experiments. [Adapted from Olson *et al.* (1980).]

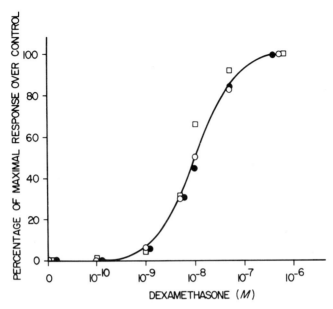

Fɪɢ. 7. Effect of steroid concentration on various parameters of tyrosine aminotransferase induction. Various concentrations of dexamethasone were added to HTC cells, and 18 hours later assays of TAT catalytic activity (O————O), the *in vivo* rate of TAT synthesis (□————□), and mRNA^{TAT} activity (●————●) were performed. The data are expressed as the percentage of the maximal response for each function. [From Olson *et al.* (1980).]

type HTC cells, and neither of these parameters increase in response to dexamethasone. When the steady-state value of mRNA^{TAT} from all these experiments was expressed against TAT activity, a straight-line function with a correlation coefficient of 0.96 was obtained (Fig. 8), and the same relationship is seen when rat liver mRNA^{TAT} activity is compared to TAT synthesis (Nickol *et al.*, 1978). Taken collectively, these data indicate the direct relationship between mRNA^{TAT} activity and the synthesis of this protein.

E. Tʜᴇ Hᴇᴘᴀᴛɪᴄ mRNA–Gʟᴜᴄᴏᴄᴏʀᴛɪᴄᴏɪᴅ Dᴏᴍᴀɪɴ

The ability to separate proteins according to size and charge by two-dimensional gel electrophoresis allows one to identify several hundred proteins in a cellular extract (O'Farrell, 1975). One can then define the response domains influenced by regulatory agents. Using this approach, Ivarie and O'Farrell (1978) showed that fewer than 1% of the proteins in hepatoma cells change in response to dexamethasone. Some of these changes may reflect

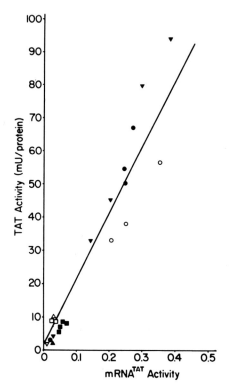

Fɪɢ. 8. Comparison of steady-state values of tyrosine aminotransferase catalytic and mRNA activities in HTC cells. Steady-state levels of mRNA^TAT activity are plotted on the abscissa, and the corresponding catalytic activities are shown on the ordinate. Values for several experiments are represented, using a different symbol (i.e., ▼, ●, ■, ○) for each experiment. The slope of the line, determined by linear regression, shows a correlation coefficient of 0.96 (Olson *et al.*, 1980).

posttranslational modification, a recently described action of glucocorticoids (Firestone *et al.*, 1982), rather than the direct action of the hormone at the genomic level. A reasonable assessment of how many mRNAs are regulated by glucocorticoids can be made by analyzing the proteins synthesized in a reticulocyte lysate system to which poly(A)⁺ RNA isolated from control or dexamethasone-treated HTC cells has been added. In this case, the proteins synthesized in the 90-minute incubation reflect the activity of specific mRNAs, since posttranslational modification presumably does not occur. The autoradiograms in Fig. 9 show that two-dimensional gel electrophoresis provides excellent resolution of several hundred peptides. Of this number, only five [labeled C,G,P,T (TAT), and M] are increased by dexamethasone,

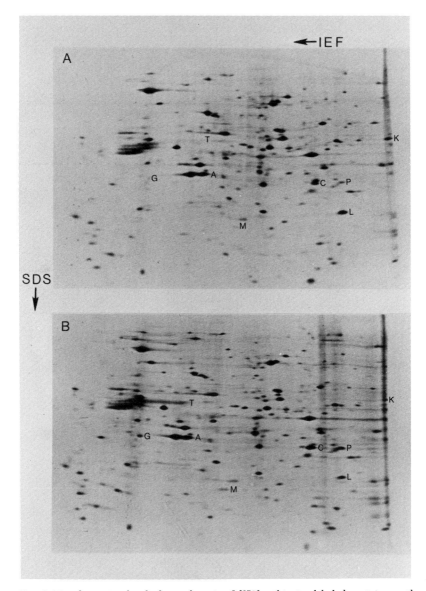

Fig. 9. Two-dimensional gel electrophoresis of [^{35}S]methionine-labeled proteins synthesized *in vitro* by whole-cell polyadenylated RNA. Polyadenylated RNA was isolated from (A) control and (B) dexamethasone-treated ($5 \times 10^{-7} M$ for 3 days) HTC cells and then translated *in vitro* in a reticulocyte lysate system. The newly synthesized [^{35}S]proteins were then electrophoresed in two dimensions by the method of O'Farrell (1975). The range of isoelectric focusing is pH 4.5–7.5 from left to right. The letters are placed to the right of proteins altered by dexamethasone treatment or by those used as a reference. Protein T is tyrosine aminotransferase; protein A is actin.

whereas two (K and L) are decreased. For reference, actin is labeled as protein A (N. B. Chrapkiewicz and D. K. Granner, unpublished observations). This technique may underestimate the number of genes affected, since those whose mRNAs are translated slowly or inefficiently in the cell-free system would not be detected. Furthermore, this technique would miss mRNAs that are not extracted equally and those lacking the polyadenylate tail. Nonetheless, the results of this experiment suggest that the mRNA domain affected by dexamethasone, like the protein domain, is very small. Coupled with the observations that hydrocortisone and dexamethasone have no effect on total poly(A)$^+$ RNA translational activity in rat liver (Diesterhaft *et al.*, 1977) or HTC cells (Olson *et al.*, 1980), it is apparent that glucocorticoids exert a very specific effect on liver and hepatoma cells.

F. THE EFFECT OF GLUCOCORTICOIDS ON mRNA^{TAT} SYNTHESIS

A direct demonstration that glucocorticoid treatment results in an increased amount of mRNA^{TAT} awaited the development of a specific cDNA^{TAT}. Scherer *et al.* (1982) isolated and identified plasmids containing cDNA^{TAT} from a library constructed from rat liver poly(A)$^+$ RNA enriched for mRNA^{TAT}. A blot hybridization analysis was performed using a ^{32}P-labeled cDNA^{TAT} as a probe. Figure 10A shows an autoradiogram in which the probe was hybridized to poly(A)$^+$ RNA isolated from the livers of adrenalectomized rats injected with dexamethazone 4 hours previously, or from control rats. When corrected for the amount of poly(A)$^+$ RNA added by using albumin mRNA as an internal standard (lanes A1–3), the data show that dexamethasone treatment (lane 6) results in a sevenfold increase of mRNA^{TAT} over the level noted in adrenalectomized rats (lane 4). Likewise, a similar increase of mRNA^{TAT} was seen in cultured hepatoma cells (Fig. 10B). Three clones of H4IIE cells were tested: Fao cells, which induce TAT in response to dexamethasone (lane B1); H5 cells, which have no basal level of TAT and show no induction of this enzyme in response to dexamethasone (lane B2); and C2 cells, a line that synthesizes a small amount of TAT (lane B3). Figure 10B shows that, following a 24-hour exposure to dexamethasone, each of these cell lines has mRNA^{TAT} in an amount proportional to the TAT catalytic activity measured in the cell. Bt$_2$cAMP results in a tenfold increase of mRNA^{TAT} (compare lane 4 with lane 5), an observation consistent with other reports that demonstrate an effect of the nucleotide on mRNA^{TAT} activity in rat liver (Ernest and Feigelson, 1978; Noguchi *et al.*, 1978; Diesterhaft *et al.*, 1980). Although an effect of dexamethasone on transcription of the *TAT* gene has not

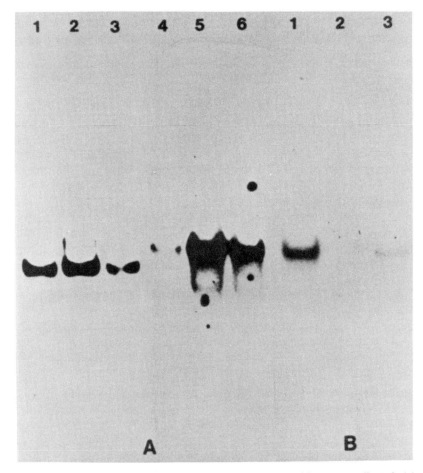

FIG. 10. Blot hybridization analysis of mRNA^{TAT} in rat liver and hepatoma cells. Poly (A)$^+$ RNA was separated on an 0.8% agarose–formaldehyde gel, transferred to nitrocellulose paper, and probed with [^{32}P]pcTAT-3, a cDNA directed against mRNA^{TAT} (lanes A4–6, B1–3), or an albumin cDNA (lanes A1–3). (A)Liver RNA isolated from adrenalectomized rats (Lanes A1–4), from rats 1 hour after injection with Bt$_2$cAMP (lanes A2 and A5), and from rats 4 hours after injection with dexamethasone (lanes A3 and A6). (B) RNA isolated from dexamethasone-treated cell lines Fao (lane B1), H5 (lane B2), and C2 (lane B3). [From Scherer *et al.* (1982).]

been reported, a fourfold enhancement of run-off transcription of mRNA^{TAT} has been noted when nuclei isolated from Bt$_2$cAMP-treated rats are compared to those isolated from control animals (G. Scherer and G. Schütz personal communication). It is very likely that a comparable effect of glucocorticoids will be demonstrated in the near future.

III. GLUCOCORTICOID REGULATION OF PHOSPHOENOLPYRUVATE CARBOXYKINASE

A. General Features of Phosphoenolpyruvate Carboxykinase

Phosphoenolpyruvate carboxykinase (GTP; EC 4.1.1.32; PEPCK) was first identified in liver mitochondria by Utter and Kurahashi (1954). Nordlie and Lardy (1963) found a cytosolic isozyme, which subsequently was shown to differ from mitochondrial PEPCK in immunochemical and physical properties (Ballard and Hanson, 1969; Diesterhaft et al., 1971). The remaining discussion deals only with the cytosolic enzyme, since this is the form that is subject to hormonal regulation (Ballard and Hanson, 1969).

Cytosolic PEPCK catalyzes the conversion of oxaloacetate to phosphoenolpyruvate and CO_2. It uses GTP as the phosphate donor and Mn^{2+} as the divalent cation. PEPCK is a single chain polypeptide of approximately 600–640 amino acids, and it has a molecular weight of 67,000–72,000 (Colombo et al., 1978; Beale et al., 1981). There is no evidence that PEPCK is subject to allosteric regulation; however, a separate protein, ferroactivator, does stimulate PEPCK activity in the presence of iron (Bentle et al., 1976). The physiological role of ferroactivator, particularly with regard to hormonal regulation, remains uncertain.

PEPCK has also been found in the cytosol of the kidney cortex and adipose tissue (Krebs et al., 1963; Ballard and Hanson, 1967). PEPCK functions as a gluconeogenic enzyme in liver and kidney, whereas in adipose tissue it is probably glyceroneogenic (Tilghman et al., 1976). The concentration of PEPCK, expressed per milligram of protein, is similar in rat liver, kidney, and adipose tissue (Tilghman et al., 1976). Its concentration in adipose tissue is ten times less when expressed by wet tissue weight, probably because of differences in the amount of cytosol (Reshef et al., 1969).

The enzymatic activity of rat liver PEPCK is increased by fasting, diabetes, glucagon, and hydrocortisone and is decreased by feeding and insulin treatment (Shrago et al., 1963). The concentration of PEPCK, expressed per milligram of tissue, ranges from 1 pmole/mg liver in fed rats to 3 pmoles/mg in fasted rats, and from 3 pmoles/mg kidney in fed rats to 7 pmoles/mg in fasted rats (Moore et al., 1982). These changes correspond to alterations in the rate of gluconeogenesis noted under the same treatment conditions (Tilghman et al., 1976). Several studies have shown that the conversion of pyruvate to phosphoenolpyruvate, catalyzed by the sequential actions of pyruvate carboxylase and PEPCK, is rate limiting in gluconeogenesis (Exton and Park, 1969; Mallette et al., 1969). These observations led to the conclusion that PEPCK and pyruvate carboxylase are rate-limiting gluconeogenic enzymes. It is thus important to determine how the activity of a critical enzyme like PEPCK is regulated by a diverse group of hormones.

The synthesis of PEPCK is under tissue-specific, multihormonal control (Tilghman *et al.*, 1976). Glucagon (with cAMP as the second messenger) and glucocorticoid hormones induce PEPCK synthesis in liver, while insulin decreases its synthesis (Gunn *et al.*, 1975b; Wicks *et al.*, 1972; Tilghman *et al.*, 1974). It is probably the concerted action of these three hormones that determines the amount of hepatic PEPCK during fasting/feeding cycles, and glucagon is probably the major inducer (Tilghman *et al.*, 1976). Similar effects of cAMP, glucocorticoids, and insulin occur in cultured H4IIE hepatoma cells (Wicks and McKibbin, 1972; Wicks *et al.*, 1974; Gunn *et al.*, 1975a), while a different situation is noted in the kidney. Renal cortex PEPCK is induced by glucocorticoids and by metabolic acidosis (Rosenzweig and Frascella, 1968; Longshaw and Pogson, 1972; Feldman, 1977), but this enzyme is unaffected by cAMP and insulin (Tilghman *et al.*, 1976). Adipose tissue presents yet another pattern as PEPCK is decreased by glucocorticoids and insulin and is increased by catecholamines and ACTH, both of which presumably act through cAMP (Reshef and Hanson, 1972; Reshef *et al.*, 1969, 1970; Gorin *et al.*, 1969).

Since the subject of this chapter is glucocorticoid action, the remainder of this discussion is directed at the mechanism by which glucocorticoids regulate PEPCK synthesis. For additional information about the general properties and regulation of PEPCK, we refer the reader to the reviews by Tilghman *et al.* (1976) and Nelson *et al.* (1981). The strategy employed in elucidating glucocorticoid control of PEPCK synthesis was essentially modeled after that used to study TAT; hence, the studies proceeded in the order illustrated in Table I. It was determined that glucocorticoids first increase PEPCK activity and then increase protein synthesis. These observations were followed in sequence by the demonstration of effects on mRNA^{PEPCK} activity, mRNA^{PEPCK} amount, and, most recently, mRNA^{PEPCK} synthesis. In general, much less work has been done on the mechanism of PEPCK regulation by glucocorticoids than on TAT regulation. However, in the past few years, primarily because a cDNA^{PEPCK} was available before cDNA^{TAT}, this situation has been reversed. In particular, the effect of glucocorticoids on transcription of the *PEPCK* gene has now been assessed (see the following discussion), whereas similar studies of the *TAT* gene remain to be completed.

B. Regulation of PEPCK Activity by Glucocorticoid Hormones

Shrago *et al.* (1963) were the first to show that glucocorticoids cause an increase in the catalytic activity of PEPCK in rat liver. This effect was not consistently observed, however, and while some investigators confirmed the finding (Foster *et al.*, 1966; Reshef *et al.*, 1970; Huttner *et al.*, 1974; Krone *et al.*, 1974), others reported a decrease in PEPCK activity in response to glucocorticoid injection (Ray *et al.*, 1964; Reshef *et al.*, 1969; Gunn *et al.*, 1975b). Two observations led to the current belief that glucocorticoids do induce hepatic PEPCK and that the repression of this enzyme noted after the injection of animals with glucocorticoids represents an indirect effect. In the first of these studies, Gunn *et al.* (1975b) demonstrated that triamcinolone induces PEPCK activity and synthesis in diabetic rats and that glucocorticoids stimulate insulin release in intact rats. Since insulin inhibits PEPCK synthesis per se in such animals (Tilghman *et al.*, 1974; Gunn *et al.*, 1975a), the amount of PEPCK probably represents the balance of the inductive action of glucocorticoids and the repressive action of insulin, hence the apparently contradictory results noted above. In the second group of experiments, glucocorticoids were shown to induce PEPCK in cultured H4IIE hepatoma cells (Wicks and McKibbin, 1972; Gunn *et al.*, 1975a). This was an important observation since it demonstrated a direct effect of glucocorticoids in a rat liver-derived cell.

Investigators have demonstrated glucocorticoid effects on PEPCK in other tissues. Gorin *et al.* (1969) and Reshef *et al.* (1969) found that these hormones repress PEPCK in adipose tissue, and Longshaw and Pogson (1972) showed that glucocorticoids induce the renal enzyme. Reshef *et al.* (1969) noted that PEPCK activity increased in adipose tissue after adrenalectomy, but this procedure had no effect on basal PEPCK activity in liver or kidney, or on the regulation of PEPCK activity by other factors in these tissues. Thus, the adipose tissue enzyme is under constant glucocorticoid regulation, while the liver and renal enzymes are not. Feldman (1977) confirmed these findings, and in an attempt to determine why renal and hepatic PEPCK responds in a manner opposite to that noted in adipose tissue, he directly compared the binding properties of the glucocorticoid receptors in liver and adipose tissue. Feldman found that the receptors in each of these tissues bound the steroid equally well and suggested that the difference in response between the two tissues must occur by a postreceptor mechanism.

The next question centered on whether the increase of hepatic PEPCK activity after glucocorticoid administration resulted from a change in the absolute amount of the protein or from an alteration of the catalytic activity of a fixed amount of PEPCK. Shrago and co-workers (1963) indirectly addressed this question by injecting puromycin and actinomycin D in conjunction with hydrocortisone. Each of these inhibitors prevented the induction of hepatic PEPCK, so they inferred that both protein and RNA synthesis were necessary, and that induction was due to a change in the amount of enzyme. At that time, a more direct assessment of the amount of PEPCK was impossible, but the conclusion proved to be correct, as will be discussed.

A direct measurement of the effect of glucocorticoids on PEPCK synthesis became possible when Ballard and Hanson (1969) purified PEPCK and developed a specific antibody. The application of immunological techniques to the study of the regulation of PEPCK by glucocorticoids was first accomplished by Gunn *et al.* (1975a,b) in rat liver and in H4IIE cells. The relative rate of PEPCK synthesis was 3.0% of total protein synthesized in livers of diabetic rats. Seven hours after injecting triamcinolone into diabetic rats, the synthesis of PEPCK had increased to 4.0% of the total protein synthesized. In contrast, the basal rate of PEPCK synthesis in H4IIE cells was 0.5% of the total protein synthesized, and 3 hours of treatment with dexamethasone increased the relative rate of synthesis to 1.4% of total protein. Iynedjian *et al.* (1975) conducted similar studies of the rat renal cortex enzyme and found that 8 hours of treatment with triamcinolone increased PEPCK synthesis from a basal rate of 3.4% of total protein to a level of 6.6%. Thus, glucocorticoids increase PEPCK synthesis in hepatic and renal tissues, but the largest effect was seen in H4IIE cells.

C. REGULATION OF mRNA^{PEPCK} ACTIVITY BY GLUCOCORTICOID HORMONES

The interval between the observation that glucocorticoid hormones increase the rate of synthesis of PEPCK and the demonstration that they also increase mRNA^{PEPCK} activity was much shorter than that in the case of TAT induction (see Table I). Within 2 years of the discovery that glucocorticoids regulate PEPCK synthesis, Iynedjian and Hanson (1977a) established an assay that was used to quantitate the activity of mRNA^{PEPCK}. They showed that triamcinolone increased renal mRNA^{PEPCK} in proportion to the increase in PEPCK synthesis (Iynedjian and Hanson, 1977b). A 7-hour treatment with triamcinolone increased renal mRNA^{PEPCK} from an average of 0.08% of total poly(A)$^+$ RNA in untreated rats to 0.21% in the treated animals. This 2.6-fold increase of mRNA^{PEPCK} compared favorably with the 2.1-fold increase of PEPCK synthesis (from 2.6% to 5.5% of total protein synthesis) noted in similarly treated rats, and led to the conclusion that glucocorticoid hormones increase renal PEPCK synthesis by increasing mRNA^{PEPCK} activity. Changes of mRNA activity have generally been associated with a corresponding alteration in the amount of the mRNA, and steroid hormones usually effect changes in mRNA concentration by regulating gene transcription. The assessment of these points required that specific cDNA and genomic DNA probes be developed.

D. Isolation of PEPCK cDNA and Genomic DNA Clones

There have been few reports concerning the mechanism of glucocorticoid regulation of PEPCK synthesis since the initial report by Iynedjian and Hanson (1977b). During this time, considerable effort was given to the construction of specific complementary DNA (cDNA^{PEPCK}) probes, since these molecules are necessary for use in the hybridization assays required to quantitate mRNA^{PEPCK} amount, for determining the nucleotide sequence of mRNA^{PEPCK} and hence the amino acid sequence of PEPCK, and for isolating and characterizing PEPCK genomic DNA as a prerequisite for structural and regulatory studies of the *PEPCK* gene. Two laboratories successfully isolated one or more cDNA^{PEPCK} molecules (Yoo-Warren *et al.*, 1981; Beale *et al.*, 1982). We will review the strategy we used to obtain cDNA^{PEPCK} and present data regarding the structure of mRNA^{PEPCK} and the *PEPCK* gene before discussing the use of the cDNA^{PEPCK} probes to quantitate the effect dexamethasone has on H4IIE cell mRNA^{PEPCK} amount and on the transcription of this RNA from the *PEPCK* gene.

mRNA^{PEPCK} normally constitutes 0.01–0.2% of total mRNA translational activity in untreated and Bt$_2$cAMP-treated rats, respectively (Iynedjian and Hanson, 1977a; Beale *et al.*, 1981). It can be further increased to 0.5% of total poly(A)$^+$ RNA activity by injecting the animals with cycloheximide, which retards mRNA^{PEPCK} degradation (Nelson *et al.*, 1980; Beale *et al.*, 1982). The highest levels achievable, however, are in the livers of diabetic rats, where mRNA^{PEPCK} constitutes 2% of total poly(A)$^+$ RNA activity (Yoo-Warren *et al.*, 1983).

Because of the relative scarceness of mRNA^{PEPCK}, we decided that the chances of successfully synthesizing a complementary DNA would be significantly enhanced if we started with partially purified mRNA^{PEPCK}. This was accomplished by polysome immunoprecipitation using a specific PEPCK antiserum (Beale *et al.*, 1982). This resulted in a marked increase in the purity of mRNA^{PEPCK} such that it represented the only major RNA species, as shown in Fig. 11. The purified mRNA^{PEPCK} was then used as a template to synthesize double-stranded cDNA^{PEPCK}, which was inserted into the unique *Pst*I site of pBR322. The recombinant plasmids were introduced into *Escherichia coli* and cloned. In order to identify the cDNA^{PEPCK}-containing clones, the transformed colonies were hybridized *in situ* to radioactive cDNA synthesized from the purified mRNA^{PEPCK}. The plasmid DNAs from the positive colonies were then tested for their ability to hybridize to, and therefore purify, mRNA^{PEPCK} by the technique of hybrid selection. The collection of cDNAs used in our studies is shown in Fig. 12. PC2, a cDNA^{PEPCK} corresponding to the 3′ end of mRNA^{PEPCK}, was described

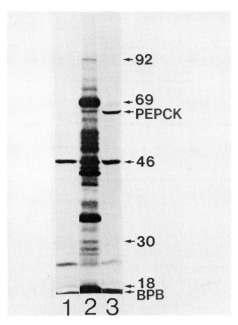

FIG. 11. Purification of mRNA[PEPCK]. Poly(A)+ RNA was extracted from rat liver polysomes before and after immunoprecipitation of polysomes with PEPCK antiserum. Translation reactions were conducted using reticulocyte lysates programmed with poly(A)+ RNA, and the [35S]methionine-labeled products were analyzed by SDS–PAGE and fluorography. Details of these procedures are described by Beale *et al.* (1982). The figure shows the products synthesized with no added RNA (lane 1), with poly(A)+ RNA extracted from total hepatic polysomes (lane 2), and with poly(A)+ RNA extracted from polysomes immunoprecipitated with antibody directed against PEPCK (lane 3). The arrows denote the location of molecular weight markers and PEPCK determined from standards on a separate lane (not shown). The standards and their molecular weights, shown at the right, are: phosphorylase *b* (92,000), bovine serum albumin (69,000), ovalbumin (46,000), carbonic anhydrase (30,000), and α-lactoglobulin A (18,000). BPB represents bromphenol blue. [From Beale *et al.* (1982).]

previously (Beale *et al.*, 1982). The other cDNAs shown in Fig. 12, PC116, PC113, and PC201, were isolated from the same cDNA library from which PC2 was obtained. The inserts from the recombinant plasmid library were fractionated by agarose gel electrophoresis to eliminate short cDNAs. *Escherichia coli* were transformed with the size-fractionated plasmids, and the library was rescreened using PC2 as the hybridization probe. PC116 and PC113 were obtained in this manner. Confirmation that PC116 is complementary to mRNA[PEPCK] was obtained using hybrid-arrested translation (Patterson *et al.*, 1977), and the results are shown in Fig. 13. The rationale behind this procedure is that cDNA[PEPCK] should form a hybrid molecule only with mRNA[PEPCK]. If the cDNA is complementary to a portion of the translated

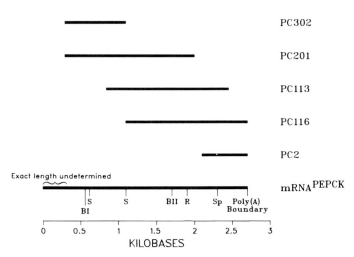

Fɪɢ. 12. The cNDA[PEPCK] library. The construction and isolation of the various cDNA[PEPCK] molecules is summarized in the text. The purified mRNA[PEPCK] (see Fig. 11) was used as the template for cDNA synthesis. The isolation and characterization of PC2 was described previously (Beale *et al.*, 1982), and PC116, PC113, and PC201 were isolated from the original cDNA library. PC302 was constructed by primer extension of the 500-bp *Sma*I/*Sma*I fragment from PC201. The locations of several restriction enzyme recognition sequences are shown for reference: BI, *Bgl*I; BII, *Bgl*II; R, *Eco*RI; S, *Sma*I; Sp, *Sph*I.

region of mRNA[PEPCK], the synthesis of PEPCK in an *in vitro* translation system will be specifically inhibited. For example, PC2 does not hybrid-arrest the translation of mRNA[PEPCK] (Beale *et al.*, 1981), because this cDNA is complementary to the 3′ nontranslated region of mRNA[PEPCK]. PC116 specifically inhibited the synthesis of PEPCK in a reticulocyte lysate; thus, it was assumed to be complementary to the coding region of mRNA[PEPCK]. This assumption was confirmed by direct sequencing of PC2 and PC116, and by identifying a single open reading frame in PC116. PC201, a cDNA that extends toward the 5′ end of mRNA[PEPCK], was discovered because it hybridized to PC116 but not to PC2. Finally, PC302 was constructed by primer extension of the 500–base pair (bp) *Sma*I/*Sma*I fragment from PC201. We have had difficulty in obtaining a cDNA[PEPCK] complementary to the remaining 5′ sequence of mRNA[PEPCK]. There may be structural features of mRNA[PEPCK] that cause reverse transcriptase to "stutter" and stop short of making a full-length transcript. Indeed, there is a potential palindromic region near the 5′ end of PC302 that closely resembles structures that can be cleaved by an endonuclease activity associated with reverse transcriptase (Duyk *et al.*, 1983). However, we have recently succeeded in using primer extension of a synthetic oligonucleotide that is complementary to a short

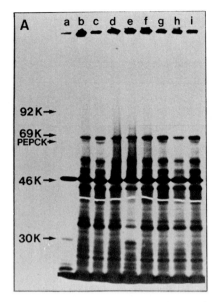
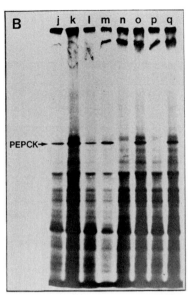

Fig. 13. pPC116 inhibits the translation of mRNA[PEPCK]. Poly(A)+ RNA was isolated from the liver of a rat treated with $N^6,O^{2'}$-dibutyryl cAMP for 90 minutes. 600 ng was hybridized to 1 μg of either pBR322 (lanes b–e and j–m) or pPC116 (lanes f–i and n–q) as described by Patterson *et al.* (1977). Following hybridization the samples were diluted with H_2O, and half of each sample (lanes c,e,g,i,k,m,o, and q) was heated to 100°C while the other half (lanes b,d,f,h,j,l,n, and p) was heated to 60°C for 1 minute. The 60°C treatment was found to minimize nonspecific inhibition of translation that occurred as a result of the hybridization, but it did not melt the hybrid molecules. Nucleic acids were precipitated with ethanol, and the mRNA was translated using a reticulocyte lysate system. Following translation, each sample was divided into two aliquots, and PEPCK was partially purified from one aliquot by immunoprecipitation with a specific antibody (Beale *et al.*, 1981). PEPCK represents less than 0.2% of the total protein synthesized in the reticulocyte lysate system using rat liver poly(A)+ RNA as template and was thus seen as a faint band in the fluorogram (A). Detection of PEPCK was enhanced by immunoprecipitation (B). We have demonstrated that this antibody is specific for PEPCK, but if the precipitate is not washed rigorously, as in this experiment, the specific PEPCK is enhanced at the expense of significant nonspecific adsorption of the other translation products (Beale *et al.*, 1981). We exploited this observation to assess with greater certainty that the translation of mRNA[PEPCK] was inhibited while the translation of other mRNAs was not. In addition, the fluorogram (B) was greatly overexposed in an effort to detect PEPCK in lanes n and p. The samples in lanes b–i correspond to the immunoprecipitated samples in lanes j–q, respectively. Lanes b–e and j–m were from RNA hybridized with pBR322, and lanes f–i and n–q were from RNA hybridized with pPC116. Each hybridization was done in duplicate. Lane a shows the products that were labeled in the absence of poly(A)+ RNA. The [14C]-protein standards and their molecular weights are: phosphorylase *b* (92,000), bovine serum albumin (69,000), ovalbumin (46,000), and carbonic anhydrase (30,000). Electrophoresis and fluorography were done as described previously (Beale *et al.*, 1981).

region in the 5′ end of PC302 to elongate the cDNA, and we are currently attempting to clone these sequences. The complete sequences of PC116 and PC302 and partial sequences for PC2, PC113, and PC201 have been determined, and they represent 2405 nucleotides of mRNA[PEPCK]. Mature cytoplasmic mRNA[PEPCK] is 2800–3000 nucleotides in length (Yoo-Warren *et al.*, 1981; Chrapkiewicz *et al.*, 1982). Assuming a poly(A) tail of approximately 200 nucleotides, the mRNA should, therefore, be 2600–2800 nucleotides in length. Hence, as noted in Fig. 12, the uncloned sequence at the 5′ end of mRNA[PEPCK] is 200–400 nucleotides in length.

These cDNA[PEPCK] probes were used to screen the rat genomic library constructed by Sargent *et al.* (1979), and 18 clones were identified. Hybridization of cDNA[PEPCK] to 12 of these was abolished by washing the filters at higher stringency, as described by Durnam *et al.* (1980). Two of the remaining six clones were subsequently shown to contain identical inserts. The structure of one of these, λPC112, is shown in Fig. 14. The genomic DNA of this clone was 15 kilobase pairs (kbp) in length and is assumed to contain the entire *PEPCK* gene plus approximately 5 kbp of 5′-flanking sequence and 4 kbp of 3′-flanking DNA. The transcription initiation site was defined by Yoo-Warren *et al.* (1983) using an *in vitro* transcription initiation assay. We located the polyadenylation site by sequencing both the cDNA and the genomic DNA in that region. The putative primary transcript is approximately 6 kbp in length, and it consists of 10 exons interrupted by 9 introns (our unpublished observations). However, Northern blot analysis of nuclear

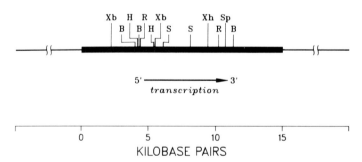

FIG. 14. Restriction map of λPC112. This PEPCK genomic DNA clone was isolated from a rat genomic DNA library that was constructed using DNA digested with *Hae*III and inserted, with *Eco*RI linkers, into the λ phage Charon 4A (Sargent *et al.*, 1979). We screened approximately 10^6 plaques by the *in situ* hybridization procedure of Benton and Davis (1977). Identification of λPC112 was accomplished by hybridizing it to a *Sma*I/*Sph*I fragment from PC116 (see Fig. 12). The λ arms are shown as thin lines, and the inserted genomic DNA is shown as a thick line. The putative transcription unit, shown as an arrow below the map, begins at the putative initiation site (Yoo-Warren *et al.*, 1983) and ends at the poly(A) site. Restriction enzyme sites are: B, *Bam*HI; H, *Hind*III; R, *Eco*RI; S, *Sma*I; Sp, *Sph*I; Xb, *Xba*I; and Xh, *Xho*I.

PEPCK RNA sequences revealed a species of approximately 6.5–6.8 kb that presumably represent the primary transcript (Cimbala *et al.*, 1982; Chrapkiewicz *et al.*, 1982; Granner *et al.*, 1983). Thus, an additional transcription initiation site that is 500–800 bp upstream from the one identified by Yoo-Warren *et al.* (1983) may be present. The availability of these cDNAs and the genomic DNA and some understanding of their structures made studies described in the remainder of this chapter possible.

E. Glucocorticoid Regulation of mRNA[PEPCK] Concentration

With the cDNA probes, it was possible to address the question of whether or not glucocorticoid hormones regulate mRNA[PEPCK] concentration. The dot blot hybridization assay adapted from the method described by Thomas (1980) was employed to measure mRNA[PEPCK]. As shown in Table II, a 24-

TABLE II
Regulation of PEPCK, mRNA[PEPCK], and *PEPCK* Gene Transcription[a]

Experiment	Treatment	PEPCK (-fold induction)	mRNA[PEPCK] (-fold induction)	Transcription (-fold induction)
I	none	1.0	1.0	1.0
	Dex-1 hours	ND	ND	5.1
	Dex-2 hours	ND	2.8	2.9
	Dex-6 hours	ND	2.1	ND
	Dex-24 hours	5.5	4.3	1.7
II	none	ND	ND	1.0
	50 n*M* Dex	ND	ND	2.5
	500 n*M* Dex	ND	ND	5.2

[a]In experiment I, 500 n*M* dexamethasone (Dex) was added to H4IIE cells and immunoassayable PEPCK, mRNA[PEPCK], and PEPCK transcription were measured at the indicated times. In experiment II, dexamethasone was present at the designated concentrations for 1 hour prior to the isolation of nuclei for measuring transcription. PEPCK was measured by a radioimmunoassay as described by Moore *et al.* (1982). mRNA[PEPCK] was measured by the dot blot hybridization assay (Thomas, 1980) as described by Beale *et al.* (1982). Transcription of the *PEPCK* gene in isolated nuclei was measured by the runoff assay described by McKnight and Palmiter (1979), as modified by Granner *et al.* (1983). All data are presented as "-fold induction," i.e., PEPCK, mRNA[PEPCK], or transcription in Dex-treated cells divided by the corresponding values in untreated cells. Values in untreated cells were typically 0.2–0.4 μg/mg protein for immunoassayable PEPCK and 100–150 ppm for transcription. Absolute concentrations of mRNA[PEPCK] are unknown since mRNA[PEPCK] is quantitated from the image density of an autoradiogram. "ND" means not determined.

hour treatment of H4IIE cells with dexamethasone caused a fourfold increase in mRNA^{PEPCK}. In other experiments, this induction ranged from four- to eightfold, and this induced steady-state level was maintained for at least 72 hours. An examination of the early induction of mRNA^{PEPCK} following the addition of dexamethasone to H4IIE cells revealed a complex pattern. An initial peak, approximately four times above the basal concentration, occurred between 2 and 4 hours (three times above basal concentration in Table II at 2 hours). mRNA^{PEPCK} then declined toward the basal level for the next 6 hours (twofold induction at 6 hours in Table II), after which it again increased to a new steady-state level, which was attained about 18 hours after the addition of the inducer (fourfold induction at 24 hours in Table II). To determine whether this induction of mRNA^{PEPCK} correlated with the induction of PEPCK itself, the enzyme was measured by a radioimmunoassay (Table II). There was a sixfold increase in PEPCK in this experiment. We have consistently noted an excellent correlation between the increase of PEPCK and mRNA^{PEPCK}.

F. REGULATION OF *PEPCK* GENE TRANSCRIPTION BY GLUCOCORTICOIDS

Although induction of mRNA^{PEPCK} by enhanced transcription might be inferred from the action of other steroids (Anderson, 1983), this mechanism could not be assumed, nor is it necessary that the entire effect of the steroid be accounted for by this means. We therefore measured transcription using a nuclear run-off assay similar to that described by McKnight and Palmiter (1979). The initiation of RNA synthesis is inefficient in this assay so that the transcription measured is primarily due to the elongation or run off of RNA chains that had initiated *in vivo*. This assay, therefore, reflects the number of RNA polymerase molecules engaged in transcription at the time the nuclei were isolated. Lamers *et al.* (1982) measured *PEPCK* gene transcription by the run-off assay in liver nuclei from dexamethasone-treated rats but saw only a 30% increase. Since the rats used by Lamers *et al.* (1982) were not diabetic, it seems likely that the full effect of glucocorticoids on transcription may have been blunted as a result of the insulin released in response to glucocorticoids (Gunn *et al.*, 1975b). Indeed, insulin is a potent inhibitor of *PEPCK* gene transcription (Granner *et al.*, 1983), and insulin inhibits dexamethasone-induced transcription in H4IIE cells (Sasaki *et al.*, 1984).

We elected to use H4IIE cells to study the mechanisms by which glucocorticoids regulate PEPCK to obviate the problem of indirect effects sometimes seen in animals. A 1-hour treatment with dexamethasone caused a fivefold increase in *PEPCK* gene transcription [from 118 to 600 ppm (Table II, Experiment I)]. The maximally effective dose of dexamethasone was 500 n*M*, which also caused a fivefold induction of transcription, from 123 to 640 ppm. The half-maximally effective concentration of dexamethasone, approximately 50 nM, increased transcription to a rate of 305 ppm (Table II, Experiment II). This correlates very well with the concentrations necessary to achieve half-maximal induction of TAT by dexamethasone (Fig. 7). Other experiments have revealed several important characteristics of this induction. First, since the induction is inhibited by α-amanitin, it can be inferred that dexamethasone increases transcription of the *PEPCK* gene by an RNA polymerase II–dependent mechanism. Second, the fact that dexamethasone does not affect total transcriptional activity indicates that glucocorticoid hormones do not alter the transcription of most genes. Third, the response to dexamethasone is rapid as measurable increases in *PEPCK* gene transcription are seen within 15 minutes of the addition of the steroid to the culture medium. Finally, *PEPCK* gene transcription reaches a peak rate, four to eight times greater than the basal transcription rate. One hour after dexamethasone is added, transcription declines rapidly, so that by 2 hours it has decreased to a new steady-state level that is about three times the control value (Table II, Experiment I). At 24 hours, the level is still two times greater than that in control cells. This is in contrast to mRNA[PEPCK] and immunoreactive PEPCK, which are also induced four- to eightfold, but these induced levels occur after 24 hours of dexamethasone treatment. Thus, dexamethasone must increase both *PEPCK* gene transcription and mRNA[PEPCK] stability. This hypothesis was tested by directly measuring the turnover rate of mRNA[PEPCK]. Untreated or dexamethasone-treated cells were labeled for 1 hour with [³H]uridine and then "chased" with 20 mM unlabled uridine. Total cellular RNA was extracted at 1-hour intervals throughout the chase period, and the radioactivity incorporated into mRNA[PEPCK] was measured using the isolation procedure employed in the transcription assay. The results showed that the $t_{1/2}$ of mRNA[PEPCK] is about 45 minutes in untreated H4IIE cells while, in cells treated for 18 hours with dexamethasone, the $t_{1/2}$ is nearly three times longer. Thus, dexamethasone has a dual effect: it increases *PEPCK* gene transcription and slows the degradation of mRNA[PEPCK]. Although effects of mRNA degradation are not generally associated with the action of glucocorticoid hormones, this is not a unique effect for steroid hormones, since estrogen stabilizes ovalbumin mRNA in chick oviduct (Palmiter and Carey, 1974) and vitellogenin mRNA in *Xenopus* liver (Brock and Shapiro, 1983).

G. Studies of the *PEPCK* Gene

The observation that dexamethasone regulates *PEPCK* gene transcription indicates that the gene itself should be the focus of studies to assess how glucocorticoid hormones regulate PEPCK. Thus, it was necessary to determine whether the *PEPCK* gene is present in a single copy or in multiple copies per haploid genome, whether there is polymorphism in *PEPCK* gene structure, and whether there are any structural changes associated with the expression and regulation of this gene. Such questions can be answered by studies of the structure of cloned DNAs and by restriction enzyme digestion of total cellular genomic DNA followed by electrophoresis, transfer to a membrane filter, and hybridization to cloned PEPCK cDNAs (Southern, 1975). Yoo-Warren *et al.* (1983) analyzed DNA isolated from rat liver and from two Reuber H35 hepatoma clones, Fao and H5, and concluded that the *PEPCK* gene is probably present as a single copy per haploid genome. Of the six restriction enzymes tested, only *Sph*I yielded DNA fragments of sizes that were not predicted from the restriction enzyme map of cloned PEPCK genomic DNA. Yoo-Warren *et al.* also concluded that there were no differences between rat liver, Fao cells, or H5 cells with respect to the structure of the *PEPCK* gene. It should be emphasized that this technique would not detect minor sequence differences unless, as with *Sph*I, these occurred within a restriction enzyme recognition site. It also might not detect minor gene rearrangements.

We conducted similar investigations using H4IIE and HTC hepatoma cells, but had an additional reason for doing the study. Specifically, HTC cells do not produce PEPCK, whereas H4IIE cells do. We reasoned that the elucidation of the molecular basis underlying this difference might provide clues about how the *PEPCK* gene is regulated by glucocorticoids and other hormones. Our first task was to determine whether there was any detectable block in the production of PEPCK and/or mRNA[PEPCK]. For example, these cells might produce an mRNA[PEPCK] that was inactive. As Table III illustrates, HTC cells do not make any mRNA[PEPCK], even in the presence of dexamethasone and dibutyryl cAMP. In contrast, dexamethasone causes a

TABLE III
mRNA[PEPCK] IN HTC AND H4IIE HEPATOMA CELLS[a]

Cell line	Treatment	mRNA[PEPCK] (densitometer units)
H4IIE	None	0.32 ± 0.04
	Dex + Bt$_2$cAMP	2.12 ± 0.10
HTC	None	None detectable
	Dex + Bt$_2$cAMP	None detectable

[a]Both cell lines were grown to confluency as attached cultures. The cells were treated for 18 hours with 500 n*M* dexamethasone (Dex) and for 3 hours with 0.5 m*M* N^6,O^2-dibutyryl cAMP (Bt$_2$cAMP) where indicated. Total RNA was extracted, and mRNA[PEPCK] was measured by dot blot hybridization to a specific cDNA[PEPCK] probe (Thomas, 1980; Beale *et al.*, 1982).

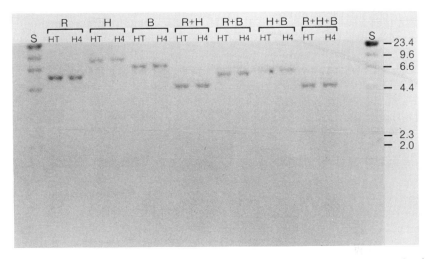

FIG. 15. Blot transfer analysis of PEPCK genomic DNA. Total genomic DNA was isolated from H4IIE and HTC cells and digested to completion with *Eco*RI, *Hind*III, or *Bam*HI used singly or in various combinations. The digestion products were resolved by electrophoresis in 0.8% agarose and analyzed by blot transfer (Southern, 1975). The blots were probed with a [32P]-labeled *Bgl*I/*Bgl*II restriction fragment from PC201 (Fig. 12). The lanes are: S, *Hind* III-digested λ DNA standards; HT, HTC cell DNA; H4, H4IIE cell DNA; R, *Eco*RI; H, *Hind*III; B, *Bam*HI.

sevenfold increase in mRNA[PEPCK] in H4IIE cells. We next investigated whether HTC cells either lacked the *PEPCK* gene or had a rearranged gene. This possibility was explored using blot-hybridization analysis and probing the genomic DNA blots with [32P]cDNA[PEPCK]. The restriction enzyme digestion patterns of genomic DNA are shown in Fig. 15. *Eco*RI, *Hind*III, and *Bam*HI were used singly and in various combinations. In all cases, DNA isolated from H4IIE and HTC cells was identical, and the restriction fragments were of the exact size predicted from the structure of λPC112 (Fig. 14). These results, and those of Yoo-Warren *et al.* (1983), indicate that the *PEPCK* gene exists as a single copy, and there is little evidence of gene polymorphism. These data also indicate that there is no gross structural reorganization of the *PEPCK* gene in HTC cells.

Since the general organization of the HTC and H4IIE cell *PEPCK* genes appears to be very similar, if not identical, the lack of inducibility with HTC cells must result from some other aspect of the structure of this gene. The extent of methylation of cytosine residues has been inversely associated with gene expression (reviewed by Razin and Riggs, 1980). The content of 5-methyl cytosine tends to be greater in genes that are not expressed than in transcribed genes, although this is not a universal finding. The extent of

DNA methylation in or around the *PEPCK* gene could thus be related to the inducibility of this gene. The observations on the glucocorticoid-sensitive metallothionein gene are of interest in this regard (Compere and Palmiter, 1981). This gene is highly methylated in W7 mouse thymoma cells and it is not subject to regulation by glucocorticoid hormones. Treatment of W7 cells with 5-azacytidine results in demethylation in the region of the metallothionein gene, and the expression of this gene in such cells is enhanced by glucocorticoid hormones. An analogous result was reported by Gasson *et al.* (1983). A line of T-lymphoma cells, designated SAK8, is normally insensitive to the lytic effect of glucocorticoid hormones (Gasson and Bourgeois, 1983). Clones that regain the normal response to glucocorticoids can be obtained by growing these cells in 5-azacytidine. Upon removal of the 5-azacytidine, there is a gradual increase of *de novo* methylation of the DNA in such clones and a corresponding return of insensitivity to glucocorticoid hormones (Gasson *et al.*, 1983).

Another set of observations may be pertinent. Since sensitivity of a gene to DNase I is an index of actual or potential gene activity (Weintraub and Groudine, 1976), and since DNase I–sensitive genes are often undermethylated (Kuo *et al.*, 1979), there may be an association between chromatin structure, DNA methylation, and transcriptional activity (Anderson, 1983). We therefore studied the methylation and the relative sensitivity to DNase I of the *PEPCK* gene in HTC and H4IIE cells.

Most 5-methyl cytosine (>90%) is present in the dinucleotide pair $^{me}C·G$ (C = cytosine, G = guanosine, me = methyl group). Several restriction enzymes, including *Msp*I and *Hpa*II, recognize sequences containing the CG pair. An estimate of the extent of methylation of CG pairs can be obtained using *Msp*I and *Hpa*II, both of which recognize the same CG-containing sequence. *Hpa*II will not digest the DNA if it is methylated, whereas the action of *Msp*I is unaffected (Razin and Riggs, 1980). Thus, these two enzymes can be used to detect differences in DNA methylation, even if the exact sequence of the DNA is unknown. We used the *Msp*I/*Hpa*II pair to probe for 5-methyl cytosine in HTC and H4IIE cells and observed clear differences in the methylation pattern of PEPCK genomic DNA (Fig. 16). Digestion with *Msp*I yielded identical fragments of approximately 500, 700, and 1000 bp in the two cell lines. When the DNA was digested with *Hpa*II, there was a single 3.0-kb restriction fragment in HTC cells, whereas in H4IIE cells the 3.0-kb fragment was much less abundant and a 2.1-kb fragment appeared. This indicates that more 5-methyl cytosine was present in the inactive *PEPCK* gene of HTC cells than in the active *PEPCK* gene in H4IIE cells. We are currently mapping the methylated sites in DNA isolated from H4IIE and HTC cells to see if this difference occurs throughout the entire *PEPCK* gene.

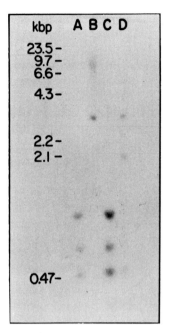

FIG. 16. Methylation of the PEPCK gene. Genomic DNA was isolated from HTC (lanes A and B) and H4IIE (lanes C and D) cells and digested to completion with *Msp*I (lanes A and C) or with *Hpa*II (lanes B and D). The digested DNA was then resolved by electrophoresis in 0.6% (w/v) agarose, transferred to a nitrocellulose filter (Southern, 1975), and hybridized to a ^{32}P-labeled 1300-bp *Sma*I/*Sph*I cDNA[PEPCK] fragment (see Fig. 12). The location of *Hind*III-digested DNA fragments is shown at the left, and the sizes of the restriction fragments are shown in kilobase pairs (kbp).

Although polymorphism is not excluded, it is tempting to conclude that differences in DNA methylation account for the different responses HTC and H4IIE cells have to glucocorticoids with respect to *PEPCK* gene expression. This must be tempered by the following observations. Hepatoma cells, which do not express α-2u globulin, have a hypomethylated α-2u globulin gene, whereas liver, which does express this protein, has a gene that contains significantly more [me]C (Makhasi *et al.*, 1982). Certain other genes are actively transcribed even though methylated. These include the genes coding for vitellogenin in *Xenopus* (Folger *et al.*, 1983) and β-globin in transformed chick erythroblasts (Weintraub *et al.*, 1982). Finally, MTV DNA sequences in both glucocorticoid-inducible and glucocorticoid-uninducible hepatoma cell lines are equally hypomethylated (Feinstein *et al.*, 1982). The fact that the correlation between DNA methylation and gene transcription is not absolute does not necessarily diminish the importance of this mechanism. Selective, site-specific demethylation could be very important (Bird *et al.*, 1981), and methylation–demethylation could interact with other mechanisms to affect gene transcription. It is likely that this issue will not be resolved until highly efficient *in vitro* transcription systems are developed.

As mentioned above, active or potentially active genes are much more sensitive to digestion by DNase I than are inactive genes (Weintraub and Groudine, 1976). We compared the rates of digestion of the *PEPCK* gene in nuclei isolated from H4IIE and HTC cells and found that, under identical conditions, the gene in the H4IIE cells was digested 5–10 times more rapidly than in HTC cells. This indicates that there are differences in the structure and/or composition of the chromatin associated with the *PEPCK* gene in these two cell lines.

Presumably, the H4IIE and HTC cell lines were both derived from normal hepatocytes that have a *PEPCK* gene that is regulated by glucocorticoids and other factors. HTC cells underwent a change that inactivated the *PEPCK* gene. The causes of this change may have been changes in DNA methylation, chromatin structure, or other unknown factors. If the inactivation can be reversed, it may be possible to elucidate the central mechanism. The example of the inactive metallothionein gene in W7 cells (Compere and Palmiter, 1981) is analogous to the inactive *PEPCK* gene in HTC cells. If, like the methallothionein gene, 5-azacytidine will cause activation and will restore glucocorticoid sensitivity to the *PEPCK* gene, it may be possible to examine the relationship between methylation and glucocorticoid regulation of PEPCK expression.

IV. CONCLUSIONS AND PERSPECTIVES

The model of steroid hormone action proposed in the early 1970s predicted that these hormones influence protein synthesis by altering the production of specific mRNAs. Experimental support for this came with the demonstrations that estrogen and/or progesterone enhance the rate of transcription of the genes coding for ovalbumin (Bellard *et al.*, 1977; Schutz *et al.*, 1977; McKnight and Palmiter, 1979) and casein (Ganguly *et al.*, 1979; Rosen *et al.*, 1980). Evidence that glucocorticoid hormones also affect gene transcription came with the observation that dexamethasone increases the production of MTV RNA in GR cells and in hepatoma cells (Ringold *et al.*, 1977). For several years, the study of MTV RNA synthesis was the only example of an effect of a glucocorticoid hormone on gene transcription. The regulation of MTV RNA synthesis offers many unique approaches to the study of glucocorticoid hormone action, yet it is a study of a pathological occurrence that might not reflect the physiological regulation of genes. This criticism was muted by a recent series of studies in which it was shown that glucocorticoid hormones increase the rate of transcription of a number of liver genes, including metallothionein I (Hager and Palmiter, 1981; Mayo and Palmiter, 1981), tryptophan oxygenase (Danesch *et al.*, 1983), and PEPCK (Sasaki *et al.*, 1984; this chapter). These observations serve several important purposes: (a) they add support to the general hypothesis regarding steroid hormone action; (b) they make the MTV system, which has several as yet unequalled experimental advantages, very relevant to studies of glucocorticoid action in normal liver; and (c) they provide a substantial base from which one can explore precisely how transcription is affected. Investigators are now confronted with at least two challenging questions: "What is involved in gene transcription?" and "How do steroid hormones affect this complex process?"

In simplest terms, mRNA transcription involves the initiation of RNA synthesis by a type II polymerase molecule followed by nascent chain elongation, termination, and processing. It is likely that each of these processes involves one or more factors, each of which in turn is a potential site of regulation. Most is known about initiation. Specific sequences of DNA located in the region 5' upstream from the RNA polymerase initiation site specify both the fidelity (site) and efficiency (frequency) of initiation (McKnight and Kingsbury, 1982). There has been some success in isolating factors involved in the initiation of class III genes (Engelke *et al.*, 1980; Manley *et al.*, 1983; Dignam *et al.*, 1983), and similar studies with class II genes are now beginning (Dynan and Tjian, 1983; Manley *et al.*, 1983; Dignam *et al.*, 1983). Much less is known about the factors involved in elongation, termination, and processing. In this regard, it may be wise initially to concentrate on RNA chain initiation, for this appears to be the step regulated by glucocorticoids in MTV RNA induction (Ucker *et al.*, 1983; Stallcup and Washington, 1983).

The sequence described above implies that gene transcription consists of an orderly, linear flow of reactions. This is almost certainly an oversimplification. Processes that enhance (Dynan and Tjian, 1982) or attenuate (Yanofsky, 1981) transcription have been described in a variety of prokaryotic and lower eukaryotic systems, and it would be most surprising if similar control mechanisms were not operative in mammalian cells. Sequences analogous to the enhancer regions of the SV40 virus have been identified in immunoglobulin genes (Chung *et al.*, 1983; Parslow and Granner, 1983), and these appear to have functional significance (Gluzman and Shenk, 1983). Yamamoto and colleagues have proposed that such regions may be the glucocorticoid-receptor binding sites, and thus may be related to the effect of this complex on MTV RNA transcription (Yamamoto, 1983). It would not be surprising if other transcription control mechanisms, as yet unidentified, are also involved.

Tremendous strides have been taken toward understanding how the steroid–receptor complex interacts with specific regions of DNA to promote transcription. Specific binding that correlates with gene expression has now been reported for glucocorticoids (Payvar *et al.*, 1981; Govindan *et al.*, 1982; Geisse *et al.*, 1982; Pfahl, 1982) and progesterone (Compton *et al.*, 1983; Savouret and Milgrom, 1983). The fact that these regions of DNA, generally in the 5′-flanking DNA near the RNA polymerase binding site, transfer hormone responsiveness when fused to other genes and transfected into appropriate host cells (Lee *et al.*, 1981; Chandler *et al.*, 1983; Dean *et al.*, 1983) adds credence to the receptor-binding studies. Still, the latter reflect a very artificial situation, in that naked DNA is used. It will be important to reconstitute steroid-sensitive genes into native chromatin and test for binding, since it is clear that local chromatin effects are very important determinants of glucocorticoid action. This statement is based on an experiment in which a mammary tumor provirus inserted into one region of the HTC cell genome is expressed and is sensitive to digestion with DNase I, while an identical provirus inserted into a different region is not expressed and is insensitive to DNase I digestion (Feinstein *et al.*, 1982). It is conceivable that effects of apparently distant regions of DNA (chromatin), either on the same or a different chromosome, brought into apposition with a specific gene because of folding of the chromosome, may also be important. Finally, trans-acting gene products may also play an important regulatory role (Glueckson-Waelsch, 1979).

Progress in the area of steroid hormone action has been extremely rapid in recent years, and while the basic hypothesis that these molecules affect gene transcription has been confirmed, the final solution to this puzzle, posed by the question mark in Fig. 1, does not appear to be in sight. In this chapter, after reviewing some of the events that made studies of enzyme regulation possible, we have summarized the knowledge currently available regarding the regulation of the synthesis of TAT and PEPCK by glucocorticoid hormones. This was done with a view toward illustrating the many fundamental questions that remain to be answered and that may well involve different aspects of the regulation of transcription of the genes that code for these proteins.

ACKNOWLEDGMENTS

We acknowledge the research done by our colleagues Joye Lynn Barnes, Debra Blair, Cathie Caldwell, Nancy Chrapkiewicz, Gerard Clancy, Martin Diesterhaft, Stuart Feinstein, Mark Granner, James Hargrove, Steve Koch, Raymond Metz, Richard Noble, Tamio Noguchi, Pam Olson, Douglas Quick, Robert Leverence, Larry Sellers, and Daniel Petersen and the secretarial assistance of Sara Paul and Cathie Kaufman. This work was supported by USPHS grants AM25295 (The Iowa Diabetes-Endocrinology Research Center), AM24037, AM20858, and by VA research funds. Daryl K. Granner is a VA Medical Investigator.

REFERENCES

Anderson, J. E. (1984). In "Biological Regulation and Development" (R. F. Goldberger and K. R. Yamamoto, eds.), Vol. 3B, Hormone Action, pp. 169–212. Plenum, New York.

Ballard, F. J., and Hanson, R. W. (1967). *Biochem. J.* **104**, 866–871.

Ballard, F. J., and Hanson, R. W. (1969). *J. Biol. Chem.* **244**, 5625–5630.

Barnabei, O., and Sereni, F. (1960). *Boll. Soc. Ital. Biol. Sper.* **36**, 1656–1658.

Baxter, J. D. (1976). *Pharmacol. Ther.* **2**, 605–659.

Baxter, J. D., and Ivarie, R. D. (1978). In "Receptors and Hormone Action" (B. W. O'Malley and L. Birnbaumer, eds.), Vol. 2, pp. 251–297. Academic Press, New York.

Baxter, J. D., and Rousseau, G. G., eds. (1979). "Glucocorticoid Hormone Action." Springer-Verlag, Berlin and New York.

Beale, E. G., Katzen, C., and Granner, D. K. (1981). *Biochemistry* **20**, 4878–4883.

Beale, E. G., Hartley, J. L., and Granner, D. K. (1982). *J. Biol. Chem.* **257**, 2022–2028.

Bellard, M., Gannon, F., and Chambon, P. (1977). *Cold Spring Harbor Symp. Quant. Biol.* **42**, 779–791.

Bentle, L. A., Snoke, R. E., and Lardy, H. A. (1976). *J. Biol. Chem.* **251**, 2922–2928.

Benton, W. D., and Davis, R. W. (1977). *Science* **196**, 180–182.

Berlin, C. M., and Schimke, R. T. (1965). *Mol. Pharmacol.* **1**, 149–156.

Bird, A., Taggart, M., and Macleod, D. (1981). *Cell* **26**, 381–390.

Brock, M. L., and Shapiro, D. J. (1983). *Cell* **34**, 207–214.

Cake, M. H., and Litwack, G. (1975). In "Biochemical Actions of Hormones" (G. Litwack, ed.), Vol. 3, pp. 317–390. Academic Press, New York.

Chandler, V. L., Maler, B. A., and Yamamoto, K. R. (1983). *Cell* **33**, 489–499.

Chrapkiewicz, N. B., Beale, E. G., and Granner, D. K. (1982). *J. Biol. Chem.* **257**, 14428–14432.

Chung, S., Folsom, V., and Wooley, J. (1983). *Proc. Natl. Acad. Sci. U.S.A.* **80**, 2427–2431.

Cimbala, M. A., Lamers, W. H., Nelson, K., Monahan, J. E., Yoo-Warren, H., and Hanson, R. W. (1982). *J. Biol. Chem.* **257**, 7629–7636.

Colombo, G., Carlson, G., and Lardy, H. (1978). *Biochemistry* **17**, 5329–5338.

Compere, S. J., and Palmiter, R. D. (1981). *Cell* **25**, 233–240.

Compton, J. G., Schrader, W. T., and O'Malley, B. W. (1983). *Proc. Natl. Acad. Sci. U.S.A.* **80**, 16–20.

Danesch, U., Hashimoto, S., Renkawitz, R., and Schutz, G. (1983). *J. Biol. Chem.* **258**, 4750–4753.

Dean, D. C., Knoll, B. J., Riser, M. E., and O'Malley, B. W. (1983). *Nature (London)* **305**, 551–554.

Diesterhaft, M., Shrago, E., and Sallach, H. (1971). *Biochem. Med.* **5**, 297–303.

Diesterhaft, M., Noguchi, T., Hargrove, J., Thornton, C., and Granner, D. (1977). *Biochem. Biophys. Res. Commun.* **79**, 1015–1022.

Diesterhaft, M., Noguchi, T., and Granner, D. K. (1980). *Eur. J. Biochem.* **108**, 357–365.

Dignam, J. D., Martin, P. L., Shastry, B. S., and Roeder, R. G. (1983). In "Methods in Enzymology" (R. Wu, L. Grossman, and K. Moldave, eds.), Vol. 101, Part C, pp. 582–598. Academic Press, New York.

Dorfman, R. (1952). *Vitam. Horm. (N.Y.)* **10**, 332–370.

Dubos, R. J. (1940). *Bacteriol. Rev.* **4**, 1–16.

Durnam, D. M., Perrin, F., Gannon, F., and Palmiter, R. D. (1980). *Proc. Natl. Acad. Sci. U.S.A.* **77**, 6511–6515.

Duyk, G., Leis, J., Longiaru, M., and Skala, A. M. (1983). *Proc. Natl. Acad. Sci. U.S.A.* **80**, 6745–6749.

Dynan, W., and Tjian, R. (1982). *TIBS* **7**, 124–125.

Dynan, W., and Tjian, R. (1983). *Cell* **35**, 79–87.

Engelke, D. R., Ng, S., Shastry, B. S., and Roeder, R. G. (1980). *Cell* **19**, 717–728.

Ernest, M. J., and Feigelson, P. (1978). *J. Biol. Chem.* **253**, 319–322.

Exton, J. H., and Park, C. R. (1969). *J. Biol. Chem.* **244**, 1424–1433.

Feigelson, P., and Greengard, O. (1962). *J. Biol. Chem.* **237**, 3714–3717.

Feinstein, S. C., Ross, S. R., and Yamamoto, K. R. (1982). *J. Mol. Biol.* **156**, 549–566.

Feldman, D. (1977). *Am. J. Physiol.* **233**, E147–E151.

Firestone, G., Payvar, F., and Yamamoto, K. (1982). *Nature (London)* **300**, 221–225.

Folger, K., Anderson, J. N., Hayward, M. A., and Shapiro, D. J. (1983). *J. Biol. Chem.* **258**, 8908–8914.

Foster, D. O., Ray, P. D., and Lardy, H. A. (1966). *Biochemistry* **5**, 555–562.

Ganguly, R., Mehta, N. M., Ganguly, N., and Banerjee, M. R. (1979). *Proc. Natl. Acad. Sci. U.S.A.* **76**, 6466–6470.

Gasson, J. C., and Bourgeois, S. (1983). *J. Cell Biol.* **96**, 409–415.

Gasson, J. C., Ryden, T., and Bourgeois, S. (1983). *Nature (London)* **302**, 621–623.

Geisse, S., Schiedereit, C., Westphal, H. M., Hynes, N. E., Groner, B., and Beato, M. (1982). *EMBO J.* **1**, 1613–1619.

Gelehrter, T. D. (1976). *N. Engl. J. Med.* **294**, 522–526, 598–595, 646–651.

Gerschenson, L. E., Andersson, M., Molson, J., and Okigaki, T. (1970). *Science* **170**, 859–861.

Glueckson-Waelsch, S. (1979). *Cell* **16**, 225–237.

Gluzman, Y., and Shenk, T., eds. (1983). "Enhancers and Eukaryotic Gene Expression." Cold Spring Harbor Lab., Cold Spring Harbor, New York.

Goldsmith, L. A., Kang, E., Bienfang, D. C., Jimbow, K., Gerald, P., and Baden, H. P. (1973). *J. Pediatr.* **83**, 798–805.

Goldsmith, L. A., Thorpe, J. M., and Marsh, R. F. (1981). *Biochem. Genet.* **19**, 687–693.

Goldstein, L., Stella, E. J., and Knox, W. E. (1962). *J. Biol. Chem.* **237**, 1723–1726.

Gorin, E., Tal-Or, Z., and Shafrir, E. (1969). *Eur. J. Biochem.* **8**, 370–375.

Govindan, M. V., Spice, E., and Majors, J. (1982). *Proc. Natl. Acad. Sci. U.S.A.* **79**, 5157–5161.

Granner, D. K. (1976). *Nature (London)* **259**, 572–573.

Granner, D. K. (1979). *In* "Glucocorticoid Hormone Action" (J. D. Baxter and G. G. Rousseau, eds.), pp. 593–612. Springer-Verlag, Berlin and New York.

Granner, D. K., and Hargrove, J. (1983). *Mol. Cell. Biochem.* **53/54**, 113–128.

Granner, D. K., Chase, L. R., Aurbach, G. D., and Tomkins, G. M. (1968a). *Science* **162**, 1018–1020.

Granner, D. K., Hayashi, S., Thompson, E. B., and Tomkins, G. M. (1968b). *J. Mol. Biol.* **35**, 291–301.

Granner, D. K., Thompson, E. B., and Tomkins, G. M. (1970). *J. Biol. Chem.* **245**, 1472–1478.

Granner, D., Andreone, T., Sasaki, K., and Beale, E. (1983). *Nature (London)* **305**, 549–551.

Greengard, O., and Acs, G. (1962). *Biochim. Biophys. Acta* **61**, 652–653.

Groner, B., Kennedy, N., Rahmsdorf, U., Herrlich, P., Van Ooyen, A., and Hynes, N. E. (1982). *Horm. Cell Regul.* **6**, 217–228.

Gunn, J. M., Tilghman, S. M., Hanson, R. W., Reshef, L., and Ballard, F. J. (1975a). *Biochemistry* **14**, 2350–2357.

Gunn, J. M., Hanson, R. W., Meyuhas, O., Reshef, L., and Ballard, F. J. (1975b). *Biochem. J.* **150**, 195–203.

Hager, C. B., and Kenney, F. T. (1968). *J. Biol. Chem.* **243**, 3296–3300.

Hager, L. J., and Palmiter, R. D. (1981). *Nature (London)* **291**, 340–342.

Hargrove, J. L., and Granner, D. K. (1984). *In* "The Transaminases" (P. Christen and D. Metzler, eds.), Wiley (Interscience), New York. In press.

Hayashi, S., Granner, D. K., and Tomkins, G. M. (1967). *J. Biol. Chem.* **242**, 3998–4006.

Huang, A. L., Ostrowski, M. C., Berard, D., and Hager, G. L. (1981). *Cell* **27**, 245–255.

Huttner, W. B., Krone, W., Seitz, H. J., and Tarnowski, W. (1974). *Biochem. J.* **142**, 691–693.

Ivarie, R. D., and O'Farrell, P. H. (1978). *Cell* **13**, 41–55.

Iynedjian, P. B., and Hanson, R. W. (1977a). *J. Biol. Chem.* **252**, 655–662.

Iynedjian, P. B., and Hanson, R. W. (1977b). *J. Biol. Chem.* **252**, 8398–8403.

Iynedjian, P. B., Ballard, F. J., and Hanson, R. W. (1975). *J. Biol. Chem.* **250**, 5596–5603.

Jacob, F., and Monod, J. (1961). *J. Mol. Biol.* **3**, 318–356.

Kenney, F. T. (1959). *J. Biol. Chem.* **234**, 2707–2712.

Kenney, F. T. (1962a). *J. Biol. Chem.* **237**, 1610–1614.

Kenney, F. T. (1962b). *J. Biol. Chem.* **237**, 3495–3498.

Kenney, F. T. (1970). *In* "Mammalian Protein Metabolism" (H. N. Munro and J. B. Allison, eds.) Vol. 4, pp. 131–176. Academic Press, New York.

King, R. J. B., and Mainwaring, W. I. P. (1974). "Steroid-Cell Interactions." University Park Press, Baltimore, Maryland.

Knox, W. E. (1951). *Br. J. Exp. Pathol.* **32**, 462–469.

Knox, W. E., and Mehler, A. H. (1951). *Science* **113**, 237–238.

Knox, W. E., Auerbach, V. H., and Lin, E. C. C. (1956). *Physiol. Rev.* **36**, 164–254.

Krebs, H. A., Bennett, D. A., deGasquet, P., Gascoyne, T., and Yoshida, T. (1963). *Biochem. J.* **86**, 22–27.

Krone, W., Huttner, W. B., Seitz, H. J., and Tarnowski, W. (1974). *FEBS Lett.* **46**, 158–161.

Kuo, M. T., Mandel, J. L., and Chambon, P. (1979). *Nucleic Acids Res.* **7**, 2105–2113.

Lamers, W. H., Hanson, R. W., and Meisner, H. M. (1982). *Proc. Natl. Acad. Sci. U.S.A.* **79**, 5137–5141.

Lee, F., Mulligan, R., Berg, P., and Ringold, G. (1981). *Nature (London)* **294**, 228–232.

Leung, K., and Munck, A. (1975). *Annu. Rev. Physiol.* **37**, 245–272.

Levine, R. (1981). *Diabetes Care* **4**, 38–44.

Lin, E. C. C., and Knox, W. E. (1957). *Biochim. Biophys. Acta* **26**, 85–88.

Lin, E. C. C., and Knox, W. E. (1958). *J. Biol. Chem.* **233**, 1186–1189.

Longshaw, I. D., and Pogson, C. I. (1972). *J. Clin. Invest.* **51**, 2277–2283.

McKnight, G., and Palmiter, R. (1979). *J. Biol. Chem.* **254**, 9050–9058.

McKnight, S., and Kingsbury, R. (1982). *Science* **217**, 316–324.

Mallette, L. E., Exton, J. H., and Park, C. R. (1969). *J. Biol. Chem.* **244**, 5713–5723.

Manley, J. L., Fire, A., Samuels, M., and Sharp, P. (1983). *In* "Methods in Enzymology" (R. Wu, L. Grossman, and K. Moldave, eds.), Vol. 101, Part C, pp. 568–582. Academic Press, New York.

Martin, D., Jr., and Tomkins, G. M. (1970). *Proc. Natl. Acad. Sci. U.S.A.* **65**, 1064–1068.

Martin, D., Jr., Tomkins, G. M., and Granner, D. K. (1969a). *Proc. Natl. Acad. Sci. U.S.A.* **62**, 248–255.

Martin, D., Jr., Tomkins, G. M., and Bresler, M. A. (1969b). *Proc. Natl. Acad. Sci. U.S.A.* **63**, 842–849.

Mayo, K., and Palmiter, R. D. (1981). *J. Biol. Chem.* **256**, 2621–2624.

Monod, J. (1947). *Growth* **11**, 223–289.

Moore, R. E., Hansen, J. D., Lardy, H. A., and Veneziale, C. M. (1982). *J. Biol. Chem.* **257**, 12546–12552.

Munck, A., and Leung, K. (1976). *In* "Receptors and Mechanism of Action of Steroid Hormones" (J. R. Pasqualini, ed.), pp. 311–397. Dekker, New York.

Nakhasi, H., Lynch, K., Dolan, K., Unterman, R., Antakly, T., and Feigelson, P. (1982). *J. Biol. Chem.* **257**, 2726–2729.

Nelson, K., Cimbala, M. A., and Hanson, R. W. (1980). *J. Biol. Chem.* **255**, 8509–8515.

Nelson, K., Cimbala, M. A., and Hanson, R. W. (1981). *In* "The Regulation of Carbohydrate Formation and Utilization in Mammals" (C. M. Veneziale, ed.), pp. 227–254. University Park Press, Baltimore, Maryland.

Nickol, J. M., Lee, K., Hollinger, T. G., and Kenney, F. T. (1976). *Biochem. Biophys. Res. Commun.* **72**, 687–699.

Nickol, J. M., Lee, K., and Kenney, F. T. (1978). *J. Biol. Chem.* **253**, 4009–4015.

Noguchi, T., Diesterhaft, M., and Granner, D. (1978). *J. Biol. Chem.* **253**, 1332–1335.

Nordlie, R. C., and Lardy, H. A. (1963). *J. Biol. Chem.* **238**, 2259–2263.

O'Farrell, P. H. (1975). *J. Biol. Chem.* **250**, 4007–4021.

O'Farrell, P. H., and Ivarie, R. D. (1979). *In* "Glucocorticoid Hormone Action" (J. D. Baxter and G. G. Rousseau, eds.), pp. 189–201. Springer-Verlag, Berlin and New York.

Olson, P. S., Thompson, E. B., and Granner, D. K. (1980). *Biochemistry* **19**, 1705–1711.

Palmiter, R. D., and Carey, N. H. (1974). *Proc. Natl. Acad. Sci. U.S.A.* **70**, 2357–2361.

Parslow, T., and Granner, D. (1983). *Nucleic Acids Res.* **11**, 4775–4792.

Patterson, B., Roberts, B., and Kuff, E. (1977). *Proc. Natl. Acad. Sci. U.S.A.* **74**, 4370–4374.

Payvar, F., Wrange, O., Carlstedt-Duke, J., Okret, S., Gustafsson, J.-A., and Yamamoto, K. R. (1981). *Proc. Natl. Acad. Sci. U.S.A.* **78**, 6628–6632.

Peterkofsky, B., and Tomkins, G. M. (1967). *J. Mol. Biol.* **30**, 49–61.

Peterkofsky, B., and Tomkins, G. M. (1968). *Proc. Natl. Acad. Sci. U.S.A.* **60**, 222–228.

Pfahl, M. (1982). *Cell* **31**, 475–482.

Pitot, H., Peraino, C., Morse, P., and Potter, V. (1964). *Natl. Cancer Inst. Monogr.* **13**, 229–245.

Pitot, H., and Yatvin, M. B. (1973). *Physiol. Rev.* **53**, 228–325.

Ray, P. D., Foster, D. O., and Lardy, H. A. (1964). *J. Biol. Chem.* **239**, 3396–3400.

Razin, A., and Riggs, A. (1980). *Science* **210**, 604–610.

Reshef, L., and Hanson, R. W. (1972). *Biochem. J.* **127**, 809–818.

Reshef, L., Ballard, F. J., and Hanson, R. W. (1969). *Biochem. J.* **244**, 5577–5581.

Reshef, L., Hanson, R. W., and Ballard, F. J. (1970). *J. Biol. Chem.* **245**, 5979–5984.

Richardson, U. I., Tashjian, A. H., Jr., and Levine, L. (1969). *J. Cell Biol.* **40**, 236–247.

Ringold, G. M., Yamamoto, K. R., Tomkins, G. M., Bishop, J. M., and Varmus, H. E. (1975). *Cell* **6**, 299–305.

Ringold, G. M., Yamamoto, K. R., Bishop, J. M., and Varmus, H. E. (1977). *Proc. Natl. Acad. Sci. U.S.A.* **74**, 2879–2883.

Roewekamp, W. G., Hofer, E., and Sekeris, C. E. (1976). *Eur. J. Biochem.* **70**, 259–268.

Rosen, J. M., Matusik, R. J., Richards, D. A., Gupta, P., and Rogers, J. R. (1980). *Recent Prog. Horm. Res.* **36**, 157–193.

Rosenzweig, S., and Frascella, D. (1968). *Bull. N.J. Acad. Sci.* **13**, 17–18.

Rousseau, G. G. (1975). *J. Steroid Biochem.* **6**, 75–89.

Rousseau, G. G., and Baxter, J. D. (1979). *In* "Glucocorticoid Hormone Action" (J. D. Baxter and G. G. Rousseau, eds.), pp. 49–78. Springer-Verlag, Berlin and New York.

Sargent, T. D., Wu, J., Sala-Trepat, J. M., Wallace, R. B., Reyes, A. A., and Bonner, J. (1979). *Proc. Natl. Acad. Sci. U.S.A.* **76**, 3256–3260.

Savouret, J. F., and Milgrom, E. (1983). *DNA* **2**, 99–104.

Sasaki, K., Cripe, T., Koch, S., Andreone, T., Petersen, D., Beale, E., and Granner, D. (1984). *J. Biol. Chem.* In press.

Scherer, G., Schmid, W., Strange, C. M., Rowekamp, W., and Schutz, G. (1982). *Proc. Natl. Acad. Sci. U.S.A.* **79**, 7205–7208.

Schimke, R. T. (1973). *Adv. Enzymol.* **37**, 135–187.

Schimke, R. T., Sweeney, E. W., and Berlin, C. M. (1965). *J. Biol. Chem.* **240**, 322–331.

Schoenheimer, R. (1942). "The Dynamic State of Body Constituents." Harvard Univ. Press, Cambridge, Massachusetts.

Schutz, G., Nguyen-Huu, M. C., Giesecke, K., Hynes, N. E., Groner, B., Wurtz, T., and Sippel, A. E. (1977). *Cold Spring Harbor Symp. Quant. Biol.* **42**, 617–624.

Sellers, L., and Granner, D. K. (1974). *J. Cell Biol.* **60**, 337–345.

Selye, H. (1946). *J. Clin. Endocrinol.* **6**, 117–230.

Shemin, D., and Rittenberg, D. (1946). *J. Biol. Chem.* **166**, 627–636.

Shrago, E., Lardy, H. A., Nordlie, R. C., and Foster, D. O. (1963). *J. Biol. Chem.* **238**, 3188–3192.

Southern, E. M. (1975). *J. Mol. Biol.* **98**, 503–517.

Spiegelman, S. (1946). *Cold Spring Harbor Symp. Quant. Biol.* **11**, 256–277.

Stallcup, M., and Washington, L. (1983). *J. Biol. Chem.* **258**, 2802–2807.

Steinberg, R. A., Levinson, B. B., and Tomkins, G. M. (1975). *Proc. Natl. Acad. Sci. U.S.A.* **72**, 2007–2011.

Talwar, G. P., Segal, S. J., Evans, A., and Davison, O. W. (1964). *Proc. Natl. Acad. Sci. U.S.A.* **52**, 1059–1066.

Thomas, P. (1980). *Proc. Natl. Acad. Sci. U.S.A.* **77**, 5201–5202.

Thompson, E. B., Tomkins, G. M., and Curran, J. F. (1966). *Proc. Natl. Acad. Sci. U.S.A.* **56**, 296–303.

Thompson, E. B., Aviv, D., and Lippman, M. (1977). *Endocrinology (Baltimore)* **100**, 406–419.

Thompson, J. F., and Mikuta, E. T. (1954). *Proc. Soc. Exp. Biol. Med.* **85**, 29–32.

Thompson, R. C., and Ballou, J. E. (1956). *J. Biol. Chem.* **223**, 795–809.

Tilghman, S. M., Hanson, R. W., Reshef, L., Hopgood, M. F., and Ballard, F. J. (1974). *Proc. Natl. Acad. Sci. U.S.A.* **71**, 1304–1308.

Tilghman, S. M., Hanson, R. W., and Ballard, F. J. (1976). *In* "Gluconeogenesis: Its Regulation in Mammalian Species" (R. W. Hanson and M. A. Mehlman, eds.), pp. 47–91. Wiley, New York.

Tomkins, G. M., Thompson, E. B., Hayashi, S., Gelehrter, T., Granner, D. K., and Peterkofsky, B. (1966). *Cold Spring Harbor Symp. Quant. Biol.* **31**, 349–360.

Ucker, D. S., Ross, S. R., and Yamamoto, K. R. (1981). *Cell* **27**, 257–266.

Ucker, D. S., Firestone, G. L., and Yamamoto, K. R. (1983). *Mol. Cell. Biol.* **3**, 551–561.

Utter, M. F., and Kurahashi, K. (1954). *J. Biol. Chem.* **207**, 787–802.

Wasserman, W. J., and Smith, L. D. (1978). *In* "The Vertebrate Ovary" (R. E. Jones, ed.), pp. 443–468. Plenum, New York.

Weintraub, H., and Groudine, M. (1976). *Science* **193**, 848–858.

Weintraub, H., Beug, H., Groudine, M., and Graf, T. (1982). *Cell* **28**, 931–940.

Wicks, W. D. (1969). *J. Biol. Chem.* **244**, 3941–3950.

Wicks, W. D., and McKibbin, J. B. (1972). *Biochem. Biophys. Res. Commun.* **48**, 205–211.

Wicks, W. D., Lewis, W., and McKibbin, J. B. (1972). *Biochim. Biophys. Acta* **264**, 177–185.

Wicks, W. D., Barnett, C. A., and McKibbin, J. B. (1974). *Fed. Proc., Fed. Am. Soc. Exp. Biol.* **33**, 1105–1111.

Yamamoto, K. R. (1983). *In* "Transfer and Expression of Eukaryotic Genes" (H. S. Ginsberg and H. J. Vogel, eds.), pp. 79–92. Academic Press, New York.

Yamamoto, K. R., Gehring, U., Stampfer, M. R., and Sibley, C. J. (1976). *Recent Prog. Horm. Res.* **32**, 3–32.

Yamamoto, K. R., Chandler, V. L., Ross, S. R., Ucker, D. S., Ring, J. C., and Feinstein, S. C. (1981). *Cold Spring Harbor Symp. Quant. Biol.* **45**, 687–697.

Yanofsky, C. (1981). *Nature (London)* **289**, 751–758.

Yoo-Warren, H., Cimbala, M. A., Felz, K., Monahan, J. E., Leis, J. P., and Hanson, R. W. (1981). *J. Biol. Chem.* **256**, 10224–10227.

Yoo-Warren, H., Monahan, J. E., Short, J., Short, H., Bruzel, A., Wynshaw-Boris, A., Meisner, H. M., Samols, D., and Hanson, R. W. (1983). *Proc. Natl. Acad. Sci. U.S.A.* **80**, 3656–3660.

CHAPTER 5

Messenger RNA Stabilization and Gene Transcription in the Estrogen Induction of Vitellogenin mRNA

*David J. Shapiro and Martin L. Brock**

Department of Biochemistry
University of Illinois
Urbana, Illinois

*Present address: Imperial Cancer Research Fund Laboratories, P.O. Box 123, Lincoln Inn Fields, London WC2A 3PX, England.

BIOCHEMICAL ACTIONS OF HORMONES, VOL. XII

I. INTRODUCTION: THE *XENOPUS* VITELLOGENIN SYSTEM

This chapter will focus on the strategies by which a eukaryotic cell can specialize to produce and accumulate large amounts of a specific mRNA. In the course of our investigations of this process, it became apparent that the estrogen induction of vitellogenin mRNA is achieved through an interrelated series of controls which include, but are not limited to, regulation of specific gene transcription.

The system we have employed as a model for steroid hormone regulation of specific gene expression is the induction by estrogen of the egg-yolk precursor protein, vitellogenin, and its cognate mRNAs in liver cells of *Xenopus laevis* (for reviews, see Shapiro *et al.*, 1983; Shapiro, 1982; Hayward *et al.*, 1982a; Wahli *et al.*, 1981; Ryffel, 1978; Tata, 1976; Shapiro and Baker, 1979; Deeley and Goldberger, 1979; Tata and Smith, 1979). *Xenopus laevis* vitellogenins are phospholipoglycoproteins with a monomer molecular weight of approximately 200,000 (Wiley and Wallace, 1978). They are encoded by a family of four closely related 6.5-kb messenger RNAs (Wahli *et al.*, 1976, 1978, 1979; Shapiro and Baker, 1977). The vitellogenin mRNAs are transcribed from a family of four genes, each of which is approximately 16–20 kb in length and contains at least 33 intervening sequences. The four expressed vitellogenin genes have been divided into two groups, designated A and B. Each group contains two closely related genes (Wahli *et al.*, 1980, 1981, 1982; Germond *et al.*, 1983). The induction of vitellogenin synthesis is accompanied by a corresponding increase in the level of vitellogenin mRNA, which indicates that it is the amount of mRNA in cells that constitutes the primary level of control over the rate of vitellogenin synthesis (Shapiro *et al.*, 1976; Shapiro and Baker, 1979). We therefore concentrated our attention on the factors regulating vitellogenin mRNA levels.

The rationale for a detailed study of the regulatory mechanisms responsible for the induction of vitellogenin mRNA was derived from experiments in which the kinetics of *in vivo* vitellogenin mRNA accumulation were examined. Three major conclusions, which are summarized in Fig. 1, emerged

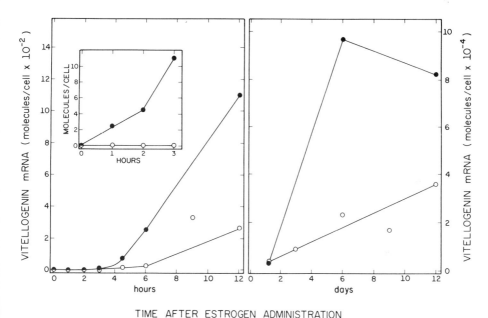

TIME AFTER ESTROGEN ADMINISTRATION

Fɪɢ. 1. Comparison of vitellogenin mRNA accumulation during primary and secondary estrogen stimulation. Male *Xenopus laevis* were either unstimulated [primary stimulation (O———O)] or injected with estrogen and withdrawn for 2 months [secondary stimulation (●———●)] prior to readministration of estrogen at zero hours. Liver RNA was isolated at the indicated times and hybridized in RNA excess to vitellogenin cDNA. The measured value of $C_r t_{1/2}$, the yield of RNA per gram of liver, and the size of vitellogenin mRNA were used to calculate the number of molecules of vitellogenin mRNA per cell, as described by Baker and Shapiro (1977, 1978). The inset in the left panel illustrates the rapid onset of vitellogenin mRNA accumulation during the first few hours of secondary (but not primary) stimulation. The data demonstrate that the accumulation of vitellogenin mRNA is several times more rapid during both early (left panel) and late (right panel) secondary estrogen stimulation than it is in primary estrogen stimulation. [From Baker and Shapiro (1978).]

from these studies (Baker and Shapiro, 1977, 1978; Shapiro and Baker, 1979; Shapiro, 1982). (a) In both unstimulated liver cells and in liver cells withdrawn from estrogen for an extended period of time, there is no detectable vitellogenin mRNA down to a level of less than 1 molecule/cell. (b) After administration of estrogen to *Xenopus* liver cells that have never expressed the vitellogenin genes before (primary stimulation), there is a lag of several hours before vitellogenin mRNA begins to accumulate in cells. When estrogen is administered to liver cells that are inactive in vitellogenin mRNA synthesis at the time of restimulation but that had previously expressed the vitellogenin genes (secondary stimulation), there is essentially no lag, and vitellogenin mRNA is detectable in cells in as little as 1 hour. (c) A major difference between the primary and secondary estrogenic responses is that the rate of vitellogenin mRNA accumulation is approximately four times greater in secondary estrogen stimulation than in primary estrogen stimulation. The elevated rate of vitellogenin mRNA accumulation is also observed in organ cultures (Felber *et al.*, 1978; Brock and Shapiro, 1983b) and in primary *Xenopus* liver monolayers (Searle and Tata, 1981).

II. NUCLEAR ACTIONS OF ESTROGEN IN VITELLOGENIN mRNA INDUCTION

A. Selective Activation of Vitellogenin Gene Transcription

In order to localize more precisely the site(s) at which estrogen regulates vitellogenin mRNA levels, it was necessary to move beyond measurement of mRNA levels and make direct measurements of the rate of vitellogenin gene transcription. The rate of vitellogenin transcription was measured by pulse labeling intact cells with [^{3}H]uridine, isolating the labeled nuclear RNA, and hybridizing it to cloned vitellogenin cDNAs immobilized on nitrocellulose. After hybridization, the filters were washed and digested under stringent conditions and counted. The ratio of the radioactivity bound to the filter, to the total radioactivity incorporated into nuclear RNA represents a measurement of the relative transcription rate and provides a direct assessment of selective estrogen regulation of vitellogenin gene transcription. This data is independent of potential effects of estrogen on overall nuclear RNA synthesis. Our measurements of relative rates of vitellogenin gene transcription indicated that the vitellogenin genes were not transcribed at a significant rate in the absence of estrogen (Brock and Shapiro, 1983a,b). The relative rate of vitellogenin transcription in secondary estrogen stimulation is greater than it is in primary estrogen stimulation (Brock and Shapiro, 1983a,b), indicating that a transcriptional event is responsible for at least part of the differences in rates of vitellogenin mRNA accumulation shown in Fig. 1. Our observation that vitellogenin transcription reaches a plateau within 24 hours and then continues at a constant rate is consistent with *in vivo* accumulation studies that demonstrated that the accumulation rate of cytoplasmic vitellogenin mRNA becomes linear within 1 day of both primary and secondary estrogen stimulation and remains linear for at least several days (Baker and Shapiro, 1977, 1978; Brock and Shapiro, 1983a,b). Our data are consistent with the view that estrogen-mediated changes in the rate of vitellogenin gene transcription represent a primary locus of control in this system.

Recent experiments (Wolffe and Tata, 1983) suggest that all four vitellogenin genes are not transcribed at the same rate. Wolffe and Tata (1983) observed that in primary estrogen stimulation, when estrogen metabolism is very rapid (Tenniswood *et al.*, 1983), the two B-group vitellogenin genes are transcribed more efficiently than the two A-group vitellogenin genes (Wolffe and Tata, 1983). They suggest that differential hormonal responsiveness of the two gene families and rapid estrogen metabolism in primary stimulation may be responsible for enhanced vitellogenin transcription in secondary estrogen stimulation.

In order to obtain a more quantitative picture of the relationship between the number of molecules of vitellogenin mRNA synthesized and the rate of accumulation of vitellogenin mRNA, it was necessary to calculate the actual amount of vitellogenin mRNA synthesized by determining the absolute gene transcription rate. Quantitation of absolute transcription rates also allowed an assessment of the relationship between overall estrogen effects on total nuclear RNA synthesis and effects on vitellogenin gene transcription. Our determination of absolute transcription rates was facilitated by the development of a simple HPLC method for separating UTP from other nucleoside triphosphates (Brock and Shapiro, 1983a). This method provided a simple and sensitive method for measuring the specific radioactivity of the cellular UTP pool. The absolute rate of vitellogenin gene transcription could then be calculated from the product of the relative transcription rate, the absolute rate of total nuclear RNA synthesis (to be described in greater detail later), and a constant derived from the size and base composition of the vitellogenin RNA transcript (Brock and Shapiro, 1983a). A comparison of the absolute transcription rates of the vitellogenin genes in primary and secondary estrogen stimulation is shown in Fig. 2. In unstimulated and withdrawn cells, the vitellogenin genes are transcribed less than once a day, demonstrating that there is no significant transcription of the vitellogenin genes in the absence of estrogen. There is an increase of at least several thousand fold in the absolute rate of vitellogenin gene transcription in both primary and secondary estrogen stimulation (Brock and Shapiro, 1983a). It is apparent that the maximum rate of vitellogenin gene transcription, which is achieved at about 6 hours, is four to five times greater in secondary stimulation than it is in primary stimulation. These data indicated that the observed fourfold increase in the rate of vitellogenin mRNA accumulation in secondary versus

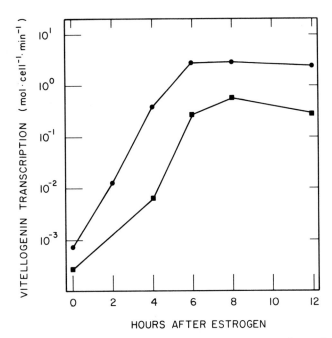

Fig. 2. Absolute rates of vitellogenin gene transcription in primary and secondary estrogen stimulation. At various times following estrogen stimulation, liver fragments were pulse labeled in organ culture with [³H]uridine. Nuclear RNA was isolated and hybridized to all four vitellogenin cDNA clones, and absolute transcription rates were calculated from the data. The absolute rate of vitellogenin gene transcription in secondary stimulation (●———●) is shown to be severalfold greater than the rate in primary estrogen stimulation (■———■). The vitellogenin gene transcription rates at time zero represent the upper limits for potential basal transcription rates. [From Brock and Shapiro (1983a).]

primary estrogen stimulation (Baker and Shapiro, 1977, 1978; Shapiro and Baker, 1979) is mediated by a specific increase in the rate of vitellogenin gene transcription.

While these data demonstrated that the vitellogenin genes are each transcribed less than once a day in unstimulated *Xenopus* liver cells, we wished to increase the sensitivity of these measurements. We therefore extended these observations to cultured *Xenopus* kidney cells in which more efficient RNA labeling is achieved. The vitellogenin genes, which are present in these cells, are each transcribed less than once a week in cultured *Xenopus* kidney cells maintained in media either containing or lacking estrogen (Brock and Shapiro, 1983a). The vitellogenin genes are not, therefore, transcribed at a low basal rate in the absence of estrogen and are transcriptionally silent in cells that are not estrogen responsive. In contrast, ovalbumin and other genes coding for egg-white proteins in hen oviduct do exhibit detectable synthesis of their mRNAs in nontarget tissues (McKnight *et al.*, 1980; Tsai *et al.*, 1979).

B. Estrogen Induction of Total Nuclear RNA Synthesis

Calculation of the absolute rate of transcription of the vitellogenin genes required the determination of the synthetic rate of total nuclear RNA (Brock and Shapiro, 1983a). This resulted in the surprising finding that estrogen regulates overall RNA synthesis independent of its specific regulation of vitellogenin gene transcription. The absolute rate of total nuclear RNA synthesis exhibits a striking 20- to 60-fold increase in primary and secondary estrogen stimulation (Fig. 3). These data demonstrate an effect of estrogen on overall liver RNA synthesis and extend earlier observations (Witliff *et al.*, 1972; Tata and Baker, 1976; Billing *et al.*, 1969) of an increased incorporation

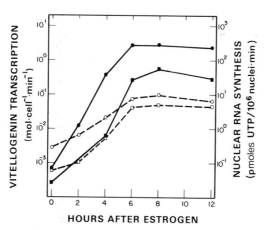

HOURS AFTER ESTROGEN

Fig. 3. Absolute rates of vitellogenin RNA synthesis in estrogen-stimulated *Xenopus* liver. The induction of total nuclear RNA synthesis in primary (□- - - -□) and secondary (○- - - -○) estrogen stimulation follows a time course similar to that shown for the induction of vitellogenin gene transcription. The extent of induction is approximately 60-fold in primary stimulation and 20-fold in secondary stimulation. The data are expressed as pmoles UTP incorporated into nuclear RNA/10^6 nuclei · minute. The induction of specific vitellogenin gene transcription (solid lines) is shown for comparison. [Data from Brock and Shapiro (1983a).]

of label into nuclear RNA following estrogen administration. The selective increase in the fraction of nuclear transcription devoted to vitellogenin RNA synthesis follows a similar time course (Fig. 3), indicating that estrogen induction of nuclear RNA synthesis is not a prerequisite for activation of vitellogenin gene transcription. This conclusion has been confirmed in several types of experiments in which estrogen effects on vitellogenin gene transcription and on total RNA synthesis have been dissociated (Hayward *et al.*, 1982b; Brock and Shapiro, 1983b). It is apparent from these data that estrogen regulates the synthesis of vitellogenin mRNA by causing both a 20- to 60-fold increase in the absolute rate of nuclear RNA synthesis and a selective increase of at least several thousand fold in the absolute rate of vitellogenin gene transcription. It is a combination of these two events that allows the rapid production of vitellogenin mRNA in cells.

C. Regulation of Nuclear Estrogen Receptor Levels

Our observation that the vitellogenin genes are not transcribed at a significant rate (<1 transcript per gene day) in the absence of estrogen was particularly striking since we had previously demonstrated that the estrogen receptor in unstimulated cells is predominantly localized in the liver cell nucleus even in the absence of estrogen (Fig. 4) (Hayward *et al.*, 1980). This surprising finding does not support the general model for steroid hormone action, in which the hormone receptor is found in the cell cytoplasm in the absence of hormone and undergoes "transformation" and translocation into the nucleus following hormone binding. Nuclear localization of the estrogen receptor in the absence of estrogen has also been reported in human MCF-7 cells (King and Green, 1984; Welshons *et al.*, 1984). The histogram shown in Fig. 4 summarizes the concentration of nuclear and cytoplasmic estrogen receptor under various conditions. In unstimulated cells, we observe 550 nuclear high-affinity estrogen binding sites and only about 100 high-affinity cytoplasmic binding sites in the absence of estrogen (Hayward *et al.*, 1980). The administration of estrogen results in the induction of nuclear estrogen receptor, which reaches a level of approximately 2000 high-affinity binding sites. Although the precise number of receptor sites observed differs significantly from those described above, Westley and Knowland (1978, 1979) have also observed a many-fold induction of nuclear estrogen receptor by estrogen. The kinetics of induction of nuclear estrogen receptor parallel those observed for activation of vitellogenin gene transcription and induction of total nuclear RNA synthesis (Hayward *et al.*, 1982a; Brock and Shapiro, 1983a). Following withdrawal of estrogen, *Xenopus* liver cells exhibit a reversal of the nuclear–cytoplasmic estrogen receptor ratio. Nuclear receptor

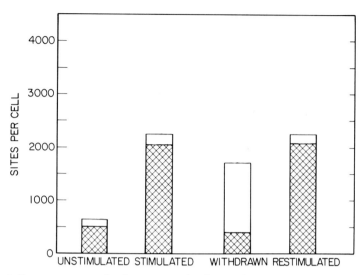

FIG. 4. Estrogen receptor levels in unstimulated, stimulated, and restimulated *Xenopus* liver cells. The level of specific high-affinity estrogen binding to cytoplasmic (open bars) and nuclear (cross-hatched bars) estrogen receptors was determined in unstimulated adult male *Xenopus* liver, 2–3 days after primary estrogen stimulation (stimulated), in animals withdrawn from estrogen for 60–70 days (withdrawn), and 2 days after restimulation of withdrawn *Xenopus* (restimulated).

levels return to the level prevailing in unstimulated cells, and the level of cytoplasmic receptor becomes elevated (Fig. 4, withdrawn).

These data also illustrate the important point that the more rapid absolute rate of vitellogenin gene transcription in secondary estrogen stimulation is not a simple function of an increased level of nuclear estrogen receptor. The level of nuclear estrogen receptor in both primary and secondary estrogen stimulation is identical. Estrogen receptor levels present in primary estrogen stimulated nuclei are sufficient to elicit a far greater rate of vitellogenin gene transcription than actually occurs.

D. ACTIVATION OF VITELLOGENIN GENE TRANSCRIPTION IS A DIRECT EFFECT OF ESTROGEN

An important question in this and other hormone-regulated systems is whether the stimulatory hormone exerts a direct early effect on gene expression or acts indirectly by eliciting the production of regulatory gene products in a fashion similar to that first clearly described in the *Drosophila* ecdysone system (Ashburner *et al.*, 1973). This question has usually been

approached through the use of protein synthesis inhibitors, such as cycloheximide, and by examination of the kinetics of the response. Since estrogen
elicits three simultaneous nuclear responses in *Xenopus* liver cells, this
problem assumes added complexity. Our examination of the kinetics of these
responses indicates that they are quite rapid for an organism that lives at 22,
not 37°C. The effect of quantitative inhibition of protein synthesis by cycloheximide on all three of these responses is summarized in Table I. Quantitative inhibition of protein synthesis blocks the estrogen-mediated increase
in nuclear estrogen receptor levels, although there is still significant receptor in the nucleus even at 12 hours after cycloheximide administration (Hayward *et al.*, 1982b).

The relative rate of vitellogenin gene transcription, which is a measure of
the ability of cells to selectively activate transcription of the vitellogenin
genes, is unimpaired following cycloheximide administration, demonstrating
that the production of new regulatory gene products is not required for this
process. However, the inhibition of protein synthesis has a very large and
striking effect on the third effect of estrogen, which is the increase in the
overall rate of nuclear RNA synthesis in these cells. The 65-fold increase in
the absolute rate of total nuclear RNA synthesis is completely blocked when
protein synthesis is inhibited, so that the rate of nuclear RNA synthesis is
actually lower than it is in control cells. In consequence, the rate of vitellogenin mRNA accumulation following inhibition of protein synthesis with
cycloheximide is very low. Since the rate of nuclear RNA synthesis has
declined approximately 100-fold, even the relatively efficient transcription of

TABLE I

INDUCTION OF VITELLOGENIN TRANSCRIPTION IN THE ABSENCE OF PROTEIN SYNTHESIS[a,b]

Treatment	Nuclear estrogen receptor (sites/cell)	Relative vitellogenin transcription (ppm)	Total RNA synthesis (pmoles UTP/10[6] nuclei · minute)	Absolute vitellogenin transcription (molecules/ cell · minute)
None	550	0	0.066	0.00026
Estrogen, 12 hours	1800	700	4.44	0.41
Estrogen and cyclo- heximide, 12 hours	450	950	0.039	0.0049

[a]Data compiled from Hayward *et al.* (1982b).

[b]Cycloheximide (10 mg/kg body weight) quantitatively inhibits protein synthesis over the
entire 12-hour time course of these experiments. Rates of vitellogenin gene transcription, total
RNA synthesis, and nuclear estrogen receptor levels were all determined at 12 hours.

the vitellogenin genes is insufficient to produce rapid accumulation of large amounts of mRNA in the cytoplasm (Hayward *et al.*, 1982b).

Interpretation of experiments involving the use of protein synthesis inhibitors has often been complicated by secondary toxic effects of these compounds. The failure to observe a biological response following administration of cycloheximide may, therefore, represent either a requirement for protein synthesis in that response or abolition of the response due to overall systemic toxicity. Only if two conditions are met can experiments involving the use of protein synthesis inhibitors be subject to straightforward interpretation. (a) The extent of inhibition of protein synthesis must be essentially quantitative so that residual protein synthesis cannot be responsible for the observed biological response. (b) The biological response must occur in the absence of protein synthesis so that alternative interpretations are not possible. Both of these criteria are met in the failure of quantitative inhibition of protein synthesis by cycloheximide to inhibit the selective activation of vitellogenin gene transcription (Table I). We therefore conclude that the activation of vitellogenin gene transcription is a direct early effect of estrogen that can be dissociated from the other nuclear effects of the hormone.

III. ESTROGEN STABILIZES CYTOPLASMIC VITELLOGENIN mRNA

A. Estrogen Regulation of Vitellogenin mRNA Stability

Several lines of indirect evidence suggested that vitellogenin mRNA might be relatively stable during estrogen induction. There was a close correspondence between the absolute rate of vitellogenin gene transcription (Brock and Shapiro, 1983a) and the rate of vitellogenin mRNA accumulation early in induction (Baker and Shapiro, 1977, 1978), indicating that vitellogenin mRNA was not undergoing significant degradation early in induction. The linear accumulation profiles during the first several days after estrogen stimulation (Fig. 5) (Shapiro *et al.*, 1976; Baker and Shapiro, 1977) are the characteristic accumulation profiles of a species that is being synthesized but not degraded (Schimke, 1970; Kafatos, 1972). Vitellogenin mRNA lost very little label during an *in vivo* labeling experiment (Wahli *et al.*, 1976). These data led us to make direct measurements of the rate of vitellogenin mRNA degradation in estrogen induction and withdrawal.

In order to examine the stability of pulse-labeled vitellogenin mRNA over long periods in liver cells, we developed an efficient primary culture system

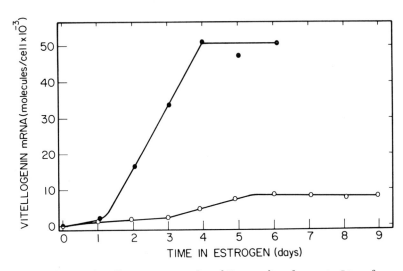

FIG. 5. Induction of vitellogin mRNA in cultured *Xenopus* liver fragments. Livers from male *X. laevis* that had never been exposed to estrogen [primary stimulation (O———O)] or from animals that had received a single dose of estrogen at least 60 days previously [secondary stimulation (●———●)] were excised, minced into liver cubes (Shapiro and Baker, 1979), and adapted to cell culture for 2 days. At that time (day zero), 17β-estradiol was added (to 10^{-6} M). At each time point, cytoplasmic RNA was isolated (Brock and Shapiro, 1983a) and levels of vitellogenin mRNA were determined by quantitative RNA dot hybridization. [From Brock and Shapiro (1983b). Copyright 1983 M.I.T.]

(Brock and Shapiro, 1983b). In this simple primary culture system for liver fragments, vitellogenin mRNA can be induced to levels as high as the 50,000 molecules per cell observed *in vivo* (Fig. 5) (Baker and Shapiro, 1977, 1978), and rates of vitellogenin gene transcription are equal to, or exceed, *in vivo* transcription rates. The complete array of cellular control mechanisms that function to achieve induction of massive amounts of vitellogenin mRNA *in vivo* must, therefore, also be operative in the cultured cells. Several other primary culture systems exhibiting estrogen induction of vitellogenin synthesis have been reported (Wangh and Knowland, 1975; Wangh *et al.*, 1979; Wangh and Schneider, 1982; Green and Tata, 1976; Felber *et al.*, 1978; Shapiro and Baker, 1979; Searle and Tata, 1981).

  Measurements of vitellogenin mRNA stability were carried out by pulse labeling liver RNA in culture. The label was chased with unlabeled uridine, and the decay of [³H]vitellogenin mRNA was quantitated by DNA excess filter hybridization. All of the data were corrected for the time-integrated specific radioactivity of the cellular UTP pool (which is negligible at all chase times beyond 24 hours), so that failure to quantitatively chase the label and reutilization of label from degraded RNA are not factors in these data. The decay of labeled vitellogenin mRNA in secondary stimulation and withdrawal is shown in Fig. 6. The data demonstrate that there is no significant degradation of vitellogenin mRNA when liver cells are maintained in medium containing estrogen ($t_{1/2} = 480 \pm 50$ hours) (Brock and Shapiro, 1983b).

When estrogen is removed from the culture medium, there is a lag period of 12–24 hours, during which residual estrogen is metabolized (Hayward and Shapiro, 1981; Croall, 1982; Tenniswood *et al.*, 1983). This is followed by a shift in the stability of vitellogenin mRNA, which begins to decay rapidly, with a half-life of 16 hours. Vitellogenin mRNA is equally stable in primary estrogen stimulation, exhibiting a half-life of approximately 500 hours in the presence of estrogen and approximately 18 hours in the absence of estrogen (Brock and Shapiro, 1983b).

The extreme stability of vitellogenin mRNA was especially striking considering its length of 6500 nucleotides (Shapiro and Baker, 1977; Wahli *et al.*, 1979). These observations were confirmed using methods that do not rely on the decay of pulse-labeled RNA. The half-life of a macromolecule such as an

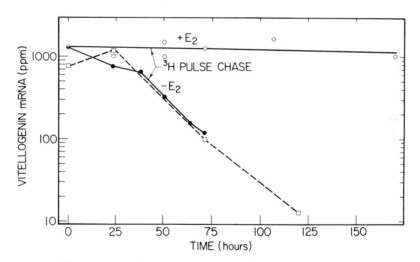

FIG. 6. Vitellogenin mRNA decay in estrogen induction ($+E_2$) and withdrawal ($-E_2$). Liver cubes were cultured for 5 days in medium containing 17β-estradiol (10^{-6} *M*), then labeled for 6 hours with 1 mCi/ml of [^{3}H]uridine. At time zero the labeled uridine was replaced with unlabeled uridine (5 m*M*), and the culture was divided into aliquots maintained in medium containing estrogen (O———O) or lacking estrogen (●———●, □- - -□). Samples were removed at the indicated times, and DNA excess filter hybridizations to cellular RNA were performed (O———O, ●———●). Data are presented as the fraction of labeled RNA in parts per million (ppm). The broken line (□——□) represents the decay of hybridizable vitellogenin mRNA in the same estrogen-withdrawn samples. [From Brock and Shapiro (1983b). Copyright 1983 M.I.T.]

mRNA can be calculated from the kinetics of its approach to a new steady state (Schimke, 1970; Kafatos, 1972). Using the most extensive data available, which describe the kinetics of vitellogenin mRNA accumulation in primary estrogen stimulation *in vivo* (Baker and Shapiro, 1977), we calculate that the half-life for vitellogenin mRNA during estrogen stimulation is 750 ± 300 hours. While the data for the induction of vitellogenin mRNA in culture (Fig. 5) are not extensive enough to ensure the reliability of this method, the fact that vitellogenin mRNA accumulates in a linear fashion (characteristic of a species that is being synthesized at a constant rate and not degraded) is in agreement with these conclusions.

We were able to confirm the half-life of 16 hours for vitellogenin mRNA during estrogen withdrawal by measuring the decay of hybridizable vitellogenin mRNA. Vitellogenin gene transcription was found to be negligible by 24 hours after removal of estrogen from the culture medium. Under conditions of hormone withdrawal, in which no vitellogenin mRNA is being synthesized, the rate of decay of hybridizable vitellogenin mRNA provides a direct measurement of half-life. The data of Fig. 6 demonstrate that the half-life of total vitellogenin mRNA in estrogen withdrawal is 16 hours, which is identical to the half-life determined from the degradation rate of pulse-labeled [³H]vitellogenin mRNA.

These data demonstrated by two independent methods that vitellogenin mRNA is essentially stable in the presence of estrogen and that it is degraded rapidly, with a half-life of 16–18 hours in the absence of estrogen.

While these data showed an estrogen-mediated stabilization of vitellogenin mRNA, they did not resolve the question of whether this represents a specific effect on the stability of vitellogenin mRNA or a general effect on the stability of all cellular mRNAs. It remained possible that estrogen had a systemic effect on RNA turnover. The specificity of this control was demonstrated by measuring the stability of total poly(A) mRNA in cells maintained in estrogen-containing or estrogen-free culture medium. The data of Fig. 7 demonstrate that the major component of total poly(A)-containing mRNA is degraded with a half-life of approximately 16 hours, both in the presence and absence of estrogen. The data also indicate that the half-life of total mRNA is very similar to the half-life of vitellogenin mRNA in hormone withdrawal. This suggests that in the absence of estrogen, vitellogenin mRNA is degraded as a typical cellular mRNA and is subject to normal degradative mechanisms. It is the selective stabilization of vitellogenin mRNA in the presence of estrogen, not the degradation of the mRNA in the absence of hormone, that represents the regulated process in this cytoplasmic control system.

These data demonstrate that the estrogen-induced stabilization of vitellogenin mRNA represents a selective rather than a general effect of estrogen, and that it is properly characterized as a specific control mechanism.

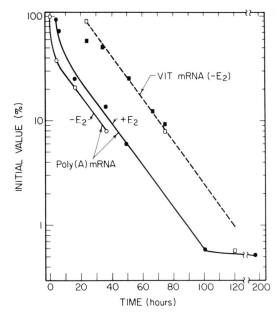

FIG. 7. Poly(A) mRNA decay in estrogen induction $(+E_2)$ and withdrawal $(-E_2)$. The samples described in the legend to Fig. 6 were subjected to two cycles of poly(U) Sepharose chromatography, and the specific radioactivity of the poly(A) mRNA was determined. The data are presented as the percentage of the initial value for poly(A) mRNA isolated from cells maintained in the presence (●———●) and absence (○———○) of estrogen. A small component of the pulse-labeled poly(A) mRNA of cells cultured in the presence of estrogen is resistant to degradation. This component presumably contains vitellogenin mRNA. The decline of label in vitellogenin mRNA estrogen sequences (■- - -■) and the decline in the abundance of vitellogenin mRNA in estrogen withdrawal (□- - -□) (data from Fig. 6) are shown for direct comparison. [From Brock and Shapiro (1983b). Copyright 1983 M.I.T.]

B. REGULATION OF mRNA STABILITY IS A COMMON CONTROL MECHANISM

Although the stabilization of vitellogenin mRNA is a particularly dramatic example of the regulation of mRNA stability, the phenomenon itself is widespread. Several types of observations indicate that the stability of mRNAs play an important role in determining their levels. Data assembled from Derman *et al.* (1981) on the rates of transcription initiation and abundance of 20 rat liver mRNAs allowed us to determine their degradation rates using the equations described below. It was clear that these RNAs, which are predominantly in the middle abundance class mRNAs, exhibit rates of gene transcription and mRNA degradation that are extremely heterogeneous, and both vary over a range of approximately 100-fold. This calculation suggests that the levels of individual mRNAs can be set by the use of specific rates of both gene transcription and mRNA degradation. Several more direct studies have also shown that the range of specific mRNA half-lives within a particular cell is extremely broad (Kafatos, 1972; Harpold *et al.*, 1979; Akusjarvi and Persson, 1981; Darnell, 1982; Derman *et al.*, 1981).

Regulation of the stability of specific mRNAs has been reported in a variety of eukaryotic systems (Table II). These data indicate that in a great many eukaryotic systems in which the level of the mRNA coding for a major differentiated cell product is regulated, regulation of mRNA stability plays a role in that process. Thus, the levels of ovalbumin, conalbumin, avian and amphibian vitellogenin casein, prostatic steroid–binding protein, histone, lactate dehydrogenase, and interferon mRNAs all appear to be modulated, at least in part, by control of mRNA stability. In addition to the examples of regulation of the stability of specific mRNAs summarized in Table II, there are several well-characterized developmental systems in which an entire developmentally regulated class of mRNAs is selectively destroyed. Aggregation of the cellular slime mold *Dictyostelium discoideum* results in the appearance of a set of 2000–3000 different aggregation-specific mRNAs. Disaggregation results in the selective degradation of this entire class of 2000–3000 different mRNA sequences (Chung *et al.*, 1981). The progressive increase in the level of globin mRNA during reticulocyte development appears to be due, in part, to selective degradation of nonglobin mRNAs (Aviv *et al.*, 1976; Bastos *et al.*, 1977).

The experimental data in Table II illustrate two important classes of regulated mRNA degradation systems. Many mRNAs are degraded very rapidly when they are not needed and are stabilized during periods of accumulation, so that they exhibit degradation kinetics comparable to those of total cell mRNAs. The mRNAs coding for the egg-white protein mRNAs, histone mRNA in cultured mammalia cells, and phage λ integrase mRNA in *E. coli* (references in Table II) all fall into this general class. The regulated process in these systems may well be the rapid destruction of the mRNA in the absence of an effector. A second class of mRNAs whose stability is regulated exhibit degradation kinetics typical of total cell mRNA in the absence of effectors and are selectively stabilized in the presence of effectors. *Xenopus* vitellogenin mRNA and casein mRNAs exhibit this type of control. Whether or not this rather arbitrary division of these systems into two different classes actually reflects the existence of two different cellular mechanisms for regulating mRNA stability remains to be established.

It has been suggested that ribosomes can protect mRNAs from degradation by cellular nucleases (Kenney *et al.*, 1972). In this model, efficient translation of the mRNA promoted by an effector would stabilize it against degradation. While this type of control may occur in a few cases in which individual mRNAs initiate translation with low efficiency (Ernest, 1982), it is unlikely to be either a general control mechanism or responsible for stabilization of vitellogenin mRNA. Translation of vitellogenin mRNA *in vivo* is no more efficient than translation of other cellular mRNAs (Berridge *et al.*, 1976; Shapiro *et al.*, 1976). Use of protein synthesis inhibitors such as cycloheximide, which slow but do not abolish elongation (Lodish, 1971; Grollman, 1968) and increase the density of ribosomes on mRNAs, produces effects on vitellogenin mRNA stability that are inconsistent with this model (Brock and Shapiro, 1983b). In addition, the specific translational control mechanisms that are central to this model have been extremely difficult to establish in eukaryotic cells (Lodish, 1971).

A simple mechanism for regulation of functional mRNA stability would be for cells to produce different mRNAs coding for the same protein. It has been proposed that isoproterenol induction of LDH mRNA in rat glioma cells results in production of a new lactate dehydrogenase A subunit mRNA with a half-life of 2.5 hours. The LDH A subunit mRNA produced in the absence of an elevated level of cAMP is thought to be produced continuously and to exhibit a half-life of approximately 50 minutes (Jungmann *et al.*, 1983). This type of model is inadequate to account for most cases of regulated mRNA stability, in which it can be shown that withdrawal of an effector, such as a hormone, can be shown to result in the accelerated degradation of preexisting mRNA.

Stabilization of Vitellogenin mRNA Is a Reversible Cytoplasmic Effect of Estrogen

This hypothesis is a specific example of the more general model that nuclear synthesis of an mRNA whose stability is regulated is accompanied by covalent modifications that render the RNA resistant to degradation. Such modifications could take the form of unusual 5' or 3' structures. In the presence or absence of an effector, these modifications would be reversed in the cytoplasm, altering the stability of the mRNA. This model predicts that a covalent and presumably irreversible modification of the mRNA is responsible for a regulated change in mRNA half-life. An alternative model is that mRNA stability is regulated through reversible protein–nucleic acid interactions in the cytoplasm. We have evaluated these models by examining the reversibility of estrogen-regulated vitellogenin mRNA degradation.

In this experiment (Brock and Shapiro, 1983b), vitellogenin mRNA was

TABLE II

BIOLOGICAL SYSTEMS THAT EXHIBIT REGULATION OF mRNA STABILITY[a]

mRNA	Tissue	Regulatory signal	Half-life		References
			+ Effector	− Effector	
Vitellogenin	*Xenopus* liver	Estrogen	+E; 500 hr	−E; 16 hr	Brock and Shapiro, 1983b
Vitellogenin	Rooster liver	Estrogen	+E; ~24 hr	−E; <3 hr	Wiskocil *et al.*, 1980 Palmiter and Carey, 1974; McKnight and Palmiter, 1979; Hynes *et al.*, 1979; Shepherd *et al.*, 1980, Thomas *et al.*, 1981
Ovalbumin, conalbumin	Hen oviduct	Estrogen, progesterone	+E; ~24 hr	−E; 2–5 hr	
Casein	Rat mammary gland	Prolactin	+Pro; 92 hr $\Delta t_{1/2} \sim 30\times$	−Pro; 5 hr	Guyette *et al.*, 1979
Prostatic steroid–binding protein	Rat ventral prostate	Androgen			Page and Parker, 1982
Lactate dehydrogenase A subunit	Rat C6 glioma cells	cAMP, isoproterenol, dibut cAMP	+Ipt; 2.5 hr	−Ipt; 45 min	Jungmann *et al.*, 1983

β-Interferon	Human fibroblasts	Poly(I·C) vs. poly(I·C) + cycloheximide or Newcastle's virus	(I·C) + ChX or (I·C) + N.V., $t_{1/2}$ > 12 hr; (I·C) $t_{1/2}$ < 30 min	Raj and Pitha, 1983
Histones	HeLa cells	DNA replication	During replication 11 hr, after 13 min	Gallwitz, 1975; Perry and Kelley, 1973
Histones	Yeast	DNA replication	During replication ~15 min, after ~5 min	Hereford et al., 1981, 1982
Adenovirus 1A (9S), 1B (14S)	HeLa cells	Early/late infection	Late, 60–100 min; early, 6–10 min	Wilson and Darnell, 1981; Babich and Nevins, 1981
L3 (ribosomal protein)	Yeast	mRNA Overproduction	$\Delta t_{1/2}$ ~ 2x	Pearson et al., 1982
γ integrase (int)	γ infected E. coli	Early/late infection (terminator read-through)	$\Delta t_{1/2}$ > 10x	Rosenberg and Schmeissner, 1982; Holmes et al., 1983

[a]We apologize to all those whose work may inadvertently have been omitted from this table. In some cases early experiments that have not been repeated with cloned DNAs have been omitted. The level of precision of these studies varies widely with the methodology available at a particular time and with the experimental constraints of each system. Those systems exhibiting developmental regulation of the stability of an entire class of mRNAs are mentioned in the text. The utility of RNase III⁻ (and RNase II⁻) mutants for the study of prokaryotic mRNA stability strongly suggests that additional examples of this class of controls will be identified in Escherichia coli.

pulse labeled early in secondary estrogen induction. Estrogen was removed from the culture medium and vitellogenin mRNA was allowed to decay rapidly for 2 days. Estrogen was then added to half the cultures, while the other half was maintained in estrogen-free medium in which continued degradation of vitellogenin mRNA occurs. The data show that estrogen quantitatively restabilizes pulse labeled vitellogenin mRNA underoing rapid degradation (Fig. 8). The restabliziation of vitellogenin mRNA coincides with the reactivation of vitellogenin gene transcription and the induction of additional vitellogenin mRNA (Fig. 8). The estrogen-induced stabilization of vitellogenin mRNA is, therefore, a reversible cytoplasmic effect of estrogen and does not involve the synthesis of mRNA species exhibiting differential stability.

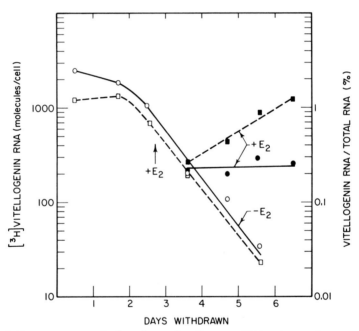

FIG. 8. Estrogen reverses the degradation of vitellogenin mRNA in *Xenopus* liver cytoplasm. Vitellogenin mRNA was labeled in estrogen-stimulated liver cubes and then transferred to estrogen-free medium (day zero). At the indicated time ($+E_2$), estrogen (10^{-6} M) was added back to half the culture. The decay of [^{3}H]vitellogenin mRNA in the presence (●———●) and absence (○———○) of estrogen was quantitated by DNA excess filter hybridization. The abundance of vitellogenin mRNA in estrogen withdrawal (□--□) and during reinduction with estrogen (■--■) was determined by quantitative RNA dot hybridization. [From Brock and Shapiro (1983b). Copyright 1983 M.I.T.]

C. STABILIZATION OF VITELLOGENIN mRNA IS NOT
MEDIATED BY THE NUCLEAR ESTROGEN RECEPTOR

The estrogen receptor complex is almost exclusively nuclear in cells maintained in estrogen (Westley and Knowland, 1978; Hayward *et al.*, 1980, 1982b). The stabilization of vitellogenin mRNA in the cytoplasm of *Xenopus* liver cells is, therefore, unlikely to be a simple estrogen receptor–mediated response. The demonstration that the stabilization of vitellogenin mRNA is reversible in the cytoplasm does not exclude the possibility that the presence or withdrawal of estrogen induces the synthesis of new proteins that control the stability of vitellogenin mRNA. This would allow indirect control of cytoplasmic vitellogenin mRNA stability through nuclear effects of the estrogen receptor. This led us to investigate the requirements for new protein synthesis in the stabilization and destabilization of vitellogenin mRNA. We chose conditions of cycloheximide inhibition of protein synthesis that maximize inhibition of protein synthesis, yet allow the liver cells to recover completely after removal of the cycloheximide. Vitellogenin mRNA pulse labeled in cells treated with cycloheximide is stable in the presence of estrogen and is destabilized in the absence of estrogen (Fig. 9). These data indicate that neither the stabilization of vitellogenin mRNA nor the transition from the stable to the unstable form of the mRNA requres the production of new protein. The cellular apparatus that is required for the destabilization of vitellogenin mRNA is present during hormone induction and is not synthesized in response to estrogen withdrawal. Since cycloheximide increases the loading density of ribosomes on mRNA and does not increase the stability of vitellogenin mRNA, it seems unlikely that the stabilization and destabilization of vitellogenin mRNA is due to changes in the translational efficiency of the mRNA or in the size of vitellogenin-synthesizing polysomes.

The reversibility of cytoplasmic vitellogenin mRNA degradation and the absence of a requirement for protein synthesis strongly suggest that the stabilization of vitellogenin mRNA is not under the direct control of the nuclear estrogen receptor. One obvious requirement for a regulated cytoplasmic mRNA degradation system is a mechanism for sensing intracellular estrogen levels. A cytoplasmic estrogen–binding protein whose properties are consistent with a role in the regulation of vitellogenin mRNA stability has been identified (Hayward and Shapiro, 1981). This estrogen-binding protein is present at sufficiently high levels in the cytoplasm of *Xenopus* liver cells to physically interact with all of the estrogen-induced mRNA in cells; if that is its function. It does not translocate into the nucleus and exhibits the same high level of specificity in estrogen binding as does the nuclear estrogen

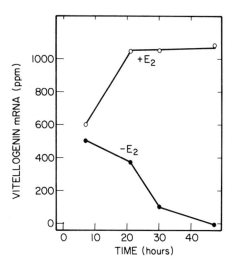

Fɪɢ. 9. Estrogen regulates vitellogenin mRNA stability in the absence of protein synthesis. Liver fragments were induced and labeled, and a level of cycloheximide sufficient to inhibit protein synthesis by 95% was added to the medium. After 1 hour the culture was divided. Half of the cultures were maintained in medium containing cycloheximide but no estrogen (●———●) and half in medium containing cycloheximide and estrogen (○———○). At the indicated times, RNA was isolated from some of the cultures, hybridized to cloned vitellogenin DNA, and used to determine the portion of the label (in ppm) in vitellogenin. [From Brock and Shapiro (1983b). Copyright 1983 M.I.T.]

receptor (Hayward and Shapiro, 1981; Hayward *et al.*, 1982a). The estrogen-binding protein has a 100-fold lower binding constant for 17β-estradiol, than the nuclear estrogen receptor. This suggests as a rather plausible working hypothesis that, in the presence of low concentrations of 17β-estradiol, the nuclear estrogen receptor may become saturated with hormone, initiating transcription of the vitellogenin genes. Since the cytoplasmic estrogen–binding protein will not be saturated under these conditions, the mRNA might not be stabilized, so that vitellogenin mRNA might only accumulate to relatively modest levels in cells. In the presence of very high levels of 17β-estradiol, the estrogen-binding protein in the cytoplasm becomes saturated with estradiol and might then mediate the stabilization of vitellogenin mRNA, allowing a further increase of up to 30-fold in the ultimate level of vitellogenin mRNA and providing great deal of flexibility in this control.

Although the 30-fold increase in the stability of vitellogenin mRNA obviously makes a major contribution to the accumulation of massive amounts of vitellogenin mRNA, it is important to emphasize the key role of activation of gene transcription in this process, since the vitellogenin genes are not transcribed at all in the absence of estrogen.

D. Modulation of Vitellogenin mRNA Levels Through
Control of the Rate of Total Nuclear RNA Synthesis

Our data on the stabilization of vitellogenin mRNA raise an interesting question. The extreme stability ($t_{1/2} \sim 3$ weeks) of *Xenopus* vitellogenin mRNA allows newly synthesized vitellogenin mRNA to accumulate in cells without undergoing significant degradation. Although hepatocyte vitellogenin mRNA remains stable for at least 1 week in the presence of estrogen (Fig. 6), it does not continue to accumulate in liver cells throughout that period. The induction profiles of Fig. 5 show that levels of vitellogenin mRNA in estrogen-stimulated liver cells eventually reach a plateau. The failure to continue accumulating vitellogenin mRNA must be caused by a shift to a more rapid rate of vitellogenin mRNA degradation or to a decrease in the rate of vitellogenin mRNA synthesis. We examined each of these parameters to determine which one was altered at the plateau of induction. Our studies clearly show that vitellogenin mRNA is stabilized by estrogen both during periods of maximum induction and during the plateau (Fig. 6) (Brock and Shapiro, 1983b). Since the induction of vitellogenin RNA synthesis results from selective activation of vitellogenin gene transcription and induction of overall nuclear RNA synthesis, we examined both of these parameters during estrogen stimulation and withdrawal. In the histogram shown in Fig. 10, the values of each parameter that we measured during periods of primary and secondary stimulation, when vitellogenin mRNA is accumulating rapidly in cells, were arbitrarily set equal to 100% and compared to values determined during the plateau stage, when vitellogenin mRNA no longer accumulates in cells. The data demonstrate that the relative rate of vitellogenin gene transcription, which represents the ratio of vitellogenin transcription to total transcription, does not decrease in the plateau stage of induction. In contrast, the absolute rate of total nuclear RNA synthesis, which increases 30- to 50-fold on induction of vitellogenin mRNA in liver cultures, declines precipitously when cells enter the plateau stage. The combination of a constant relative rate of vitellogenin transcription superimposed on a decline by a factor of 4 to 10 in overall nuclear RNA synthesis produces a corresponding decline in the absolute rate of vitellogenin RNA synthesis.

Our data are consistent with the view that the absolute rate of vitellogenin RNA synthesis is indirectly controlled through estrogen regulation of the overall rate of total nuclear RNA synthesis. This work also suggests a mechanism for this novel regulatory process. The estrogen induction of total nuclear RNA synthesis is accompanied by approximately tenfold increases in the intracellular levels of the nucleoside triphosphates (Brock and Shapiro, 1983a,b). The close correlation between the absolute rate of total nuclear RNA synthesis and the intracellular levels of all four nucleoside triphos-

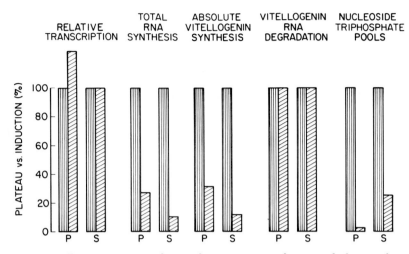

FIG. 10. Vitellogenin mRNA production during estrogen induction and plateau. The regulatory processes that lead to induction of vitellogenin mRNA were measured during induction (vertical lines) and during the plateau period (diagonal lines). Plateau values are compared to values during induction, which were set equal to 100% for both primary (P) and secondary (S) estrogen stimulation in culture. The actual values for each measured parameter are given as follows. Relative rate of vitellogenin transcription: P, 2110 ppm; S, 3830 ppm. Total RNA synthesis: P, 11.1 pmoles UTP/10^6 nuclei $\cdot$ min; S, 41.1 pmoles UTP/10^6 nuclei $\cdot$ min. Absolute vitellogenin transcription: P, 3.2 molecules/cell/minute; S, 21.5 molecules/cell/minute. Vitellogenin RNA degradation $t_{1/2}$: P, 500 hours; S, 485 hours. Nucleoside triphosphate pools are in arbitrary units for ATP and UTP, since precise values for the extent of hydrolysis during isolation and the volume of a *Xenopus* hepatocyte in culture are unknown.

phates strongly suggests a cause-and-effect relationship. For example, inhibition of protein synthesis by cycloheximide completely blocks the estrogen-mediated increase in nucleoside triphosphate levels and abolishes the increase in the absolute rate of total nuclear RNA synthesis (M. L. Brock and D. J. Shapiro, unpublished observations; Hayward *et al.*, 1982a). The decline in total RNA synthesis when cells enter the plateau stage is also accompanied by a sharp decline in intracellular nucleoside triphosphate levels (Fig. 10). Addition of high levels of uridine to the culture medium elevates intracellular nucleoside triphosphate levels and increases the absolute rate of total nuclear RNA synthesis (Brock, 1983). While correlation does not necessarily imply causation, taken together, these data strongly suggest that the estrogen-mediated increase in nucleoside triphosphate pool sizes results in saturation of the cellular transcription complex with substrate, and thereby increases the absolute rate of nuclear RNA synthesis.

The selective estrogen activation of vitellogenin gene transcription is not brought about by changes in nucleoside triphosphate pools, since it occurs in cycloheximide-treated cells in which nucleoside pools and total RNA synthesis do not increase (Table I). Nevertheless, changes in nucleoside triphosphate pools could conceivably affect the efficiency with which specific *Xenopus* liver promoters are transcribed. Blumenthal and Hill (1980) have shown that Qβ replicase transcribes only Qβ and other favored templates at low GTP concentrations. At high GTP concentrations, Qβ replicase efficiently transcribes a variety of prokaryotic templates. At this time it is not known whether estrogen regulation of the levels of other *Xenopus* liver mRNAs is mediated by changes in nucleoside triphosphate pools.

Although hormonal control of total RNA synthesis was apparently observed during estrogen stimulation of uterine development in the rat more than 10 years ago (Billing *et al.*, 1969), it has been generally ignored. It is likely that this control mechanism is widespread and has been overlooked in other systems. The increase in nucleoside triphosphate pool size dilutes the radioactive label and masks this effect. If nuclear RNA synthesis is measured by simply quantitating the incorporation of radioactive label into nucleic acid, without reference to the specific radioactivity of the nucleoside triphosphate pools, only a minimal increase in the rate of total nuclear RNA synthesis is observed in *Xenopus* liver cells.

IV. METHODS FOR DETERMINATION OF RATES OF GENE TRANSCRIPTION AND mRNA DEGRADATION

Our methods for measurement of the absolute rate of vitellogenin gene transcription and mRNA degradation entail pulse labeling of nuclear or cytoplasmic RNA, hybridization to cloned DNA, and determination of the specific radioactivity of the cellular nucleoside triphosphate pool. Since cloned probes complementary to a variety of eukaryotic genes are available, it may seem surprising that such measurements have been rare. The paucity of data from other systems is caused in part by the fact that our measurement were greatly facilitated by two special features of the vitellogenin system. Vitellogenin is a major differentiated cell product. Vitellogenin mRNA is the most abundant mRNA in these cells, and the genes exhibit an extremely high relative rate of transcription (up to 4000 ppm in secondary stimulation; see Fig. 10) (Brock and Shapiro, 1983b). Efficient labeling of the mRNA is facilitated by the long half-life of the mRNA, which also simplifies pulse-chase experiments. The approach-to-equilibrium (Schimke, 1970; Greenberg, 1972; Perry and Kelley, 1973) and pulse-chase methods, while enormously useful, suffer from several limitations. The approach-to-equilibrium method is an indirect method that assumes constant rates of synthesis and degradation. In pulse-labeling techniques, it is assumed that degradation is slow relative to pulse labeling. For many species, however, decay is rapid. Application of this methodology to mRNAs that are degraded rapidly or are transcribed at relatively low rates has been difficult. In order to allow a new approach to this problem, we derived a series of equations that extend the classical approaches.

These equations allow determination of the absolute synthetic rate or rate of decay if the steady-state level of the macromolecule and either the synthetic rate or the rate of decay are known (Brock, 1983). This allows the use of extended pulse-labeling times, which are long relative to the decay rate, and makes possible the incorporation of sufficient label into many mRNAs to allow reliable quantitation of their rates of synthesis and degradation. A brief description of the derivation of these expressions is given below.

In labeling a species undergoing synthesis and decay, whether or not it is at a steady state, the kinetics of label incorporation will follow an asymptotic approach to equilibrium. The labeling time is usually chosen to be rapid relative to the rate of decay, so *synthesis* can be defined as the fraction of labeled precursor incorporated per unit time:

$$S' = \text{label in species}/T$$

where T is the labeling time. However, even in rapid labeling, decay may be significant. A correction is applied to S' in order to achieve the true synthetic rates S, by measuring the decay rate D.

$$S = [DT/(1 - e^{-DT})]S' \tag{1}$$

which allows the determination of synthesis even after long labeling times, on the order of several half-lives. The origin of this equation comes from a consideration of the relationships between synthesis and degradation.

$$-d(Sdt)/dt = DSdt \tag{2}$$

Integrating this over the labeling period T, the above formulation is derived (for details, see Brock, 1983).

A measurement of D may necessitate considerable fortitude. Fortunately, most measurements are in a steady-state mode, in which species abundance is constant. In such a steady-state situation, $S = DA$, where A is the species abundance (Kafatos, 1972), so

$$S = -(A/T)\ln[1 - (S'T/A)] \tag{3}$$

Equations that are related but not identical to Eq. (3) have been described (Zak *et al.*, 1979; Galau *et al.*, 1977; Chung *et al.*, 1981). Equation (3) and related expressions (Brock, 1983) allow an accurate determination of the synthetic rate of any species in any labeling time if, in addition to the amount of label incorporated, *either* the degradation rate or the species abundance can be independently measured. Since it is straightforward to measure mRNA levels, this equation should be useful in a broad range of studies. Use of this equation requires that the intranuclear pool of label has rapidly reached equilibrium or that the time-integrated specific activity of the labeled pool is known.

V. POTENTIAL MECHANISMS FOR THE REGULATION OF mRNA DEGRADATION

Observations demonstrating that the stability of specific mRNAs are regulated have not been reflected by the acquisition of comparable mechanistic data. The recent description of some potential models for regulated mRNA degradation lends plausibility to certain essentially speculative ideas.

At this time, the site of mRNA degradation in eukaryotic cells is unclear. Schlessinger and his colleagues (Sameshima *et al.*, 1981) have demonstrated that increased RNA degradation in confluent cell monolayers is blocked by poisoning lysosomal function. It is possible that the regulated step in mRNA degradation is entry into the lysosomal compartment. The basis for this type of discrimination between mRNAs is completely obscure. Lysosomal poisoning experiments that entail raising the intralysosmal pH through the addition of amines to the culture medium have, in general, not been performed on systems exhibiting regulation of the stability of individual mRNAs. One plausible role for lysosomal degradation mechanisms is the selective destruction of entire classes of developmentally regulated mRNA—a process observed during slime mold morphogenesis and red blood cell maturation (Chung *et al.*, 1981; Aviv *et al.*, 1976; Bastos *et al.*, 1977).

Several types of experiments indicate that the poly(A) tract at the 3'-OH of most eukaryotic mRNAs may play a role in their degradation. It has been shown that poly(A) has no nuclear function and that poly(A)$^-$ mRNA can be found correctly spliced and is found on polyribosomes (Zeevi *et al.*, 1981). Since cordycepin, an inhibitor of poly(A) addition, prevented cytoplasmic accumulation of RNA, it was argued that poly(A) was involved in nuclear export. However, Zeevi *et al.* (1982) showed that this could be accounted for by the rapid cytoplasmic turnover of poly(A)$^-$ mRNA. They conclude that the role of poly(A) is to stabilize mRNA against degradation.

Deadenylated globin mRNA microinjected into *Xenopus* oocytes (Marbaix *et al.*, 1975; Huez *et al.*, 1975) or HeLa cells (Huez *et al.*, 1978) was degraded more rapidly than the polyadenylated RNA. Histone mRNA, which is not polyadenylated in most eukaryotes, is degraded extremely rapidly under most circumstances (Hereford *et al.*, 1982; Perry and Kelley, 1973; Gallwitz, 1975). One plausible hypothesis for regulated mRNA degradation is that a site-specific cleavage that results in deadenylation is followed by rapid degradation of the mRNA. Regulation of mRNA stability would be achieved by protein–nucleic acid interactions that either alter secondary structure and nuclease recognition near the poly(A) addition site or physically block access to the cleavage site. Recent experiments demonstrating the existence of a similar mechanism in prokaryotic cells demonstrate the feasibility of this regulatory strategy. RNase III in *E. coli* produces specific cleavages at hairpin loops and can be used to regulate the level of specific mRNAs. Rosenberg and Schmeissner (1982) found that bacteriophage λ integrase mRNA levels are regulated by selective degradation of an integrase mRNA that reads through a transcription termination signal t_I. This read-through mRNA forms a large hairpin loop in its 3′ region, which is recognized by RNase III, and is cleaved. The RNase III–cleaved mRNA is degraded very rapidly by cellular nucleases. Late in infection, the integrase transcript is initiated from a second promoter, terminates at T_I, and produces functional mRNA, which contains a smaller stem and loop and is not subject to rapid degradation (Rosenberg and Schmeissner, 1982; Holmes *et al.*, 1983). Although RNases whose specificity parallels that of RNase III have not been identified in the cytoplasm of eukaryotic cells, this nevertheless remains an attractive mechanism for regulated mRNA degradation.

A related possibility is that the presence of a hairpin near the 3′ end of a eukaryotic mRNA blocks degradation by exonucleases similar to RNase II, which degrades RNA from the 3′-OH end. Regions of secondary structure in the 3′-untranslated region of the mRNA would block sequential degradation of the mRNA. A prediction of this model is that degradation and removal of the poly(A) at the 3′ end would occur, since degradation would proceed until the region of secondary structure is encountered. Although a general shortening of poly(A) sequences in the cytoplasm is usually observed over time (Darnell, 1982; Brawerman, 1981), there is no evidence to support the proposition that the degradation of specific mRNAs is blocked as precessive RNases encounter regions of secondary structure. Vitellogenin mRNA, when it is stabilized in the presence of estrogen ($t_{1/2} \sim 3$ weeks) and when it is rapidly degraded in the absence of estrogen ($t_{1/2} \sim 16$ hours), exhibits similar binding to and elution from oligo(dT) cellulose, indicating the presence of poly(A) tracts very similar in length.

The 5′ cap on most eukaryotic mRNAs probably serves as a barrier to exonuclease attack. Mechanisms for specific removal of the 5′ cap would render the mRNA susceptible to nucleolytic cleavage. Removal of the cap would also diminish the translational efficiency of the mRNA, perhaps increasing its susceptibility to endonuclease attack. Experimental support for mechanisms of regulated mRNA degradation based on removal of the 5′ cap are lacking, and they appear to have received less attention than mechanisms based on events at the 3′ end of the mRNA.

Additional support for the view that sequences in the 3′-untranslated region of the mRNA control mRNA stability is obtained from recent experiments of Wickens (1984). He cloned a 220-bp fragment of SV40 DNA containing the last 8 codons of the late virion protein, the 115 bases constituting the 3′-untranslated region, and some flanking DNA. When this clone is microinjected into *Xenopus* oocyte nuclei, it is processed to form a correct 3′ end, polyadenylated, and transported to the cytoplasm. In a 1-day incubation, the same amount of processed mRNA accumulates in the cytoplasm using the 3′-untranslated region sequence clone, as is observed on microinjection of wild-type SV40 DNA. This suggests that the sequences in the 3′-untranslated region contained all of the information necessary to specify the stability of the RNA, and that of the presence of a functional, translatable mRNA sequence was not very important in controlling mRNA degradation.

Most models for regulation of specific mRNA degradation are based on the interaction of cytoplasmic components with regions of secondary structure on the mRNA. The available evidence to support this proposition is modest. Adenovirus early mRNAs are rapidly degraded only in cells that contain a functional DNA-binding protein (Babich and Nevins, 1981). Preliminary evidence suggests that the protein affects the stability of the mRNA through a direct interaction (Nevins, 1983). Obviously, attempts to identify both the proteins and the regions and structures on the mRNA with which they interact represent a major focus for future research.

The demonstration that RNA can act in an autocatalytic way to mediate its own processing (Kruger *et al.*, 1982) raises the possibility that RNA-catalyzed cleavage events may be involved in the degradation of eukaryotic mRNAs. These events could be intramolecular autocatalytic cleavages or intermolecular cleavages catalyzed by small RNAs, whose potential roles may be in sequence recognition and/or cleavage. The roles of small RNA molecules (in SnRNP particles and in RNase P) in RNA processing will be of great interest to studies of mRNA degradation also.

Whether these hypothetical constructs have any basis in physical reality remains to be established. Most of these models make specific predictions that may be amenable to experimental testing. An important problem in this area is the current lack of a functional assay for regulated mRNA degradation that is amenable to manipulation of the RNA and protein components. In the absence of such an assay or of genetic approaches, a correlation between a particular mRNA structure or protein and RNA degradation is all that can be achieved. Most of the possible models for regulated mRNA degradation require at least the beginning of an understanding of mRNA secondary structure. If the structures involved in protein mRNA interaction are more complex than simple stem-and-loop structures, they may be extremely difficult to identify in these relatively large RNAs.

VI. ESTROGEN ACTION IN *XENOPUS* LIVER

The central observation made in these studies is that estrogen has direct and well-defined effects on both the specific transcription of the vitellogenin genes and on the cytoplasmic stability of vitellogenin mRNA. In addition, estrogen has a series of effects on total nuclear RNA synthesis. These three effects can account for the major features of the regulation of vitellogenin mRNA levels by estrogen in *Xenopus* liver.

The data show that vitellogenin RNA synthesis is absolutely dependent on the presence of estrogen. When estrogen is present, vitellogenin gene transcription is activated quite rapidly. Our data suggest that vitellogenin gene transcription can be accounted for by a two-state process, in which the genes are either transcribed at a high rate relative to other genes or are not transcribed at all. This view is supported by our observation that the relative rate of vitellogenin gene transcription remains constant when cells shift from the period of vitellogenin mRNA induction to the plateau phase (Fig. 10) (Brock and Shapiro, 1983b) and when protein synthesis is inhibited by cycloheximide (Table I) (Hayward *et al.*, 1982a). Selective transcription of the vitellogenin genes is not a process susceptible to fine regulatory control. The only reproducible difference in relative vitellogenin transcription rates is that observed in primary versus secondary estrogen stimulation (Fig. 10).

Vitellogenin mRNA stabilization also seems to be a two-state system. The mRNA is extremely stable ($t_{1/2} \sim 3$ weeks) throughout induction in the presence of estrogen and exhibits a degradation rate characteristic of total-cell mRNA ($t_{1/2} = 16$ hours) in the absence of estrogen. There is no significant difference between the stability of the mRNA in primary and secondary stimulation (Brock and Shapiro, 1983b).

These relatively simple on/off responses are insufficient to account for the levels of vitellogenin mRNA during the accumulation and plateau stages of induction. The effects of estrogen on nucleoside triphosphate pools and on total RNA synthesis are required to explain the vitellogenin RNA accumulation profiles. The effects of estrogen on total RNA synthesis are under fine control, with maximum induction of total RNA synthesis observed during periods of maximal vitellogenin mRNA accumulation and minimum rates of total RNA synthesis observed during the plateau period, when levels of vitellogenin mRNA remain essentially constant (Fig. 10).

The half-life of vitellogenin mRNA in estrogen-stimulated liver cells is approximately 3 weeks. This is several times longer than the half-life of any other eukaryotic mRNA whose stability is regulated. Our data on RNA synthetic rates provides a persuasive rationale for the biological utility of this extreme stability. The level of egg-yolk protein production is obviously one of the constraints on the reproductive capacity of *X. laevis*. In order to maximize seasonal vitellogenin production, it is necessary for liver cells to respecialize for high-level production of vitellogenin. A major constraint on this process is that the fully induced rate of RNA synthesis in *Xenopus* cells (which normally exist at 18–22°C) is approximately five times lower than it is in mammalian and avian cells (Brock and Shapiro, 1983a; McKnight and Palmiter, 1979). In order to achieve the same mRNA levels as those of major differentiated products such as globin and ovalbumin, it is necessary for *Xenopus* liver cells to achieve either a higher relative rate of vitellogenin gene transcription or to stabilize vitellogenin mRNA to levels beyond those normally observed in avian or mammalian cells. The relative rate of vitellogenin gene transcription in secondary estrogen stimulation is approximately 4000 ppm (Fig. 10) (Brock and Shapiro, 1983b). This is equal to or higher than relative rates of transcription observed for other regulated eukaryotic genes and may approach the upper limit for selective transcription of a regulated gene. In contrast, vitellogenin mRNA is produced seasonally, and no deleterious consequences attend extreme stabilization of its mRNA. This allows retention of virtually all of the vitellogenin mRNA synthesized during induction and permits accumulation of approximately 50,000 molecules of vitellogenin mRNA per cell.

It is clear that *Xenopus* must regulate the stability of vitellogenin mRNA rather than synthesize an mRNA with extremely high intrinsic stability under all physiologic conditions. Female *Xenopus* synthesize vitellogenin during a 2-month period each year (Deucher, 1975). If vitellogenin mRNA exhibited an intrinsic half-life of 3 weeks under all conditions, it would persist for months after it was needed. The rapid degradation of vitellogenin mRNA after oogenesis allows the liver to devote its full metabolic capacity to normal functions and prevents serum accumulation of a potentially deleterious protein.

VII. SUMMARY

The accumulation of massive amounts of vitellogenin mRNA in estrogen-stimulated *Xenopus* liver cells is not simply the consequence of the activation of vitellogenin gene transcription. The selective activation of vitellogenin gene transcription represents only one of a hierarchy of at least four estrogen-mediated effects. It is only through the interaction of these processes—selective vitellogenin gene transcription, induction of nuclear estrogen receptor, induction of total nuclear RNA synthesis, and stabilization of vitellogenin mRNA against cytoplasmic degradation—that induction of high levels of vitellogenin mRNA in *Xenopus* liver cells is achieved. Now that the identification of these sites of estrogen action has been achieved, the next phase of research in this system will surely focus on elucidation of the mechanism(s) of these processes.

ACKNOWLEDGMENT

The research described in this chapter was supported by grants from the National Science Foundation (PCM 79-20671 and PCM 83-02451) and the American Cancer Society (NP-196). David J. Shapiro was a Research Career Development Awardee from the National Heart Lung and Blood Institute, and Martin L. Brock was a Predoctoral Trainee of the National Institutes of Health.

REFERENCES

Akusjarvi, G., and Persson, H. (1981). *Nature (London)* **292**, 420–426.

Ashburner, M., Chihara, D., Meltzer, P., and Richard, G. (1973). *Cold Spring Harbor Symp. Quant. Biol.* **38**, 655–662.

Aviv, H., Volloch, Z., Bastos, R., and Levis, L. (1976). *Cell* **8**, 493–503.

Babich, A., and Nevins, J. R. (1981). *Cell* **26**, 371–379.

Baker, H. J., and Shapiro, D. J. (1977). *J. Biol. Chem.* **252**, 8434–8438.

Baker, H. J., and Shapiro, D. J. (1978). *J. Biol. Chem.* **253**, 4521–4524.

Bastos, R. N., Volloch, Z., and Aviv, H. (1977). *J. Mol. Biol.* **110**, 191–203.

Berridge, M. V., Farmer, S. R., Green, C. D., Henshaw, E. C., and Tata, J. R. (1976). *Eur. J. Biochem.* **62**, 161–171.

Billing, R. J., Barbiroli, B., and Smellie, R. M. S. (1969). *Biochim. Biophys. Acta* **190**, 60–65.

Blumenthal, T. (1980). *Proc. Natl. Acad. Sci. U.S.A.* **77**, 2601–2605.

Blumenthal, T., and Hill, D. (1980). *J. Biol. Chem.* **258**, 5449–5455.

Brawerman, G. (1981). *CRC Crit. Rev. Biochem.* **10**, 1–38.

Brock, M. L. (1983). Ph.D. Thesis, University of Illinois, Urbana.

Brock, M. L., and Shapiro, D. J. (1983a). *J. Biol. Chem.* **258**, 5449–5455.

Brock, M. L., and Shapiro, D. J. (1983b). *Cell* **34**, 207–214.

Chung, S., Landfear, S. M., Blumberg, D. D., Cohen, N. S., and Lodish, H. F. (1981). *Cell* **24**, 795–797.

Croall, D. E. (1982). *Biochim. Biophys. Acta* **714**, 200–208.

Darnell, J. E. (1982). *Nature (London)* **297**, 365–371.

Deeley, R. G., and Goldberger, R. F. (1979). *In* "Ontogeny of Receptors and Reproductive Hormone Action" (T. H. Hamilton, J. H. Clark, and W. A. Sadler, eds.), pp. 291–307. Raven Press, New York.

Derman, E., Krauter, K., Walling, L., Weinberger, C., Ray, M., and Darnell, J. E., Jr. (1981). *Cell* **23**, 731–739.

Deucher, E. M. (1975). "Xenopus: The South African Clawed Frog." Wiley, London.

Ernest, M. J. (1982). *Biochemistry* 21, 6761–6767.

Felber, B. K., Ryffel, G. U., and Weber, R. W. (1978). *Mol. Cell. Endocrinol.* 12, 151–166.

Galau, G. A., Lipson, E. D., Britten, R. J., and Davidson, E. H. (1977). *Cell* 10, 415–432.

Gallwitz, D. (1975). *Nature (London)* 257, 247–249.

Germond, J. E., ten Heggeler, B., Schubiger, J.-L., Walker, P., Westley, B., and Wahli, W. (1983). *Nucleic Acids Res.* 11, 2979–2997.

Green, C. D., and Tata, J. R. (1976). *Cell* 7, 131–139.

Greenberg, J. B. (1972). *Nature (London)* 240, 102–104.

Grollman, A. P. (1968). *J. Biol. Chem.* 243, 4089–4093.

Guyette, W. A., Matusik, R. J., and Rosen, J. M. (1979). *Cell* 17, 1013–1023.

Harpold, M. M., Evans, R. M., Salditt-Georgieff, M., and Darnell, J. E. (1979). *Cell* 17, 1025–1035.

Hayward, M. A., and Shapiro, D. J. (1981). *Dev. Biol.* 88, 333–340.

Hayward, M. A., Mitchell, T. A., and Shapiro, D. J. (1980). *J. Biol. Chem.* 255, 11308–11312.

Hayward, M. A., Brock, M. L., and Shapiro, D. J. (1982a). *Am. J. Physiol.* 243(12) C1–C6.

Hayward, M. A., Brock, M. L., and Shapiro, D. J. (1982b). *Nucleic Acids Res.* 10, 8273–8284.

Hereford, L. M., Osley, M. A., Ludwig, J. R., and McLaughlin, C. S. (1981). *Cell* 24, 367–375.

Hereford, L. M., Bromley, S., and Osley, M. A. (1982). *Cell* 30, 305–310.

Holmes, W. M., Platt, T. P., and Rosenberg, M. (1983). *Cell* 32, 1029–1032.

Huez, G., Marbaix, G., Hubert, E., Cleuter, Y., LeClercq, M., Chantrenne, H., Devos, R., Soreq, H., Nudel, U., and Littauer, U. Z. (1975). *Eur. J. Biochem.* 59, 589–592.

Huez, G., Marbaix, G., Gallwitz, D., Weinberg, E., Devos, R., Hubert, E., and Cleuter, Y. (1978). *Nature (London)* 271, 572–573.

Hynes, N. E., Groner, B., Sippel, A. E., Jeep, S., Wurtz, T., Ngu, Y.-H., Giesecke, K., and Schutz, G. (1979). *Biochemistry* 18, 616–624.

Jungmann, R. A., Kelley, D. C., Miles, M. F., and Milkowski, D. M. (1983). *J. Biol. Chem.* 258, 5312–5318.

Kafatos, F. (1972). *Acta Endocrinol. (Copenhagen), Suppl.* 168, 319–345.

Kenney, F. T., Lee, K., and Stiles, C. D. (1972). *Acta Endocrinol. (Copenhagen) Suppl.* 168, 369–376.

King, W. J., and Green, G. L. (1984). *Nature (London)* 307, 745–747.

Kruger, J., Grabowski, P. J., Zaug, A. J., Sands, J., Gottschling, D. E., and Cech, T. R. (1982). *Cell* 31, 147–157.

Lodish, H. F. (1971). *J. Biol. Chem.* 246, 7131–7138.

McKnight, G. S., and Palmiter, R. D. (1979). *J. Biol. Chem.* 254, 9050–9058.

McKnight, G. S., Lee, D. C., and Palmiter, R. D. (1980). *J. Biol. Chem.* 255, 148–153.

Marbaix, G., Huez, G., Burny, A., Cleuter, Y., Hubert, E., LeClercq, M., Chantrenne, H., Soreq, H., Nudel, U., and Littauer, U. Z. (1975). *Proc. Natl. Acad. Sci. U.S.A.* 72, 3065–3067.

Nevins, J. R. (1983). *Annu. Rev. Biochem.* 52, 462.

Page, M. J., and Parker, M. G. (1982). *Mol. Cell. Endocrinol.* 27, 343–355.

Palmiter, R. D., and Carey, N. H. (1974). *Proc. Natl. Acad. Sci. U.S.A.* 71, 2357–2361.

Pearson, N. J., Fried, H. M., and Warner, J. R. (1982). *Cell* 29, 347–355.

Perry, R. P., and Kelley, D. E. (1973). *J. Mol. Biol.* 79, 681–696.

Raj, N. B. K., and Pitha, P. M. (1983). *Proc. Natl. Acad. Sci. U.S.A.* 80, 3923–3927.

Rosenberg, M., and Schmeissner, V. (1982). *In* "Interaction of Translational and Transcriptional Controls in the Regulation of Gene Expression" (M. Grunberg-Manago and B. Safer, eds.), p. 1–25. Am. Elsevier, New York.

Ryffel, G. U. (1978). *Mol. Cell. Endocrinol.* 12, 237–246.

Sameshima, M., Liebhaber, S. A., and Schlessinger, D. (1981). *Mol. Cell. Biol.* 1, 75–81.

Schimke, R. T. (1970). *In* "Mammalian Protein Metabolism" (H. N. Munro and J. B. Allison, eds.), Vol. 4, pp. 117–227. Academic Press, New York.

Searle, P. F., and Tata, J. R. (1981). *Cell* **23**, 741–746.

Shapiro, D. J. (1982). *CRC Crit. Rev. Biochem.* **12**, 187–203.

Shapiro, D. J., and Baker, H. J. (1977). *J. Biol. Chem.* **252**, 5244–5250.

Shapiro, D. J., and Baker, H. J. (1979). *In* "Ontogeny of Receptors and Reproductive Hormone Action" (T. H. Hamilton, J. H. Clark, and W. A. Sadler, eds.), pp. 309–330. Raven Press, New York.

Shapiro, D. J., Baker, H. J., and Stitt, D. T. (1976). *J. Biol. Chem.* **251**, 3105–3111.

Shapiro, D. J., Brock, M. L., and Hayward, M. A. (1983). *In* "Gene Regulation by Steroid Hormones II" (A. K. Roy and J. H. Clark, eds.), pp. 61–78. Springer-Verlag, Berlin and New York.

Shepherd, J. H., Mulvihill, E. R., Thomas, P. S., and Palmiter, R. D. (1980). *J. Cell Biol.* **87**, 142–151.

Tata, J. R. (1976). *Cell* **9**, 1–14.

Tata, J. R., and Baker, B. (1976). *Biochem. J.* **150**, 345–355.

Tata, J. R., and Smith, D. F. (1979). *Recent Prog. Horm. Res.* **35**, 47–95.

Tenniswood, M. P. R., Searly, P. F., Wolffe, A. P., and Tata, J. R. (1983). *Mol. Cell. Endocrinol.* **30**, 329–345.

Thomas, P. S., Shepherd, J. H., Mulvihill, E. R., and Palmiter, R. D. (1981). *J. Mol. Biol.* **150**, 143–166.

Tsai, S. Y., Tsai, M. J., Lin, C. T., and O'Malley, B. W. (1979). *Biochemistry* **18**, 5726–5731.

Wahli, W., Wyler, T., Weber, R., and Ryffel, G. U. (1976). *Eur. J. Biochem.* **66**, 457.

Wahli, W., Ryffel, G. U., Wyler, T., Jaggi, R. B., Weber, R., and Dawid, I. B. (1978). *Dev. Biol.* **67**, 371–383.

Wahli, W., Dawid, I. B., Wyler, T., Jaggi, R. B., Weber, R., and Ryffel, G. U. (1979). *Cell* **16**, 535–549.

Wahli, W., Dawid, I. B., Wyler, T., Weber, R., and Ryffel, G. U. (1980). *Cell* **20**, 107–117.

Wahli, W., Dawid, I. B., Ryffel, G. U., and Weber, R. (1981). *Science* **212**, 298–304.

Wahli, W., Germond, J.-E., ten Heggeler, B., and May, F. E. B. (1982). *Proc. Natl. Acad. Sci. U.S.A.* **79**, 6832–6836.

Wangh, L. J., and Knowland, J. (1975). *Proc. Natl. Acad. Sci. U.S.A.* **72**, 3172–3175.

Wangh, L. J., and Schneider, W. (1982). *Dev. Biol.* **89**, 287–293.

Wangh, L. J., Osborne, J. A., Hentschel, C. C., and Tilly, R. (1979). *Dev. Biol.* **70**, 479–499.

Welshons, W. V., Lieberman, M. E., and Gorski, J. (1984). *Nature* **307**, 747–748.

Westley, B., and Knowland, J. (1978). *Cell* **15**, 367–374.

Westley, B., and Knowland, J. (1979). *Biochem. Biophys. Res. Commun.* **88**, 1167–1172.

Wickens, M. (1984). In preparation.

Wiley, W. H., and Wallace, R. A. (1978). *Biochem. Biophys. Res. Commun.* **85**, 153–159.

Wilson, M. C., and Darnell, J. E., Jr. (1981). *J. Mol. Biol.* **148**, 231–251.

Wiskocil, R., Bensky, P., Dower, W., Goldberger, R. F., Gordon, J. I., and Deeley, R. G. (1980). *Proc. Natl. Acad. Sci. U.S.A.* **77**, 4474–4478.

Witliffe, J. L., Lee, K., and Kenney, F. T. (1972). *Biochim. Biophys. Acta* **269**, 493–504.

Wolffe, A. P., and Tata, J. R. (1983). *Eur. J. Biochem.* **130**, 365–372.

Zak, R., Martin, A. F., and Blough, R. (1979). *Physiol. Rev.* **59**, 407–447.

Zeevi, M., Nevins, J. R., and Darnell, J. E. (1981). *Cell* **26**, 39–46.

Zeevi, M., Nevins, J. R., and Darnell, J. E. (1982). *Mol. Cell. Biol.* **2**, 517–525.

CHAPTER 6

Regulation of Growth Hormone and Prolactin Gene Expression by Hormones and Calcium*

Carter Bancroft, Gregory G. Gick, Marcia E. Johnson, and Bruce A. White†

Molecular Biology and Virology Department
Sloan Kettering Institute
New York, New York

*Abbreviations: T_3, triiodothyronine; GRF, human pancreatic growth hormone–releasing factor; TRH, thyrotropin-releasing hormone; EGF, epidermal growth factor; EGTA, ethylene glycol bis (β-aminoethyl ether)-N,N,N',N'-tetraacetic acid.

†Present address: Department of Anatomy, University of Connecticut Health Center, Farmington, Connecticut 06032.

BIOCHEMICAL ACTIONS OF HORMONES, VOL. XII

I. INTRODUCTION

For studies of hormonal regulation of specific gene expression, it is useful to have available homogeneous populations of hormonally responsive cells. The GH cells are related clonal lines of rat pituitary tumor cells that produce the pituitary polypeptides growth hormone and prolactin. In addition, the GH cells have a property that is quite unusual among functional cell lines: synthesis of these two polypeptide hormones can be strongly regulated by adding to the culture medium a variety of hormones and other factors that regulate pituitary function in the intact animal (Bancroft, 1981). In this chapter, we first (Section II) describe the origins and properties of the various GH cell lines that are currently employed for hormonal regulation studies. In Section III, we describe the development of a convenient cytoplasmic dot hybridization technique for the simultaneous analysis of relative levels of a specific mRNA sequence in multiple samples. In the following section (Section IV), we describe studies of the regulation by glucocorticoid and thyroid hormones of growth hormone gene expression in GH cells, with particular emphasis on the question of the dependence of glucocorticoid action on the presence of thyroid hormones and insulin. Finally (Section V), we describe our recent investigations of the role of calcium ion, both as a regulator of prolactin gene expression and as a mediator of the action of peptide hormones on expression of the prolactin gene.

II. CELL LINES CURRENTLY EMPLOYED TO STUDY REGULATION OF GROWTH HORMONE AND PROLACTIN

A number of related cell lines that produce growth hormone and/or prolactin (designated collectively as GH cells) are currently employed for hormonal regulation studies. Differences among these cell lines may account, to some extent, for differences in the results by various groups, described in the following sections. The origins and properties of these various lines have been described (Bancroft, 1981). Briefly, the GH_3 and GH_1 cells were cloned from pituitary tumor cells transferred twice or four times, respectively, between animal and tissue culture. The GC and GH_4C_1 cells are cloned variants of the GH_3 cells, which produce low or undetectable amounts of prolactin and growth hormone, respectively. Because the GH_3 cells are not variant cell lines and thus are presumably one step closer to their normal counterparts, and because they produce both growth hormone and prolactin, we have employed these cells for all of our regulation studies. It should also be noted that our regulation studies have been performed with GH_3 cells incubated in suspension culture, whereas many such studies by other groups with GH cells have employed monolayer culture conditions.

In the past, indirect evidence has indicated that growth hormone and prolactin are produced by different pituitary cell types, designated somatotropes and mammotropes, respectively (Daughaday, 1981). Since the GH_3 cells produce both of these hormones, it has been suggested that the normal precursors of these cells produce only one of these hormones, and that production of the other represents an inappropriate function induced by the neoplastic state of the cells (Bancroft, 1981; Ivarie and Morris, 1983). However, Frawley and Neil (1983) have recently employed a newly developed reverse hemolytic plaque assay to show that pituitaries contain a large number of cells that secrete both growth hormone and prolactin, which they designate *somatomammotropes*. In light of this evidence, it now appears more likely that the GH_3 cells are derived from normal somatomammotropes and have thus retained the normal ability of this cell type to produce both growth hormone and prolactin.

A number of hormones and other factors have opposite effects on prolactin and growth hormone mRNA levels in GH cells (Bancroft, 1981). It has been suggested previously that this observation might be simply explained if the corresponding genes were adjacent and coordinately regulated (Bancroft, 1981). However, we have recently employed direct hybridization *in situ* with ^{125}I-labeled cDNA plasmids to show that the prolactin and growth hormone genes in the rat reside on different chromosomes (Gerhard *et al.*, 1984). This observation clearly rules out any such simple model for coordinate regulation of expression of these two genes.

III. DEVELOPMENT OF A CYTOPLASMIC DOT HYBRIDIZATION TECHNIQUE FOR STUDIES OF mRNA REGULATION

For many types of regulation studies, it would be useful to have available a convenient technique for the simultaneous analysis of relative levels of a specific mRNA sequence in multiple samples. For example, in endocrine studies at the molecular level, such a technique would be useful for carrying out replicate determinations of the time course or dose–response curve of the effect of single or multiple hormones on levels of one or more specific mRNAs. In this section, we describe the development and characterization of such a technique. Experimental details are described in White and Bancroft (1982).

It has been shown previously that RNA will bind efficiently to nitrocellulose in the presence of a high concentration of salt ($3M$ NaCl), and that this RNA will hybridize efficiently to a complementary probe (Thomas, 1980). Since one of the more time-consuming and possibly variable steps in the analysis of relative levels of an mRNA in the cytoplasm of a cell is isolation of the RNA, we investigated whether the analysis could be performed with unfractionated cytoplasmic preparations. Cytoplasmic samples were prepared by treatment of GH_3 cells with a nonionic detergent, NP-40 (Borun *et al.*, 1967), followed by pelleting of the nuclei. The samples were then heated (65°C, 15 minutes) in the presence of high salt and formaldehyde or glyoxal, dotted onto nitrocellulose, and baked (80°C, 90 minutes) to attach the RNA irreversibly. The nitrocellulose was then hybridized with

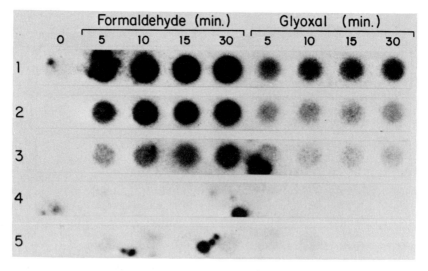

FIG. 1. Detection by cytoplasmic dot hybridization of prolactin mRNA in GH_3 cells. Rows 1–3: cytoplasm prepared from 4, 2, and 1×10^5 GH_3 cells, respectively, were either untreated (0) or heated with formaldehyde or glyoxal as described in the text. Row 4: same as row 1, except that samples were treated with RNase. Row 5: same as row 1, except that GC cells were substituted for GH_3 cells. Dotting of samples and hybridization analysis were as described in the text. [From White and Bancroft (1982).]

[32]P-labeled prolactin cDNA plasmid, employing a standard hybridization protocol (Dobner *et al.*, 1981).

Figure 1 shows that prolactin mRNA can be readily detected in cytoplasmic preparations from $1-4 \times 10^5$ GH$_3$ cells, but only if the preparations are denatured first by heating in the presence of formaldehyde or glyoxal. It is not presently clear why this treatment increases the signal so dramatically, but it may result from release of mRNA from macromolecular complexes by these denaturing agents. Since formaldehyde treatment yielded a larger signal, it has been employed in our standard procedure. With this procedure, cytoplasmic dot hybridization appears to be as sensitive as RNA dot

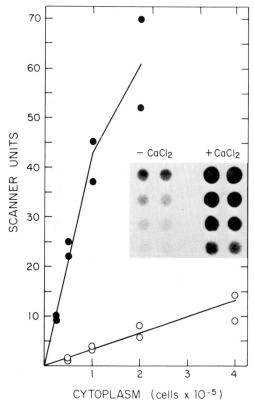

FIG. 2. Quantitation by cytoplasmic dot hybridization of prolactin mRNA induction in GH$_3$ cells. GH$_3$ cells were incubated in serum-free medium for 5 days plus (●———●) or minus (○———○) CaCl$_2$ (0.4 m*M*). Cytoplasmic aliquots from the indicated number of cells from each culture were analyzed in duplicate. The inset shows the autoradiographic spots employed for the analysis. [From White and Bancroft (1982).]

hybridization for detecting prolactin mRNA in the GH_3 cells (White and Bancroft, 1982). Figure 1 also demonstrates the specificity of the technique, since the signal was virtually abolished if the samples were RNase-treated (row 4) or if the prolactin mRNA-deficient GC cells (Bancroft, 1973, 1981) were substituted for GH_3 cells (row 5).

Figure 2 illustrates the use of this technique to quantitate an induction: the stimulation by Ca^{2+} of prolactin mRNA (see Section V). At a sufficiently low input of cytoplasm, the spot intensities were proportional to the amount of cytoplasm for cells incubated plus or minus Ca^{2+}, so that the stimulation of prolactin mRNA (14-fold) could be calculated from the slopes of the lines shown. Figure 2 also shows that this technique can be employed to detect the prolactin mRNA sequences in cytoplasm prepared from 10^5 GH_3 cells incubated under these conditions, or about 0.1–0.2 ml of a suspension culture of these cells.

The use of this technique to detect prolactin mRNA in cytoplasm prepared from pituitary glands is shown in Fig. 3. The prolactin mRNA present in 1/50 or 1/100 of a male or female rat pituitary (about 100–200 µg of tissue) can be readily detected.

Thus cytoplasmic dot hybridization can be employed for the convenient analysis of relative prolactin mRNA levels in multiple samples of cytoplasm prepared from very small amounts of pituitary cells or tissue. As described in the following sections, we have employed this technique in our recent regulation studies to follow relative levels of prolactin and growth hormone mRNA sequences in cultures of GH_3 cells and normal pituitary cells. Recent

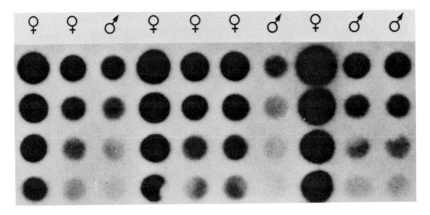

FIG. 3. Analysis by cytoplasmic dot hybridization of prolactin mRNA in rat hemipituitaries. Cytoplasmic aliquots were prepared from cultured hemipituitaries from single male (♂) or female (♀) rats. Rows 1–4 received cytoplasmic aliquots corresponding to approximately 1/12.5, 1/25, 1/50, and 1/100, respectively, of a rat pituitary. [From White and Bancroft, (1982).]

reports indicate that the technique can be employed in analogous regulation studies with other systems (Burch *et al.*, 1983; Cochran *et al.*, 1983).

IV. REGULATION BY GLUCOCORTICOID AND THYROID HORMONES OF GROWTH HORMONE GENE EXPRESSION

A. INTRODUCTION

The regulation of growth hormone production by glucocorticoid and thyroid hormones appears to be mediated by specific intracellular receptors located in the cytoplasm and nucleus, respectively (Samuels *et al.*, 1983). The regulation by these hormones of growth hormone production *in vivo* has been recently reviewed by Samuels *et al.* (1983).

The first studies of hormone action with GH cells involved the demonstration that cortisol increased growth hormone production by either GH_3 cells (Bancroft *et al.*, 1969) or GH_1 cells (Kohler *et al.*, 1969). Shortly thereafter, an inhibition by cortisol of prolactin production by GH_3 cells was reported (Tashjian *et al.*, 1970). Studies of thyroid hormone action on protein hormone production by the GH cells began with the demonstration by Tsai and Samuels (1974) that, when GH_1 cells are incubated in a medium containing hypothyroid serum, T_3 increases growth hormone production and cellular growth and decreases prolactin production.

Subsequently, studies were carried out of the regulation by these hormones of growth hormone synthesis by GH cells. Growth hormone synthesis was assayed by briefly exposing GH cells to [^{3}H]leucine, followed by immunoprecipitation of intracellular growth hormone with a highly specific antiserum raised in baboons (Bancroft, 1973). Pulse and pulse-chase studies showed that newly synthesized growth hormone is not degraded intracellularly or extracellularly by GH_3 cells (Yu *et al.*, 1977; Samuels and Shapiro, 1976). A synthetic glucocorticoid, dexamethasone, was shown to stimulate relative growth hormone synthesis (growth hormone synthesis ÷ total protein synthesis) by GH_3 cells incubated in a medium containing normal fetal calf serum, to a maximum of 8- to 14-fold by 48 hours (Yu *et al.*, 1977). Similar experiments with GH_1 cells incubated in a medium containing hypothyroid calf serum showed that T_3 stimulates relative growth hormone synthesis to a maximum of about threefold by 21 hours (Samuels and Shapiro, 1976), and that cortisol is unable to stimulate growth hormone synthesis during a 48-hour incubation period unless T_3 is also present (Samuels *et al.*, 1977).

In experiments involving detection and quantitation of growth hormone mRNA by translation *in vitro*, it was shown that dexamethasone stimulates growth hormone mRNA levels in GH_3 cells incubated in a medium containing normal fetal calf serum, and that the size of growth hormone mRNA was about 1060 nucleotides (Tushinski *et al.*, 1977). Analysis of the translation product of growth hormone mRNA showed that growth hormone is synthesized in the form of a precursor, designated *pregrowth hormone* (Sussman *et al.*, 1976; Bancroft *et al.*, 1980a). Similar *in vitro* translation experiments with RNA isolated from either GC cells (Martial *et al.*, 1977) or GH_1 cells (Samuels *et al.*, 1979) incubated in a medium containing hypothyroid serum showed that, under these incubation conditions, glucocorticoids will not stimulate growth hormone mRNA levels unless T_3 is also present. However, in one of these studies (Samuels *et al.*, 1979), it was observed that cortisol alone yielded a moderate (two- to threefold) increase in growth hormone synthesis, which was detectable only after 48 hours of incubation of GH_1 cells in medium containing hypothyroid, hyposteroid medium, or in serum-free medium.

Quite recently, we have carried out studies of the regulation by human pancreatic growth hormone–releasing factor (GRF) of growth hormone and prolactin gene expression, both in primary cultures of rat pituitary cells and in the GH_3 cells. We have observed that, in primary pituitary cell cultures, exposure to GRF causes a 2.0 to 2.5-fold increase in growth hormone mRNA levels, with no detectable effect on prolactin mRNA levels (Gick *et al.*, 1984). Thus, in normal pituitary cells, GRF functions not only as a secretogogue for growth hormone, but also as a regulator of growth hormone gene expression. By contrast, in experiments performed under a number of different conditions, we have been unable to detect any effect of GRF on either growth hormone secretion or mRNA levels in the GH_3 cells (Zeytin *et al.*, 1984). It thus appears that, although the GH_3 cells respond to a variety of stimuli, they are unable to respond to this important physiological regulator of growth hormone production. This is probably due to a lack of GRF receptors in these cells. It has not yet been technically possible to assay GRF receptors. However, the recent evidence for GRF receptors associated with pituitary secretory granules (Lewin *et al.*, 1983), together with the observation that a GH cell line (GC) is virtually devoid of secretory granules (Masur *et al.*, 1974), supports this concept.

B. GLUCOCORTICOID AND THYROID HORMONES CAN INDEPENDENTLY REGULATE GROWTH HORMONE GENE EXPRESSION

As discussed in the previous section, investigations by a number of groups showed that glucocorticoid and thyroid hormones stimulate growth hormone synthesis by various GH cell lines, and that this stimulation is accompanied by corresponding increases in translatable growth hormone mRNA. Reports by two groups also suggested that glucocorticoid hormones cannot induce a significant stimulation of either growth hormone synthesis or growth hormone mRNA levels in the GH cells unless thyroid hormone is also present.

We have investigated further the regulation by glucocorticoid and thyroid hormones of growth hormone gene expression by the GH_3 cells. For these studies we employed a low serum "induction medium" containing a serum supplement (Bauer *et al.*, 1976) modified by omitting all hormones, plus 1% fetal calf serum. The serum employed was extracted first with Dowex 1-X10 to remove thyroid hormones (Samuels *et al.*, 1979) and then with activated charcoal to remove steroid hormones (Yu *et al.*, 1977). Analysis with added radioactive hormones showed that this protocol removed from the serum 98.2% and 97.6% of the endogenous thyroid and glucocorticoid hormones, respectively; analysis by radioimmunoassay showed that T_3 levels in the serum were reduced to undetectable levels (<5 ng/100 ml) (Dobner *et al.*, 1981). Hormonal effects were studied by incubating suspension cultures of GH_3 cells in this medium for 3 days to remove glucocorticoid and thyroid hormones from the cells and to lower cellular levels of growth hormone RNA sequences; they were then incubated an additional 3 days in the presence or absence of T_3 (50 nM) and/or dexamethasone (80 nM). Relative growth hormone synthesis and translatable growth hormone mRNA were assayed as described (Dobner *et al.*, 1981). A rat growth hormone cDNA plasmid, pBR322-GH_1 (Harpold *et al.*, 1978), was employed to assay directly hormonal regulation of cytoplasmic and nuclear growth hormone RNA sequence levels.

Table I shows that T_3, dexamethasone, or both hormones together yielded stimulations of growth hormone synthesis of 3-, 14-, and 9-fold, respectively. The stimulation of translatable growth hormone mRNA in these cultures closely paralleled the stimulation of growth hormone synthesis (Table I). In a number of similar experiments, we have consistently observed that dexamethasone alone yields a large stimulation of growth hormone synthesis. Furthermore, we have detected no consistent difference between the stimulation by dexamethasone alone and by dexamethasone plus T_3. Although the presence of both hormones usually yielded a somewhat greater stimulation than did dexamethasone alone, we have occasionally observed, as in the experiment analyzed in detail in Table I, that the stimulation of growth hormone synthesis by T_3 plus dexamethasone was actually lower than that obtained with dexamethasone alone. Thus, under our experimental conditions, dexamethasone is capable of causing a large stimulation of growth hormone synthesis that is apparently independent of T_3.

An RNA gel blot hybridization procedure was employed to investigate whether the hormonal stimulations described previously arose from increase

Carter Bancroft et al.

TABLE I

STIMULATION BY DEXAMETHASONE AND T_3 OF GROWTH HORMONE SYNTHESIS
AND mRNA LEVELS IN GH_3 CELLS[a,b,c]

Condition	Relative GH synthesis (hormone/control)	pGH mRNA (hormone/control)		
		Translation	RNA gel	RNA dot
Control	1	1	1	1
+ T3	3.3	2.2	3.4	4.5
+ dex	13.9	15.7	22.5	21.3
+ T3 + dex	9.3	10.1	11.4	15.4

[a]From Dobner et al. (1981).

[b]For each experimental condition, cytoplasmic RNA was extracted and relative GH synthesis was measured simultaneously in aliquots of cells from the same suspension culture. In control cells, relative GH synthesis was 0.8%; when assayed by translation, pGH mRNA was 1.8% of total cytoplasmic RNA.

[c]Abbreviations: Dex, dexamethasone; pGH mRNA, pregrowth hormone mRNA; RNA gel, RNA gel blot hybridization; RNA dot, RNA dot hybridization.

in cytoplasmic growth hormone mRNA sequences (Dobner et al., 1981). Figure 4 illustrates that total cytoplasmic RNA isolated from control cells (lanes a, b, and c) contained a single 1.0-kilobase (kb) growth hormone mRNA band, and that increased amounts of growth hormone mRNA, indistinguishable in size from that observed in control cells, were observed in cells incubated with T_3 (lanes d, e, and f), dexamethasone (lanes g, h, and i), or T_3 plus dexamethasone (lanes j, k, and l). Quantitative analysis of the results illustrated in Fig. 4 showed that the stimulation of cytoplasmic growth hormone mRNA paralleled the stimulation of growth hormone synthesis (Table I). In addition, quantitation of relative levels of cytoplasmic growth hormone mRNA by an RNA dot hybridization procedure (Dobner et al., 1981) yielded results in good agreement with those obtained by RNA gel blot hybridization (Table I).

To investigate further the regulation by T_3 and dexamethasone of growth hormone gene expression, the hormonal regulation of the accumulation of nuclear growth hormone RNA sequences was examined by RNA gel blot hybridization. Figure 5 illustrates that incubation of GH_3 cells with either T_3 (lanes d and e), dexamethasone (lanes g and h), or T_3 plus dexamethasone (lanes j and k) led to increased accumulation of two nuclear growth hormone RNA sequences about 1.0 and 2.7 kb in size respectively. As discussed further in Dobner et al. (1981), it is possible that some of the material in the 1.0-kb band arose from slight cytoplasmic contamination of our nuclear preprarations. However, it is clear that the 2.7-kb band is entirely a nuclear RNA species, since it is not detected in cytoplasm from the same cells (see

Fig. 5, lanes c, f, i, and l). Figure 5 shows that accumulation of the 2.7-kb band paralleled accumulation of cytoplasmic growth hormone mRNA under the three conditions of hormonal stimulation examined. Since the apparent size of this band approximates the size of the rat growth hormone gene (about 2.1 kbp) (Chien and Thompson, 1980; Barta *et al.*, 1981; Page *et al.*, 1981), we assume that the 2.7-kb band represents the primary transcript of the growth hormone gene. Thus, the results in Fig. 5 strongly imply that T_3 and dexamethasone can regulate expression of the growth hormone gene at

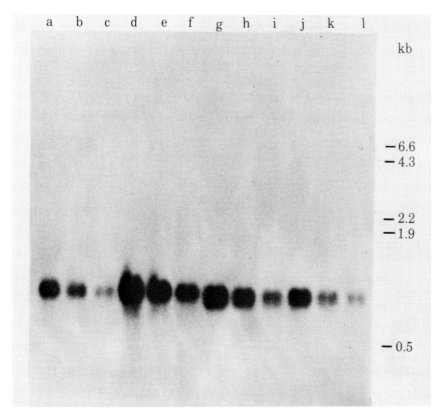

FIG. 4. Analysis of growth hormone mRNA sequences in total cytoplasmic RNA from control and hormone-treated GH_3 cells. RNA was subjected to gel electrophoresis under denaturing conditions, hybridized to a ^{32}P-labeled GH cDNA plasmid, and autoradiographed. The lanes contained RNA from control cells (a, 10 μg; b, 5 μg; c, 2.5 μg) or from cells grown in the presence of T_3 (d, 10 μg; e, 5 μg; f, 2.5 μg), dexamethasone (g, 1 μg; h, 0.5 μg; i, 0.25 μg), or T_3 plus dexamethasone (j, 1 μg; k, 0.5 μg; l, 0.25 μg). Note that the amounts of RNA applied from cells grown under the first two conditions were tenfold higher than for cells grown under the second two conditions. [From Dobner *et al.* (1981).]

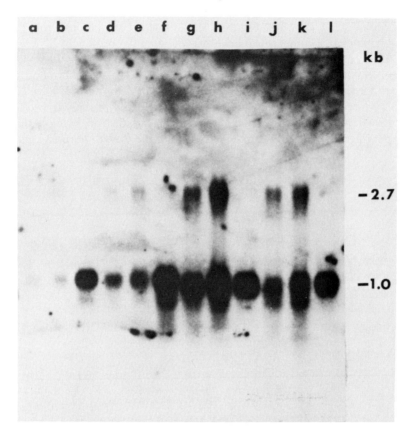

FIG. 5. Analysis of growth hormone mRNA sequences in total nuclear RNA from control and hormone-treated GH_3 cells. Nuclear RNA was isolated from the cultures described in Fig. 4 and analyzed as in Fig. 4. The lanes contained nuclear RNA from control cells (a, 10 μg; b, 20 μg) or from cells grown in the presence of T_3 (d, 10 μg; e, 20 μg), dexamethasone (g, 10 μg; h, 20 μg), or T_3 plus dexamethasone (j, 10 μg; k, 20 μg). For comparison, total cytoplasmic RNA from control cells (c, 10 μg), or from cells grown in the presence of T_3 (f, 10 μg), dexamethasone (i, 1 μg), or T_3 plus dexamethasone (l, 1 μg) was analyzed. [From Dobner *et al.* (1981).]

the level of transcription. Recent experiments by two groups (Spindler *et al.*, 1982; Evans *et al.*, 1982), employing a nuclear run-on transcription assay, have confirmed the ability of T_3 and dexamethasone to regulate growth hormone gene transcription in the GC cells. One of these studies (Evans *et al.*, 1982) employed a low-serum medium similar to the induction medium described above. In agreement with our observations, Evans *et al.* (1982) found that under these conditions T_3 and dexamethasone act independently to regulate growth hormone gene expression.

It should be noted finally that the GC cells have been reported to contain nuclear growth hormone RNA species as large as six to seven kb (Maurer *et al.*, 1980), i.e., considerably larger than the known size of the growth hormone gene. Hence, the size of the primary transcript of the growth hormone gene is at present unclear. This issue can be resolved definitively only by a kinetic analysis of the precursor–product relationship between these various large nuclear growth hormone RNA species and mature cytoplasmic growth hormone mRNA. To date, such an analysis has not been technically feasible.

C. Inability of Insulin to Block the Stimulation by Dexamethasone of Growth Hormone mRNA or Synthesis

In the preceding sections, we have shown that, when GH_3 cells are incubated in a low-serum (1%) medium, dexamethasone alone is capable of causing a large stimulation of growth hormone synthesis and mRNA. This finding is discordant with previous results, which showed that, when GH- cells are incubated in a medium containing 10% hypothyroid serum, a significant glucorticoid hormone stimulation of growth hormone synthesis or mRNA is not observed unless T_3 is also present (Samuels *et al.*, 1977, 1979; Martial *et al.*, 1977; Shapiro *et al.*, 1978). It could be that these differences arise from the presence of high serum concentrations in the culture medium employed for the latter investigations compared to the low serum concentration in our induction medium. Thus, serum might contain a component that inhibits the stimulation by glucocorticoids of growth hormone synthesis, and this inhibition could itself be blocked by T_3. A report by Ivarie *et al.* (1981) supported this concept and suggested that the proposed component is insulin (or an associated or insulinlike activity). These workers employed medium quite similar to our induction medium, but lacking serum. In agreement with the results described in the previous section, they found that under these conditions dexamethasone alone causes a substantial stimulation of growth hormone synthesis by GH_3 cells. However, when insulin was present at a high concentration (10 µg/ml, 24 units/mg) in the medium, dexamethasone was unable to affect the synthesis of growth hormone. No effect of insulin itself on growth hormone synthesis was observed (Ivarie *et al.*, 1981).

This is an attractive hypothesis, since it could explain the discordant observations described previously. In addition, it suggests a role in growth hormone gene expression for the insulin receptors on GH_3 cells that have recently been identified and characterized (Corin *et al.*, 1983). Hence, we have investigated whether insulin can block the stimulation by dexametha-

sone of growth hormone mRNA sequences or growth hormone synthesis in
GH_3 cells incubated in a serum-free medium.

Insulin at various final concentrations (1 ng/ml to 10 μg/ml) was added to
cultures 2 days prior to addition of dexamethasone $(10^{-7}\ M)$. Figure 6 is an
autoradiograph of the result of analyzing such an experiment by cytoplasmic
dot hybridization, and Fig. 7 shows the quantitation of the results. Consistent with the observations of Ivarie *et al.* (1981), in a serum-free medium
dexamethasone alone causes a large stimulation of growth hormone mRNA
in GH_3 cells. However, at no concentration of insulin tested was there a
marked inhibition of the stimulation by dexamethasone of growth hormone
mRNA. At the high insulin concentration (10 μg/ml) examined by Ivarie *et
al.* (1981), there was a slight (27%) inhibition of the dexamethasone induc-

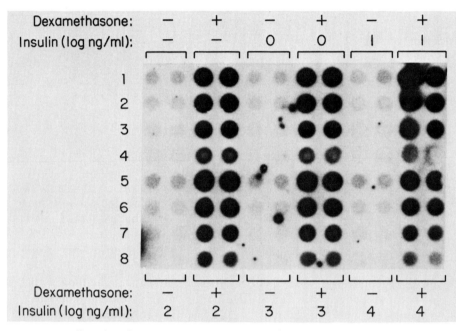

FIG. 6. Effect of insulin at various concentrations on the stimulation by dexamethasone of
growth hormone mRNA. GH_3 cells were incubated for 2 days in serum-free medium (White *et
al.*, 1981) containing 0.4 mM $CaCl_2$ plus the indicated concentrations of insulin [Bovine pancreas (Sigma), 26.4 I.U. per mg] and then incubated for an additional 3 days in the presence or
absence of dexamethasone $(10^{-7}\ M)$. Relative growth hormone mRNA levels were then analyzed by cytoplasmic dot hybridization (White and Bancroft, 1982).

Rows 1–4 and 5–8 represent, respectively, twofold serial dilutions of cytoplasm from cells
treated as shown above and below the dots. Rows 1 and 5 received cytoplasm from equal
aliquots of suspension culture containing 3 to 5 × 10^5 cells. The duplicate dots under each
condition correspond to cells from duplicate cultures.

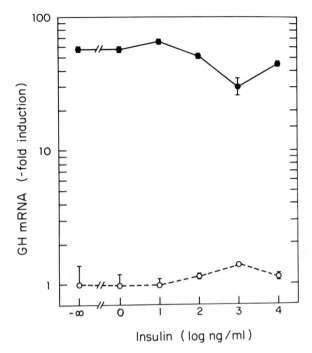

FIG. 7. Quantitation of the results shown in Fig. 6. Quantitation of relative prolactin mRNA per cell was performed as described (White and Bancroft, 1982), and is expressed relative to control cells, which received neither hormone. The mean and range of duplicate cultures are shown, except for the two points without error bars, where quantitation of results with only one culture could be performed. (O- - -O, −dexamethasone; ●———●, +dexamethasone.)

tion. However, this slight inhibition was not observed in a number of other similar experiments performed (data not shown). Consistent with the results of Ivarie *et al.* (1981), insulin itself had no effect on growth hormone mRNA levels in the GH$_3$ cells.

It seemed possible that the results of Ivarie *et al.* (1981) could be due to an inhibition by insulin of translation of growth hormone mRNA, which would then be detectable when growth hormone synthesis was assayed, but not when growth hormone mRNA sequences were assayed. To investigate this possibility, the ability of insulin to block the dexamethasone stimulation of growth hormone synthesis by GH$_3$ cells was examined. Table II shows that insulin at concentrations of 1, 10, or 100 μg/ml yielded no detectable inhibition of the stimulation by dexamethasone (10^{-7} *M*) of growth hormone synthesis.

We thus conclude, in agreement with Ivarie *et al.* (1981), that dexamethasone alone can strongly stimulate growth hormone synthesis and

TABLE II

EFFECT OF INSULIN AT VARIOUS CONCENTRATIONS
ON THE STIMULATION BY DEXAMETHASONE
OF GROWTH HORMONE SYNTHESIS[a]

Additions	Growth hormone synthesis
None	1.0
Insulin (1 μg/ml)	1.0
Dex[b]	4.8
Insulin (1 μg/ml) + dex	4.8
Insulin (10 μg/ml)	1.0
Insulin (10 μg/ml) + dex	5.0
Insulin (100 μg/ml)	1.4
Insulin (100 μg/ml) + dex	5.0

[a]GH_3 cells were incubated in the presence or absence of dexamethasone ($10^{-7} M$) or insulin as in Fig. 6. Relative growth hormone synthesis was measured as described (Bancroft *et al.*, 1980b) and is expressed relative to control cells, which received neither hormone. Relative growth hormone synthesis in the control cells was 1.5%.

[b]Dex, dexamethasone.

mRNA levels in GH_3 cells incubated in a serum-free medium lacking insulin. However, we find that insulin cannot block the stimulation by dexamethasone of either growth hormone mRNA or synthesis by GH_3 cells under the conditions. The reason for the discordance between our results and those of Ivarie *et al.* (1981) is not clear, but it may result from differences in either the cells or the culture conditions employed. However, the results presented above argue against a physiological role for insulin in the regulation by glucocorticoid and thyroid hormones of growth hormone gene expression.

V. REGULATION AND MEDIATION BY CALCIUM OF SPECIFIC GENE EXPRESSION

A. INTRODUCTION

As discussed in Section IV, studies on the hormonal regulation of growth hormone gene expression by GH_3 cells have concentrated on the action of thyroid and glucocorticoid hormones, which exert their action by binding to intracellular receptors. In contrast, corresponding studies with these cells of the hormonal regulation of prolactin gene expression have concentrated on the action of peptide hormones such as thyrotropin-releasing hormone (TRH) or epidermal growth factor (EGF), which exert their actions by binding to specific receptors on the cell surface. As a consequence, studies of the mechanisms of action of TRH or EGF generally fall into two categories: (1) studies of the translocation of either TRH (Laverriere *et al.*, 1981) or EGF (Johnson *et al.*, 1980) into the nucleus, and (2) studies of cellular events other than internalization of hormone–receptor complexes, which occur as a result of binding of either hormone to its receptor. The latter studies have concentrated on identifying cellular mediators or "second messengers" of the action of these hormones and characterizing their mechanisms of action.

Studies by a number of groups have provided evidence that Ca^{2+} can act as such a mediator in the stimulation by TRH of prolactin *secretion* by GH_3 cells (Kidokoro, 1975; Taraskevitch and Douglas, 1977; Tashjian *et al.*, 1978; Dufy *et al.*, 1979; Ozawa and Kimura, 1979; Moriarty and Leuschen, 1981; Ronning *et al.*, 1982; Sobel and Tashjian, 1983; Gershengorn and Thaw, 1983). In addition, previous studies have shown that incubation of the GH_3 cells with the Ca^{2+} chelator EGTA inhibited both the basal synthesis of prolactin and growth hormone and the ability of dexamethasone and TRH to stimulate the synthesis by these cells of growth hormone and prolactin, respectively (Gautvik and Tashjian, 1973).

We therefore decided to investigate first whether Ca^{2+} itself can regulate the expression of the prolactin and growth hormone genes by GH_3 cells and normal pituitary cells. The results of these studies are described in Section V,B. Then, to investigate the physiological significance of these findings, we have begun to examine whether Ca^{2+} acts as a mediator of the actions of TRH and EGF on prolactin gene expression and of dexamethasone on growth hormone gene expression by the GH_3 cells. These studies are described in Section V,C.

B. Calcium Regulation of Prolactin Gene Expression

For our initial studies in this area, it was important to be able to distinguish direct effects of Ca^{2+} on the GH_3 cells from effects arising from the ability of Ca^{2+} to act as a hormonal stimulus–response coupler. Thus, we decided to employ a chemically defined medium that contains no added Ca^{2+}, serum, or hormones (White *et a.*, 1981). This serum-free medium consists of the induction medium described in Section III, from which the serum was omitted. The Ca^{2+} content of this medium, as assayed by flameless atomic absorption spectrophotometry, is less than 2.5 μM (White and Bancroft, 1983). Because both known and unknown hormones are absent, results observed upon addition of Ca^{2+} can be attributed directly to an effect of this ion on the cells. Viability of the GH_3 cells, as assayed by Trypan blue exclusion, is at least 80–90% for at least 8 days in this medium. The cells seldom exhibit any growth when incubated under these conditions. Recent studies employing flow cytometry have shown that, under this condition of incubation, the cells contain about 50% as much total RNA per cell as cells grown in the presence of serum. Preliminary studies with this technique indicate that the cells are blocked in G_1.

1. Ca^{2+} Stimulates Prolactin Synthesis by GH_3 Cells

Transfer of the GH_3 cells in suspension culture from their normal serum-containing growth medium to serum-free medium reduced relative prolactin and growth hormone synthesis (hormone synthesis ÷ total protein synthesis) from about 2.5% to 0.2–0.3% after about 3–4 days (White and Bancroft, 1984). Figure 8 shows that addition of 0.4 mM Ca^{2+} at this time leads to a large stimulation of prolactin synthesis that reaches a maximum (about 48-fold) by about 4 days.

The specificity of this effect of Ca^{2+} on prolactin synthesis in the GH_3 cells is demonstrated by the following observations. First, as shown in Fig. 8, there was no detectable effect of Ca^{2+} under these conditions on the synthesis of growth hormone. It should be noted, however, that we have subsequently found that Ca^{2+} does consistently yield a slight (1.5- to 2-fold) stimulation of growth hormone mRNA in the GH_3 cells (see Figs. 11 and 17). Furthermore, neither total protein synthesis (White *et al.*, 1981) nor total RNA synthesis (G. Gick, unpublished observations) by the GH_3 cells are significantly altered by exposure to Ca^{2+}. Finally, Sobel and Tashjian (1983) have recently reported the use of two–dimensional polyacrylamide gel electrophoresis to examine effects of the Ca^{2+} chelator EGTA on the synthesis of individual cytoplasmic proteins by a variant of the GH_3 cell line, termed GH_4C_1. They observed that EGTA markedly reduced the prolactin spot, while affecting the synthesis of almost no other protein visible on the two-dimensional gels. The latter results imply that Ca^{2+} exhibits a high degree of specificity in its stimulation of prolactin synthesis by GH cells.

Investigation of the dose–response stimulation of prolactin synthesis by $CaCl_2$ showed that half-maximal and maximal stimulations were achieved at $CaCl_2$ concentrations of 0.07 and 0.2–0.4 mM, respectively (White *et al.*, 1981). The same studies showed that it is the Ca^{2+} ion that is responsible for this stimulation, since neither $MgCl_2$ nor KCl at 0.4 mM yielded a detectable stimulation of prolactin synthesis (White *et al.*, 1981).

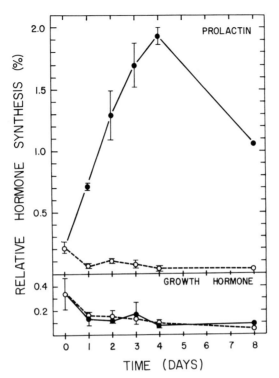

Fɪɢ. 8. Stimulation by Ca^{2+} of prolactin synthesis. GH_3 cells were incubated for 4 days in serum-free medium and then for various times in the presence (●———●) or absence (○- - -○) of $CaCl_2$ (0.4 mM). Relative hormone synthesis was measured as described (Bancroft *et al.*, 1980b). The mean and range of values obtained with duplicate cultures (except for day 8) are shown. [From White *et al.* (1981).]

2. Ca^{2+} *Stimulates Prolactin RNA Levels in* GH_3 *Cells*

Figure 9 illustrates the effect of Ca^{2+} on prolactin synthesis (A) and on cytoplasmic prolactin mRNA levels assayed either by cell-free translation (B) or by RNA gel blot hybridization (C). Panels (B) and (C) show that Ca^{2+} stimulates prolactin mRNA. Furthermore, quantitation of the results in Fig. 2 showed that Ca^{2+} increased relative prolactin synthesis, translatable poly(A^+) prolactin mRNA, and poly(A^+) prolactin mRNA sequences by 7.3-, 5.5-, and 6.8-fold, respectively (White *et al.*, 1981). The agreement among these quantities suggests that the Ca^{2+} regulation of prolactin synthesis is exerted entirely at a pretranslational level.

The early kinetics of the induction by Ca^{2+} of prolactin mRNA sequences are shown in Fig. 10. For these studies, relative prolactin mRNA levels were

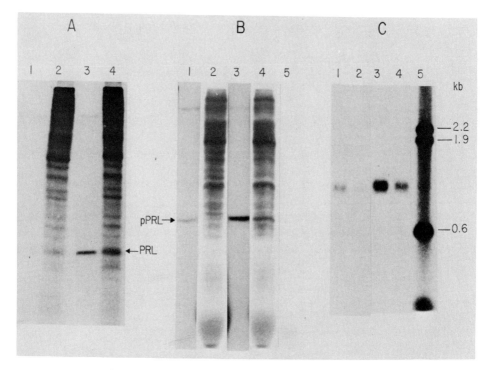

FIG. 9. Stimulation by Ca^{2+} of prolactin mRNA levels. GH_3 cells were incubated for 3 days with or without $CaCl_2$ as in Fig. 8. (A) Synthesis of prolactin (PRL) (lanes 1 and 3) or total proteins (lanes 2 and 4) in cells incubated without (lanes 1 and 2) or with (lanes 3 and 4) $CaCl_2$. (B) Synthesis of preprolactin (pPRL) (lanes 1 and 3) or total products (lanes 2 and 4) of translation in reticulocyte lysates of poly(A+) RNA from cells incubated without (lanes 1 and 2) or with (lanes 3 and 4) $CaCl_2$. Lane 5, endogenous products. (C) Analysis by RNA gel blot hybridization of prolactin mRNA from $-CaCl_2$ cells (lanes 1 and 2, 950 and 425 ng, respectively) or from $+CaCl_2$ cells (lanes 3 and 4, 500 and 250 ng, respectively) was analyzed. [From White *et al.* (1981).]

assayed by the cytoplasmic dot hybridization procedure described in Section III. There was a lag period of 6–9 hours, after which prolactin mRNA levels in the Ca^{2+}-treated cells rapidly increased. In other similar experiments, a lag period as short as 3 hours has been observed. This lag period may represent a time during which Ca^{2+} induces a cellular event(s) requisite for the increase in prolactin mRNA; i.e., Ca^{2+} regulation of prolactin mRNA may not represent a primary induction. Alternatively, Ca^{2+} may prove to have a more rapid effect on prolactin gene transcription in these cells, in which case the lag observed could represent the time before a subsequent increased accumulation of cytoplasmic mRNA is detectable.

The specificity of the action of Ca^{2+} in stimulating prolactin mRNA is illustrated in Fig. 11 (A–C). Suboptimal (0.1 mM) and optimal (0.4 mM) Ca^{2+} concentrations yielded inductions of prolactin mRNA of 93- and 198-fold, respectively. By contrast, these two concentrations of Ca^{2+} yielded increases in growth hormone mRNA of only 10% and 60%, respectively. It should be noted that the stimulation by Ca^{2+} of growth hormone mRNA, although quite small compared to the stimulation of prolactin mRNA, has been reproducibly observed in a number of similar experiments (for example, see Fig. 17). Figure 11 (B and D) also illustrates an example of the opposite effects by a hormone on growth hormone and prolactin gene expression in GH cells. Thus, dexamethasone causes a 35-fold increase in growth hormone mRNA sequences in the GH_3 cells while causing a 7-fold decrease in prolactin mRNA sequences. However, dexamethasone is apparently unable to totally block the Ca^{2+} induction of prolactin mRNA sequences (Fig. 11, D).

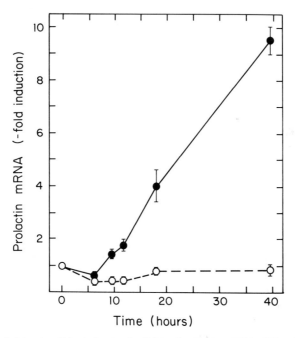

FIG. 10. Early kinetics of the induction by Ca^{2+} of prolactin mRNA. GH_3 cells were preincubated for 3 days in serum-free medium and then for the indicated times plus (●———●) or minus (○- - -○) $CaCl_2$ (0.4 mM). Relative prolactin mRNA levels were assayed by cytoplasmic dot hybridization. The mean and range of results with duplicate cultures are shown. [From White and Bancroft (1983).]

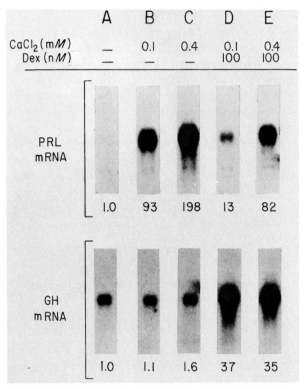

FIG. 11. Effects of Ca^{2+} and dexamethasone on prolactin and growth hormone mRNA sequences. GH_3 cells were incubated for 4 days ±$CaCl_2$ and then for 3 days ±dexamethasone (Dex). Relative prolactin (PRL) and growth hormone (GH) mRNA levels were analyzed by RNA gel blot hybridization as in Fig. 4. The quantitation of the results is shown beneath each lane. [From White *et al.* (1981).]

The effect of Ca^{2+} on cytoplasmic and nuclear prolactin RNA sequence levels in the GH_3 cells is illustrated in Fig. 12. Incubation of GH_3 cells in the absence or presence of 0.4 mM Ca^{2+} for 5 days yielded a typical induction by Ca^{2+} of cytoplasmic 1.0 kb prolactin mRNA of about 14-fold (lanes A and B). Total nuclear RNA isolated from the same cells was analyzed on the same gel (lanes C and D). RNA from the Ca^{2+}-treated cells (lane D) contained, in addition to an intense band at the position of mature 1.0-kb prolactin mRNA, at least seven larger bands ranging in size from about 2.0 kb up to about 14.5 kb. The number and sizes of these large presumptive precursors of cytoplasmic prolactin mRNA are similar to those reported by other investigators (Hoffman *et al.*, 1981; Potter *et al.*, 1981). Comparing lane C ($-Ca^{2+}$) with lane D ($+Ca^{2+}$) shows that incubation of GH_3 cells with Ca^{2+} caused sizable increases in all of these large nuclear prolactin RNA species. It should be noted that the sizes of the two largest nuclear prolactin RNA bands (about 12.0 and 14.5 kb) are apparently larger than the rat prolactin gene, which is reported to be about 10 kb long (Chien and Thompson, 1980; Cooke and Baxter, 1982). Hence, the size and identity of the primary transcript of this gene remains to be determined. However, the observation that Ca^{2+} increased the levels of all detectable nuclear prolactin RNA sequences argues strongly that Ca^{2+} regulates transcription of the prolactin gene. Because the transcription rate of the prolactin gene in GH_3 cells incubated under the conditions described here is below the level of detection, we have

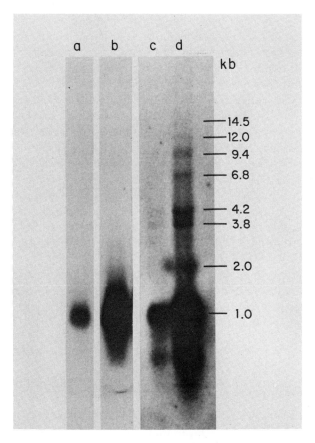

FIG. 12. Regulation by Ca^{2+} of cytoplasmic and nuclear prolactin RNA sequences. GH_3 cells were preincubated as in Fig. 10 and then for 5 days $\pm CaCl_2$ (0.4 mM). Prolactin RNA in total cytoplasmic RNA from $-CaCl_2$ cells (lane a) or $+CaCl_2$ cells (lane b) and total nuclear RNA from $-CaCl_2$ (lane c) or $+CaCl_2$ cells (lane d) were analyzed by RNA gel blot hybridization as in Fig. 4. [From White and Bancroft (1983).]

not yet been able to employ the nuclear run-on transcription assay (Mc-Knight and Palmiter, 1979) to investigate regulation by Ca^{2+} of prolactin gene transcription in these cells. However, the results obtained when this assay was employed with primary cultures of normal rat pituitary cells, described in Section V,B,4, provide direct evidence that Ca^{2+} does regulate transcription of the prolactin gene.

3. Ca^{2+} Regulation of Prolactin mRNA in GH_3 Cells Incubated in a Serum-Containing Medium

The experiments described in the previous section were performed with cells incubated in a serum-free medium. It seemed possible that the Ca^{2+} induction of prolactin mRNA might be limited to cells incubated under this condition. For example, the induction might be limited to a particular stage of the cell cycle. To investigate this possibility, the effect of Ca^{2+} on prolactin mRNA in GH_3 cells grown in a serum-containing medium was examined.

Ca^{2+} was removed from the serum by extraction with Chelex 100 resin as described by Brennan *et al.* (1975). The iminodiacetic acid residues attached to a styrene–divinylbenzine copolymer matrix in this resin have a high affinity for Ca^{2+}, Mg^{2+}, and heavy metal ions (Bio-Rad Laboratories Product Information, 1981). When assayed with the metallochromic Ca^{2+} indicator arsenazo III (Scarpa *et al.*, 1978), medium containing the standard concentrations (15% horse serum, 2.5% fetal calf serum) of untreated or Chelex-treated serum contained Ca^{2+} concentrations of 530 μM and 17 μM, respectively. When serum that had been preincubated with ^{45}Ca was treated with Chelex, 99.2% of the ^{45}Ca was removed.

The generation times of GH_3 cells incubated 3–4 days in medium prepared with Chelex-treated serum, in the absence or presence of Ca^{2+} (0.5 mM) were, respectively, 2.0 and 2.5 days. When the cells were incubated in a normal serum-containing medium, this value was 2.0. Thus, Chelex-treated serum appears to support cell growth as well as normal serum, whether Ca^{2+} is added or not. Furthermore, total RNA synthesis in cells incubated in the presence of Chelex-treated serum, plus or minus Ca^{2+}, is the same as that in cells incubated in the presence of untreated serum (Table III).

The results of two indpendent experiments with GH_3 cells incubated in the presence of Chelex-treated serum are shown in Table III. Under these conditions, Ca^{2+} stimulates prolactin mRNA levels in the cells. Although the induction kinetics appear to be slower than those observed under serum-free conditions (cf. Fig. 10), by 72 hours Ca^{2+} had stimulated prolactin mRNA levels eight- to ninefold. Hence, Ca^{2+} can also stimulate prolactin mRNA in GH_3 cells growing in a serum-containing medium.

TABLE III

Ca^{2+} Regulation of Prolactin mRNA in GH$_3$ Cells Incubated
in a Serum-Containing Medium[a]

Experiment	Relative prolactin mRNA (fold induction)		
	24 hours	48 hours	72 hours
#1	0.85	4.5	8.3
#2	1.4	4.2	9.1

[a]GH$_3$ cells were transferred from their normal serum-containing growth medium (Dobner *et al.*, 1981) to this medium containing serum extracted with Chelex 100. Three days later, cultures received either nothing (control), or CaCl$_2$ (0.5 mM). At various times thereafter, relative prolactin mRNA levels (experimental/control) were assayed by cytoplasmic dot hybridization. Results of two independent experiments are shown.

Total RNA synthesis under the conditions of this experiment was measured by trichloroacetic acid extraction of cells that had been incubated 30 minutes with [³H]uridine. RNA synthesis in cells preincubated, then incubated 3 days −Ca^{2+} or +Ca^{2+} in the presence of Chelex-treated serum was 92% and 101%, respectively, of the value in cells incubated in normal growth medium.

4. Ca^{2+} Regulation of Prolactin and Growth Hormone Gene Expression in Primary Cultures of Rat Pituitary Cells

The results described in the previous section show that Ca^{2+} stimulates prolactin mRNA levels in GH$_3$ cells incubated under either serum-free conditions or in the presence of suitably treated serum. As described in Section II, the GH$_3$ cells are a line of pituitary tumor cells. It thus seemed important to investigate whether Ca^{2+} also regulates prolactin mRNA in normal pituitary cells.

Primary cultures of retired female breeder rat pituitary cells were prepared and exposed to Ca^{2+} in serum-free medium as described in Section V,B,2. However, in preliminary experiments in which cells were exposed to Ca^{2+} concentrations up to 1.0 mM, no significant stimulation by Ca^{2+} of either prolactin or growth hormone mRNA sequences was observed (Table IV; G. Gick, unpublished observations). Measurements with arsenazo III of the Ca^{2+} content of the serum-free medium employed have yielded values in the range of 10–40 μM. It seemed possible that the presence of Ca^{2+} at these extracellular concentrations was capable of stimulating prolactin mRNA levels in the pituitary cells, thus preventing an induction by exogenously added Ca^{2+}. The effect of exposure of the pituitary cells to EGTA concentrations in this range was therefore examined. Table IV shows that incubation of pituitary cells for 3 days with 10–50 μM EGTA led to a large,

TABLE IV

EFFECT OF EGTA ON PROLACTIN AND GROWTH HORMONE mRNA LEVELS
IN PRIMARY CULTURES OF RAT PITUITARY CELLS[a]

	Percentage of control		
EGTA (μM)	Prolactin mRNA	Growth hormone mRNA	Total RNA synthesis
0	100 ± 2	100 ± 10	100 ± 30
10	59 ± 28	83 ± 7	N.D.[b]
20	7 ± 2	25 ± 11	N.D.
50	2 ± 0.4	11 ± 0.4	120 ± 2
50, plus Ca^{2+} (1 mM)	111 ± 12	100 ± 10	N.D.

[a]Primary cultures of pituitary cells were prepared from retired female breeder rats as described (Hymer *et al.*, 1973). The cells were then plated in 35-mm tissue culture petri dishes (1.0×10^6 cells/dish) in serum-free medium and incubated 15 minutes at 37°C in a CO_2 (2.5%) incubator and then overnight in fresh medium. Following incubation for 3 days in fresh medium with the indicated additions, prolactin and growth hormone mRNA levels, relative to controls, were measured by cytoplasmic dot hybridization. Where indicated, total RNA synthesis was measured as in Table III. The mean and range of results with duplicate cultures is shown.
[b]N.D., not determined.

dose-dependent decrease in the levels of the mRNAs for both prolactin and growth hormone. The complete inhibition by 1 mM Ca^{2+} of the effects of 50 μM EGTA shows that removal of Ca^{2+} was responsible for the observed effects of EGTA. Table IV also shows that, at each EGTA concentration tested, prolactin mRNA levels were reduced to a considerably greater extent than growth hormone mRNA levels. This is consistent with the results obtained in this serum-free medium with GH_3 cells, in which Ca^{2+} caused a considerably larger stimulation of prolactin mRNA than of growth hormone mRNA (see Section V,B,2). The decreases in prolactin and growth hormone mRNA induced by exposure to EGTA do not arise simply from inhibition by EGTA of overall RNA synthesis by pituitary cells, since this parameter was not inhibited by 50 μM EGTA (Table IV). Finally, these effects of EGTA are not limited to pituitary cells from retired female breeder rats, since quite similar results have been observed in primary cultures of pituitary cells from normal male rats (G. Gick, unpublished observations).

The kinetics of the reduction by EGTA of prolactin and growth hormone mRNA levels in pituitary cells is illustrated in Fig. 13. Over a 6-day period, there was a gradual decrease in the levels of both mRNAs in control cultures incubated in serum-free medium alone. Incubation of parallel cultures with 50 μM EGTA for 1 day led to reductions, relative to controls, of about twofold in both mRNAs. By 3 days, prolactin and growth hormone mRNAs in the EGTA-treated cultures were reduced 45-fold and 9-fold, respectively, relative to controls. Between 3 and 6 days, EGTA caused a further threefold decrease in the relative level of growth hormone mRNA. Whether EGTA also caused a further decrease in prolactin mRNA during this period could not be determined accurately, since prolactin mRNA levels in the EGTA-treated cells were close to the limit of detection.

To investigate the reversibility of these effects of EGTA, pituitary cells were incubated in the presence or absence of EGTA (20 μ*M*) for 3 days, after

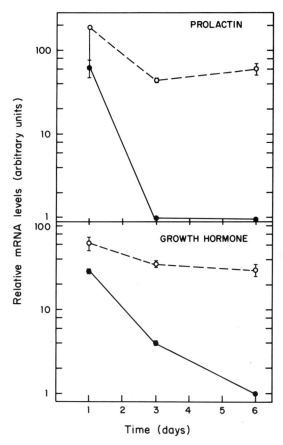

Fig. 13. Time course of the decrease of prolactin and growth hormone mRNA levels in rat pituitary cell cultures treated with EGTA. Primary cultures of pituitary cells were prepared and preincubated as in Table IV. Then, beginning on day zero, they were incubated with or without EGTA (50 μ*M*). At various times thereafter, relative prolactin and growth hormone mRNA levels were assayed as in Table IV. The mean and range of results with duplicate cultures are shown. (O- - -O, −EGTA; ●———●, +EGTA.)

which some of the EGTA-treated cultures received Ca^{2+} (0.4 mM). Table V shows that incubation of pituitary cells with EGTA for 6 days caused prolactin and growth hormone mRNA sequences to decrease to 4% and 11%, respectively, of the levels in control cultures. Addition of Ca^{2+} to EGTA-treated cultures after 3 days led, by 6 days, to increases of both mRNAs to about 30–35% of the levels in the control cultures. Table V also shows that none of these treatments significantly affected either total RNA synthesis or ribosomal RNA levels in the pituitary cells. The ability of Ca^{2+} to stimulate prolactin and growth hormone mRNA levels in cultures pretreated with EGTA shows that the EGTA effects observed are not due simply to irreversible inactivation of the pituitary cells that produce growth hormone and prolactin mRNA. Furthermore, the results of the measurements of RNA synthesis and ribosomal RNA content show that, under the conditions of these experiments, EGTA is not grossly altering overall RNA metabolism in these cultures.

The results described previously show that Ca^{2+} stimulates both prolactin and growth hormone mRNA levels in normal rat pituitary cells incubated in culture. To begin to elucidate the mechanisms involved in these effects, we have investigated whether Ca^{2+} regulates expression of the corresponding genes at the level of transcription. Nuclei isolated either from control cells or from cells incubated with EGTA $\pm Ca^{2+}$ were incubated with [^{32}P]UTP under conditions permitting elongation of preinitiated transcripts. Synthesis of prolactin or growth hormone RNA was then assayed by hybridization of

TABLE V

Ability of Ca^{2+} to Reverse the EGTA-Induced Decrease of Prolactin and Growth Hormone mRNA in Rat Pituitary Cell Cultures[a]

	Percentage of control			
Additions	Prolactin mRNA	Growth hormone mRNA	Total RNA synthesis	18 S rRNA
None (6 days)	100 ± 8	100 ± 61	100	100 ± 4
20 μM EGTA (6 days)	4 ± 1	11 ± 3	84	104 ± 4
20 μM EGTA (3 days), then 0.4 mM Ca^{2+} (3d)	31 ± 3	35 ± 4	96	116 ± 13

[a]Primary cultures of pituitary cells were prepared and preincubated as in Table IV. They were then incubated for 6 days with the indicated additions. Relative prolactin and growth hormone mRNA levels in duplicate cultures and total RNA synthesis in single cultures were measured as in Table IV. Relative levels of 18 S ribosomal RNA (rRNA) were measured in the same cultures employed for the prolactin and growth hormone mRNA assays by using an 18 S ribosomal DNA probe (Katz *et al.*, 1983) in the cytoplasmic dot hybridization technique.

total nuclear RNA to the corresponding cDNA hybrid plasmids immobilized on nitrocellulose filters. Table VI shows that the transcription rates of the prolactin and growth hormone genes in cells incubated 4 days without EGTA were greater by 6.9- and 2.7-fold, respectively, than those in cells incubated in the presence of EGTA (50 μM). For each gene, nearly identical transcription rates, relative to the EGTA controls, were observed in cells incubated 1 day in EGTA and then 3 days in the presence of added Ca^{2+} (50 μM). Overall transcription was essentially identical under the three conditions examined (Table VI). These results show that Ca^{2+} regulates expression of both the prolactin and growth hormone genes in pituitary cells at the level of transcription. The observation that prolactin gene transcription is stimulated to a greater degree than growth hormone gene transcription is consistent with the differential stimulation by Ca^{2+} of the corresponding mRNA levels shown in Table IV. Finally, measurements by arsenazo III of the medium Ca^{2+} concentrations under the experimental conditions employed (Table VI) suggest that transcription of these genes is sensitive to external Ca^{2+} concentrations as low as about 20 μM. However, it should be emphasized that the corresponding intracellular Ca^{2+} concentrations of the pituitary cells that produce prolactin and growth hormone mRNA are not known and may not be directly related to the external Ca^{2+} concentration.

Measurements of relative prolactin and growth hormone mRNA levels in the cells employed for the transcription assays showed that the stimulation of both mRNAs by Ca^{2+} was greater than the stimulation of transcription of the corresponding genes (Table VI). This difference was especially pronounced for prolactin, with which the stimulation of the level of the mRNA was seven to nine times greater than the stimulation of transcription. The differences between these quantities cannot readily be interpreted without a detailed kinetic analysis of the synthesis, processing, and accumulation of transcripts of these genes in the presence or absence of Ca^{2+}. However, the differences observed suggest that, in addition to regulating transcription of the prolactin and growth hormone genes, Ca^{2+} may also regulate stability of the corresponding mRNAs.

C. THE ROLE OF CALCIUM IN HORMONAL REGULATION OF PROLACTIN GENE EXPRESSION

As described in Section V,A, Ca^{2+} has been implicated as a mediator of the stimulation by TRH of prolactin secretion and synthesis by GH_3 cells. The growth factor EGF has also been shown to stimulate prolactin synthesis in these cells (Schonbrunn *et al.*, 1980; Johnson *et al.*, 1980). Furthermore, Ca^{2+} has been implicated in the mechanism of action of a number of serum

TABLE VI

Regulation by Ca^{2+} of Prolactin and Growth Hormone Gene Transcription in Primary Cultures[a]

Additions	Ca^{2+} in medium (μM)	Total RNA synthesis (cpm × 10^{-6})	Fold increase			
			PRL RNA synthesis	GH RNA synthesis	PRL mRNA	GH mRNA
50 μM EGTA (4 days)	0.1	4.2	1.0 ± 0.1	1.0 ± 0.1	1.0 ± 0.1	1.0 ± 0.2
None (4 days)	18	5.1	6.9 ± 1.3	2.7 ± 0.1	64 ± 13	6.3 ± 1.3
50 μM EGTA (1 day), then 50 μM CaCl$_2$ (3 days)	44	4.4	7.6 ± 0.1	2.7 ± 0.0	49 ± 8	3.7 ± 0.4

[a] Primary cultures of pituitary cells were prepared and preincubated as in Fig. 4. Groups of 11 plates were then incubated 4 days with the indicated additions. Three plates from each group were employed for determinations in triplicate cultures of relative levels of prolactin and growth hormone mRNA as in Table IV. Mean values ±SE are shown. Medium from the remaining eight cultures was pooled and employed for assays of Ca^{2+} by the arsenazo III assay. Transcription of the prolactin and growth hormone genes in nuclei isolated from these latter cultures was assayed as described (Evans et al., 1981), employing rat prolactin or growth hormone cDNA plasmids affixed to nitrocellulose filters and the hybridization conditions described by McKnight and Palmiter (1979). In the controls treated with 50 μM EGTA, the prolactin and growth hormone gene transcription rates were 21 and 7 parts per million (ppm), respectively. All transcription rates have been corrected for a 34–48% hybridization efficiency and a background hybridization to filters containing pBR322 DNA of 2–3 ppm. The mean and range of duplicate hybridization reactions are shown.

growth factors including EGF (Sawyer and Cohen, 1981; Owen and Villareal, 1982a,b). Hence, to investigate the role of Ca^{2+} in hormonal regulation of prolactin gene expression, we have examined the effect on prolactin synthesis and mRNA levels of incubating GH_3 cells in the presence or absence of Ca^{2+}, TRH, or EGF.

In the first series of experiments, GH_3 cells were preincubated in serum-free medium and then incubated with optimal concentrations of either $CaCl_2$ (0.4 mM), TRH (10^{-7} M), or both. Figure 14 illustrates the effect of the incubation on relative prolactin synthesis by the cells. Incubation with $CaCl_2$, TRH, or $CaCl_2$ plus TRH yielded stimulations of prolactin synthesis of 56-, 13- and 141-fold, respectively. Thus, TRH alone yielded a significant stimulation, which was smaller than the stimulation by Ca^{2+} alone. Both factors together yielded a considerably larger stimulation than either alone, suggesting that they were acting synergistically.

To determine whether these effects on prolactin synthesis were due to changes in prolactin mRNA levels, cytoplasmic dot hybridization was em-

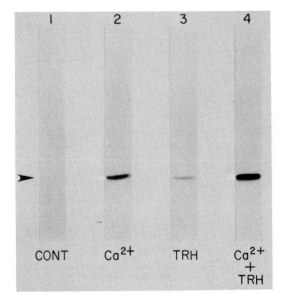

FIG. 14. Effect of incubation with Ca^{2+} and/or TRH on prolactin synthesis. Cells were incubated for 4 days in serum-free medium and then for 3 days with nothing (lane 1), with 0.4 mM $CaCl_2$ (lane 2), with 10^{-7} M TRH (lane 3), or with $CaCl_2$ and TRH (lane 4). Relative prolactin synthesis was then measured by analysis on SDS polyacrylamide gels of immunoprecipitates of [³H]leucine-labeled cells as described (White *et al.*, 1981). The arrow shows the position of prolactin.

ployed to examine the effects of $CaCl_2$ (0.4 mM), EGF (5 nM), and TRH (100 nM), alone or in combination, on relative levels of prolactin mRNA (Fig. 15). Ca^{2+} alone yielded a 15-fold stimulation, while EGF or TRH alone yielded stimulations of 7.5- and 11-fold, respectively. Either EGF plus Ca^{2+} or TRH plus Ca^{2+} yielded stimulations of 60 to 70-fold. Thus, either EGF or TRH acts synergistically with Ca^{2+} in regulating prolactin mRNA, since the stimulation with either peptide plus Ca^{2+} is considerably larger than the stimulation with either peptide alone or with Ca^{2+} alone.

The results of the experiments described above show that either EGF or TRH require extracellular Ca^{2+} in order to achieve maximal stimulation of prolactin mRNA levels. However, the observation that either peptide alone was capable of causing a significant stimulation of prolactin mRNA suggested the possible existence of a Ca^{2+}-independent mechanism of action for either peptide. However, it also seemed possible that the stimulation with either peptide alone was mediated by small amounts of residual Ca^{2+} present in the medium and/or the cells. To examine this possibility, the regulation of prolactin mRNA by various concentrations of EGF or TRH in the presence or absence of Ca^{2+} (0.4 mM) was examined in GH_3 cells incubated in serum-free medium containing EGTA (Fig. 16). Under these conditions, Ca^{2+} alone yielded an 18-fold stimulation, and either EGF or TRH in the pres-

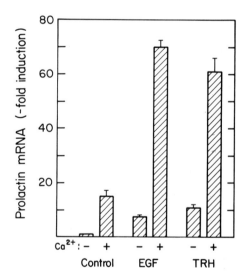

Fig. 15. Regulation of prolactin mRNA by EGF and TRH in the presence and absence of added Ca^{2+}. GH_3 cells were preincubated for 3 days in serum-free medium and then for 3 days with or without Ca^{2+} (0.4 mM), TRH (100 nM), or EGF (5 nM). Relative prolactin mRNA levels were assayed by cytoplasmic dot hybridization. The mean and range of results with duplicate cultures are shown. [From White and Bancroft (1983).]

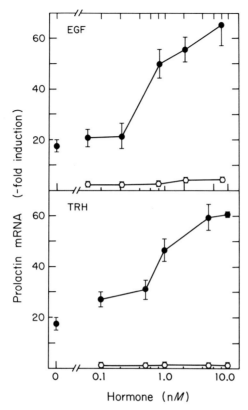

FIG. 16. Ability of various concentrations of EGF or TRH to stimulate prolactin mRNA in cells incubated in EGTA with or without added Ca^{2+}. GH_3 cells were preincubated as in Fig. 15, with EGTA (5 μM) present the last day. They were then incubated for 3 days in EGTA (5 μM), plus (●————●) or minus (○————○) $CaCl_2$ (0.4 mM). Relative prolactin mRNA levels were assayed as in Fig. 15. The mean and range of results with duplicate cultures are shown. [From White and Bancroft (1983).]

ence of Ca^{2+} yielded dose-dependent stimulations of prolactin mRNA, resulting in maximal increases of 66-fold and 61-fold, respectively, in good agreement with the results of the previous experiment. However, in the presence of EGTA, EGF yielded a small (fourfold) stimulation of prolactin mRNA at the highest concentration tested, while TRH alone failed to stimulate prolactin mRNA at any concentration tested. Thus, TRH appears to be absolutely dependent on Ca^{2+} for its regulation of prolactin mRNA. However, the question of whether this is also true for EGF was not resolved by this experimental approach.

It seemed possible that the inability of TRH to regulate prolactin mRNA in the absence of Ca^{2+} could be a reflection of a more general inability of Ca^{2+}-deprived GH_3 cells to respond to hormonal stimulation. To examine this possibility, the ability of dexamethasone to stimulate growth hormone mRNA levels in GH_3 cells incubated with or without Ca^{2+} was examined (Fig. 17). The inductions by dexamethasone of GH mRNA in cells incubated plus or minus Ca^{2+} were 25- and 20-fold, respectively. The slightly higher induction in the Ca^{2+}-treated cells was probably due to the ability of Ca^{2+} itself to cause a small (twofold) stimulation of growth hormone mRNA (Fig. 17) (see also Section V,A). Although in the experiment shown here EGTA was not present to chelate residual Ca^{2+}, similar experiments performed in the presence of 20 μM EGTA have yielded results similar to those shown in Fig. 17. Thus, GH_3 cells incubated under the Ca^{2+}-free conditions described here are quite capable of exhibiting a hormonal response. Furthermore, these results imply that the induction by dexamethasone of growth hormone mRNA in GH_3 cells is entirely independent of Ca^{2+}.

The results shown in Fig. 16 indicate that it is difficult to resolve the question of the dependence of EGF upon Ca^{2+} for its regulation of prolactin mRNA by experiments involving the removal of extracellular Ca^{2+}. Experi-

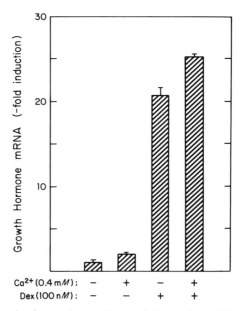

FIG. 17. Regulation by dexamethasone (Dex) and Ca^{2+} of growth hormone mRNA. GH_3 cells were preincubated for 3 days in serum-free medium and then for 3 days plus or minus Ca^{2+} or dexamethasone. Relative growth hormone mRNA levels were assayed by cytoplasmic dot hybridization, employing as probe a growth hormone cDNA plasmid pBR322-GH[1] (Dobner et al., 1981). The mean and range of results with duplicate cultures are shown.

ments in which ^{45}Ca-loaded GH_3 cells were transferred to serum-free medium have shown that about 95% of intracellular Ca^{2+} is lost from the cells within about 1 hour (White and Bancroft, 1984). Thus, when the cells are incubated in serum-free medium, a new equilibrium must be reached among intracellular stores of Ca^{2+} (i.e., Ca^{2+} sequestered in mitochondria and endoplasmic reticulum), cytosolic Ca^{2+}, and extracellular and plasma membrane–bound Ca^{2+}. Even though the Ca^{2+} levels in all cellular compartments are probably decreased by incubation in serum-free medium, high-affinity Ca^{2+} transport proteins (e.g., mitochondrial Ca^{2+} ATPase) probably ensure a degree of Ca^{2+} retention by the cells. Although this cellular retention of Ca^{2+} undoubtedly contributes to the viability of GH_3 cells incubated in serum-free medium, it also can make it difficult to assess whether Ca^{2+} plays a crucial role in the ability of a particular hormone to regulate specific gene expression in these cells.

A different experimental approach to studies of Ca^{2+}–hormone interactions with the GH_3 cells involves the use of inhibitors of the Ca^{2+}-binding protein calmodulin. It is well established that Ca^{2+} regulates a large domain of cellular processes via a Ca^{2+}–calmodulin complex (Chafouleas *et al.*, 1982). By incubating the GH_3 cells with appropriate calmodulin inhibitors, it should be possible to investigate both the general question of the involvement of calmodulin in regulation of gene expression and specific questions concerning the Ca^{2+} requirement for the actions of hormones such as EGF and TRH on prolactin gene expression.

The ability of a naphthalene sulfonamide derivative calmodulin inhibitor W-7 (Hidaka *et al.*, 1979) to block the induction by EGF plus Ca^{2+} or TRH plus Ca^{2+} of prolactin mRNA is illustrated in Fig. 18. W-7 inhibited in a dose-dependent fashion the induction of prolactin mRNA in GH_3 cells incubated under either of these conditions. This effect was not due simply to an inhibition by W-7 of overall RNA synthesis by the cells, since this parameter was not inhibited at either W-7 concentration tested (Fig. 18, inset). At the higher concentration tested (30 μM), W-7 totally inhibited the induction by either EGF plus Ca^{2+} or TRH plus Ca^{2+} of prolactin mRNA. The results with EGF plus Ca^{2+} are particularly striking since, unlike the Ca^{2+}-depletion experiments illustrated in Figs. 15 and 16, they imply an absolute dependence on a functional Ca^{2+}–calmodulin complex for the ability of EGF to regulate prolactin mRNA.

Similar experiments with two other calmodulin inhibitors, W-13 (Chafouleas *et al.*, 1982) and calmidazolium (compound R-24571) (Van Belle, 1981), have yielded comparable results. As illustrated in Fig. 19, both drugs totally inhibited the ability of EGF plus Ca^{2+} to stimulate prolactin mRNA in the GH_3 cells. The specificity of the results with W-13 is indicated by the fact that W-12 at the same concentration scarcely inhibited the stimulation by

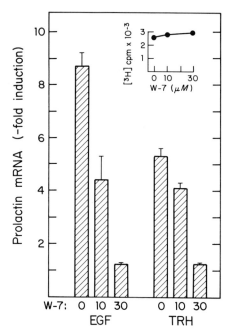

Fig. 18. Effect of calmodulin antagonist W-7 on the stimulation by EGF plus Ca^{2+} or TRH plus Ca^{2+} of prolactin mRNA. GH_3 cells were preincubated for 3 days in serum-free medium and then for 24 hours with either EGF (5 nM) or TRH (100 nM), plus $CaCl_2$ (0.4 mM), plus various concentrations (0, 10, or 30 μM) of W-7. The W-7 was added 1 hour before the other additions. Prolactin mRNA levels were analyzed by cytoplasmic dot hybridization and are expressed relative to controls receiving no additions. The mean and range of results with duplicate cultures are shown. The inset shows the effect of W-7 on RNA synthesis by GH_3 cells incubated with W-7 as above. RNA synthesis was measured as in Table III.

EGF plus Ca^{2+} of prolactin mRNA (Fig. 19). Preliminary experiments have indicated that W-13 is also more effective than W-12 in blocking the induction by EGF alone of prolactin mRNA (data not shown). W-12 is a suitable control for results obtained with W-13, since the naphthalene sulfonamide derivatives W-13 and W-12 have similar structures and hydrophobicity indices, but W-12 has only 20% of the anticalmodulin activity of W-13 (Chafouleas *et al.*, 1982). The specificity of the results with calmidazolium is indicated by the observation that treatment of GH_3 cells with this compound under the conditions of the experiment shown in Fig. 19, at concentrations up to 1.0 μM, caused no inhibition of overall synthesis by the cells of either RNA or protein (data not shown).

The results with calmodulin inhibitors described above imply a central role for calmodulin in the regulation by EGF, TRH, and Ca^{2+} of expression of the prolactin gene. However, it should be noted that some caution needs to be exercised in interpreting this type of experiment, since other "calmodulin inhibitors" have been shown to interact with cellular proteins other than calmodulin, such as the glucocorticoid receptor (Van Bohemen and Rousseau, 1982) and the Ca^{2+}-phospholipid-dependent kinase (Wise *et al.*, 1982).

As described in Section V,A, there is extensive evidence for an involvement of Ca^{2+} in the regulation by TRH of prolactin secretion by the GH_3 cells. Thus, it is perhaps not surprising that TRH also requires Ca^{2+} for its regulation of prolactin gene expression in these cells. By contrast, studies of the interaction of EGF with GH cells have been more limited. However, both TRH and EGF produce similar effects on shape and growth of GH cells (Schonbrunn *et al.*, 1980), induce identical changes in protein phosphorylation in these cells (Sobel and Tashjian, 1983), and stimulate prolactin gene expression at a nuclear level (Potter *et al.*, 1981; Murdoch *et al.*, 1982). Furthermore, the results in Fig. 16 show that the two peptides exhibit quite similar dose–response curves and maximal stimulations of prolactin mRNA. These observations, plus the similar effects of calmodulin inhibitors on the

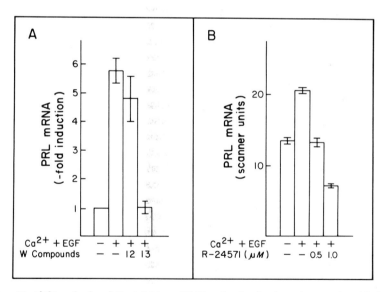

Fig. 19. Ability of calmodulin inhibitors W-13 and calmidazolium (R-24571) to block the induction by EGF plus Ca^{2+} of prolactin mRNA. GH_3 cells were incubated for 2 days in serum-free medium and then for 24 hours in the presence or absence of EGF (40 ng/ml) plus Ca^{2+} (0.4 mM), plus or minus W-13 or W-12 (10 µM) (Panel A), or R-24571 (Panel B). Prolactin mRNA levels were determined by cytoplasmic dot hybridization. The mean and range of duplicate determinations are shown.

ability of these two peptides to regulate prolactin mRNA (Figs. 18 and 19), suggest that their intracellular pathways of action may converge at some point, possibly at a step requiring a functional Ca^{2+}–calmodulin complex.

VI. SUMMARY

The GH cell lines have proven to be useful model systems for studies by a number of groups of the regulation of growth hormone and prolactin synthesis. We have developed a cytoplasmic dot hybridization technique that has proven useful in GH cells and other experimental systems for multiple analyses of regulation of cellular levels of specific mRNAs. Employing this and related techniques, we have shown that a thyroid hormone, T_3, regulates cytoplasmic and nuclear levels of growth hormone RNA in GH_3 cells. We have also found that a glucocorticoid hormone, dexamethasone, can regulate growth hormone synthesis and RNA sequences in the GH_3 cells, via a mechanism that does not require the presence of either thyroid hormone or Ca^{2+} and that is not inhibited by insulin.

In experiments employing a serum-free medium containing no added Ca^{2+}, we have observed that Ca^{2+} causes a large stimulation of cytoplasmic and nuclear prolactin RNA sequences in the GH_3 cells and a considerably smaller stimulation of growth hormone mRNA sequences. Experiments with primary cultures of rat pituitary cells have yielded similar results and have shown that Ca^{2+} regulates expression of the prolactin and growth hormone genes at the level of transcription. Investigations have been carried out of the Ca^{2+} requirement for two known peptide regulators of prolactin gene expression in the GH_3 cells, TRH and EGF. Experiments involving removal of extracellular Ca^{2+} from the incubation medium showed that TRH absolutely requires Ca^{2+} for its regulation of prolactin mRNA, but did not resolve the question of the dependence of EGF action upon Ca^{2+}. However, experiments employing a number of calmodulin inhibitors implied an absolute dependence on a functional Ca^{2+}–calmodulin complex for the ability of either TRH plus Ca^{2+} or EGF plus Ca^{2+} to regulate prolactin mRNA. These results imply that both of these peptides require Ca^{2+} for their regulation of prolactin gene expression. However, the results presented do not distinguish between two possible models for the involvement of Ca^{2+} in the actions of these peptides: (1) requirement for Ca^{2+} as a co-factor in prolactin gene expression per se, and/or in some step(s) in the pathways of action of the peptides on prolactin gene expression, and (2) changes in Ca^{2+} levels in some cellular compartment as a result of exposure of the GH_3 cells, under physiological Ca^{2+} conditions, to either of these peptides, which then leads to changes in expression of the prolactin gene. The second model would correspond most closely to the concept of Ca^{2+} as a mediator of the actions of these two peptides on prolactin gene expression. In experiments currently in progress, we are attempting to distinguish which of these models is correct.

ACKNOWLEDGMENTS

The work from our laboratory reported in this chapter was supported by National Institutes of Health Grant GM-24442, American Cancer Society Grant NP-271, and Core Grant CA-08748 from the National Cancer Institute. G. G. G. was supported by Postdoctoral Fellowship AM-06851; M. E. J. and B. A. W., by Endocrine Research Training Grant AM-07313; and B. A. W., by Postdoctoral Fellowship AM-06770, all from the National Institutes of Health. We thank Colette Brown for typing the manuscript.

REFERENCES

Bancroft, F. C. (1973). *Endocrinology (Baltimore)* **92,** 1014–1021.
Bancroft, F. C. (1981). *In* "Functionally Differentiated Cell Lines" (G. Sato, ed.), pp. 47–60. Alan R. Liss, Inc., New York.
Bancroft, F. C., Levine, L., and Tashjian, A. H., Jr. (1969). *J. Cell Biol.* **43,** 432–441.
Bancroft, F. C., Sussman-Berger, P., and Dobner, P. R. (1980a). *Ann. N.Y. Acad. Sci.* **343,** 56–68.
Bancroft, F. C., Dobner, P. R., and Y, L.-Y. (1980b). *In* "Synthesis and Release of Adenohypophyseal Hormones" (M. Justisz and K. M. McKerns, eds.), pp. 311–333. Plenum, New York.
Barta, A., Richards, R. I., Baxter, J. D., and Shine, J. (1981). *Proc. Natl. Acad. Sci. U.S.A.* **78,** 4867–4871.
Bauer, R. F., Arthur, L. O., and Fine, D. L. (1976). *In Vitro* **12,** 558–563.
Bio-Rad Laboratories Production Information (1981). No. 2020.
Borun, T. W., Scharff, M. D., and Robbins, E. (1967). *Biochim. Biophys. Acta* **149,** 302–304.
Brennan, J. K., Mansky, J., Roberts, G., and Lichtman, M. A. (1975). *In Vitro* **11,** 354–360.
Burch, J. B. E., and Weintraub, H. (1983). *Cell* **33,** 65–76.
Chafouleas, J. G., Bolton, W. E., Hidaka, H., Boyd, A. E., III, and Means, A. R. (1982). *Cell* **28,** 41–50.
Chien, Y.-H., and Thompson, E. B. (1980). *Proc. Natl. Acad. Sci. U.S.A.* **77,** 4583–4587.
Cochran, B. H., Reffel, A. C., and Stiles, C. D. (1983). *Cell* **33,** 939–947.
Cooke, N. E., and Baxter, J. D. (1982). *Nature (London)* **297,** 603–607.
Corin, R. E., Bancroft, F. C., Sonenberg, M., and Donner, D. B. (1983). *Biochim. Biophys. Acta* **762,** 503–511.
Daughaday, W. H. (1981). *In* "Textbook of Endocrinology" (R. H. Williams, ed.), pp. 73–116. Saunders, Philadelphia, Pennsylvania.
Dobner, P. R., Kawasaki, E. S., Yu, L.-Y., and Bancroft, F. C. (1981). *Proc. Natl. Acad. Sci. U.S.A.* **78,** 2230–2234.
Dufy, B., Vincent, J., Fleury, H., Du Pasquier, P., Gourdji, D., and Tixier-Vidal, A. (1979). *Science* **204,** 509–511.
Evans, M. I., Hager, L. J., and McKnight, G. S. (1981). *Cell* **25,** 187–193.

Evans, R. M., Birnberg, N. C., and Rosenfeld, M. G. (1982). *Proc. Natl. Acad. Sci. U.S.A.* **79**, 7659–7663.

Frawley, L. S., and Neill, J. D. (1983). *Program 65th Annu. Meet. Endocr. Soc., Abstract 918.*

Gautvik, K. M., and Tashjian, A. H., Jr. (1973). *Endocrinology (Baltimore)* **92**, 573–583.

Gerhard, D. S., Szabo, P., Kawasaki, E., and Bancroft, F. C. (1984). *DNA* **3**, 139–145.

Gershengorn, M. C., and Thaw, C. (1983). *Endocrinology (Baltimore)* **113**, 1522–1524.

Gick, G. G., Zeytin, F. N., Brazeau, P., Ling, N. C., Esch, F. S., and Bancroft, F. C. (1984). *Proc. Natl. Acad. Sci. U.S.A.* **81**, 1553–1555.

Harpold, M. M., Dobner, P. R., Evans, R. M., and Bancroft, F. C. (1978). *Nucleic Acids Res.* **5**, 2039–2054.

Hidaka, H., Yamaki, T., Totsuka, T., and Asano, M. (1979). *Mol. Pharmacol.* **15**, 49–59.

Hoffman, L. M., Fritsch, M. K., and Gorski, J. (1981). *J. Biol. Chem.* **256**, 2597–2600.

Hymer, W. C., Evans, W. H., Kraicer, J., Mastro, A., Davis, J., and Griswold, E. (1973). *Endocrinology (Baltimore)* **92**, 275–287.

Ivarie, R. D., and Morris, J. A. (1983). *DNA* **2**, 113–120.

Ivarie, R. D., Baxter, J. D., and Morris, J. A. (1981). *J. Biol. Chem.* **256**, 4520–4528.

Johnson, L. K., Vlodarsky, I., Baxter, J. D., and Gospodarowicz, D. (1980). *Nature (London)* **287**, 340–343.

Katz, R. A., Erlanger, B. F., and Guntaka, R. B. (1983). *Biochim. Biophys. Acta* **739**, 258–264.

Kidokoro, Y. (1975). *Nature (London)* **258**, 741–742.

Kohler, P. O., Frohman, L. A., Bridson, W. E., Vanha-Pertulla, T., and Hammond, J. M. (1969). *Science* **166**, 633–634.

Lavarriere, J. N., Gourdji, D., Picart, R., and Tixier-Vidal, A. (1981). *Biochem. Biophys. Res. Commun.* **103**, 833–840.

Lewin, M. J., Reyl-Desmars, and Ling, N. (1983). *Proc. Natl. Acad. Sci. U.S.A.* **80**, 6538–6541.

McKnight, S. G., and Palmiter, R. D. (1979). *J. Biol. Chem.* **254**, 9050–9058.

Martial, J. A., Baxter, J. D., Goodman, H. M., and Seeburg, P. H. (1977). *Proc. Natl. Acad. Sci. U.S.A.* **74**, 1816–1820.

Masur, S. K., Holtzman, E., and Bancroft, F. C. (1974). *J. Histochem. Cytochem.* **22**, 385–394.

Maurer, R. A., Gubbins, E. J., Erwin, C. R., and Donelson, J. E. (1980). *J. Biol. Chem.* **255**, 2243–2246.

Moriarty, C. M., and Leuschen, M. P. (1981). *Am. J. Physiol.* **240**, E705–E711.

Murdoch, G. H., Potter, E., Nicholaisen, A. K., Evans, R. M., and Rosenfeld, M. G. (1982). *Nature (London)* **300**, 192–194.

Owen, N. E., and Villereal, M. L. (1982a). *Proc. Natl. Acad. Sci. U.S.A.* **79**, 3537–3541.

Owen, N. E., and Villereal, M. L. (1982b). *Biochem. Biophys. Res. Commun.* **109**, 762–768.

Ozawa, S., and Kimura, N. (1979). *Proc. Natl. Acad. Sci. U.S.A.* **76**, 6017–6020.

Page, G. S., Smith, S., and Goodman, H. M. (1981). *Nucleic Acids Res.* **9**, 2087–2104.

Potter, E., Nicolaisen, K. A., Ong, E. S., Evans, R. M., and Rosenfeld, M. G. (1981). *Proc. Natl. Acad. Sci. U.S.A.* **78**, 6662–6666.

Ronning, S. A., Heatley, G. A., and Martin, T. F. J. (1982). *Proc. Natl. Acad. Sci. U.S.A.* **79**, 6294–6298.

Samuels, H. H., and Shapiro, L. E. (1976). *Proc. Natl. Acad. Sci. U.S.A.* **73**, 3369–3373.

Samuels, H. H., Horowitz, Z. D., Stanley, F., Casanova, J., and Shapiro, L. E. (1977). *Nature (London)* **268**, 254–257.

Samuels, H. H., Stanley, F., and Shapiro, L. E. (1979). *Biochemistry* **18**, 715–721.

Samuels, H. H., Casanova, J., Horowitz, Z. D., Raaka, B. M., Shapiro, L. E., Stanley, F., Tsai, J. S., and Yaffe, B. M. (1983). *In* "Biochemical Actions of Hormones" (G. Litwak, ed.), Vol. 10, pp. 115–161. Academic Press, New York.

Sawyer, S. T., and Cohen, S. (1981). *Biochemistry* **20**, 6280–6286.

Scarpa, A., Brinley, F. J., Tiffert, T., and Dubyak, G. R. (1978). *Ann. N.Y. Acad. Sci.* **307**, 86–112.

Schonbrunn, A., Krasnoff, M., Westendorf, J. M., and Tashjian, A. J., Jr. (1980). *J. Cell Biol.* **85**, 786–797.

Shapiro, L. E., Samuels, H. H., and Yaffe, B. M. (1978). *Proc. Natl. Acad. Sci. U.S.A.* **75**, 45–49.

Sobel, A., and Tashjian, A. J., Jr. (1983). *J. Biol. Chem.* **258**, 10312–10324.

Spindler, S. R., Mellon, S. H., and Baxter, J. D. (1982). *J. Biol. Chem.* **257**, 11627–11632.

Sussman, P. M., Tushinski, R. J., and Bancroft, F. C. (1976). *Proc. Natl. Acad. Sci. U.S.A.* **73**, 29–33.

Taraskevitch, P. S., and Douglas, W. W. (1977). *Proc. Natl. Acad. Sci. U.S.A.* **74**, 4064–4067.

Tashjian, A. H., Jr., Bancroft, F. C., and Levine, L. (1970). *J. Cell Biol.* **47**, 61–70.

Tashjian, A. H., Jr., Lomedico, M. E., and Maina, D. (1978). *Biochem. Biophys. Res. Commun.* **81**, 798–806.

Thomas, P. S. (1980). *Proc. Natl. Acad. Sci. U.S.A.* **77**, 5021–5025.

Tsai, J. S., and Samuels, H. H. (1974). *Biochem. Biophys. Res. Commun.* **59**, 420–428.

Tushinski, R. J., Sussman, P. M., Yu, L.-Y., and Bancroft, F. C. (1977). *Proc. Natl. Acad. Sci. U.S.A.* **74**, 2357–2361.

Van Belle, H. (1981). *Cell Calcium* **2**, 483–494.

Van Bohemen, G. C., and Rousseau, G. G. (1982). *J. Biol. Chem.* **257**, 10613–10616.

White, B. A., and Bancroft, F. C. (1982). *J. Biol. Chem.* **257**, 8569–8572.

White, B. A., and Bancroft, F. C. (1983). *J. Biol. Chem.* **258**, 4618–4622.

White, B. A., and Bancroft, F. C. (1984). *In* "Prolactin" (M. Flavio, ed.). Academic Press, New York.

White, B. A., Bauerle, L. R., and Bancroft, F. C. (1981). *J. Biol. Chem.* **256**, 5942–5945.

Wise, B. C., Glass, D. B., Chou, J. C.-H., Raynor, R. L., Katoh, N., Scharzman, R. C., Turner, R. S., Kibler, R. F., and Kuo, J. F. (1982). *J. Biol. Chem.* **257**, 8489–8495.

Yu, L.-Y., Tushinski, R. J., and Bancroft, F. C. (1977). *J. Biol. Chem.* **252**, 3870–3875.

Zeytin, F. N., Gick, G. G., Brazeau, P., Lling, N., McLaughlin, M., and Bancroft, C. (1984). *Endocrinology (Baltimore)* **114**, 2054–2059.

CHAPTER 7

Mechanisms Involved in the Actions of Calcium-Dependent Hormones

Peter F. Blackmore and John H. Exton

Howard Hughes Medical Institute and Department of Physiology
Vanderbilt University School of Medicine
Nashville, Tennessee

I. INTRODUCTION

It is becoming clear that the actions of a very large number of hormones, neurotransmitters, and related agents involve an increase in cytosolic ionized calcium. This is demonstrated by the facts that their actions are

BIOCHEMICAL ACTIONS OF HORMONES, VOL. XII

impaired in calcium-deficient media or when intracellular calcium pools are depleted, that their effects can be mimicked by agents that increase cytosolic Ca^{2+} such as A23187, and that they alter cell or tissue Ca^{2+} fluxes.

The mechanisms by which calcium-dependent hormones alter cell Ca^{2+} fluxes and thereby raise cytosolic Ca^{2+} have been studied in some detail in liver, smooth muscle, salivary gland, platelets, and pituitary. The two basic mechanisms for increasing cytosolic Ca^{2+} are (1) a mobilization of Ca^{2+} from intracellular Ca^{2+} pools such as those in the mitochondria or endoplasmic reticulum or those associated with the plasma membrane or other intracellular membranes, and (2) an alteration in plasma membrane Ca^{2+} permeability and/or Ca^{2+}, Mg^{2+}-ATPase (Ca^{2+} pump) activity such that there is a net influx of extracellular Ca^{2+}. Mobilization of intracellular Ca^{2+} is usually the initial response to Ca^{2+}-dependent hormones, whereas increased Ca^{2+} influx and/or decreased Ca^{2+} efflux across the plasma membrane usually occurs later to sustain the biological effects.

In this chapter, attention will be focused on the liver, since the molecular mechanisms involved in the actions of the calcium-dependent hormones have been studied in greatest detail in this tissue.

II. CHANGES IN CYTOSOLIC Ca^{2+} INDUCED BY CALCIUM-DEPENDENT HORMONES

The demonstration that calcium-dependent hormones actually increase cytosolic Ca^{2+} is crucial to current hypotheses of how these hormones act. Murphy *et al.* (1980). first presented direct evidence that the α-adrenergic agonist phenylephrine increased cytosolic Ca^{2+} in rat hepatocytes. They employed a "null point" method in which the Ca^{2+} concentration of the extracellular medium was varied until it was equal to that in the cytosol as shown by the fact that there was no change in arsenazo III absorption upon disruption of the plasma membrane with digitonin. They calculated that the basal cytosolic Ca^{2+} was 0.19 μM and that it was increased with α-adrenergic stimulation by two- to threefold at 2 minutes. There was also a good correlation between the dose responses for phenylephrine on cytosolic Ca^{2+} and phosphorylase *a* levels.

More recently, Charest *et al.* (1983, 1984) have employed the acetoxymethyl ester of Quin 2, a fluorescent Ca^{2+} chelator with a quinoline ring system (Tsien, 1980; Tsien *et al.*, 1982), to continuously measure the changes in cytosolic Ca^{2+} in rat hepatocytes. The ester is uncharged and can penetrate into the cells, whereupon intracellular esterases release the free compound, which accumulates in the cytosol but does not penetrate into intracellular organelles. When excited at 340 nm, the free compound emits fluorescence at 500 nm in a Ca^{2+}-dependent manner and thus can be used to measure cytosolic Ca^{2+}.

Figure 1 from Charest *et al.* (1983) shows the increase in cytosolic Ca^{2+}, monitored by fluorescence emitted at 500 nm in Quin 2–loaded hepatocytes incubated with maximally effective concentrations of epinephrine, phenylephrine, vasopressin, and glucagon. The two α-adrenergic agonists produce a rapid rise in cytosolic Ca^{2+} within 2 seconds, and vasopressin produces the same change after a slight lag. In contrast, the rise in Ca^{2+} with glucagon (10^{-8} M) is slower and occurs after a longer lag. With more physiological concentrations of glucagon ($10^{-10}-10^{-9}$ M), the response is greatly delayed and is of much smaller magnitude (Charest *et al.*, 1984). There is no evidence that the rise in cytosolic Ca^{2+} plays any role in the metabolic actions of glucagon, which can be attributed entirely to the rise in cAMP (e.g., Assimacopoulos-Jeannet *et al.*, 1977; Blackmore *et al.*, 1979a,b).

The rise in cytosolic Ca^{2+} induced by epinephrine or vasopressin is from

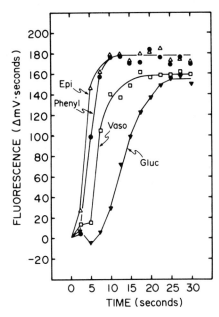

FIG. 1. Time course of change in fluorescence of Quin 2–loaded hepatocytes following addition of epinephrine (Epi, 10^{-5} M), phenylephrine (Phenyl, 10^{-5} M), vasopressin (Vaso, 10^{-8} M), and glucagon (Gluc, 10^{-8} M). The results are presented as the change in fluorescence from time zero with each point being the mean from triplicate incubations from a representative experiment. Fluorescence measurements were collected every 0.5 seconds after the addition of hormones at time zero. Free cytosolic Ca^{2+} increased from a resting level of 0.2 μM to a maximum of 0.6 μM. [From Charest *et al.* (1983).]

approximately 0.2 to 0.6 μM, in agreement with the findings of Murphy *et al.* (1980), and precedes the rise in phsophorylase *a* (Charest *et al.*, 1983, 1984). This is consistent with Ca^{2+} stimulation of phosphorylase *b* kinase (see Section V) (Blackmore and Exton, 1981), which converts phosphorylase *b* to the active form phosphorylase *a*. There is also a very close correlation between the concentration dependence of epinephrine, vasopressin, and phenylephrine effects on cytosolic Ca^{2+} and phosphorylase *a* (Blackmore *et al.*, 1978; Charest *et al.*, 1983, 1984). Consistent with earlier findings, the effects of epinephrine and phenylephrine on both parameters are blocked by α-adrenergic antagonists (Blackmore *et al.*, 1978; Charest *et al.*, 1983). Addition of an α-antagonist to liver cells incubated with phenylephrine causes an abrupt fall in cytosolic Ca^{2+} (Charest *et al.*, 1983) consistent with this process being under dynamic control.

III. MOBILIZATION OF INTRACELLULAR Ca^{2+} BY CALCIUM-DEPENDENT HORMONES

There is much evidence that Ca^{2+}-dependent hormones raise cytosolic Ca^{2+} initially by mobilizing intracellular Ca^{2+} stores. The strongest evidence comes from the fact that these hormones cause a rapid, large decrease in total cell calcium measured by atomic absorption spectroscopy in hepatocytes (Blackmore *et al.*, 1978; Chen *et al.*, 1978) or a large release of Ca^{2+} from livers perfused with nonrecirculating medium (Blackmore *et al.*, 1979b). Since the decrease in cell Ca^{2+} is much larger than the pool of cytosolic Ca^{2+}, this implies that Ca^{2+} must have been mobilized from intracellular stores. More evidence for the importance of intracellular mobilization of Ca^{2+} comes from the fact that the biological effects of the hormones and their ability to increase cytosolic Ca^{2+} are unaltered on a short-term basis when the extracellular Ca^{2+} concentration is decreased by EGTA to 30 nM, i.e., the net influx of Ca^{2+} in hepatocytes is abolished (Blackmore *et al.*, 1978, 1982; Charest *et al.*, 1984). On the other hand, extensive washing and incubation of hepatocytes with EGTA will deplete intracellular Ca^{2+} pools, leading to an inhibition of all responses (Blackmore *et al.*, 1978).

Further support for intracellular Ca^{2+} mobilization comes from measurements of the calcium content of intracellular organelles. Several studies using atomic absorption spectrometry and $^{45}Ca^{2+}$ have shown that Ca^{2+}-dependent hormones cause a reduction in mitochondrial calcium (Blackmore *et al.*, 1979b; Dehaye *et al.*, 1980, 1981; Barritt *et al.*, 1981b; Murphy *et al.*, 1980; Babcock *et al.*, 1979; Studer and Borle, 1983), and most workers agree that these organelles are a major source of mobilized Ca^{2+}. Efforts to show changes in "microsomal" calcium have yielded variable results (Blackmore *et al.*, 1979b; Murphy *et al.*, 1980; Dehaye *et al.*, 1981; Morgan *et al.*, 1983b). This is because it is difficult to prevent redistribution of Ca^{2+} during the isolation of these structures. Recent data suggest that the Ca^{2+} load of the hepatocyte alters the distribution of Ca^{2+} between the mitochondria and endoplasmic reticulum and thus influences the relative contributions of these organelles toward Ca^{2+} mobilization by hormones (Joseph and Williamson, 1983; Joseph *et al.*, 1983).

Some groups have suggested that mitochondria are not the major source of Ca^{2+} mobilized in hepatocytes by Ca^{2+}-dependent hormones (Poggioli *et al.*, 1980; Althaus-Salzmann *et al.*, 1980). These groups reported increased uptake of $^{45}Ca^{2+}$ by mitochondria in hepatocytes or perfused liver following α-adrenergic stimulation. However, the possibility of artifactual posthomogenization $^{45}Ca^{2+}$ uptake and other problems have been noted with these studies (Williamson *et al.*, 1981).

Due to technical problems, it has not been possible to observe changes in mitochondrial calcium earlier than 30 seconds after addition of Ca^{2+}-dependent hormones, and it is therefore possible that these organelles may not be the immediate source of Ca^{2+} mobilized by these hormones (Blackmore *et al.*, 1983b). Several groups have suggested that the plasma membrane may be the initial source of Ca^{2+} (Blackmore *et al.*, 1983b; Poggioli *et al.*, 1980), but efforts to demonstrate this have given variable results (Burgess *et al.*, 1983).

IV. STIMULATION OF Ca^{2+} INFLUX OR INHIBITION OF Ca^{2+} EFFLUX BY CALCIUM-DEPENDENT HORMONES

As noted previously, short-term reduction of extracellular Ca^{2+} to the submicromolar range does not alter the *initial* effects of calcium-dependent hormones on cytosolic Ca^{2+} or phosphorylase *a* in hepatocytes, i.e., those changes occurring during the first 30 seconds (Blackmore *et al.*, 1978; Charest *et al.*, 1984). However, if prolonged, the reduction in extracellular Ca^{2+} leads to the depletion of intracellular Ca^{2+} stores and attenuation of the responses (Blackmore *et al.*, 1978). These findings indicate that influx of extracellular Ca^{2+} is not *necessary* for the *initial* actions of the hormones, but do not exclude that it is involved in later events.

In any consideration of hormone effects on cell Ca^{2+}, it is important to recognize that the release of Ca^{2+} from intracellular stores is of limited magnitude and duration (e.g., Blackmore *et al.*, 1979b). Thus, hormone effects at the plasma membrane to alter efflux or influx of Ca^{2+} will be necessary to maintain an elevated cytosolic Ca^{2+} concentration and thereby prolong the hormone actions. Furthermore, influx of extracellular Ca^{2+} will be a necessary event to restore intracellular Ca^{2+} stores following their depletion by Ca^{2+}-dependent hormones (Morgan *et al.*, 1982).

Studies utilizing the perfused rat liver or isolated hepatocytes have consistently failed to show net influx of Ca^{2+} during the initial stages of epinephrine or vasopressin action, despite the presence of $\sim$1 mM Ca^{2+} in the extracellular medium (e.g., Morgan *et al.*, 1982; Blackmore *et al.*, 1978). As illustrated in Fig. 2, these hormones cause a rapid, large, but transient efflux of Ca^{2+}, which lasts approximately 5 minutes and is followed by no net change in medium Ca^{2+} until the hormone is removed or degraded. Withdrawal of the hormone is followed by Ca^{2+} uptake to restore the liver calcium content to normal levels (Blackmore *et al.*, 1982; Morgan *et al.*, 1982). Analogous experiments with isolated hepatocytes show that in media

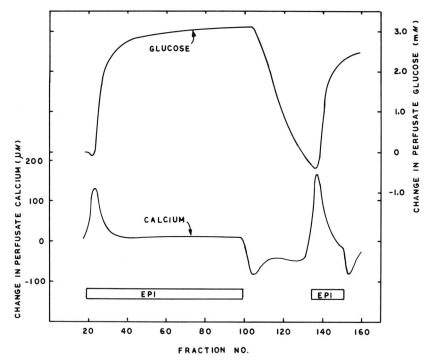

Fig. 2. Effects of prolonged epinephrine (Epi) stimulation on the ability of a subsequent epinephrine stimulus to increase glucose output and stimulate Ca^{2+} efflux in the perfused rat liver. Livers of rats 200–250 g body weight were perfused, and samples were collected every 18 seconds. The erythrocytes were removed by centrifugation, and aliquots were taken for the measurement of glucose and Ca^{2+}. Basal values for perfusate Ca^{2+} and glucose were 1.02 $\pm$ 0.012 mM and 2.1 $\pm$ 0.6 mM, respectively.

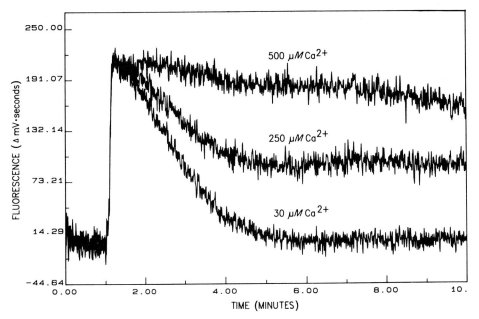

FIG. 3. Effect of various extracellular Ca^{2+} concentrations on the increase in cystolic Ca^{2+} induced by 10^{-8} M vasopressin. Quin 2 and non-Quin 2–loaded hepatocytes were washed and resuspended in medium containing either 500, 250, or 30 μM Ca^{2+} for 5 minutes before fluorescence measurements were made. The values shown are the differences between Quin 2 and control fluorescence changes and are the means from four separate experiments. Vasopressin was added at 1 minute.

containing physiological levels of Ca^{2+}, vasopressin induces a prolonged rise in cytosolic Ca^{2+} and activation of phosphorylase (Charest *et al.*, 1984). However, if the experiments are carried out with low Ca^{2+} media, the cytosolic Ca^{2+} rise and phosphorylase activation induced by the hormones decline after about 1 minute, and a second dose of hormone is ineffective (Charest *et al.*, 1983, 1984). With readdition of Ca^{2+} to the media, the hormone responses are restored. Although these data could have been interpreted as indicating a hormone effect stimulating Ca^{2+} influx, the alternative explanation that hormone-sensitive cell Ca^{2+} stores have been repleted is equally likely.

Stronger evidence for a hormone effect at the plasma membrane comes from the experiments illustrated in Fig. 3. These show the changes in cytosolic Ca^{2+} in hepatocytes incubated in medium containing either 30, 250, or 500 μM Ca^{2+} and then exposed to vasopressin. The rise in cytosolic Ca^{2+} with vasopressin is transient in the presence of low Ca^{2+} but is maintained in the presence of 500 μM Ca^{2+}. These findings suggest that the hormone also controls the level of cytosolic Ca^{2+} by altering the transmembrane flux of Ca^{2+}. However, the effect is not discernible before 1 minute.

These data do not distinguish between possible effects of vasopressin on plasma membrane Ca^{2+} permeability or Ca^{2+} pump activity. However, there have been reports of a small inhibitory effect of vasopressin on plasma membrane Ca^{2+},Mg^{2+}-ATPase in hepatocytes (Lin *et al.*, 1983; Prpić *et al.*, 1983). A large inhibition of Ca^{2+} transport into inside-out plasma membrane vesicles, isolated from vasopressin-treated perfused livers, has been observed by Prpić *et al.* (1984). The effect is maximal (50% inhibition) after 3–6 minutes of exposure but not significant before 1 minute. A half-maximal effect is obtained with 5×10^{-10} M vasopressin (Fig. 4), which compares favorably with the concentration required to half-maximally increase cytosolic Ca^{2+} and activate phosphorylase (Charest *et al.*, 1984). The other Ca^{2+}-mobilizing hormones, epinephrine and angiotensin II, also inhibit Ca^{2+} transport by 24 and 21%, respectively, at 3 minutes, whereas 10^{-8} M glucagon is without effect (Prpić *et al.*, 1984). Inhibition of the plasma membrane Ca^{2+} pump would maintain cytosolic Ca^{2+} at a higher-than-basal

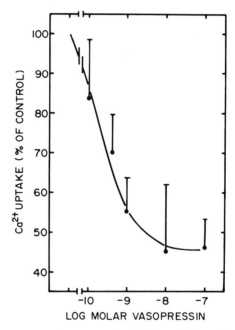

Fig. 4. Dose–response curve for vasopressin inhibition of liver plasma membrane Ca^{2+} pump activity. Rat livers were perfused for 3 minutes with the concentrations of vasopressin shown. Ca^{2+} uptake into plasma membrane vesicles prepared from the livers was measured as described by Prpić *et al.* (1984).

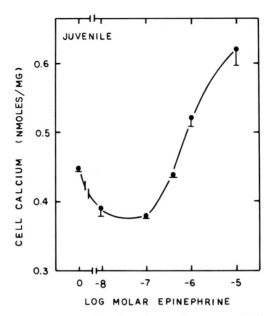

Fᴵɢ. 5. Dose–response curve for the effects of epinephrine on total cell calcium content in hepatocytes from juvenile rats. Hepatocytes from juvenile male rats (80–110 g) were incubated with epinephrine for 4 minutes, and then cell Ca^{2+} was determined by atomic absorption spectroscopy. Values are means ±SEM from triplicate incubations from a representative experiment.

level beyond the time at which intracellular Ca^{2+} mobilization ceases, provided extracellular Ca^{2+} is available to maintain influx of Ca^{2+} into the cell (Fig. 3).

Under certain circumstances, the Ca^{2+}-mobilizing hormones markedly stimulate influx of Ca^{2+} into the liver, namely, when cAMP levels are elevated simultaneously with the application of the Ca^{2+}-mobilizing hormone. This can be achieved by adding high concentrations of epinephrine to hepatocytes isolated from female rats or juvenile male rats (Fig. 5), since these hepatocytes contain functional β_2-adrenergic receptors that elevate cAMP up to tenfold and α_1-adrenergic receptors that mobilize Ca^{2+} (Morgan *et al.*, 1983a,b). Calcium influx can also be achieved by combining glucagon or exogenously added cAMP with the Ca^{2+}-mobilizing hormones vasopressin, epinephrine, and angiotensin II (Morgan *et al.*, 1983b).

When hepatocyte cAMP is elevated during the stimulation with α_1-adrenergic agonists, vasopressin, and angiotensin II, total cell Ca^{2+} can increase up to fivefold (Morgan *et al.*, 1983b), and most of this Ca^{2+} ·is sequestered into mitochondria. Once sequestered into mitochondria, the Ca^{2+} becomes tightly bound, such that further stimulation with the Ca^{2+}-mobilizing hormones in the absence of elevated cAMP fails to promote release of Ca^{2+}.

V. ROLE OF CYTOSOLIC Ca^{2+} IN THE PHYSIOLOGICAL RESPONSES TO CALCIUM-DEPENDENT HORMONES

As described previously, there is strong evidence that the activation of phosphorylase by Ca^+-dependent hormones is a consequence of a rise in cytosolic Ca^{2+}, which stimulates phosphorylase b kinase. This enzyme has been purified to homogeneity from rat liver and contains the Ca^{2+}-dependent regulatory protein calmodulin as the δ subunit (Chrisman et $al.$, 1982). It shows an increase in activity when the Ca^{2+} concentration is raised from 0.1 μM to 1 μM (Fig. 6), which is the range through which Ca^{2+}-dependent hormones increase cytosolic Ca^{2+} in liver (Charest et $al.$, 1983).

Ca^{2+}-dependent hormones also inactivate glycogen synthase in liver (Strickland et $al.$, 1980), but it is not certain which Ca^{2+}-sensitive enzyme or enzymes are involved. Phosphorylase b kinase can phosphorylate and inactivate liver glycogen synthase in $vitro$ (Imazu et $al.$, 1984) and can also act indirectly by increasing phosphorylase a, which is an inhibitor of liver glycogen synthase phosphatase (Strickland et $al.$, 1983).

A Ca^{2+}–calmodulin-dependent protein kinase has been purified from rat liver (Schworer et $al.$, 1983), and similar, if not identical, enzymes have been identified in muscle and brain (Woodgett et $al.$, 1982; Kennedy et $al.$, 1983). Several physiological substates for these enzymes have been identified, including liver and muscle glycogen synthase. However, evidence has been presented that this enzyme is not responsible for the inactivation of rat liver glycogen synthase elicited by the Ca^{2+}-dependent hormones (Blackmore et $al.$, 1981; Strickland et $al.$, 1983). Another Ca^{2+}-sensitive protein kinase present in liver is the calcium–phospholipid-dependent protein kinase discovered by Nishizuka and associates (Inoue et $al.$, 1977; Takai et $al.$, 1979). This kinase phosphorylates liver glycogen synthase and may alter its activity (Imazu et $al.$, 1984; Roach and Goldman, 1983).

The molecular mechanisms involved in the effects of Ca^{2+}-dependent hormones on other physiological responses in liver are much less clear. They include the stimulation of gluconeogenesis (e.g., Kneer et $al.$, 1979), respiration (e.g., Sugano et $al.$, 1980; Dehaye et $al.$, 1981; Blackmore et $al.$, 1983a,b), fatty acid oxidation (Sugden et $al.$, 1980), amino acid transport (Pariza et $al.$, 1977; LeCam and Freychet, 1978) and K^+ fluxes (Haylett and Jenkinson, 1972; Jakob and Diem, 1975; Blackmore et $al.$, 1979b), inhibition of branched-chain α-keto acid oxidation (Buxton et $al.$, 1982), and changes in

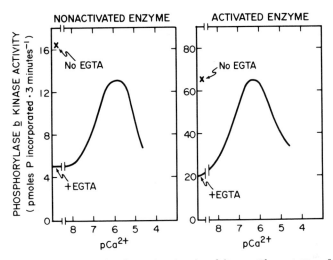

FIG. 6. Ca^{2+} requirement of rat liver phosphorylase b kinase. The activities of the nonactivated and activated enzymes were measured as a function of pCa^{2+} using Ca^{2+} −EGTA buffers at pH 7.4 with MgATP being 1 mM. (Reprinted by permission of the publisher from Mechanisms involved in the actions of calcium-dependent hormones in liver, Chapter IX, Subcellular Calcium Distribution and Calcium-mediated Hormone Action, by R. A. Harris and N. W. Cornell, eds., "Isolation, Characterization, and Use of Hepatocytes," p. 402. Copyright 1983 by Elsevier Science Publishing Co., Inc.)

lipogenesis (Assimacopoulos-Jeannet *et al.*, 1981). Most of these effects have been shown to require Ca^{2+}, but the basis of this requirement is unclear in most instances.

In the case of the stimulation of gluconeogenesis from reduced substrates such as lactate and glycerol, Ca^{2+} may be acting in part by stimulating the mitochondrial oxidation of cytosolic-reduced pyridine nucleotide through an effect on mitochondrial glycerol-3-P dehydrogenase (Wernette *et al.*, 1981). Ca^{2+}-dependent hormones also phosphorylate and inhibit pyruvate kinase (Garrison *et al.*, 1979), and this contributes to the stimulation of gluconeogenesis. Phosphorylation of pyruvate kinase has been reported to be Ca^{2+} dependent, but the protein kinase or phosphoprotein phosphatase involved is unknown. Another change involved in the stimulation of gluconeogenesis by Ca^{2+}-dependent hormones is an increase in mitochondrial pyruvate carboxylation (Garrison and Borland, 1979). The role of Ca^{2+} in this effect is undefined, although it is known that pyruvate carboxylase is inhibited by high concentrations of Ca^{2+} (e.g., Foldes and Barritt, 1977).

The stimulation of respiration by the Ca^{2+}-dependent hormones could be due in part to the increased oxidation of cytosolic NADH via Ca^{2+} stimulation of the glycerol-3-P dehydrogenase reaction alluded to above. Other possibilities are Ca^{2+} activation of the 2-oxoglutarate and pyruvate dehydrogenase complexes and of NAD^+-linked isocitrate dehydrogenase (Denton *et al.*, 1981). These effects would require that the mitochondrial matrix/free Ca^{2+} concentration be increased by the hormones. It has been demonstrated that pyruvate dehydrogenase activity is increased in hepatocytes by Ca^{2+}-dependent hormones and the Ca^{2+} ionophore A23187 (Denton *et al.*, 1981; Blackmore *et al.*, 1983a; Assimacopoulos-Jeannet *et al.*, 1983), but the postulated changes in the other two enzymes are speculative. Pyruvate dehydrogenase is activated between 20 and 40 seconds, with maximal activation at 1 minute and a return to basal activity at 4 minutes (Blackmore *et al.*, 1983a). The activation is not observed in Ca^{2+}-depleted hepatocytes (Blackmore *et al.*, 1983a), but it is not clear that it can be attributed solely or partly to Ca^{2+} stimulation of pyruvate dehydrogenase phosphatase since the complex can be regulated by a large number of factors that could be altered indirectly by Ca^{2+} (Roche and Cate, 1977).

The above findings, with respect to regulation of pyruvate dehydrogenase in hepatocytes, differ from those obtained in studies with the perfused liver (Sies *et al.*, 1983), in which the activity of the enzyme was monitored by measuring $^{14}CO_2$ production from [1-^{14}C]pyruvate. These studies show that vasopressin and α-adrenergic agonists cause a transient inhibition of $^{14}CO_2$ production that is maximal within 1–2 minutes (Sies *et al.*, 1983) and followed by more sustained stimulation. Since these changes are not associated with decreases in the assayed activity of active pyruvate dehydrogenase (Sies *et al.*, 1983), they are probably due to changes in allosteric effectors of the enzyme rather than increases in its phosphorylation state. The reasons for the discrepancies between these findings and those obtained with hepatocytes are unclear. One explanation is that the transient inhibition of pyruvate dehydrogenase activity observed in the perfused liver is due to a rise in mitochondrial $NADH/NAD^+$ (see following discussion). This change may not have been preserved in the mitochondria isolated from the hepatocytes. With respect to the assayed activities of pyruvate dehydrogenase, it is of note that vasopressin increased these in both experimental systems.

The stimulation of fatty acid oxidation to CO_2 induced by Ca^{2+}-dependent hormones in hepatocytes from fed rats (Sugden and Watts, 1983) may explain their antiketogenic action (Sugden *et al.*, 1980). The effect is not due to alterations in fatty acid esterification or β-oxidation, but is apparently due to increased citric acid cycle activity (Sugden and Watts, 1983). The specific mitochondrial enzyme reactions involved are unknown, but it has been speculated that they are 2-oxoglutarate dehydrogenase and NAD^+-linked isocitrate dehydrogenase (Sugden and Watts, 1983).

Although Ca^{2+}-dependent hormones stimulate mitochondrial respiration as described previously, they also cause an initial transient increase in the reduction state of mitochondrial pyridine nucleotides (Balaban and Blum, 1982; Buxton *et al.*, 1982), implying that increased generation of reduced coenzyme transiently exceeds mitochondrial oxidation. The increase in mitochondrial $NADH/NAD^+$ is Ca^{2+} dependent and is probably the major factor responsible for the transient inhibition of pyruvate and branched-chain α-keto acid oxidation caused by Ca^{2+}-dependent hormones (Sies *et al.*, 1983; Buxton *et al.*, 1982).

Variable effects of Ca^{2+}-dependent hormones on lipogenesis have been reported (Assimacopoulos-Jeannet *et al.*, 1981; Ly and Kim, 1981). α-Adrenergic agonists have been reported to be inhibitory (Ly and Kim, 1981) or without effect (Assimacopoulos-Jeannet *et al.*, 1981) on hepatic fatty acid synthesis, whereas vasopressin has been reported to be stimulatory. Likewise, acetyl-CoA carboxylase has been found to be inhibited by α-agonists and stimulated by vasopressin (Ly and Kim, 1981; Assimacopoulos-Jeannet *et al.*, 1981). The inactivation of the enzyme by α-agonists in hepatocytes is correlated with its phosphorylation (Ly and Kim, 1981). A possible resolution of these differences is that the effects of the α-agonists are due mainly to the increase in cAMP (Chan and Exton, 1977; Kemp and Clark, 1978; Blair *et al.*, 1979; Blackmore *et al.*, 1979a). In this regard, α_1-adrenergic agonists increase cAMP in the livers of mature rats as opposed to juvenile rats (Morgan *et al.*, 1983a), and it has been shown that glucagon and dibutyrul cAMP phosphorylate and inactivate hepatic acetyl-CoA carboxylase (Witters *et al.*, 1979a,b).

Ca^{2+}-dependent hormones have different effects on K^+ fluxes in liver, depending on the species. In guinea pig, K^+ efflux is observed, and this is attributed to a Ca^{2+}-dependent increase in plasma membrane K^+ permeability (Haylett and Jenkinson, 1972). In rat, there is a transient influx of K^+ (Jacob and Diem, 1975; Blackmore *et al.*, 1979b), which due to a Ca^{2+}-dependent stimulation of Na^+,K^+-ATPase activity (Becker and Jakob, 1982; Capiod *et al.*, 1982 Radominskia-Pyrek *et al.*, 1982).

VI. INTRACELLULAR SIGNALING MECHANISMS OF CALCIUM-DEPENDENT HORMONES

The hepatic receptors for the Ca^{2+}-dependent hormones are located in the plasma membrane as revealed by radioligand binding studies (El-Refai *et al.*, 1979; Dehaye *et al.*, 1980; Campanile *et al.*, 1982; Cantau *et al.*, 1980). A major question is how activation of these receptors is linked to the cellular Ca^{2+} fluxes induced by the hormones. As discussed previously, a major factor in the initial rise in cytosolic Ca^{2+} is the release of Ca^{2+} from mitochondria and other intracellular calcium reservoirs. Thus, there must be communication between the plasma membrane receptors and these calcium storage sites. In addition, it is speculated that there may be a release of Ca^{2+} from the inner surface of the plasma membrane (Blackmore *et al.*, 1983b; Burgess *et al.*, 1983). There is also an inhibition of plasma membrane Ca^{2+}, Mg^{2+}-ATPase/Ca^{2+} transport activity, although this inhibition appears to be a relatively late event and may be secondary to the rise in cytosolic Ca^{2+} (Prpić *et al.*, 1984).

Many candidates have been proposed for the putative "second messenger" that is generated by activation of the plasma membrane receptors for the Ca^{2+}-dependent hormones and that acts on intracellular Ca^{2+} stores. As we will discuss, these include certain products of phosphoinositide metabolism. In addition, ions such as Na^+ and H^+ and nucleotides such as cyclic GMP have been proposed. However, there is much evidence against a role for Na^+ (Hughes *et al.*, 1980), and no changes in cytosolic or mitochondrial pH have been detected (Strzelecki *et al.*, 1983). Data on the effects of Ca^{2+}-dependent hormones on cyclic GMP levels in liver are inconsistent (Pointer *et al.*, 1976; Hems *et al.*, 1978), and observations in other tissues indicate that an increase in this nucleotide may be a result rather than a cause of a rise in Ca^{2+}.

VII. EFFECTS OF CALCIUM-DEPENDENT HORMONES ON PHOSPHOINOSITIDE METABOLISM

There is much evidence that Ca^{2+}-dependent hormones stimulate the turnover of phosphatidylinositol and phosphatidylinositol-4,5-P_2 in liver (Prpić *et al.*, 1982; Rhodes *et al.*, 1983; Thomas *et al.*, 1983; Creba *et al.*, 1983; Joseph *et al.*, 1984; Charest *et al.*, 1984). The key question is whether this turnover plays a primary causal role in the cell Ca^{2+} changes induced by the hormones. Vasopressin and epinephrine stimulate the breakdown of phosphatidylinositol as indicated by studies employing isotopic labeling of the phospholipid or by chemical measurements. However, the breakdwon is not detectable during the first minute (e.g., Prpić *et al.*, 1982), whereas Ca^{2+} is mobilized within 2 seconds (Charest *et al.*, 1983, 1984). The breakdown is also Ca^{2+}-dependent and requires higher hormone concentrations than do Ca^{2+} mobilization and phosphorylase activation (Charest *et al.*, 1984). Thus, it seems unlikely that phosphatidylinositol hydrolysis plays a primary role in the initial changes in Ca^{2+}.

More recently, much attention has been turned to phosphatidylinositol-4,5-P_2, since this compound breaks down more rapidly in hepatocytes in response to Ca^{2+}-dependent hormones than does phosphatidylinositol. It has been proposed that the breakdown increases the permeability of the plasma membrane to Ca^{2+} ("opens Ca^{2+} gates") and/or generates a second messenger that releases intracellular Ca^{2+} (e.g., Thomas *et al.*, 1983; Downes and Michell, 1982; Blackmore *et al.*, 1983b). Two suggested second messengers are *myo*-inositol-1,4,5-P_3 and diacylglycerol, which are the immediate products of phosphatidylinositol-4,5-P_2 breakdown by phosphodiesterase. Others are phosphatidate derived from diacylglycerol by the action of diacylglycerol kinase, and arachidonate and its further metabolites derived from diacylglycerol through lipase action. Several lines of evidence against phosphatidate and arachidonate playing a second messenger role in liver have been presented (Barritt *et al.*, 1981a; Whiting and Barritt, 1982). On the other hand, as discussed below, there is strong evidence that *myo*-inositol-1,4,5-P_3 plays a messenger role to mobilize intracellular Ca^{2+} and that diacylglycerol acts on a specific protein kinase to increase the phosphorylation of specific proteins.

As illustrated in Fig. 7, vasopressin (10^{-7} M) and epinephrine (10^{-5} M) very rapidly increase *myo*-inositol-P_3 in hepatocytes. The effect is detectable

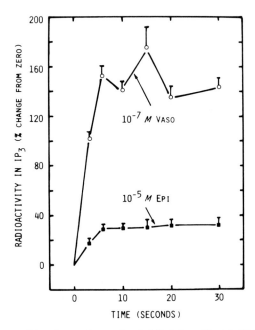

FIG. 7. Time course of the changes in *myo*-inositol-P_3 induced by 10^{-7} M vasopressin (Vaso) and 10^{-5} M epinephrine (Epi). Hepatocytes were incubated with [2-^{3}H]*myo*-inositol for 90 minutes to label phosphoinositides. Aliquots were removed at the times indicated, and the trichloroacetic acid–soluble products were chromatographed on Dowex 1 formate form resin to separate the inositol phosphate. The data shown are means ±SE from three separate incubations.

within 3 seconds and persists for 5–10 minutes with high concentrations of hormone (Charest *et al.*, 1984). Thus, the time course of phosphatidylinositol 4,5-P_2 hydrolysis as measured by *myo*-inositol-P_3 accumulation is consistent with its playing a role in Ca^{2+} mobilization. However, studies of the con- centration-dependence of phosphatidylinositol-4,5-P_2 breakdown on vaso- pressin have been interpreted differently (Charest *et al.*, 1984). In three reports, the breakdown was observed to be not significantly affected by hormone concentrations (10^{-10}–10^{-9} M) that cause near-maximal mobiliza- tion of cell Ca^{2+} and activation of phosphorylase (Rhodes *et al.*, 1983; Charest *et al.*, 1984; Creba *et al.*, 1983). In another report, there was a good corre- spondence between the dose response for the rate of breakdown of the phospholipid and for the rate of activation of phosphorylase (Thomas *et al.*, 1983). An explanation for these different findings would be that it only requires an extremely small breakdown of phosphatidylinositol-4,5-P_2 to elicit Ca^{2+} mobilization.

Support for a functional role for phosphatidylinositol-4,5-P_2 turnover in the initial actions of Ca^{2+} hormones in liver comes from the increasing evidence that *myo*-inositol-P_3 acts as a second messenger for the release of intracellular Ca^{2+} (Charest *et al.*, 1983). As shown in Fig. 8 and reported recently by several groups, this compound releases Ca^{2+} from saponin- or digitonin-permeabilized hepatocytes and other cells (Streb *et al.*, 1983; Joseph *et al.*, 1984; Putney, 1984; Berridge, 1984; Thiyagarajah *et al.*, 1984). Furthermore, direct effects to release Ca^{2+} from isolated microsomes and mitochondria by *myo*-inositol-P_3 have been observed (Thiyagarajah *et al.*, 1984). The half-maximally effective dose of *myo*-inositol-P_3 was 0.15 μM, with maximum effects being observed with 0.4 μM *myo*-inositol-P_3 (Thiya- garajah *et al.*, 1984). The effect on Ca^{2+} release from permeabilized cells, isolated mitochondria, and microsomes occurred without a lag (<1 second) and was transient, due to a rapid dephosphorylation to *myo*-inositol-P_2 and *myo*-inositol-P_1 (Thiyagarajah *et al.*, 1984). In addition to generating *myo*- inositol-P_3, hormone-induced hydrolysis of phosphatidylinositol-4,5-P_2 could possibly also affect cytosolic Ca^{2+} because of inhibition of the plasma membrane Ca^{2+},Mg^{2+}-ATPase (Buckley and Hawthorne, 1972; Penniston, 1983; Prpić *et al.*, 1983).

As noted previously, phosphoinositide breakdown generates 1,2-di- acylglycerol in addition to inositol phosphates, and diacylglycerol has been shown to activate a Ca^{2+}–phospholipid-dependent protein kinase by reduc- ing its requirement for Ca^{2+} to near the cytosolic range (Kaibuchi *et al.*, 1982). This enzyme is present in liver (Kuo *et al.*, 1980) and appears to play some role in the hepatic actions of the Ca^{2+}-dependent hormones (Garrison *et al.*, 1984). The effects of diacylglycerol to stimulate the kinase can be mimicked by tumor-promoting phorbol esters (Castagna *et al.*, 1982), and

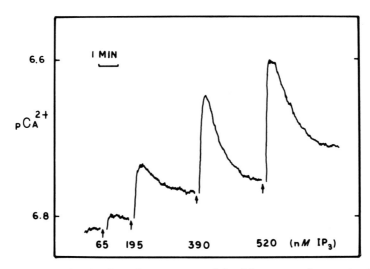

FIG. 8. Release of Ca^{2+} from digitonin permeabilized hepatocytes by *myo*-inositol-P_3. Hepatocytes were permeabilized with digitonin essentially as described by Becker *et al.* (1980). The recorder trace shows the effect of sequential additions of increasing concentrations of *myo*-inositol-P_3 to the free Ca^{2+} in the medium measured using Quin 2.

addition of these esters to hepatocytes has been reported to inactivate glycogen synthase (Roach and Goldman, 1983) and to increase the phosphorylation of three unidentified cytosolic proteins (Garrison *et al.*, 1984).

In summary, it appears very likely that the breakdown of phosphatidylinositol-4,5-P_2 induced in liver by Ca^{2+}-dependent hormones is responsible for the initial Ca^{2+} changes and protein phosphorylations that cause the biological responses.

VIII. SUMMARY

Calcium-dependent hormones such as epinephrine (acting via α_1-adrenergic receptors), vasopressin, and angiotensin II elicit their biological responses in liver by increasing cytosolic Ca^{2+}. Phosphorylase *b* kinase is the Ca^{2+}-stimulated, calmodulin-containing enzyme responsible for the activation of glycogen phosphorylase induced by these hormones. Other Ca^{2+}-sensitive proteins probably involved in the other physiological changes include a calmodulin-sensitive protein kinase and a phospholipid-sensitive protein kinase.

The hormones increase cytosolic Ca^{2+} initially by causing release of the cation from mitochondria and other intracellular stores. They later reduce the transmembrane efflux of Ca^{2+} by inhibiting the plasma membrane Ca^{2+},Mg^{2+}-ATPase pump, and this functions to prolong the biological responses.

Changes in polyphosphoinositide metabolism appear to play a fundamental role in the biological responses to the Ca^{2+}-dependent hormones. These hormones rapidly stimulate the breakdown of phosphatidylinositol-4,5-P_2, resulting in increased levels of *myo*-inositol-1,4,5-P_3 and 1,2-diacylglycerol. *Myo*-inositol-1,4,5-P_3 acts on mitochondria and components of the endoplasmic reticulum to release Ca^{2+} and thus may represent the intracellular second messenger for these hormones. 1,2-Diacylglycerol activates calcium–phospholipid-dependent protein kinase, which probably also mediates some of the biological response to the hormones.

REFERENCES

Althaus-Salzmann, M., Carafoli, E., and Jakob, A. (1980). *Eur. J. Biochem.* **106**, 241–248.

Assimacopoulos-Jeannet, F., Blackmore, P., and Exton, J. H. (1977). *J. Biol. Chem.* **252**, 2662–2669.

Assimacopoulos-Jeannet, F., Denton, R. M., and Jeanrenaud, B. (1981). *Biochem. J.* **198**, 485–490.

Assimacopoulos-Jeannet, F., McCormack, J. G., and Jeanrenaud, B. (1983). *FEBS Lett.* **159**, 83–88.

Babcock, D. F., Chen, J.-L. J., Yip, B. P., and Lardy, H. A. (1979). *J. Biol. Chem.* **254**, 8117–8120.

Balaban, R. S., and Blum, J. J. (1982). *Am. J. Physiol.* **242**, C182–C187.

Barritt, C. G., Dalton, K. A., and Whiting, J. A. (1981a). *FEBS Lett.* **125**, 137–140.

Barritt, G. J., Parker, J. C., and Wadsworth, J. C. (1981b). *J. Physiol. (London)* **312**, 29–55.

Becker, G. L., Fiskum, G., and Lehninger, A. L. (1980). *J. Biol. Chem.* **255**, 9009–9012.

Becker, J., and Jakob, A. (1982). *Eur. J. Biochem.* **128**, 293–296.

Berridge, M. J. (1984). *In* "Proceedings of Chilton Conference on Inositol and Phosphoinositides" (J. Bleasdale, ed.). Humana Press, Clifton, New Jersey (in press).

Blackmore, P. F., and Exton, J. H. (1981). *Biochem. J.* **198**, 379–383.

Blackmore, P. F., Brumley, F. T., Marks, J. L., and Exton, J. H. (1978). *J. Biol. Chem.* **253**, 4851–4858.

Blackmore, P.F., Assimacopoulos-Jeannet, F., Chan, T. M., and Exton, J. H. (1979a). *J. Biol. Chem.* **254**, 2828–2834.

Blackmore, P. F., Dehaye, J.-P., and Exton, J. H. (1979b). *J. Biol. Chem.* **254**, 6945–6950.

Blackmore, P. F., El-Refai, M. F., Dehaye, J.-P., Strickland, W. G., Hughes, P. F., and Exton, J. H. (1981). *FEBS Lett.* **123**, 245–248.

Blackmore, P. F., Hughes, B. P., Shuman, E. A., and Exton, J. H. (1982). *J. Biol. Chem.* **257**, 190–197.

Blackmore, P. F., Hughes, B. P., and Exton, J. H. (1983a). *In* "Isolation, Characterization and Use of Hepatocytes" (R. A. Harris and M. W. Cornell, eds.), pp. 433–438. Elsevier/North-Holland Biomedical Press, Amsterdam.

Blackmore, P. F., Hughes, B. P., Charest, R., Shuman, E. A., and Exton, J. H. (1983b). *J. Biol. Chem.* **258**, 10488–10494.

Blair, J. B., James, M. E., and Foster, J. L. (1979). *J. Biol. Chem.* **254**, 7579–7584.

Buckley, J. T., and Hawthorne, J. N. (1972). *J. Biol. Chem.* **247**, 7218–7223.

Burgess, G. M., Giraud, F., Poggioli, J., and Claret, M. (1983). *Biochim. Biophys. Acta* **731**, 387–396.

Buxton, D., Barron, L. L., and Olson, M. S. (1982). *J. Biol. Chem.* **257**, 14318–14323.

Campanile, C. P., Crane, J. K., Peach, M. J., and Garrison, J. C. (1982). *J. Biol. Chem.* **257**, 4951–4958.

Cantau, B., Keppens, S., DeWulf, H., and Jard, S. (1980). *J. Recept. Res.* **1**, 137–168.

Capiod, T., Berthon, B., Poggioli, J., Burgess, G. M., and Claret, M. (1982). *FEBS Lett.* **141**, 49–52.

Castagna, M., Takai, Y., Kaibuchi, K., Sano, K., Kikkawa, U., and Nishizuka, Y. (1982). *J. Biol. Chem.* **257**, 7847–7851.

Chan, T. M., and Exton, J. H. (1977). *J. Biol. Chem.* **252**, 8645–8651.

Charest, R., Blackmore, P. F., Berthon, B., and Exton, J. H. (1983). *J. Biol. Chem.* **258**, 8769–8773.

Charest, R., Prpić, V., Exton, J. H., and Blackmore, P. F. (1984). *Biochem. J.* (accepted subject to revision).

Chen, J.-L. J., Babcock, D. F., and Lardy, H. A. (1978). *Proc. Natl. Acad. Sci. U.S.A.* **75**, 2234–2238.

Chrisman, T. D. C., Jordan, J. E., and Exton, J. H. (1982). *J. Biol. Chem.* **257**, 10798–10804.

Creba, J. A., Downes, C. P., Hawkins, P. T., Brewster, G., Michell, R. H., and Kirk, C. J. (1983). *Biochem. J.* **212**, 733–747.

Dehaye, J.-P., Blackmore, P. F., Venter, J. C., and Exton, J. H. (1980). *J. Biol. Chem.* **255**, 3905–3910.

Dehaye, J.-P., Hughes, B. P., Blackmore, P. F., and Exton, J. H. (1981). *Biochem. J.* **194**, 949–956.

Denton, R. M., McCormack, J. G., and Oviasu, O. A. (1981). *In* "Short-term Regulation of Liver Metabolism" L. Hue and G. Van de Werve, eds.), pp. 159–174. Elsevier/North-Holland, Amsterdam.

Downes, P., and Michell, R. H. (1982). *Cell Calcium* **3**, 467–502.

El-Refai, M. F., Blackmore, P. F., and Exton, J. H. (1979). *J. Biol. Chem.* **254**, 4375–4386.

Foldes, M., and Barritt, G. J. (1977). *J. Biol. Chem.* **252**, 5372–5380.

Garrison, J. C., and Borland, M. K. (1979). *J. Biol. Chem.* **254**, 1129–1133.

Garrison, J. C., Borland, M. K., Florio, V. A., and Twible, D. A. (1979). *J. Biol. Chem.* **254**, 7147–7156.

Garrison, J. C., Johnsen, D. E., and Campanile, C. P. (1984). *J. Biol. Chem.* **259**, 3283–3292.

Haylett, D. G., and Jenkinson, D. H. (1972). *J. Physiol. (London)* **255**, 751–772.

Hems, D. A., Davies, C. J., and Siddle, K. (1978). *FEBS Lett.* **87**, 196–199.

Hughes, B. P., Blackmore, P. F., and Exton, J. H. (1980). *FEBS Lett.* **121**, 260–264.

Imazu, M., Strickland, W. G., Chrisman, T. D., and Exton, J. H. (1984). *J. Biol. Chem.* **259**, 1813–1821.

Inoue, M., Kishimoto, A., Takai, Y., and Nishizuka, Y. (1977). *J. Biol. Chem.* **254**, 7610–7616.

Jakob, A., and Diem, S. (1975). *Biochim. Biophys. Acta* **404**, 57–66.

Joseph, S. K., and Williamson, J. R. (1983). *J. Biol. Chem.* **258**, 10425–10432.

Joseph, S. K., Coll, K. E., Cooper, R. H., Marks, J. S., and Williamson, J. R. (1983). *J. Biol. Chem.* **258**, 731–741.

Joseph, S. K., Thomas, A. P., Williams, R. J., Irvine, R. F., and Williamson, J. R. (1984). *J. Biol. Chem.* **259**, 3077–3081.

Kaibuchi, K., Sano, K., Woshijima, M., Takai, Y., and Nishizuka, Y. (1982). *Cell Calcium* **3**, 323–335.

Kemp, B. E., and Clark, M. G. (1978). *J. Biol. Chem.* **253**, 5147–5154.
Kennedy, M. B., McGuinness, T., and Greengard, P. (1983). *J. Neurosci.* **3**, 818–831.
Kneer, N. M., Wagner, M. J., and Lardy, H. A. (1979). *J. Biol. Chem.* **254**, 12160–12168.
Kuo, J. F., Anderson, R. G. G., Wise, B. C., Mackerlova, L., Salomonsson, I., Brackett, N. L., Katoh, N., Shoji, M., and Wrenn, R. W. (1980). *Proc. Natl. Acad. Sci. U.S.A.* **77**, 7039–7043.
LeCam, L., and Freychet, P. (1978). *Endocrinology (Baltimore)* **102**, 379–385.
Lin, S.-H., Wallace, M. A., and Fain, J. N. (1983). *Endocrinology (Baltimore)* **113**, 2268–2275.
Ly, S., and Kim, K.-H. (1981). *J. Biol. Chem.* **256**, 11585–11590.
Morgan, N. G., Shuman, E. A., Exton, J. H., and Blackmore, P. F. (1982). *J. Biol. Chem.* **257**, 13907–13910.
Morgan, N. G., Blackmore, P. F., and Exton, J. H. (1983a). *J. Biol. Chem.* **258**, 5102–5109.
Morgan, N. G., Blackmore, P. F., and Exton, J. H. (1983b). *J. Biol. Chem.* **258**, 5110–5116.
Murphy, E., Coll, K., Rich, T. L., and Williamson, J. R. (1980). *J. Biol. Chem.* **255**, 6600–6608.
Pariza, M. W., Butcher, F. R., Becker, J. E., and Potter, V. R. (1977). *Proc. Natl. Acad. Sci. U.S.A.* **74**, 234–237.
Penniston, J. T. (1983). *Ann. N.Y. Acad. Sci.* **402**, 296–303.
Poggioli, J., Berthon, B., and Claret, M. (1980). *FEBS Lett.* **115**, 243–246.
Pointer, R. H., Butcher, F. R., and Fain, J. N. (1976). *J. Biol. Chem.* **251**, 2987–2992.
Prpić, V., Blackmore, P. F., and Exton, J. H. (1982). *J. Biol. Chem.* **257**, 11323–11331.
Prpić, V., Rhodes, D., Blackmore, P. F., and Exton, J. H. (1983). *Fed. Proc., Fed. Am. Soc. Exp. Biol.* **42**, 2228.
Prpić, V., Green, K. C., Blackmore, P. F., and Exton, J. H. (1984). *J. Biol. Chem.* **259**, 1382–1385.
Putney, J. W. (1984). *In* "Proceedings of Chilton Conference on Inositol and Phosphosinositides" (J. Bleasdale, ed.). Humana Press, Clifton, New Jersey (in press).
Radominska-Pyrek, A., Kraus-Friedmann, N., Lester, R., Little, J., and Denkins, Y. (1982). *FEBS Lett.* **141**, 56–58.
Rhodes, D., Prpić, V., Exton, J. H., and Blackmore, P. F. (1983). *J. Biol. Chem.* **258**, 2770–2773.
Roach, P. J., and Goldman, M. (1983). *Proc. Natl. Acad. Sci. U.S.A.* **80**, 7170–7172.
Roche, T. E., and Cate, R. L. (1977). *Arch. Biochem. Biophys.* **183**, 664–677.
Schworer, C. M., Payne, M. E., Williams, A. T., and Soderling, T. R. (1983). *Arch, Biochem. Biophys.* **224**, 77–86.
Sies, H., Graf, P., and Crane, D. (1983). *Biochem. J.* **212**, 271–278.
Streb, H., Irvine, R. F., Berridge, M. J., and Schultz, I. (1983). *Nature (London)* **306**, 67–69.
Strickland, W. G., Blackmore, P. F., and Exton, J. H. (1980). *Diabetes* **29**, 617–622.
Strickland, W. G., Imazu, M., Chrisman, T. D., and Exton, J. H. (1983). *J. Biol. Chem.* **258**, 5490–5497.
Strzelecki, T., Lanoue, K. F., and Thomas, J. A. (1983). *In* "Isolation, Characterization and Use of Hepatocytes" (R. A. Harris and N. W. Cornell, eds.), pp. 303–310. Elsevier/North-Holland Biomedical Press, Amsterdam.
Studer, R. K., and Borle, A. B. (1983). *Biochim. Biophys, Acta* **762**, 302–314.
Sugano, T., Shiota, M., Khono, H., Shimada, M., and Oshino, N. (1980). *J. Biochem. (Tokyo)* **87**, 465–472.
Sugden, M. C., and Watts, D. I. (1983). *Biochem. J.* **212**, 85–89.
Sugden, M. C., Ball, A. J., Ilic, V., and Williamson, D. H. (1980). *FEBS Lett.* **116**, 37–40.
Takai, Y., Kishimoto, A., Iwasa, Y., Kawahara, Y., Mori, T., and Nishizuka, Y. (1979). *J. Biol. Chem.* **254**, 3692–3695.

Thiyagarajah, P., Charest, R., Exton, J. H., and Blackmore, P. F. (1984). *J. Biol. Chem.* (accepted subject to revision).

Thomas, A. P., Marks, J. S., Coll, K. E., and Williamson, J. R. (1983). *J. Biol. Chem.* **258**, 5716–5725.

Tsien, R. Y. (1980). *Biochemistry* **19**, 2396–2404.

Tsien, R. Y., Pozzan, T., and Kirk, T. J. (1982). *J. Cell Biol.* **94**, 325–334.

Wernette, M. E., Ochs, R. S., and Lardy, H. A. (1981). *J. Biol. Chem.* **256**, 12767–12771.

Whiting, J. A., and Barritt, G. J. (1982). *Biochem. J.* **206**, 121–129.

Williamson, J. R., Cooper, R. H., and Hoek, J. B. (1981). *Biochim. Biophys. Acta* **639**, 243–295.

Witters, L. A., Kowaloff, E. M., and Avruch, J. (1979a). *J. Biol. Chem.* **254**, 245–248.

Witters, L. A., Moriarity, D., and Martin, D. B. (1979b). *J. Biol. Chem.* **254**, 6644–6649.

Woodgett, J. R., Tonks, N. K., and Cohen, P. (1982). *FEBS Lett.* **148**, 5–11.

CHAPTER 8

Steroid and Polypeptide Hormone Interaction in Milk-Protein Gene Expression

Mihir R. Banerjee and Michael Antoniou

Tumor Biology Laboratory
School of Biological Sciences
University of Nebraska-Lincoln
Lincoln, Nebraska

BIOCHEMICAL ACTIONS OF HORMONES, VOL. XII

I. INTRODUCTION

In female mammals, the mammary glands present a major endocrine target organ. At the onset of pregnancy, the ductal mammary organ undergoes a number of hormonally programmed developmental changes, such as lobuloalveolar morphogenesis (mammogenesis), functional differentiation (lactogenesis), and regression of the alveolar structures (involution) to a ductal parenchyma after weaning. The principal hormones required for this sequential regulatory process are different combinations of several steroid and polypeptide hormones, including estrogen, progesterone, aldosterone, glucocorticoid (cortisol or corticosterone), and prolactin (Lyons *et al.*, 1958; Nandi, 1958, 1959). Involvement of the growth hormone and the thyroid hormone in this complex process also has been suggested (Singh *et al.*, 1969, 1970; Tucker, 1974; Vonderhaar, 1975). Moreover, when exposed to an oncogenic agent, the mammary cells are also prone to neoplastic transformation (Nandi and McGrath, 1973; Medina, 1978). The hormones required for regulation of the normal developmental cycle are also conducive to mammary carcinogenesis, apparently acting as promoting agents (Nandi, 1978).

During developmental processes, regulated expression of specific genes is believed to be key to differentiation (Davidson, 1976). On the other hand, pathogenesis of the neoplastic disease is associated with alterations of the state of differentiation of the tissue. This suggests an escape of the transformed cell population from the normal regulatory mechanisms of gene expression. Thus, understanding of the biochemical pathways of hormone-regulated gene expression leading to mammary cell differentiation has been of much interest to the molecular endocrinologists. Functional differentiation of the mammary cells is characterized by the hormone-stimulated production of several specific proteins, including the caseins, which constitute the major group of the proteins in milk (Jeness, 1974). Prolactin and a glucocorticoid are the principal hormones required for the expression of functional differentiation of the mammary cells (Lyons *et al.*, 1958; Nandi, 1959), and progesterone acts as an antagonist in this process (Assairi *et al.*, 1974). Studies in our laboratory are centered on the elucidation of the mechanisms of action of the polypeptide and the steroid hormone on the regulation of selective expression of the milk-protein genes in murine mammary glands. In this chapter, we will briefly review the present status of our knowledge of the mechanisms of the hormonal regulation of the genes coding for the caseins, a complex group of acidic phosphoproteins.

II. HORMONAL STIMULATION OF MILK-PROTEIN SYNTHESIS IN MAMMARY TISSUE *IN VITRO*

Topper (1970) and his associates were first to demonstrate that mammary tissue explants obtained from midpregnant mice synthesize the caseins during short-term incubation in a chemically defined medium containing prolactin, cortisol, and insulin (Juergens *et al.*, 1965). This observation opened a new perspective to the concept of hormone-inducible gene expression, revealing that interaction of multiple hormones may be involved in regulation of specific gene expression. Recently, requirements of glucocorticoid and thyroid hormone for growth hormone gene expression have been observed (Spindler *et al.*, 1982). On the other hand, the emphasis of contemporary studies at that time was centered on the mechanisms of action of a single hormone, particularly a steroid hormone–regulating specific gene expression in the target tissues. Notable among these are regulation of ecdysone-induced dopa-carboxylase in *Drosophila* (Karlson, 1963), estrogen- or progesterone-induced expression of the egg-white proteins in chick oviduct (Schimke *et al.*, 1975; O'Malley *et al.*, 1977a), estrogen regulation of egg-yolk protein in liver (Tata, 1976; Tata and Smith, 1979), and glucocorticoid-induced expression of tyrosine aminotransferase (TAT) also in liver cells (Tomkins, 1974).

In the mammary glands, knowledge about the requirement of prolactin and cortisol for lactogenesis prompted the studies concerning elucidation of the role of the polypeptide and the steroid hormone in the regulatory pathways of the expression of the milk-protein genes (Denamur, 1974; Banerjee, 1976). It has been over a decade since the studies on hormone regulation of milk-protein gene expression were reviewed (Turkington, 1972) in Volume

II of this treatise. Thus, a brief discussion of the findings of those studies is included to provide the necessary background information. Earlier studies in the animal attempted to determine the influence of the polypeptide and the steroid hormone, acting individually or in combination, on macromolecular biosynthesis, particularly the nucleic acids in the mammary glands of various species, and the findings have been extensively reviewed at regular intervals (Turkington *et al.*, 1973; Denamur, 1974; Topper and Oka, 1974; Banerjee, 1976; Topper and Freeman, 1980). Briefly, measurements of the incorporation of radioactive precursors into the macromolecules have shown that RNA, protein, and DNA synthesis, including DNA polymerase activity, remain elevated during morphogenesis of the mammary glands in the pregnant animals. Exogenous hormone treatment of the ovariectomized virgin mice further revealed that estrogen and progesterone can significantly influence synthesis of these macromolecules during morphogenesis of the mammary glands (Banerjee and Rogers, 1971; Banerjee and Banerjee, 1973). This indicates that during pregnancy lobuloalveolar development of the mammary parenchyma is responsive to the ovarian steroid hormones and/or to the elevated levels of prolactin, conceivably stimulated by estrogen treatment of the animals (Tucker, 1974). Estrogen is stimulatory to prolactin gene expression (Maurer, 1982). Characterization of the mammary gland RNA by sedimentation in sucrose gradient and by agarose gel-electrophoresis further revealed that the hormone-stimulated synthesis of RNA includes both rRNA and heterogenous nuclear RNA (hnRNA) (Banerjee and Banerjee, 1973).

In the postpartum animal, RNA content of the mammary glands rises markedly, and this corresponds to a tenfold rise of RNA synthesis in early lactating mice (Banerjee, 1976) over that in virgin animals, and the newly synthesized RNA represents mostly α_s-casein mRNA (Denamur, 1974; Banerjee, 1976). The processing of the rRNA precursors and cytoplasmic migration of 28 S and 18 S rRNA in lactating mammary cells is similar to that in other eukaryotic cells. The increase in the level of RNA in postpartum mammary glands is responsive to adrenal ablation and cortisol treatment of the animal (Banerjee *et al.*, 1971; Banerjee, 1976). Prolactin also enhances the levels of mammary gland RNA synthesis in postpartum animals (Denamur, 1974). Studies *in vivo* have further shown that glucocorticoid and/or prolactin stimulation of RNA synthesis is accompanied by increased secretory activity in the mammary glands of lactating animals. However, in the absence of information about the biochemical properties of the secretory products, a relationship between the hormone-induced RNA and the milk proteins remained unclear in these studies. Moreover, complexity of the hormone environment in the animal also prevented reliable interpretation of these results, particularly with respect to their significance in the specific regulatory processes in the mammary gland. Nevertheless, the studies *in vivo* did show that the concentrations of mammary cell RNA are sensitive to the levels of the lactogenic hormones, prolactin and cortisol, in the animals. Our studies *in vivo* also showed that transition of the animal from pregnancy to lactation is marked by a pronounced increase of ribosomal aggregation, forming larger polysomes, and maintenance of these polysomes is sensitive to both cortisol and prolactin (Banerjee *et al.*, 1977).

III. STUDIES IN EXPLANTS OF MAMMARY TISSUE *IN VITRO*

Several laboratories also attempted to establish a temporal relationship between the hormonal stimulation of RNA and casein synthesis in explant cultures of mammary tissue from pregnant mice (Topper, 1970; Turkington, 1972; Forsyth, 1971). In these studies, casein was measured in Ca^{2+}, rennin precipitate of tissue extract. The results again showed that both prolactin and cortisol are required for maximal stimulation of RNA synthesis, including hnRNA in the explants in medium containing insulin. Attempts were also made to ascertain whether prolactin or cortisol alone can stimulate RNA and casein synthesis in the explants *in vitro* (Turkington *et al.*, 1973). The explants were first incubated with insulin and cortisol, and this failed to stimulate RNA synthesis. However, the explants preincubated with insulin and cortisol were capable of increased RNA and casein synthesis during subsequent culture in medium containing insulin and prolactin. Actinomycin D, an inhibitor of RNA synthesis, blocked hormonal stimulation of casein synthesis in the explants. Based on these observations, it was interpreted that prolactin acts as an inducer for the mRNAs coding for the caseins. However, actinomycin D at the concentration used acts as a nonspecific inhibitor of total cellular RNA synthesis (Perry, 1967). Consequently, it was not possible to explain whether the blockage of casein synthesis was due to inhibition of rRNA synthesis, ribosome biogenesis, or specific inhibition of synthesis of the milk-protein mRNA itself.

RNA synthesis was also measured (Turkington *et al.*, 1973) in isolated nuclei *in vitro* at high ionic condition, which is believed to enhance hnRNA synthesis (Tata, 1966). Results showed that RNA synthesis in the isolated nuclei from mammary explants incubated with insulin, prolactin, and cortisol was 300% greater than that in the nuclei from the explants incubated with insulin and cortisol, and these observations were correlated with a high level of casein synthesis in the explants cultured under similar conditions. These observations were considered evidence that transcription of the casein genes is regulated by prolactin. Reliability of this interpretation, however, remained subject to several experimental limitations. Mammary tissue of pregnancy is exposed to the elevated levels of circulating glucocorticoid (Gala and Westphal, 1965), and sequential incubation of the explants first with insulin, cortisol followed by insulin, and prolactin is likely to reflect a synergistic action of residual endogenous glucocorticoid in the explants and of prolactin in the medium. Although at high ionic condition isolated nuclei are believed to synthesize hnRNA (presumably mRNA) more efficiently, a substantial amount of rRNA is also synthesized during the same reaction (Tata, 1970). Thus, in the absence of a specific characterization of the RNA synthesized in the isolated nuclei, it remained unclear how much of the 300% increase represents milk-protein mRNA, if any.

Despite the limitations discussed above, the studies in the explant cultures provided important information about a temporal relationship between the lactogenic hormone–induced RNA and casein synthesis in the mammary glands. Measurements of precursor uptake into the cellular macromolecules, their sedimentation properties, and their responses to inhibitors provided some clues in that the protein synthesis apparatus of the mammary cells is responsive to the lactogenic hormone stimulation, resulting in synthesis of the milk proteins determined in Ca^{2+} rennin precipitate of tissue extract. However, limitations of knowledge about the eukaryotic mRNAs and the molecular pathways of their regulation prevented determination of the specific nature of the responses at transcriptional and/or posttranscriptional levels of control of the milk-protein genes. Moreover, it was also evident from the studies in the explant culture that a mammary cell culture system that can mimic the hormone-regulated developmental stages of the mammary glands in a control environment *in vitro* is more desirable for these studies.

IV. ADVANCES IN MOLECULAR AND CELL BIOLOGY OF PROTEIN SYNTHESIS

Meanwhile, remarkable advances in the areas of molecular and cell biology of the eukaryotic cells (Perry, 1976) and the concept of receptor-mediated action of the hormones, specifically the steroid hormones (Jensen and DeSombre, 1972), allowed innovated studies on the problems of hormonal regulation of specific gene expression. The discovery of the presence of the polyadenylic acid [poly(A)] residues on the 3′-OH terminal of the eukaryotic mRNAs allowed isolation of the mRNA by oligo(dT) cellulose affinity chromatography (Brawerman, 1974). Improved knowledge of the eukaryotic protein synthesis apparatus (Lodish, 1976; Weissbach and Ochoa, 1976) promoted the development of cell-free protein synthesis sytems derived from homologous or heterologous ribosomes. These cell-free protein synthesis systems then permitted faithful translation of the poly(A) mRNA and immunological determination of the specific peptides coded by the exogenous mRNA in the cell-free protein synthesis reaction mixture. These advances made it feasible to measure influence of the hormones directly on the mRNAs coding for the milk proteins.

V. MEASUREMENTS OF CASEIN mRNA ACTIVITY

Using a cell-free protein synthesis system derived from reticulocyte lysates, Denamur and his associates were first to obtain cell-free translation of

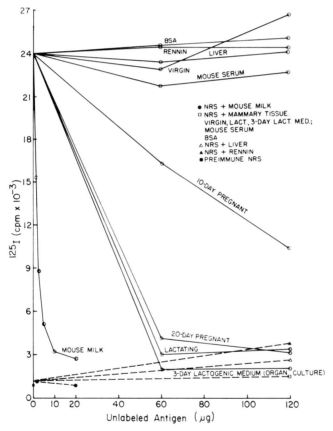

FIG. 1. Results of an indirect radioimmunoassay for mouse casein using casein antibody and 125I-labeled mouse casein. Immunologically detectable casein is present in milk, lactating mammary tissue extract, and extract of mammary tissue cultivated in organ culture with insulin, prolactin, and cortisol. A modest amount of casein is also detectable in mammary tissue of midpregnancy. NRS, normal rabbit serum; BSA, bovine serum albumin. [From Banerjee *et al.* (1977).]

the casein (α-casein) mRNA from lactating ewe mammary glands (Gaye *et al.*, 1973). This report was followed by the accomplishment of faithful translation of the murine casein mRNAs in an ascites ribosome system supplemented with rabbit reticulocyte factors (0.5 *M* KCl 5–30 wash) and tRNA (Terry *et al.*, 1975a). Casein in the reaction mixture was determined by immunoprecipitation with a specific antibody to mouse casein (Terry *et al.*, 1975b). Subsequently, specific cell-free translation of the milk-protein mRNAs from the lactating mammary glands of rats (Rosen, 1976), rabbits (Devinoy *et al.*, 1978), guinea pigs (Craig *et al.*, 1976), cows (Willis *et al.*, 1982), and humans (Hall *et al.*, 1979) also has been accomplished in different laboratories. Radioimmunoassay of the mouse mammary tissue with the specific antibody to caseins at different stages of development also revealed (Banerjee *et al.*, 1977) that little casein is present in the mammary glands of virgin mice, and the milk proteins are readily measurable on the tenth day of gestation, reaching a maximal level after parturition (Fig. 1).

VI. HORMONE RESPONSES OF MAMMARY CELL POLYSOMES ACTIVE IN CASEIN SYNTHESIS

The patterns of the ribosomal aggregates in the mammary glands at various stages of development have been discussed in detail in recent reviews (Banerjee, 1976; Banerjee *et al.*, 1977; Rosen *et al.*, 1980), and a brief account particularly concerning the studies in mouse mammary glands is included in this section. Since the polysomes constitute the cellular site of protein synthesis or translation of the mRNAs, a possible influence of cortisol and prolactin on the polysomal aggregation pattern in murine mammary cell ribosomes was of interest in our earlier studies (Banerjee, 1976; Terry *et al.*, 1977b). Sedimentation analysis in sucrose gradient revealed that the ribosomes in the mammary glands of virgin and pregnant mice resolve mostly as monomers, with some dimers and trimers. Immediately prior to parturition, the ribosomes sediment as larger aggregates, and the enriched population of the larger polysomes dissociate after mild RNase treatment, indicating that the polysomes represent the ribosomal aggregates carrying the mRNA (Fig. 2). Specific mRNA translation assays in the homologous ribosome system also indicated that the mammary polysomes most active in casein synthesis are aggregates of 6–10 ribosomes, the enriched cellular concentration of the larger polysomes is reduced after adrenalectomy of the lactating mouse, and the adverse effect of adrenal ablation is less pronounced in the animals nursing larger numbers of pups (Terry *et al.*, 1977b). Exogenous cortisol therapy of adrenalectomized mice stimulates enrichment of the larger polysomes in the lactating animals. Thus, influence of the

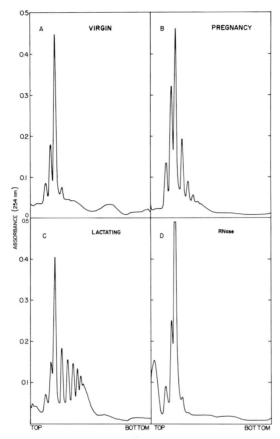

FIG. 2. Sedimentation characteristics of mammary gland ribosomes of BALB/c mice. (A) Virgin, (B) 20-day pregnancy, (C) 6-day lactation, and (D) lactating mammary gland polysomes after mild ribonuclease (RNase) treatment (5 μg RNase/ml). The polysomes were prepared by a modification of a procedure described by Bonanou-Tzedaki and Arnstein (1972). Frozen mammary tissue was homogenized in buffer containing TKM (50 mM Tris-HCl, pH 7.6; 25 mM KCl; 5 mM MgCl$_2$), 6 mM β-mercaptoethanol, 0.25 M sucrose, 100 μg/ml heparin (Schechter, 1974), and 1% Triton X-100. The homogenate was then centrifuged at 17,000 g for 10 minutes at 0°C. The supernatant was layered over 4.5 ml of buffer (TKM + 20% sucrose, 50 μg/ml heparin, and 6 mM β-mercaptoethanol) and centrifuged 2 hours in a Spinco Ti 50 rotor at 45,000 rpm and 4°C. The polysome pellet was then rinsed and suspended in buffer (20 mM K HEPES, pH 7.5; 0.12 M KCl, 5 mM Mg acetate, 6 mM β-mercaptoethanol). The suspension was centrifuged at 17,000 g for 10 minutes at 0°C to pellet-insoluble residues. The polysome suspension was then analyzed for sedimentation characteristics in a 15–60% linear sucrose gradient in TKM buffer containing 50 μg/ml heparin. After centrifugation for 60 minutes in a Spinco S.W. 41 rotor at 39,000 rpm and 4°C, the gradients were analyzed using an ISCO (Lincoln, Nebraska) 640 density gradient fractionator equipped with a recording spectrophotometer. Absorbance was recorded at 254 nm. [From Banerjee *et al.* (1977).]

glucocorticoid on the maintenance of the larger polysomes, presumably active in casein mRNA translation, is indicated by results of the studies *in vivo*. A stimulatory influence of cortisol on the rough-endoplasmic reticulum (RER) was also observed in mouse mammary explants in culture in medium containing insulin and prolactin (Oka and Topper, 1971). Adrenalectomy of lactating mice also results in a loss of RER in the mammary cells *in vivo* (Banerjee and Banerjee, 1971). Thus, the findings show that glucocorticoid exerts a modulatory influence on the formation of the lactating mammary cell polysomes, both in the animal and in the mammary explants *in vitro*. Our observations more than 10 years ago also showed that an enriched glucocorticoid environment is needed to maintain the high levels of RNA and casein synthesis in the mammary gland of lactating mice (Banerjee and Banerjee, 1971). In these studies, casein synthesis was measured in the Ca^{2+} rennin–precipitable material of mouse mammary glands *in vivo*. These findings may tempt one to conclude that the role of glucocorticoid in milk-protein gene expression is exerted at the translational level by modulation of the protein synthesis apparatus of the mammary cell. On the other hand, it is also conceivable that the cortisol-mediated dramatic changes in the translational apparatus of the mammary cells reflect a consequence of the modulatory action of the steroid hormone on cellular concentration of the specific mRNAs.

Assessment of this possibility by cell-free translation of the lactating mammary cell RNA in the heterologous ribosome system (Terry *et al.*, 1977b) showed that casein mRNA translation is 85–90% lower in adrenalectomized animals than the level present in sham-operated or nonoperated nursing mice. Treatment of adrenalectomized animals with exogenous cortisol can prevent this adverse effect of adrenal ablation, indicating that cortisol in postpartum mice can modulate the translational activity of the casein mRNA itself, possibly by regulating concentration of the translatable casein mRNA in the mammary cells.

Interestingly, these studies *in vivo* further revealed that the number of pups nursed by the mother is directly related to the level of casein mRNA activity in the glands, although the relative level of the adverse effect of adrenal ablation remains similar, regardless of the number of pups nursed. Since the intensity of suckling increases the circulating prolactin level in the animal (Mena *et al.*, 1976), it appears that, in addition to cortisol, prolactin is also involved in modulation of the cellular concentration of the milk-protein mRNAs.

Thus, the findings of the specific translational assay in the heterologous ribosome system indicate that an enriched glucocorticoid environment is needed to maintain the high levels of the translationally active casein mRNAs in the lactating animals. As indicated by the indirect evidence that enrichment of the prolactin level in the animal is caused by intensity of suckling, suckling can also cause variations in the levels of casein mRNA activity. This then raises the questions about the role of the steroid and the polypeptide hormone at the transcriptional level of control of the milk-protein genes.

VII. SPECIFIC TRANSCRIPTION OF CASEIN mRNAs

A. SYNTHESIS OF THE SPECIFIC cDNA PROBE

Measurement of gene transcription requires the use of a sensitive molecular hybridization probe for monitoring the specific mRNA transcripts. The procedures of mRNA isolation on oligo(dT) cellulose column, cell-free mRNA translation in the heterologous ribosome (wheat-germ) system, and specific immunological determination of the translational product were utilized to isolate from the lactating mammary gland RNA a 15 S mRNA fraction highly enriched (95%) in casein mRNA activity (Ganguly *et al.*, 1979; Banerjee *et al.*, 1981). A ^{3}[H]cDNA to the 15 S casein mRNA was then synthesized using the avian myeloblastosis virus (AMV)–reverse transcriptase. It should be mentioned that the 15 S casein mRNA includes the total casein mRNA complex, and, after electrophoresis in agarose, the 15 S casein mRNA resolves as a doublet (Fig. 3). Sedimentation analysis of the ^{3}[H]cDNA in alkaline sucrose gradient showed that most of the cDNA bands, corresponding to 1000–1200 nucleotide regions, as determined by sedimentation of marker DNA in parallel gradients. Complexity of the 15 S casein mRNA is estimated as $4.0–4.5 \times 10^5$ M_r, and this corresponds to approximately 1300 nucleotides. Thus, the cDNA to the 15 S mouse casein mRNA synthesized essentially represents a complete copy of the 15 S mouse casein mRNA complex. The cDNA hybridizes to the purified 15 S casein mRNA 114-fold faster than does the total RNA from lactating mammary glands, and the pseudo first-order kinetics of the reaction reaches a 90% level of completion with a single transition. No hybridization of mouse liver RNA to the cDNA to 15 S mammary RNA is detectable even at eR_0t values greater than 1000 moles · seconds · liters^{-1}. Thus, the [^{3}H]cDNA to the 15 S casein mRNA provides a sensitive hybridization probe for quantitative measurement of the mRNA casein concentration in the total mammary cell RNA. Hereafter, the 15 S casein mRNA complex and the cDNA to the 15 S casein mRNA will be abbreviated as mRNA$_{csn}$ and cDNA$_{csn}$, respectively. The details of the procedures used for isolation of the 15 S mRNA$_{csn}$ fraction and synthesis of the cDNA$_{csn}$ have been described previously (Ganguly *et al.*, 1979; Banerjee *et al.*, 1981).

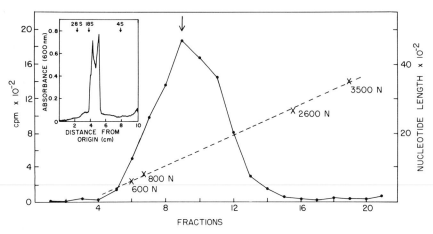

FIG. 3. Alkaline sucrose gradient centrifugation of [³H]cDNA$_{csn}$. cDNA, made against mRNA$_{csn}$, was centrifuged in an 8–18% alkaline sucrose gradient in 0.1 *M* NaOH/0.9 *M* NaCl/5 m*M* EDTA at 5°C for 24 hours at 38,000 rpm in a Spinco S.W. 41 rotor, and an aliquot of each gradient fraction was assayed for radioactivity. X indicates the position of the ³H-labeled viral marker DNAs centrifuged on a parallel gradient. The arrow shows the peak fraction of the synthesized cDNA, which has a nucleotide length (N) of about 1250. (Inset) Agarose gel electrophoresis of purified casein mRNA. After purification of RNA, 10 μg of RNA from the 15 S region of the sucrose gradient was electrophoresed on a 2.5% agarose gel in 0.025 *M* citric acid, pH 3.5/6 *M* urea for 4 hours at 3.5 mA per gel tube. Stained (1% methylene blue) gels were scanned at 600 nm. The marker RNAs (arrows) were electrophoresed in parallel gels. [From Ganguly *et al.* (1979).]

B. RNA SYNTHESIS IN ISOLATED MAMMARY CELL NUCLEI *IN VITRO*

One of the primary events of eukaryotic split-gene expression is regulated transcription of the pre-mRNA, which is then processed as the mature mRNA through a complex series of splicing reactions, associated with the cleavage of intron sequences present in the primary transcript (Leder *et al.*, 1980; Breathnach and Chambon, 1981). In the mammary cells, the hormones may play a significant regulatory role in this process. Thus, an efficient cell-free RNA synthesis system is essential for measuring the influence of the steroid and the polypeptide hormones at the transcriptional level of regulation of the milk-protein genes. *In vitro* RNA synthesis systems derived from isolated chromatin have been used for measuring hormone-induced mRNA transcription, in presence of bacterial RNA polymerase (O'Malley *et al.*, 1977b). However, the *in vitro* RNA synthesis system derived from isolated nuclei is considered more desirable for measuring eu-karyotic gene transcription, because a nuclear RNA synthesis system per-mits measurement of transcription in the presence of endogenous RNA polymerases (Chambon, 1977). In eukaryotic cells, the relationship between the type of RNA polymerase and the molecular species of RNA being synthe-sized is known to be specific. For example, among the three eukaryotic RNA polymerases, the interaction of the RNA polymerase II with the DNA tem-plate is involved in mRNA transcription (Chambon *et al.*, 1974).

Thus, an RNA synthesis system in isolated nuclei from the murine mam-mary cells was developed in our laboratory (Ganguly and Banerjee, 1978). In this *in vitro* system, RNA synthesis in the isolated nuclei at high ionic condition remains linear for 180 minutes. Over 90% and 68% of the reaction is sensitive to actinomycin D and α-amanitin, respectively, indicating a DNA-dependent, RNA polymerase II (mRNA polymerase)–directed RNA synthesis. Moreover, oligo(dT) cellulose affinity chromatography of the RNA in the reaction product showed that a portion of the RNA is polyadenylated *in vitro*, and sedimentation analysis in sucrose gradients revealed that the transcripts include the 15 S RNA. This indicates that the RNA synthesis in the isolated nuclei in the presence of homologous RNA polymerases from the mammary cells represents a faithful *in vitro* transcription system.

C. Isolation of the Purified Transcripts Synthesized *In Vitro*

One of the major problems of *in vitro* RNA synthesis systems derived from isolated chromatin or nuclei has been the presence of an excess level of endogenous RNA, including mRNA in the reaction mixture. Thus, isolation of the purified fraction of the newly synthesized RNA from the endogenous RNA has restricted the measurement of specific mRNA transcription. This was overcome after the finding that, in the *in vitro* systems, RNA poly-merase reaction remains unaltered when mercury-labeled nucleotides are used as substrates, and the newly synthesized HgRNA can be isolated from the endogenous RNA by affinity chromatography of the reaction product on sulfhydryl (SH)–agarose column, eluted with a mercaptan (Dale *et al.*, 1973). The purified transcripts thus obtained hybridize to the specific cDNAs to the respective mRNAs (Nguyen-Huu *et al.*, 1978; Orkin and Swerdlow, 1977). Figure 4 shows that the kinetics of RNA synthesis in the isolated nuclei from the mammary cells remains virtually identical in pres-ence of HgCTP or unmodified nucleotides, and 85% of the reaction is inhib-ited by α-amanitin, indicating that the HgRNA synthesized in the isolated nuclei is product of RNA polymerase II–directed DNA-dependent RNA

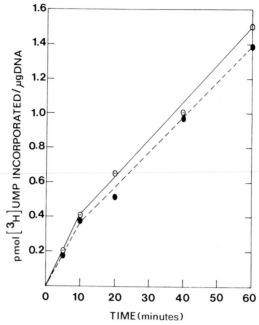

Fɪɢ. 4. Kinetics of RNA synthesis in isolated nuclei from mammary cells in presence of unmodified nucleotides or HgCTP. Nuclei were transcribed for 60 minutes in the presence of [³H]UTP and in the presence of unmodified CTP (⊙—⊙) or HgCTP (●— — —●). Aliquots were removed for counting at various time points. [From Banerjee *et al.* (1982b). Reprinted by permission of Eden Press.]

synthesis and that the HgRNA also includes the 15 S RNA (Fig. 5). Furthermore, the purified HgRNA synthesized in the isolated mammary cell nuclei from lactating mice hybridizes to the $cDNA_{csn}$, at a relatively low $eR_ot_{1/2}$ value, whereas HgRNA synthesized in the isolated nuclei from liver cells of lactating mice fails to hybridize to the $cDNA_{csn}$ probe (Ganguly *et al.*, 1979; Banerjee *et al.*, 1981). This demonstrates that transcription of the milk-protein genes is measurable in the HgRNA synthesized in the isolated nuclei. Quantitative analysis of the $eR_ot_{1/2}$ values of hybridization showed that 0.09% of the HgRNA was $mRNA_{csn}$, and the estimated level of $mRNA_{csn}$ in total nuclear RNA of lactating mammary cells was 0.07%. Additional control experiments showed that RNA extracted from the isolated nuclei, initially incubated *in vitro* in the absence of any nucleotide substrate, after SH–agarose chromatography fails to hybridize to the $cDNA_{csn}$ probe, indicating that the non-HgRNA does not bind to the SH–agarose column. These findings thus made it feasible to obtain a reliable measure of the influence of the hormones on transcription of the milk-protein genes.

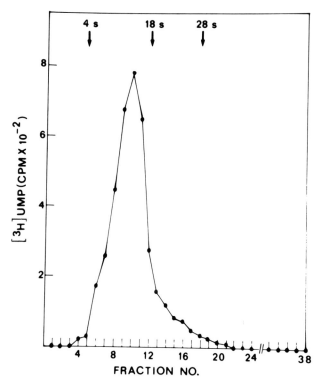

FIG. 5. Formamide–sucrose density gradient sedimentation analysis of the HgRNA synthesized in the isolated nuclei of lactating mammary cells. [From Banerjee *et al.* (1982b). Reprinted by permission of Eden Press.]

VIII. QUANTITATIVE MEASUREMENT OF HORMONAL INFLUENCE ON CASEIN GENE EXPRESSION IN MURINE MAMMARY GLAND *IN VIVO*

A. CELLULAR ACCUMULATION OF mRNA$_{csn}$

As measured by the cDNA$_{csn}$ probe, molecular hybridization of the mammary gland RNA to the cDNA$_{csn}$ done in RNA excess condition failed to show a detectable level of mRNA$_{csn}$ in the mammary glands of young virgin mice. In midpregnant animals, mRNA$_{csn}$ constitutes 0.09% of the total mammary gland RNA and, as expected, the highest concentration (2.5%) of mRNA$_{csn}$ is present in the lactating mammary gland of the mouse (Banerjee *et al.*, 1982b).

TABLE I

INFLUENCE OF HYDROCORTISONE ON ACCUMULATION OF THE $mRNA_{csn}$
SEQUENCES IN POSTPARTUM MAMMARY GLAND[a,b]

Animals	$mRNA_{csn}$ (%)	Fold increase over 5-day adrenalectomized animals
10-day lactating	1.56	—
5 days after adrenalectomy	0.25	—
Hours after hydrocortisone injection		
1	0.25	—
3	0.25	—
6	0.74	3.0
12	1.10	4.4
24	0.50	2.0

[a] Data from Ganguly *et al.* (1979).

[b] For each determination, mammary glands from 4–6 animals were pooled, total RNA was extracted, and $mRNA_{csn}$ sequences were measured by RNA excess-$cDNA_{csn}$ hybridization.

Table I shows that, 5 days after adrenalectomy of the lactating mouse, there is a marked reduction of $mRNA_{csn}$ accumulation in the total mammary RNA, and this loss is substantially replenished within hours after injections of exogenous cortisol (Ganguly *et al.*, 1979). A single injection of cortisol given 5 days after adrenalectomy stimulates a 4.4-fold increase of $mRNA_{csn}$ accumulation in the glands of postpartum mice at 12 hours. These results, obtained by quantitative measurement of the modulatory influence of glucocorticoids on $mRNA_{csn}$ concentration in the gland, are consistent with the similar findings of earlier translation assays (Terry *et al.*, 1977b). These quantitative measurements also confirm that the glucocorticoid plays a significant role in regulating cellular accumulation of $mRNA_{csn}$ in murine mammary gland.

B. HORMONAL MODULATION OF $mRNA_{csn}$ TRANSCRIPTION *IN VIVO*

In one set of these studies (Ganguly *et al.*, 1979), lactating mice 5 days after adrenalectomy were given a single injection of cortisol. Nuclei isolated from the mammary glands were allowed to synthesize HgRNA *in vitro* as described in the preceding section. The HgRNA synthesized *in vitro* was then isolated by SH–agarose affinity chromatography. Hybridization of the purified HgRNA to the $cDNA_{csn}$ probe showed that 5 days after adrenalectomy there is a 75% reduction in $mRNA_{csn}$ transcription, as compared to the nuclear transcripts of unoperated control animals (Fig. 6). Six hours after the single injection of cortisol, the $mRNA_{csn}$ sequences in the transcripts increased more than twofold above the level in the nuclei of 5-day adrenalectomized mice. These results demonstrate that glucocorticoids exert a regulatory influence on transcription of the casein genes in murine mammary glands, suggesting that cortisol stimulation of cellular accumulation of $mRNA_{csn}$ reflects an action of the steroid hormone at the genomic level of control of expression of the milk-protein genes.

Attempts were then made (Ganguly *et al.*, 1979) to ascertain the action of

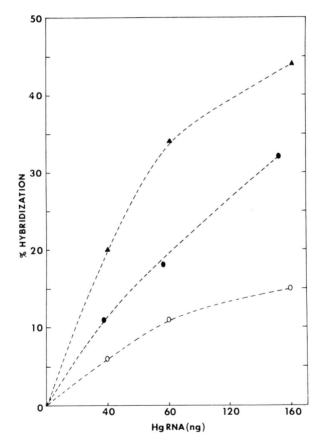

FIG. 6. Effect of adrenalectomy and cortisol treatment on $mRNA_{csn}$ transcription *in vitro*. Hybridization of $[^3H]cDNA_{csn}$ to RNA from 10-day unoperated lactating mice (▲- - -▲), 5 days after adrenalectomy (○- - -○), 5 days after adrenalectomy and 6 hours after a single injection of hydrocortisone (●- - -●).[From Banerjee *et al.* (1982b). Reprinted by permission of Eden Press.]

prolactin on transcription of the casein genes in animals treated with the specific prolactin inhibitor 2-bormo-α-ergocryptin (CB-154) (Welsch *et al.*, 1971). Serum prolactin levels of the lactating mouse were reduced 80% by injecting the animals with CB-154. Isolated mammary cell nuclei from the CB-154–treated and untreated lactating mice were allowed to synthesize HgRNA in the *in vitro* RNA synthesis system. After SH–agarose chromatography, the purified HgRNA synthesized in the nuclei *in vitro* was hybridized to the cDNA$_{csn}$ probe. The CB-154 treatment failed to show an alteration of mRNA$_{csn}$ transcription compared to nontreated control mice, even though the serum prolactin level in the CB-154 treated mice was reduced 80%. However, the negative results of these studies done in the animal do not permit a conclusion that prolactin exerts little or no influence on casein gene transcription *in vivo*, because the residual 20% prolactin in CB-154–treated mice may be sufficient to support casein gene transcription in the nursing animals in the presence of endogenous circulating glucocorticoid. Serum prolactin level in nursing animals is known to be much higher than is necessary to induce lactogenesis (Tucker, 1974). Furthermore, studies in our laboratory have also shown that intensity of suckling, a known stimulus for pituitary prolactin synthesis and release, also stimulates mRNA$_{csn}$ accumulation in the mammary gland, as measured by translation assays in a heterologous ribosome system (Terry *et al.*, 1977b).

Therefore, it is likely that the rise in mRNA$_{csn}$ transcription in adrenalectomized mice treated with cortisol reflects a synergistic action of cortisol with endogenous prolactin. The endogenous endocrine environment in the animal is further complicated by the fact that suckling may also stimulate pituitary ACTH release, which in turn elevates the serum glucocorticoid level (Tucker, 1974). The increased glucocorticoid level then can reduce the levels of serum prolactin. Thus, the complexities of endocrine environment in the animal make it virtually impossible to obtain a reliable measurement of the influence of the polypeptide or the steroid hormone on the expression of the milk-protein genes and mammary cell differentiation.

IX. MILK-PROTEIN GENE EXPRESSION IN MAMMARY TISSUE *IN VITRO*

A. Explant Culture of Pieces of Mammary Tissue

The serious limitations of the *in vivo* system were appreciated by earlier investigators studying the complex multihormonal regulation of mammary gland physiology. Thus, a culture model derived from pieces of mammary tissue from pregnant mice was developed, and the mammary cells in the explant culture respond to the lactogenic action of cortisol and prolactin and elicit milklike secretory material during 48- to 72-hour incubation (Elias, 1957; Rivera and Bern, 1961). Subsequently, this short-term explant culture in a chemically defined medium was used to demonstrate that prolactin and cortisol induce casein synthesis in the explants in the presence of insulin (Juergens *et al.*, 1965). However, important shortcomings associated with the mammary explant culture model often limit reliable interpretation of the results. Mammary glands of pregnant mice contain casein (Terry *et al.*, 1975b), and the mammary cells rich in prolactin and glucocorticoid receptor are exposed to the increased circulating levels of the hormones (Tucker, 1974; Shyamala, 1973). Consequently, responses of the explants to the hormones in the medium after short-term culture are likely also to reflect actions of the residual endogenous hormones present in the explants.

B. Culture of the Whole Mammary Organ

It is evident from the discussion in the preceding section that an improved culture model of the mammary tissue in controlled hormonal environment *in vitro* is needed for the elucidation of the mechanisms of multiple hormonal regulation of mammary cell differentiation. A culture model that mimics the developmental cycle of the mammary glands in hormonally defined serum-free medium would be most desirable for these studies. Prop (1966) initially attempted to obtain morphogenesis of the murine mammary parenchyma in the isolated whole organ in culture. Subsequently, using an innovative manipulation of the endocrine environment of the animal, Ichinose and Nandi (1964) were first to accomplish hormonal induction of pregnancylike lobuloalveolar morphogenesis *in vitro* in an isolated whole mammary organ obtained from immature female mice. Responses of the parenchyma to the hormones in the chemically defined serum-free medium are dependent on estrogen and progesterone stimulation of the donor animal. Subsequently, our laboratory has shown that the whole mammary organ obtained from an immature female mouse can sequentially mimic the stages of mammogenesis, lactogenesis, and alveolar regression (involution) in a serum-free medium containing an appropriately controlled *in vitro* hormone environment (Wood *et al.*, 1975). Moreover, the ductal parenchyma in the regressed glands *in vitro* can also complete a second round of morphogenesis in medium containing the hormones and the epidermal growth factor (Tonelli and Sorof, 1980).

This unique culture model of the whole mammary organ has been extensively described (Mehta and Banerjee, 1975; Lin *et al.*, 1976; Banerjee *et al.*,

1976; Banerjee and Antoniou, 1984). Briefly, as a prerequisite to the culture procedure, 3–4 week old BALB/c female mice (used in our studies) are primed by daily injections of a mixture of 17β-estradiol and progesterone for 9 days. The whole second thoracic mammary gland from these animals is excised on a dacron raft under sterile conditions. The gland resting on the

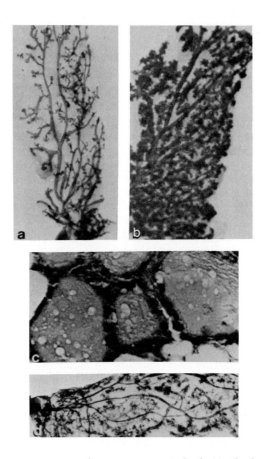

FIG. 7. Whole-mount preparation of mouse mammary gland. (a) Gland at beginning of culture. (b) Extensive alveolar growth after 5-day cultivation in a medium with insulin, prolactin, and aldosterone. (c) After initial 5-day cultivation in a growth-promoting medium, the alveolar gland [as in (b)] was then cultivated for 6 days in the lactogenic medium containing insulin, prolactin, and cortisol. Note the presence of extensive milklike secretory material. (d) After 12-day cultivation of the lobuloalveolar gland [as in (b)] in a medium with insulin and aldosterone. Note regression of the lobuloalveolar structure. Cultivation of the lobuloalveolar gland in a medium with insulin alone also results in similar alveolar regression. [From Banerjee (1976).]

raft is then transferred into a plastic petri dish containing Waymouth's synthetic medium MB/751 supplemented with appropriate combinations of the steroid and the polypeptide hormones. The glands are then incubated at 37°C in an atmosphere of 95% oxygen and 5% carbon dioxide in a humidified chamber (Rivera, 1971). Incubation of the gland first in a mammogenic hormone–containing medium induces full lobuloalveolar morphogenesis within 5–6 days. The parenchyma containing the secretory structures during subsequent culture in medium containing insulin, prolactin, and cortisol produces abundant milklike secretory material, including the caseins (Wood *et al.*, 1975; Terry *et al.*, 1975b). Continued culture in a prolactin-free medium causes the alveolar structures to undergo complete regression, leaving only the ductal parenchyma (Fig. 7). The different combinations of the polypeptide and the steroid hormones needed to obtain mammogenesis, lactogenesis, and alveolar regression *in vitro* have been described in detail (Banerjee *et al.*, 1976). The mammary glands of strains of mice other than BALB/c mice also can complete lobuloalveolar development in the whole organ in culture (Singh *et al.*, 1970).

The mammary gland during its morphogenesis *in vitro*, when exposed to a carcinogenic chemical, also undergoes neoplastic transformation *in vitro* (Telang *et al.*, 1979; Banerjee *et al.*, 1981), and the transformed cells *in vitro* are morphologically detectable as nodulelike alveolar lesions (Banerjee *et al.*, 1974; Lin *et al.*, 1976). The transformed cells, after transplantation into syngeneic hosts, initially produce hyperplastic outgrowth and mammary tumors, and then appear in the outgrowth tissue (Iyer and Banerjee, 1981; Banerjee, 1984).

X. DISSOCIATION OF MAMMOGENESIS AND LACTOGENESIS IN A TWO-STEP CULTURE MODEL

In the animal, the mammary parenchyma during gestation is exposed to the elevated levels of the circulating glucocorticoid and prolactin, and the milk proteins are measurable in these glands (Tucker, 1974; Banerjee *et al.*, 1977). This overlap of the morphogenetic and functional differentiation of the mammary glands makes it difficult to determine the role of the steroid and the polypeptide hormones in regulation of the expression of the milk-protein genes. Thus, it was necessary to dissociate the stages of morphogenesis and functional differentiation of the glands in a two-step culture model so that influence of prolactin and glucocorticoid could be measured in the glands not preexposed to the steroid hormone, which can be retained by the mammary cells for extended periods of time (Strobl and Lippman, 1979).

A. Mammary Gland Morphology *in Vitro*

In the two-step culture model (Terry *et al.*, 1977a), the immature parenchyma develops pregnancylike lobuloalveolar structures after 6 days of step I incubation in a corticosteroid-free medium containing insulin, prolactin, growth hormone, estrogen, and progesterone. During step II culture, the lobuloalveolar glands are incubated in a corticosteroid-free medium containing insulin, prolactin, growth hormone, estrogen, and progesterone. During step II culture, the lobuloalveolar glands are incubated in a medium containing the lactogenic hormone mixture, insulin, prolactin, and cortisol. No secretory material is detectable in the histology of the lobuloalveolar glands after 6 days of incubation in the corticosteroid-free, step I mammogenic medium (Fig. 8). In step II, abundant milklike material is present (Fig. 8) in the alveolar lumen after 6 days of incubation in medium contain-

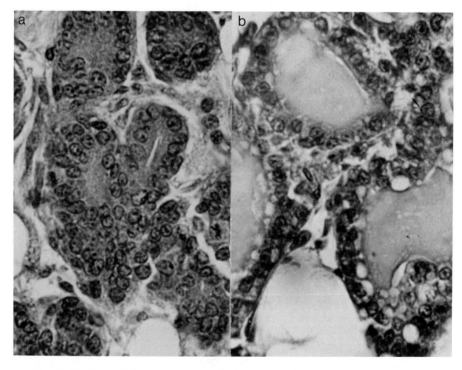

Fig. 8. Histology of the mammary gland after organ culture. (a) Six days in the step I medium with insulin, prolactin, growth hormone, 17β-estradiol, and progesterone. (b) After additional 6 days in the step II medium with insulin, prolactin, and cortisol. 400X [From Banerjee *et al.* (1982b). Reprinted by permission of Eden Press.]

ing insulin, prolactin, and cortisol. Thus, the two-step culture model dissociates the developmental stages of morphogenesis and lactogenesis of the gland into two distinct, nonoverlapping compartments. Absence of cortisol in the medium seems to accomplish this separation.

B. Casein mRNA Translation Activity

The two-step culture model of the whole mammary organ was then used in the following studies on the assessment of the action of prolactin and cortisol individually in stimulating the expression of the casein genes (Terry *et al.*, 1977a). The glands were incubated in step I culture with insulin, prolactin, growth hormone, estrogen, and progesterone for 6 days to obtain the lobuloalveolar structures. Culture of the lobuloalveolar glands was then done in the step II medium containing insulin, prolactin, and cortisol for an additional 6 days. RNA extracted from these glands was analyzed in the cell-free translational system drived from heterologous ribosomes (Terry *et al.*, 1975b, 1977a). Virtually no $mRNA_{csn}$ activity was measurable immunologically in the glands after step I culture, even though the glands contained the secretory structures. On the other hand, RNA from the glands after 6 days of step II culture with insulin, prolactin, and cortisol showed abundant $mRNA_{csn}$ activity, also determined immunologically. Consistent with the results of the translational assays, radioimmunoassay of tissue extracts with antibody to mouse casein also failed to show any measurable casein in the gland after step I culture, whereas abundant casein was present in the gland at the end of step II culture (Terry *et al.*, 1975b, 1977a).

C. Quantitative Measurement of $mRNA_{csn}$ Accumulation Measured by Molecular Hybridization

The cell-free translation assays described above thus showed that prolactin in the corticosteroid-free mammogenic medium fails to stimulate expression of the casein genes in the whole mammary organ *in vitro*, but the combination of polypeptide and the steroid hormone (cortisol) stimulates the appearance of $mRNA_{csn}$ activity. However, results of translation assays do not provide a quantitative measure of this stimulatory action. Therefore, in the following set of studies (Mehta *et al.*, 1980) the more sensitive molecular hybridizations were done using the $cDNA_{csn}$ probe. Figure 9 shows that the $cDNA_{csn}$ fails to detect a measurable level of $mRNA_{csn}$ in the mammary glands of the estrogen–progesterone primed animals or nonprimed animals. RNA from the lobuloalveolar glands, obtained after 6 days of step I incuba-

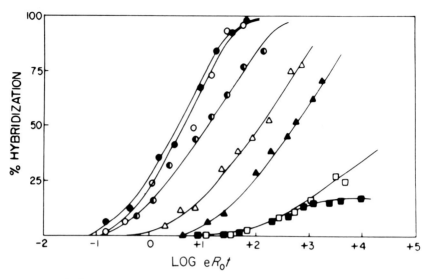

FIG. 9. Hybridization of cDNA$_{csn}$ to total RNA from glands at different stages of organ culture. RNA from glands of nonprimed virgin mice (■———■); RNA from glands of primed mice (□———□); RNA from glands after 6 days of culture in step I mammogenic medium (▲———▲); RNA from glands after 1 day (△———△), 3 days (◐———◐), 6 days (○———○), and 9 days (●———●) in step II culture medium with insulin, prolactin, and cortisol. [From Banerjee *et al.* (1982b). Reprinted by permission of Eden Press.]

tion in the corticosteroid-free mammogenic medium, hybridized to the cDNA$_{csn}$ to above the 50% level but at a rather high eR_ot value. The concentration of mRNA$_{csn}$ sequences in total RNA of these glands was only 0.00067%. Quantitative estimates further revealed a concentration of only 147 molecules of mRNA$_{csn}$ per epithelial cell. This low level of mRNA$_{csn}$ remains unaltered after subsequent three days of incubation of the glands in prolactin or ovarian steroid-free step I medium, indicating that 147 molecules/cell represents a basal level of the mRNA$_{csn}$ concentration in the lobuloalveolar glands in the corticosteroid-free mammogenic medium. In chick oviduct, the uninducted tubular gland cells *in vitro* contain a basal level of 40 and 500 molecules of ovalbumin and conalbumin mRNAs per cell, respectively (McKnight, 1978). The maintenance of the basal level of the mRNA$_{csn}$ in the lobuloalveolar mammary gland thus indicates that the mammary glands after step I culture remain in an uninduced state, and this is in contrast to the relatively high concentrations (0.09%) of mRNA$_{csn}$ and caseins present in the lobuloalveolar mammary glands of pregnant mice. In the pregnant animal, the accumulation of mRNA$_{csn}$ corresponds to a rise in the level of circulating glucocorticoids and prolactin. Consistent with the events *in vivo,* our studies have also shown that, when the mammogenic hormone mixture is supplemented with aldosterone (a corticoid having some glucocorticoid activity), the glands *in vitro* elicit both $mRNA_{csn}$ and caseins (Terry *et al.*, 1977a). Moreover, addition of cortisol in the step I mammogenic medium results in greater than a twofold increase of $mRNA_{csn}$ over the basal level after 3 days (Ganguly *et al.*, 1982). Thus, glucocorticoid deficiency of the step I mammogenic medium appears to prevent the expression of the casein genes in the glands *in vitro*, and the presence of prolactin in the medium is not sufficient to provide the needed stimulating action.

The same studies (Mehta *et al.*, 1980) also showed (Table II) that, during step II culture of the lobuloalveolar glands in the lactogenic medium with insulin, prolactin, and cortisol, $mRNA_{csn}$ rises ninefold over the basal level within 24 hours. This marked stimulatory action as early as 24 hours also indicates that an antagonistic action of residual progesterone (carried over from step I medium), if any, is of little significance. Progesterone is antagonistic to lactogenesis in the mammary glands *in vivo* (Assairi *et al.*, 1974). During 9 days of incubation of the glands in step II medium containing prolactin and cortisol, accumulation of $mRNA_{csn}$ progressively rises from 0.00067 to 0.09% of the total RNA of the gland (Table II). The cellular concentration of $mRNA_{csn}$ during the same period rises from the basal level of 147 molecules to 37,524 molecules/cell, a 255-fold increase. The number of epithelial cells during the 9-day step II incubation period remains essentially unaltered, indicating that the 255-fold rise of the cellular accumulation of $mRNA_{csn}$ over the basal level represents a net increase in cellular con-

TABLE II

NUMBER OF CASEIN mRNA MOLECULES PER CELL AT DIFFERENT STAGES OF
MORPHOGENESIS AND DIFFERENTIATION OF THE MAMMARY GLAND IN CULTURE[a]

Culture medium	$R_0t_{1/2}$	Casein mRNA (%)	Number of casein mRNA molecules per cell	Fold increase over IPrlEPGH[b] (molecules/cell)
6 day IPrlEPGH	524.8	0.00067	147	—
6 day IPrlEPGH + 1 day IPrlF	104.7	0.0033	1,366	9.3
6 day IPrlEPGH + 3 day IPrlF	12.0	0.029	4,826	32.8
6 day IPrlEPGH + 6 day IPrlF	5.1	0.068	23,699	161.2
6 day IPrlEPGH + 9 day IPrlF	3.9	0.09	37,524	255.2

[a] From Mehta *et al.* (1980).

[b] Abbreviations: I, insulin; Prl, prolactin; GH, growth hormone; E, 17β-estradiol; P, progesterone; F, cortisol.

centration of the $mRNA_{csn}$, very likely as a result of *de novo* transcription of the casein genes in the glands *in vitro*. Cortisol in the medium containing prolactin and insulin thus appears to exert this stimulatory action during the step II incubation. A concomitant increase of the translational activity of $mRNA_{csn}$ assayed in the wheat-germ ribosome system (Banerjee *et al.*, 1981, 1982b) further suggests that the milk-protein RNAs are translated in the glands *in vitro* as they accumulate in the cells. These findings strongly indicate that in the murine mammary glands the requirement of the glucocorticoid is essential for the induction of the casein genes in the presence of prolactin (Banerjee *et al.*, 1983a). Thus, the findings in the mammary glands in culture are consistent with the observations that, within 12 hours after a single injection, hydrocortisone can stimulate a fourfold replenishment of the loss of $mRNA_{csn}$ in the mammary gland caused by adrenalectomy, and this increased accumulation of the $mRNA_{csn}$ is concomitant with glucocorticoid stimulation of specific transcription of the casein genes (Banerjee *et al.*, 1982b).

XI. SIMULTANEOUS OCCURRENCE OF MORPHOGENESIS AND CASEIN GENE EXPRESSION

It is clear from the results discussed in Section X that the loculoalveolar mammary glands *in vitro* accumulate abundant $mRNA_{csn}$ only when exposed to the step II lactogenic medium containing both prolactin and cortisol. However, under physiological conditions in the animal, the lobuloalveolar morphogenesis of the mammary gland during gestation is accompanied by accumulation of $mRNA_{csn}$, indicating that the expression of the casein genes ensues prior to parturition. Moreover, the simultaneous occurrence of morphogenesis and functional differentiation of the mammary gland *in vivo* becomes increasingly evident as the circulating levels of glucocorticoid and prolactin also rise during the advanced stages of gestation, reaching the maximal level at parturition (Banerjee, 1976; Tucker, 1974).

Thus, experiments were done to ascertain whether similar simultaneous occurrence of morphogenesis and functional differentiation can be obtained in the mammary organ in culture, by modification of the hormone mixture that mimics the hormone environment in the pregnant animal. In these studies (Ganguly *et al.*, 1981), estrogen–progesterone primed mammary glands were incubated in a medium containing insulin, aldosterone, cortisol, and growth hormone. In this medium, the immature ductal glands develop pregnancylike lobuloalveolar structures after 6 days of incubation. During this morphogenetic process, cellular accumulation of $mRNA_{csn}$ increased progressively 17-fold on the sixth day over day-zero level, whereas the rise in cell number in the glands during the same period is only 2-fold (Fig. 10), indicating a net increase of cellular concentration of the $mRNA_{csn}$ in the glands *in vitro*. Omission of aldosterone from the medium does not alter $mRNA_{csn}$ levels in the gland, showing that the hormone combination of insulin, cortisol, and growth hormone is sufficient to maintain the simultaneous occurrence of morphogenesis and functional differentiation of the gland *in vitro*. Presence of aldosterone in the medium favors increased lobuloalveolar development in the gland (Mehta and Banerjee, 1975).

Growth hormone is believed to be nonlactogenic (Tucker, 1974). Thus, the accumulation of $mRNA_{csn}$ in the mammary gland in prolactin-free medium with growth hormone and the adrenal steroids may tempt the interpretation that the growth hormone in combination with the adrenal steroids in the absence of prolactin is stimulatory to casein gene expression. However, the batch of National Institues of Health (NIH) bovine growth hormone prepara-

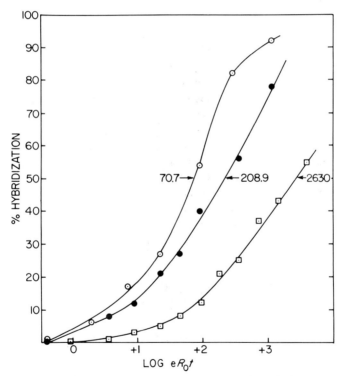

FIG. 10. Casein mRNA accumulation in the glands during 6 days of culture in medium with insulin, prolactin, aldosterone, and cortisol. Concentration of casein RNA in total RNA of the gland after 1 day (□———□), 3 days (●———●), and 6 days (⊙—⊙) of culture as measured by hybridization to the $[^3H]cDNA_{csn}$ probe. [From Banerjee *et al.* (1982b). Reprinted by permission of Eden Press.]

TABLE III

mRNA$_{csn}$ Level in the Glands Incubated in Different
Hormonal Combinations *in Vitro*[a]

Culture condition[b]	$R_o t_{1/2}$[c]	% mRNA$_{csn}$
6 day IGHAF	70.7 ± 3.0[c]	0.005 ± 0.0002[d]
6 day IAF + 80 ng/ml Prl	39.8 ± 2.0	0.0083 ± 0.0004
6 day IGHF	15.9 ± 2.0	0.021 ± 0.003

[a] From Ganguly *et al.* (1981).

[b] Abbreviations: I, insulin; GH, growth hormone; A, aldosterone; F, cortisol; Prl, prolactin.

[c] $R_o t_{1/2}$ of purified mRNA$_{csn}$ = 0.0003 molecules · seconds · liters^{-1}.

[d] Mean ± range of duplicate determination.

tion used in these experiments contained 80 ng of contaminating prolactin per 5 μg of growth hormone added in the medium (Ganguly *et al.*, 1981). Thus, the expression of the casein genes during morphogenesis in the medium with NIH growth hormone is very likely due to a synergistic action between the contaminating prolactin and the adrenal steroid hormones in the medium. This possibility was confirmed by incubating the glands in medium containing insulin, aldosterone, cortisol, and 80 ng prolactin (Ganguly *et al.*, 1981), and mRNA$_{csn}$ accumulation at a measurable (0.0083%) level was observed in these glands (Table III). The results described in this section demonstrate that the simultaneous occurrence of alveolar morphogenesis and casein gene expression as known to occur during pregnancy can be mimicked in the gland *in vitro* by modifying the prolactin- and glucocorticoid-enriched hormone mixture that mimics hormonal environment during gestation.

XII. GLUCOCORTICOID AND PROLACTIN INTERACTION IN MILK-PROTEIN GENE EXPRESSION

The results of the studies discussed in the preceding sections clearly demonstrate the remarkable ability of the mammary epithelium in the whole organ *in vitro* to faithfully express the characteristics in response to the stimulatory actions of selective combinations of the hormones. Moreover, in the two-step culture model, mammogenesis is completed in medium containing a modified hormone mixture that does not promote expression of the milk-protein genes, but the secretory structures remain highly sensitive to the complete lactogenic hormone mixture. This accomplishment for the first time made it feasible to test individually the stimulatory effects of prolactin or cortisol in the glands not preexposed to the glucocorticoid, and the uninduced mammary cells *in vitro* contain a basal level of the milk-protein mRNAs (Mehta *et al.*, 1980; Banerjee *et al.*, 1982a,b).

In these studies (Ganguly *et al.*, 1980), whole mammary organs obtained from immature female mice were incubated for 6 days in the step I corticosteroid-free mammogenic medium containing insulin, prolactin, estradiol, progesterone, and growth hormone to stimulate lobuloalveolar development. Virtually no mRNA$_{csn}$ is present in these lobuloalveolar glands, although the secretory structures are highly sensitive to the complete lactogenic hormone mixture. When these lobuloalveolar glands were transferred to step II medium containing insulin and prolactin or insulin and cortisol, no increase in mRNA$_{csn}$ over the basal levels was observed. However, the glands remain competent to respond to the complete lactogenic hormone mixture, because subsequent 3-day incubation in the medium containing insulin, cortisol, and prolactin stimulates a significant increase in the level of mRNA$_{csn}$ in the glands. These findings for the first time provided the demonstration that in a control hormonal environment neither prolactin nor cortisol alone can induce expression of the casein genes, even though functionally competent secretory structures are present in the gland (Table IV).

The same studies also revealed that, when incubation of the lobuloalveolar glands for 3 days with insulin and prolactin was followed by an additional 3 days in the medium containing insulin and cortisol, mRNA$_{csn}$ levels in the glands also remained at the basal level (Table IV). On the other hand, when incubation of the lobuloalveolar glands in step II culture with insulin and cortisol was followed by incubation in medium containing insulin and prolactin, an 18-fold increase in mRNA$_{csn}$ concentration was observed (Ganguly *et al.*, 1980). This pronounced increase cannot be attributed to a stimulatory action of prolactin alone, because observations described above have shown that the glands fail to accumulate mRNA$_{csn}$ above the basal levels when incubated in the step II medium containing insulin and prolactin. Therefore, one may ask whether the stimulatory action of the polypeptide hormone is synergistic with residual cortisol retained in the lobuloalveolar gland during the prior 3 days of incubation with the steroid hormone. Steroid hormones are retained by the mammary glands for extended periods of time (Strobl and Lippman, 1979).

The hypothesis was tested using the following experimental protocol (Ganguly *et al.*, 1980; Banerjee *et al.*, 1982a,b). At the end of the 6-day step I culture, the lobuloalveolar glands were incubated for 48 hours in medium with insulin and cortisol. One batch of the glands during this incubation period was incubated in the presence of [³H]cortisol during the last 24

TABLE IV

EFFECTS OF STEROID HORMONE ON mRNA ACCUMULATION[a]

A. $mRNA_{csn}$ in mammary gland after incubation with insulin plus
glucocorticoid or insulin plus prolactin

Culture condition[b]	$R_o t_{1/2}$[c]	% $mRNA_{csn}$
6 days I, Prl, E, P, GH	417	0.0009
3 days I, F	832	0.0005
3 days I, F → 3 days I, Prl, F	5.02	0.076
3 days I, Prl	n.m.[d]	n.m.
3 days I, Prl → 3 days I, Prl, F	10	0.038

B. Effect of preincubation of the lobuloalveolar glands with cortisol
or prolactin on the accumulation of $mRNA_{csn}$

Culture condition[b]	$R_o t_{1/2}$[c]	% $mRNA_{csn}$
3 days I, Prl	n.m.	n.m.
3 days I, Prl → 3 days I, F	316	0.0012
3 days I, F	832	0.0005
3 days I, F → 3 days I, Prl	23.4	0.016

[a] Data from Ganguly *et al.* (1980).
[b] I, insulin (5 μg/ml); Prl, prolactin (5 μg/ml); E, 17β-estradiol (0.001 μg/ml); P, progesterone (1 μg/ml); GH, growth hormone (5 μg/ml); F, cortisol (5 μg/ml). All glands were first incubated for 6 days in I, Prl, E, P, and GH medium.
[c] $R_o t_{1/2}$ of purified $mRNA_{csn}$ is 0.0038 moles/liter × seconds.
[d] n.m., not measurable.

hours. The glands were then transferred to a medium with insulin and prolactin. Batches of glands exposed to [³H]cortisol were analyzed at different times and were examined for the levels of residual cortisol during incubation with insulin and prolactin. The glands cultured with unlabeled cortisol were used for assessment of the $mRNA_{csn}$ levels. The results showed that a measurable level of [³H]cortisol radioactivity is present in the glands preincubated with the radioactive steroid hormone, indicating that the steroid hormone is retained in the lobuloalveolar gland during subsequent incubation in the medium containing insulin and prolactin, and the residual cortisol depletes progressively during the 48-hour incubation period (Fig. 11). The concentration of $mRNA_{csn}$ in the glands in parallel cultures increased from 0.006 to 0.016% during the initial 2 days in the glucocorticoid-free medium containing insulin and prolactin. Corresponding to the loss of residual cortisol, $mRNA_{csn}$ concentration in the glands also declined, reaching a near-basal level after 6 days of culture. After addition of cortisol on the sixth day in the medium containing insulin and prolactin, mRNA$_{csn}$ levels in the glands showed a dramatic 25-fold increase after only 3 days of incubation.

Thus, the preceding observations obtained under a controlled hormonal environment *in vitro* clearly demonstrate that (a) neither prolactin nor glucocorticoid alone is sufficient to initiate expression of the casein genes in murine mammary glands, (b) the mammary glands preexposed to glucocorticoid take up and retain the steroid hormone for an extended period of time, (c) the residual cortisol can promote mRNA$_{csn}$ accumulation in medium with prolactin, and (d) continuous presence of glucocorticoid in the medium is essential for induction of casein gene expression in murine mammary glands. These controlled studies further reveal that preincubation of the mammary tissue with cortisol introduces the residual steroid hormone effect during subsequent incubation in presence of prolactin. Unawareness of this problem may result in erroneous interpretation of the results concerning the

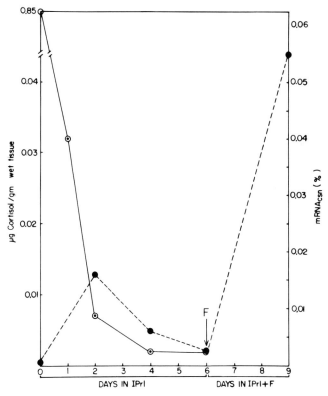

Fig. 11. Relationship between residual cortisol retained (○—○) and the mRNA$_{csn}$ accumulation (●- - -●) in the glands. [From Banerjee *et al.* (1982b). Reprinted by permission of Eden Press.]

regulatory role of the polypeptide and the steroid hormone in milk-protein gene expression. Similar residual glucocorticoid effect on casein synthesis in rat mammary explant culture in experiments using a virtually identical protocol has also been observed (Bolander *et al.*, 1979).

XIII. ROLE OF PROGESTERONE IN CASEIN GENE EXPRESSION

Since progesterone acts as an antagonist to lactogenesis (Assairi *et al.*, 1974), the mechanism of the action of the ovarian steroid hormone in the complex processes of mammary cell differentiation has been of interest to molecular endocrinologists. However, since the serum concentration of progesterone is reduced to a basal level (Tucker, 1974) at parturition, the involvement of progesterone on functional differentiation of the mammary cells is likely to remain limited to the gestation period. Nevertheless, understanding of the mechanisms of action of the ovarian steroid hormone is important for the overall elucidation of the multiple steroid and polypeptide hormone involvement in regulation of selective expression of the milk-protein genes.

Several recent reports (Houdebine, 1980; Rosen *et al.*, 1980) have suggested that progesterone may act as an inhibitor of casein gene expression by interfering with the stimulatory action of prolactin, although no mechanism of a progesterone–prolactin interaction has yet been postulated. On the other hand, it is known that the ability of the mammary gland to produce caseinlike proteins in ovariectomized pregnant rats is impaired when the animals are also adrenalectomized (Tucker, 1974). This observation suggests that progesterone may act by interfering with the lactogenic action of the adrenal steroid hormone. In pregnant animals, serum progesterone levels remain reasonably high through most of the gestation period (Tucker, 1974). The circulating levels of the adrenal steroid(s) also rise progressively with the advance of pregnancy (Gala and Westphal, 1965). Thus, it is conceivable that the maintenance of a restricted level of lactogenic activity, including expression of the casein genes, in the prepartum mammary gland may reflect a progesterone-mediated interference on the stimulatory action of glucocorticoid. This possibility appears likely also because progesterone, in addition to specific binding to its own receptor, also interacts with the cytoplasmic glucocorticoid receptor in the mammary cells (Shyamala and Dickson, 1976; Shyamala, 1982). Thus, a possible mode of a receptor-mediated antagonistic action of progesterone appears to be present in the mammary cells. This hypothesis was tested in the two-step culture model of the whole mammary organ of the mouse (Ganguly *et al.*, 1982; Banerjee *et al.*, 1982a).

As usual, the mammary glands from the immature female mice were stimulated to lobuloalveolar development after 6 days of incubation in the corticosteroid-free step I mammogenic medium. The lobuloalveolar glands were then incubated for another 3 or 6 days with the same mammogenic hormone mixture plus cortisol, in the medium with or without progesterone. RNA isolated from these glands was assessed for the concentration of mRNA$_{csn}$ by the cDNA$_{csn}$ probe. Results showed that, when cortisol is present in the mammogenic medium without progesterone, the mRNA$_{csn}$ level increases progessively and its concentration remains essentially similar in medium with 1 or 5 μg/ml of cortisol. In contrast, when progesterone is added to the mammogenic medium, the concentration of the mRNA$_{csn}$ is significantly reduced. This suggests that, while cortisol is capable of promoting casein gene expression in the mammogenic medium that includes prolactin, the presence of progesterone can restrict the stimulatory action of the glucocorticoid.

Furthermore, the glucocorticoid-stimulated progressive rise in the level of mRNA$_{csn}$ in the progesterone-free medium containing cortisol is interrupted after addition of progesterone to the medium on the third day. The rise in accumulation of mRNA$_{csn}$ in the glands is arrested at approximately the 45% level, and no further increase is evident between the third and sixth days of culture. The observation that the ovarian steroid causes a partial inhibition of the mRNA$_{csn}$ accumulation suggests a sustained stimulatory action of cortisol in the medium, although at a reduced level. This possibility was examined by measuring the concentrations of the mRNA$_{csn}$ at different molar ratios of progesterone and cortisol in the culture medium. The results showed that, while the mRNA$_{csn}$ concentration reached 0.01% in medium with 3 μM cortisol and no progesterone after 3 days of incubation, mRNA$_{csn}$ levels in the glands progressively decrease as the progesterone–cortisol ratio in the medium is increased. At equimolar concentrations of progesterone and glucocorticoid, the level of inhibition reaches 85%. These results clearly show that the degree of the antagonistic action of progesterone is limited by the concentration of glucocorticoid present in the medium. Thus, the inhibitory action of progesterone on expression of the casein genes appears to be associated with some adverse interaction of the ovarian steroid hormone with the stimulatory function of the glucocorticoid. Moreover, the extent of this unfavorable action of progesterone is dependent upon concentration of cortisol in the medium. Addition of an excess amount (5 μg/ml) of cortisol in the prolactin-containing medium stimulates mRNA$_{csn}$ accumulation in the gland in the presence of progesterone. Progesterone is known to compete for the glucocorticoid cytoplasmic receptors in the mammary cells, although the progesterone–receptor complex is not translocated into the nuclei of the mammary cells (Shyamala and Dickson, 1976; Shymala, 1982). Thus, the mechanism of progesterone-mediated adverse action may be related to the competitive binding of the ovarian steroid hormone for the glucocorticoid receptors in the cytoplasm of the mammary cells.

For an assessment of this possibility, glucocorticoid cytosol receptors in the mammary cells in organ culture were determined by measuring the specific [³H]dexamethasone binding in the mammary cytosol (Ganguly *et al.*, 1982). As expected, the mammary cells in the whole organ *in vitro* contain a specific glucocorticoid cytoplasmic receptor. The ligand–receptor interaction represents a single class of high-affinity binding with an apparent dissociation constant (K_d) of 4.31×10^{-8} M (Fig. 12). Consistent with the earlier findings (Shyamala and Dickson, 1976), results further showed that progesterone competes for the glucocorticoid-receptor sites in the cytosol of the mammary cells in organ culture. At higher progesterone–glucocorticoid molar ratio in the culture medium, the reduced $mRNA_{csn}$ level in the glands is accompanied by a corresponding reduction of glucocorticoid binding to cytosol receptors in the mammary glands *in vitro* (Fig. 13). This finding thus indicates that progesterone antagonism on expression of the milk-protein genes is associated with reduced glucocorticoid binding to the mammary cytosol receptor, apparently caused by competitive binding of progesterone to the same receptors. Thus, it appears likely that the mechanism of progesterone antagonism to milk-protein gene expression is related to a reduced

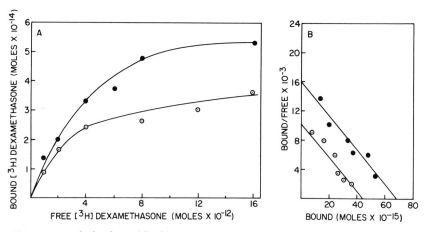

FIG. 12. Specific binding of [³H]dexamethasone to cytosol of murine mammary glands *in vitro*. (A) Saturation binding kinetics of [³H]dexamethasone binding to glucocorticoid receptors. Step I incubation (6 days) with insulin, prolactin, growth hormone, 17β-estradiol, and progesterone (○—○); 6 days of step I incubation followed by 3 days in step II medium with insulin, prolactin, and cortisol (●———●); (B) Scatchard-plot analysis of the data shown in (A). [From Banerjee *et al.* (1982a).]

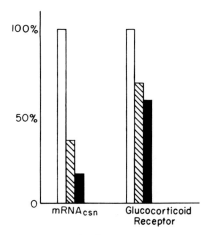

FIG. 13. The levels of mRNA$_{csn}$ and [^{3}H]dexamethasone receptors in mammary gland in medium containing different progesterone (P)/cortisol (F) ratios. The mammary glands were incubated in medium containing P/F molar ratios. [^{3}H]Dexamethasone binding to the cytosol receptors in these glands was assayed *in vitro*. The levels of mRNA$_{csn}$ and glucocorticoid receptor in the glands at P/F ratio = 0 were considered the 100% value. Open bars, P/F = 0; stippled bars, P/F = 0.21; shaded bars, P/F = 1. [From Ganguly *et al.* (1982).]

glucocorticoid binding to its receptors in the mammary cells. Recent results in our laboratory have further shown that progesterone competition for the glucocorticoid binding sites in the mammary cytosol also results in a reduced nuclear binding of the ligand–receptor complex (P. K. Majumder and M. R. Banerjee, unpublished), an event believed to be crucial for steroid hormone–induced specific gene transcriptions (Yamamoto and Albert, 1976).

XIV. NUCLEAR BINDING OF GLUCOCORTICOID RECEPTOR AND MILK-PROTEIN GENE EXPRESSION

Pyridoxal-5'-phosphate (PALP), a vitamin B$_6$ derivative, can inhibit nuclear binding of the steroid hormone receptors including the glucocorticoid receptor by interacting with the lysine residue(s) of the receptor molecule (Litwack, 1979). PALP then can act as a potential physiological modulator of steroid hormonal induction of specific gene expression. Moreover, PALP also inhibits the synthesis of TAT in the liver cells (Disorbo and Litwack, 1981). Thus, studies (Majumder *et al.*, 1983) were done to determine whether the regulatory influence of glucocorticoid on the expression of the milk-protein genes involves receptor-mediated nuclear interaction of the steroid hormone in the mammary cells (Banerjee *et al.*, 1983b).

As usual, the mammary glands from immature female mice were initially incubated in the step I medium containing the corticosteroid-free mammogenic hormone mixture to obtain the lobuloalveolar structures. Step II incubation of the lobuloalveolar glands was then done in medium containing the lactogenic hormone combination of cortisol, prolactin, and insulin. After incubation with 2 mM or 5 mM PALP in the step II medium for 3 days, the concentration of PALP in the mammary tissue increased 4- and 12-fold, respectively, over the basal levels (Table V). The increased tissue concentration of PALP at 2 mM was accompanied by a 52% inhibition of specific [3H]dexamethasone nuclear binding in the glands after 3 days of step II incubation with the lactogenic hormones. [3H]Dexamethasone nuclear binding reached a 92% inhibition with 5 mM PALP in the step II medium containing the same hormones (Table V).

Figure 14 also shows that RNA from the glands not exposed to PALP hybridized to the $cDNA_{csn}$ probe at $eR_0t_{1/2}$ of 11.64 moles · seconds · liters^{-1}, indicating a 0.03% concentration of $mRNA_{csn}$ sequences in the total RNA from the glands incubated for 3 days in the step II medium containing cortisol, prolactin, and insulin. The RNA from the glands exposed to 2 mM PALP showed an increased $eR_0t_{1/2}$ value of 83.95 moles · seconds · liters^{-1}, reflecting a reduced $mRNA_{csn}$ concentration of 0.0041%. In glands incubated with 5 mM PALP under similar culture conditions, the $mRNA_{csn}$ concentration was further reduced to 0.0026%. These results demonstrate that a dose-dependent inhibition of nuclear binding of the glucocorticoid–receptor complex is correlated with a marked loss of $mRNA_{csn}$ accumulation in the mammary glands *in vitro*.

The inhibitory action of PALP is reversible; withdrawal of the vitamin B_6 derivative from the medium restores nuclear binding of the steroid–receptor complex as well as the $mRNA_{csn}$ levels in the glands (Fig. 15). These results

TABLE V

LEVELS OF NUCLEAR BINDING OF [3H]-DEXAMETHASONE AND $mRNA_{csn}$ CONCENTRATION AT DIFFERENT EXPERIMENTAL CONDITIONS[a]

Hormones	[3H]-dexamethasone bound[b] (fmoles/μg DNA)	Cell tissue (no./g)	Total RNA (μg)	$mRNA_{csn}$ $eR_0t_{1/2}$	%
Insulin, prolactin, cortisol	0.53	2.9×10	777	11.64	0.0026
+ 2 mM Pyridoxal-5'-phosphate	0.25	2.3×10	650	83.95	0.0041
+ 5 mM Pyridoxal-5'-phosphate	0.06	n.m.[c]	525	135.50	0.0026

[a] From Majumder *et al.* (1983).
[b] The glands were incubated with [3H]-dexamethasone for 60 minutes.
[c] Not measurable.

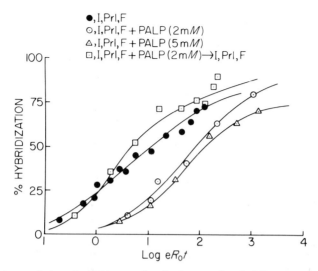

Fig. 14. Accumulation of mRNA$_{csn}$ in the glands treated with different concentrations of PALP in the medium containing the lactogenic hormones insulin, prolactin, and cortisol. mRNA was measured by molecular hybridization of the RNA from the glands *in vitro* to the cDNA$_{csn}$ probe. Abbreviations: I, insulin; Prl, prolactin; F, cortisol; PALP, pyridoxal-5'-phosphate. [From Majumder *et al.* (1983).]

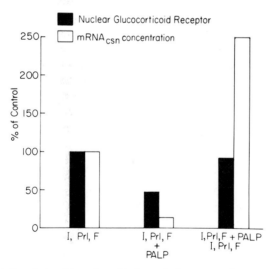

Fig. 15. Correlation between nuclear binding of glucocorticoid–receptor complex and mRNA$_{csn}$ accumulation at 2 mM concentration of PALP. The first column shows the control values of the glands (0.51 fmoles/μg of DNA glucocorticoid bound and 0.030% mRNA$_{csn}$ concentration) used as 100%. The second column shows the levels in the gland treated with 2 mM PALP, and the third column shows the levels after withdrawal of 2 mM PALP from the medium. Abbreviations: I, insulin; Prl, prolactin; F, hydrocortisone; PALP, pyridoxal-5'-phosphate. [From Majumder *et al.* (1983).]

also demonstrate that PALP at the concentrations used does not alter the specific hormone responsiveness of the mammary cells *in vitro*. Correlation between the inhibition of nuclear binding of the glucocorticoid–receptor complex and the corresponding loss of mRNA$_{csn}$ strongly indicates that the modulatory role of the glucocorticoid on the expression of the milk-protein genes in the murine mammary gland is associated with nuclear interaction of the steroid hormone–receptor complex. Since interaction of the steroid hormone–receptor complex with the nuclear acceptor sites is considered essential for the onset of hormone-inducible gene transcription (O'Malley and Means, 1974; Yamamoto and Albert, 1976), the results described above further indicate that glucocorticoid as a component of the lactogenic hormones very likely acts at the genomic level of control of the milk-protein genes. This contention is in agreement with our earlier finding (Ganguly *et al.*, 1979) on glucocorticoid modulation of transcription of the casein genes in the mammary gland of postpartum mice.

XV. HORMONAL REGULATION OF MILK-PROTEIN GENE EXPRESSION IN RATS AND RABBITS

The regulatory role of prolactin and cortisol on milk-protein gene expression also has been investigated in rats using the explant culture model of mammary tissue from pregnant animals (Rosen *et al.*, 1980). Mammary tissue of pregnant rats normally contains a high concentration of mRNA$_{csn}$. Therefore, in these studies, the explants needed to be preincubated for 48 hours in a prolactin-free culture medium containing insulin and cortisol to reduce the endogenous mRNA$_{csn}$ to a near-basal level, measured also by a cDNA probe to 15S rat mRNA$_{csn}$. Subsequent 48-hour incubation of the explants in the serum-free medium containing insulin and prolactin was found to stimulate a 13-fold increase of mRNA$_{csn}$ accumulation over the basal level. Furthermore, preincubation of the explants with insulin and cortisol followed by 24-hour incubation with insulin and prolactin increased casein mRNA transcription two- to fourfold over the basal level. Half-life of the mRNAs estimated in the medium containing insulin and cortisol was only 5 hours, whereas, after addition of prolactin in the medium, it increased to 92 hours. Based on these results it was concluded that (a) prolactin induces transcription of the milk-protein mRNAs, (b) the peptide hormone also regulates cellular accumulation of the mRNAs by extending their half-life, and (c) continuous presence of the glucocorticoid is not needed, although addition of cortisol can "potentiate" the stimulatory action of prolactin. A 3.3-fold increase of transcription in medium with insulin and cortisol was explained as due to a better maintenance of the explants in presence of the glucocorticoid. Recently, the hormonal stimulation of the accumulation of individual rat casein mRNAs (α, β, γ) and the whey acidic protein (PC-32) mRNA in rat mammary tissue were measured using cloned cDNA probes to the individual milk-protein mRNAs (Hobbs *et al.*, 1982). Results showed that a maximal expression of the individual casein mRNAs occurs in a coordinated manner in medium with insulin, prolactin, and hydrocortisone. In the animal, expression of the casein mRNAs is also coordinated during pregnancy and lactation. Accumulation of the whey protein PX-32 (whey acidic protein) mRNA showed a greater sensitivity to cortisol. It has been stated that, because of the residual cortisol effect inherent to the mammary explant culture model used, it is not possible to conclude that there is an absolute requirement of the glucocorticoid for accumulation of the mRNAs. Prolactin stimulation of the mRNAs was observed in explants obtained from pregnant rats 2 days after adrenalectomy, although at a much reduced level.

On the other hand, a more recent study (Kulski *et al.*, 1983) measuring accumulation of the mRNAs for 42K and 25K rat caseins, also using cloned cDNA probes, reported that mRNA for the 42K casein in the mammary explants from adrenalectomized rats is highly dependent upon exogenous cortisol in the medium containing prolactin, and expression of the 25K casein mRNA is almost entirely dependent upon the glucocorticoid. These authors explain that the much-reduced dependence on glucocorticoid observed in the earlier study (Hobbs *et al.*, 1982) may be due to the effects of the residual glucocorticoid present in the explants, and the same explanation is also applicable for the experiments in which explants were obtained from pregnant rats adrenalectomized only 2 days prior to using the tissue for explant culture. Thus, based on the studies on the measurement of the accumulation of the mRNAs for 42K and 25K rat caseins, Kulski *et al.* (1983) have concluded that expression of the casein genes in rats is highly, perhaps entirely, dependent on the glucocorticoid, and absence of the steroid hormone does not affect viability of tissue *in vitro*.

Consideration of the findings discussed above thus seems to prompt the following comments: (a) mammary tissue of pregnant rats and mice rich in glucocorticoid receptors is exposed to the elevated levels of endogenous glucocorticoids (Gala and Westphal, 1965), (b) mammary tissue of mice and rats can retain the steroid hormone for prolonged period (Bolander *et al.*, 1979; Ganguly *et al.*, 1980), and (c) preincubation with cortisol to deplete the endogenous $mRNA_{csn}$ is likely to further enrich the glucocorticoid concentration in the explants. Therefore, the stimulation of milk-protein gene expression (transcription and accumulation) observed in the rat mammary explant cultures in medium containing insulin and prolactin very likely reflects a synergistic action of prolactin in the medium, with the residual glucocorticoid retained in the tissue. Bolander *et al.* (1979) have confirmed this possibility in rats, and these findings are also consistent with similar observations in the mouse mammary organ *in vitro*. The action of the steroid hormone is dose dependent. The level of residual glucocorticoid in the explant may not be optimal, and addition of cortisol (5 μg/ml) in the medium containing prolactin should stimulate a dose-depenedent maximal increase of accumulation of the mRNAs in insulin- and prolactin-containing medium. It appears that this added stimulatory action has been interpreted to indicate that glucocorticoid potentiates the action of prolactin. Thus, the current status of our knowledge on hormonal regulation of milk-protein gene expression in the mammary glands may be summarized as follows.

1. The milk-protein genes are hormone inducible; both prolactin and glucocorticoid are needed to stimulate this response of the mammary cells.
2. The glucocorticoid can modulate transcription and accumulation of the milk-protein mRNAs in presence of prolactin, indicating that the steroid hormone acts at the genomic level. However, neither the glucocorticoid nor prolactin alone can support mRNA$_{csn}$ accumulation, and elucidation of the specific mode of action of prolactin and the glucocorticoid on transcription of the milk-protein genes in this complex process must come from future investigations.
3. In the mouse, binding of the glucocorticoid–receptor complex to the nuclear acceptor site is associated with casein mRNA accumulation in the mammary glands *in vitro*.
4. Progesterone acts as a down-regulator, reducing glucocorticoid binding to mammary cell receptors, and consequently limits glucocorticoid stimulation of milk-protein gene expression. This mode of action of progesterone is also likely to influence milk-protein gene transcription by reducing the level of nuclear glucocorticoid–receptor interaction.
5. At this time, our knowledge is based mostly on measurement of cellular accumulation of the mRNA$_{csn}$.

The regulation of expression of the milk-protein genes also has been investigated in rabbits, mostly using pseudopregnant animals (Houdebine, 1980). Based on the results of these studies, it has been concluded that expression of the casein genes measured by a cDNA probe is regulated by prolactin. While cortisol alone does not stimulate transcription or accumulation of the mRNAs for the milk-proteins, the glucocorticoid can potentiate the action of prolactin, although a mechanism of this "potentiating" interaction between the steroid and the polypeptide hormone remains unclear. Nevertheless, as in the mouse, a modulatory role of the glucocorticoid on transcription of the casein genes in prolactin-stimulated pseudopregnant rabbits has been observed. Thus, at this time it may not be appropriate to conclude that the glucocorticoid plays only a marginal role in regulation of the milk-protein genes. The response of the mammary cells to prolactin in presence of low levels of cortisol may indicate greater sensitivity of the rabbit mammary cells to the steroid hormones. Part of the difficulty in elucidation of the role of the glucocorticoid in the regulation of milk-protein gene expression may relate to the endocrine complexities of the pseudopregnant rabbits used as an experimental model.

XVI. POSSIBLE MECHANISMS OF PROLACTIN ACTION

Despite the contention that prolactin is the principal regulatory hormone for casein synthesis and milk-protein gene expression, very little is known about the mechanisms of milk-protein gene induction by the polypeptide hormone (Rilema, 1982; Rosen *et al.*, 1980; Oka *et al.*, 1982). Numerous attempts to ascertain whether the cAMP or cGMP, prostaglandins, BucAMP, BuGMP, and polyamines may be involved in the pathway of prolactin stimulation of milk-protein gene expression have failed to reveal any correlation. Nonetheless, interaction of the polypeptide hormone with the steroid (glucocorticoid) hormone is required for the expression of the milk-protein genes. Preliminary studies have also indicated that antibody to prolactin can inhibit casein synthesis in explants of rabbit mammary glands (Shiu and Friesen, 1976). Thus, it is important to learn about the mechanisms of the action of prolactin during its regulatory influence on morphogenesis and functional differentiation of the mammary cells. Recently, Teyssot *et al.* (1981) have postulated an intriguing concept of a membrane receptor–mediated pathway of prolactin action in the mammary cells. It has been reported that incubation of prolactin receptor–positive mammary cell membranes with prolactin or other lactogenic peptide hormones results in the appearance of a small oligopeptide (1000 daltons), which is capable of stimulating casein gene transcription in the isolated mammary cell nuclei *in vitro*. Membranes without the prolactin receptor or the nonlactogenic hormones fail to elicit this stimulatory factor. Based on these observations, it has been suggested that the membrane-derived oligopeptide may act as "second messenger" in stimulating the nuclear event. Confirmation of this intriguing idea must await future studies, including elucidation of the question concerning the mode of the mitogenic action of prolactin associated with morphogenesis of the mammary parenchyma.

XVII. ACTION OF INSULIN

Studies in the mammary tissue *in vitro* have clearly shown that insulin is involved in this complex multiple-hormone regulatory process. Although it is known that the metabolic hormone is required for viability of the mammary parenchyma *in vitro* (Mehta and Banerjee, 1975) and that insulin acts as a permissive hormone supporting the mitogenic action of prolactin in the mammary tissue (Mukherjee *et al.*, 1973), its direct involvement, if any, in milk-protein gene expression still remains unclear. Possible roles of insulin in regulation of mammary gland development were recently reviewed in Volume XI of this treatise (Topper *et al.*, 1984).

XVIII. MILK-PROTEIN cDNA CLONES AND CONCLUDING REMARKS

In recent years, recombinant cDNA clones for the milk proteins of several mammalian species have been described. These include the rat (Richards *et al.*, 1981a,b; Dandekar and Qasba, 1981), mouse (Mehta *et al.*, 1981; Hennighausen and Sippel, 1982a), guinea pig (Craig *et al.*, 1981), rabbit (Suard *et al.*, 1982), bovine (Willis *et al.*, 1982), and human (Hall *et al.*, 1981) species. These cDNA clones have allowed two major types of study. First, sequence determination of the clones has made it possible to predict the primary amino acid sequence of the corresponding milk proteins. As a result, some insight into the structure and function of the proteins has been obtained. In addition, a comparison of DNA sequences had led to some interesting findings with regard to the evolution of the milk-protein genes. Second, the cDNA clones have been used to prepare pure hybridization probes for mRNAs. These probes have allowed the accumulation of individual milk-protein mRNAs to be measured during the hormonally induced growth and differentiation of the mammary gland.

A. SEQUENCE ANALYSIS OF cDNA CLONES

A comparison of the cDNA sequences of the rat (Blackburn *et al.*, 1982; Hobbs and Rosen, 1982) and bovine (Willis *et al.*, 1982) caseins and the mouse ε-casein (Hennighausen *et al.*, 1982a) has shown extensive homology in specific areas, namely the 5'-noncoding region, the signal peptides, and sequences coding for possible protein phosphorylation sites. These results indicate that the casein genes may have evolved into a small multigene family by intragenic duplication of a sequence containing the primitive serine phosphorylation site $(Ser)_{an}$-Glu-Glu. This hypothesis is supported by the finding that the mouse casein genes exist as a cluster on a single chromosome (Gupta *et al.*, 1982). A unique feature of the rat α-casein sequence is an insertion in the coding region containing 10 repeated elements of 18 nucleotides each (Hobbs and Rosen, 1982).

Human and guinea pig α-lactalbumin mRNAs have been shown to exhibit a high degree of sequence homology in both coding and 3'-noncoding regions (Hall *et al.*, 1982). An interesting finding from the sequence analysis of guinea pig (Hall *et al.*, 1982) and rat (Dandekar and Qasba, 1981) α-lactalbumin cDNA clones is the existence of a carboxy-terminal, hydrophobic extension of 17 and 19 amino acids in the rat and guinea pig proteins, respectively. These results imply the existence of a minor mRNA coding for an α-lactalbumin variant. Although such a protein has not yet been demonstrated in the guinea pig, rat α-lactalbumin has been known to exist in a minor and abundant form for a number of years (Qasba and Chakrabartty, 1978).

Clones for the novel whey acidic protein (WAP) for mouse (Hennighausen and Sippel, 1982b) and rat (Hennighausen *et al.*, 1982b) have also been sequenced. Whey acidic protein is rich in cysteine. The results from the sequence analysis show that the majority of the cysteine residues are present in two groups of six arranged in an identical pattern. Thus, WAP appears to be composed of two domains. In this respect, WAP resembles the family of four disulfide core proteins that includes wheat germ agglutinin, and neurophysin (Hennighausen and Sippel, 1982b).

A comparison of rat and mouse WAP (Hennighausen *et al.*, 1982b) shows extensive homology both at the cDNA sequence and amino acid levels in the signal peptide, first cysteine domain, and 3'-noncoding regions. In conclusion, the caseins and whey proteins from a number of different mammals show homology in only a few distinct regions. Presumably this reflects functionally important domains that are under high evolutionary selective pressure. Apart from these areas, the milk proteins exhibit a large degree of divergence.

B. Developmental Studies

The first application of milk-protein cDNA clones to the study of mammary gland development was reported by Burditt *et al.* (1981). Pure radiolabeled cDNA probes for the caseins and α-lactalbumin were used to measure the accumulation of the corresponding mRNAs in the guinea pig mammary gland during pregnancy and lactation. α-Lactalbumin mRNA sequences were present late in pregnancy and reached maximum concentrations at parturition. Casein gene transcripts were absent late in pregnancy but by parturition had reached the levels observed throughout lactation. In the same study, differential rates of casein and α-lactalbumin synthesis and secretion were observed. These results indicated that milk production is regulated at several subcellular sites.

Similar studies in the rat (Hobbs *et al.*, 1982) showed a steady increase in the concentrations of α-, β-, and γ-casein and WAP during pregnancy. A very sharp rise in the rate of accumulation of these milk-protein mRNAs occurred at parturition, and this increase continued through 18 days of lactation. In organ culture of mammary explants from midpregnant rats (Hobbs *et al.*, 1982), all four milk-protein mRNAs required both prolactin and cortisol for maximum accumulation. Interestingly, cortisol alone had little effect on the accumulation of the three casein mRNAs but increased the amount of WAP mRNA 68-fold during a 24-hour period of culture.

Recently, Kulski *et al.* (1983) have used mammary explants from adrenal-ectomized virgin rats to demonstrate the importance of glucocorticoids for casein gene expression. It was found that α-casein mRNA accumulation was 20-fold higher in the presence of insulin, prolactin, and hydrocortisone than in the presence of insulin and prolactin alone. The induction of β-casein gene expression was found to be totally dependent on the presence of the steroid hormone in medium containing insulin and prolactin.

In our own laboratory, we have used a number of different milk protein cDNA clones to study mammary gland development both *in vivo* and *in vitro*. Clones for murine α_1-casein, β_2-casein, ε-casein, and WAP were isolated from a cDNA library constructed from poly(A)-containing mRNA of lactating mouse mammary gland. The cloning strategy employed insertion of the double-stranded cDNA into the *Pst*I site of the plasmid vector pBR322 by GC-tailing.

In one series of experiments, the two-step culture system of the whole murine mammary gland described earlier was used to study the hormonal regulation of WAP and α-lactalbumin gene expression. Mammary glands were initially grown for 6 days in mammogenic medium containing insulin, prolactin, estrogen, progesterone, and growth hormone. The glands were then further cultured in the presence of various combinations of insulin, prolactin, and hydrocortisone for up to 6 days. The RNA extracted from the mammary tissue was analyzed for WAP and α-lactalbumin mRNA sequences by dot blot hybridization (Thomas, 1980) using cDNA clones radiolabeled with [^{32}P] by nick translocation (Rigby *et al.*, 1977). The autoradiograms obtained were scanned with a densitometer (Fig. 16). The semiquantitative nature of this type of analysis prevents an accurate determination of the rates of accumulation for WAP and α-lactalbumin mRNA. However, the hormonal dependence of WAP and α-lactalbumin gene expression was clearly demonstrated (Table VI). A low level of both WAP and α-lactalbumin mRNA was detectable at the end of the initial 6 days of alveolar morphogenesis. The maximum increase in both WAP and α-lactalbumin mRNA sequences oc-

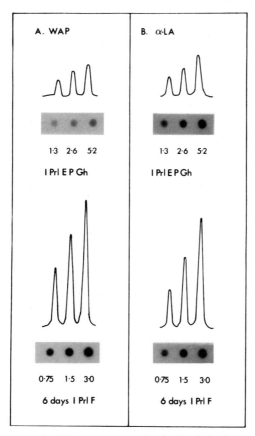

FIG. 16. Measurement of mRNA concentration by dot blot hybridization and densitometric scanning. Total RNA from murine mammary glands cultured in the presence of different hormone combinations was assayed for (A) whey acidic protein (WAP) and (B)α-lactalbumin (α-LA) mRNA by dot blot hybridization using ^{32}P-labeled cloned DNA probes as described in Section XVIII,B. The autoradiograms of the dots and their corresponding densitometric scans are shown. The numbers below the dots refer to the micrograms of RNA spotted. The dots from the following hormone treatments are illustrated: 6 days in mammogenic medium containing insulin (I), prolactin (Prl), estrogen (E), progesterone (P), and growth hormone (Gh) (top row); 6 days in I, Prl, E, P, and Gh plus 6 days in the presence of I, Prl, and hydrocortisone (F) (bottom row).

curred during the subsequent culture of the glands in the presence of insulin, prolactin, and hydrocortisone. It was also observed that a significant amount of α-lactalbumin mRNA accumulation took place in medium containing only insulin and the glucocorticoid.

We have used the same experimental techniques to measure the accumulation of the mRNAs for the murine milk proteins during different

TABLE VI

HORMONAL DEPENDENCE OF WHEY ACIDIC PROTEIN (WAP)
AND α-LACTALBUMIN (α-LA) GENE EXPRESSION[a]

| Hormone treatment | Fold increase over I, Prl, E, P, GH | |
	WAP	α-LA
3 days I, P	0.0	0.0
3 days I, F	1.35	1.5
6 days I, F	1.35	2.2
3 days I, Prl, F	1.75	1.5
6 days I, Prl, F	5.0	3.85

[a] Murine mammary glands were cultured for 6 days in mammogenic medium containing insulin (I), prolactin (Prl), estrogen (E), progesterone (P), and growth hormone (GH). The glands were then incubated in the presence of various combinations of insulin, prolactin, and hydrocortisone (F) for up to 6 days. Total RNA extracted from this tissue was assayed for WAP and α-LA mRNA sequences by dot blot hybridization using cloned DNA probes (see Section XVIII, B). The autoradiograms of the dots were quantitated by densitometric scanning as illustrated in Fig. 16. The results are expressed as the fold increase in the intensity of the spots over that obtained for the mammogenic period of culture (I, Prl, E, P, GH).

stages of pregnancy and lactation (Table VII). The mammary gland of the mouse, like that of the rat and rabbit, undergoes gradual development through pregnancy (Anderson, 1974). Thus, despite extensive growth of the mammary gland even by midpregnancy, a significant increase in the accumulation of α_1- and β_2-casein and WAP mRNAs was not detected until 18 days of gestation. The amount of these mRNAs continued to rise up to midlactation. The pattern of α-lactalbumin mRNA accumulation was contrastingly different. α-Lactalbumin mRNA was not observed to rise significantly until parturition and by 8 days of lactation had decreased to the levels observed prepartum.

The results from the developmental studies described previously indicate a differential expression among the milk-protein genes during mammary gland development. This is particularly evident between α-lactalbumin and the caseins in both the guinea pig and the mouse.

Tissue culture experiments have shown that maximum accumulation of the milk-protein mRNAs is generally observed to take place in the presence of both prolactin and glucocorticoids in insulin-containing medium. However, some genes appear to be particularly sensitive to the steroid hormone, namely those for WAP (Hobbs *et al.*, 1982) and β-casein (Kulski *et al.*, 1983) in the rat and α-lactalbumin in the mouse. Future studies utilizing recombinant DNA probes should reveal the role(s) of prolactin and cortisol at transcriptional and posttranscriptional levels of gene regulation.

The availability of cDNA clones also makes it possible to isolate the genomic milk-protein genes. The characterization of the rat γ-casein gene was reported (Yu-Lee and Rosen, 1983). This subsequently allowed distinct DNA methylation sites to be detected within the gene; they become demethylated when γ-casein is expressed during lactation (Johnson *et al.*, 1983). As more genomic milk-protein sequences are characterized, it will be possible to ascertain whether they share common genetic elements that are essential for steroid hormone–receptor interaction as has been demonstrated for the chicken egg-white protein genes (Mulvihill *et al.*, 1982; Compton *et al.*, 1983). Furthermore, it will be interesting to see whether the DNA sequence necessary for glucocorticoid regulation of the milk-protein genes is homologous with that delineated to be essential for mammary tumor virus expression induced by the same hormone (Groner *et al.*, 1982; Buetti and Diggelmann, 1983; Scheidereit *et al.*, 1983). Thus, as the detailed structure of the milk-protein genes is uncovered, it should become possible to determine the fine molecular mechanisms of the hormonal regulation of mammary differentiation in both normal and neoplastic tissues.

TABLE VII

ACCUMULATION OF THE mRNAs FOR THE MURINE MILK PROTEINS
DURING MAMMARY GLAND DEVELOPMENT[a]

Stage of development	Fold increase over virgin							
	α_1		β_2		WAP		α-LA	
Virgin	—	(7.6)[b]	—	(9.5)	—	(13)	—	(33)
5 days' pregnancy	0	(6.6)	1.85	(14.1)	0	(9.8)	1.1	(36)
11 days' pregnancy	0	(8.4)	1.85	(17)	0	(9.4)	0	(36)
18 days' pregnancy	6.2	(48)	4.5	(45.2)	2.4	(29)	0	(28)
Parturition	7	(54)	5.8	(57)	3.5	(43)	3.1	(100)
8 days' lactation	14	(100)	10.8	(100)	8.3	(100)	1.1	(36)

[a] Total RNA from mammary gland at different stages of pregnancy and lactation was assayed for α_1- and β_2-casein, whey acidic protein (WAP), and α-lactalbumin (α-LA) mRNAs by dot blot hybridization as described in the text (Section XVIII, B). The results are expressed as the fold increase in the intensity of the spots over that obtained for the RNA from tissue of virgin female mice.

[b] The values in parentheses are expressed as percentages and are the fraction of the maximum observed level of expression.

NOTE ADDED IN PROOF

Recently (June 1984) Dr. Houdebine has publicly retracted the "second messenger" theory of prolactin activation of the milk-protein genes (see p. 277), because the results published from his laboratory supporting this theory were found to be not reproducible. Consequently at this time the regulatory pathway(s) of action of the polypeptide hormone in milk-protein gene expression in the mammary gland remains unknown.

ACKNOWLEDGMENTS

We thank Dr. Padman Qasba, National Institutes of Health, for kindly providing us with the mouse α-lactalbumin cDNA clone. We acknowledge the research assistance of Dr. Ravi Menon, and Mr. Scott McDowell. We also thank Arvilla Kirchhoff and Dana Scheele for secretarial assistance in preparation of this manuscript. Research in our laboratory is supported by Grants CA11058 and CA25304 from the Department of Health and Human Services, National Cancer Institute.

REFERENCES

Anderson, R. R. (1974). *In* "Lactation: A Comprehensive Treatise" (B. L. Larson and V. R. Smith, eds.), Vol. 1, pp. 97–140. Academic Press, New York.

Assairi, L., Delouis, C., Gaye, P., Houdebine, L. M., Olliver-Bousquet, M., and Denamur, R. (1974). *Biochem. J.* **144**, 245–252.

Banerjee, M. R. (1976). *Int. Rev. Cytol.* **46**, 1–97.

Banerjee, M. R. (1984). *In* "*In Vitro* Model for Cancer Research" (M. Weber and L. Sekely, eds.), CRC Press, Boca Raton, Florida (in press).

Banerjee, M. R., and Antoniou, M. (1984). *In* "Methods in Molecular and Cellular Biology" Vol. 2 (D. Barnes, D. Sirbasku, and G. Sato, eds.), pp. 143–169. Alan R. Liss, Inc., New York.

Banerjee, M. R., and Banerjee, D. N. (1971). *Exp. Cell Res.* **64**, 307–316.

Banerjee, D. N., and Banerjee, M. R. (1973). *J. Endocrinol.* **56**, 145–154.

Banerjee, M. R., and Rogers, F. M. (1971). *J. Endocrinol.* **49**, 39–49.

Banerjee, M. R., Rogers, F. M., and Banerjee, D. N. (1971). *J. Endocrinol.* **50**, 281–291.

Banerjee, M. R., Wood, B. G., and Washburn, L. L. (1974). *J. Natl. Cancer Inst. (U.S.)* **53**, 1387–1393.

Banerjee, M. R., Wood, B. G., Lin, F. K., and Crump, L. R. (1976). *Tissue Cult. Assoc. Man.* **2**, 457–462.

Banerjee, M. R., Terry, P. M., Sakai, S., and Lin, F. K. (1977). *Horm. Res.* **3**, 281–306.

Banerjee, M. R., Ganguly, N., Mehta, N. M., Iyer, A. P., and Ganguly, R. (1981). *In* "Cell Biology of Breast Cancer" (C. M. McGrath, M. J. Brennan, and M. A. Rich, eds.), pp. 485–516. Academic Press, New York.

Banerjee, M. R., Mehta, N. M., Ganguly, R., Majumder, P. K., Ganguly, N., and Joshi, J. (1982a). *In* "Growth of Cells in a Hormonally Defined Medium" (D. A. Sirbasku, G. H. Sato, and A. B. Pardee, eds.), Vol. 9, pp. 789–805. Cold Spring Harbor Lab., Cold Spring Harbor, New York.

Banerjee, M. R., Ganguly, R. Mehta, N. M., and Ganguly, N. (1982b). *In* "Hormonal Regulation of Mammary Tumors" (B. Leung, ed.), Vol. 2, pp. 229–283. Eden Press, Montreal.

Banerjee, M. R., Antoniou, M., Joshi, J., and Majumder, P. K. (1983a). *In* "Understanding Breast Cancer: Hormone-Inducible Selective Gene Expression in the Mammary" (A. Rich, J. Hager, and P. Furmanoki, eds.), pp. 335–364. Marcel Dekker, New York.

Banerjee, M. R., Majumder, P. K., Antoniou, M., and Joshi, J. (1983b). *In* "Hormonally Defined Media" (G. Fischer and R. J. Weiser, eds.), pp. 234–249. Springer-Verlag, Berlin.

Blackburn, D. E., Hobbs, A. A., and Rosen, J. M. (1982). *Nucleic Acids Res.* **10,** 2295–2307.

Bolander, F. F., Jr., Nicholas, K. R., and Topper, Y. J. (1979). *Biochem. Biophys. Res. Commun.* **91,** 247–252.

Bonanou-Tzedaki, S. A., and Arnstein, R. (1972). *In* "Subcellular Components, Preparation and Fractionation" (G. Bernie, ed.), pp. 215–234. University Park Press, Baltimore, Maryland.

Brawerman, G. (1974). *Annu. Rev. Biochem.* **43,** 621–642.

Breathnach, R., and Chambon, P. (1981). *Annu. Rev. Biochem.* **50,** 349–383.

Buetti, E., and Diggelmann, H. (1983). *EMBO J.* **2,** 1423–1429.

Burditt, L. J., Parker, D., Craig, R. K., Getova, T., and Campbell, P. N. (1981). *Biochem. J.* **194,** 999–1006.

Chambon, P. (1977). *Cold Spring Harbor Symp. Quant. Biol.* **42,** 1209–1234.

Chambon, P., Gissinger, F., Kedinger, C., Mandel, J. L., and Meilhac, M. (1974). *In* "The Cell Nucleus" (H. Busch, ed.), Vol. 3, pp. 270–308. Academic Press, New York.

Compton, J. G., Schrader, W. T., and O'Malley, B. W. (1983). *Proc. Natl. Acad. Sci. U.S.A.* **80,** 16–20.

Craig, R. K., Brown, P. A., Harrison, O. S., Mollreavy, D., and Campbell, P. N. (1976). *Biochem. J.* **160,** 57–74.

Craig, R. K., Hall, L., Parker, D., and Campbell, P. (1981). *Biochem. J.* **194,** 989–998.

Dale, R. M. K., Livingston, D. C., and Ward, D. C. (1973). *Proc. Natl. Acad. Sci. U.S.A.* **70,** 2238–2242.

Dandekar, A. M., and Qasba, P. K. (1981). *Proc. Natl. Acad. Sci. U.S.A.* **77,** 4853–4857.

Davidson, E. H. (1976). "Gene Activity in Early Development," 2nd ed. Academic Press, New York.

Denamur, R. (1974). *In* "Lactation: A Comprehensive Treatise" (B. L. Larson and V. R. Smith, eds.), Vol. 1, pp. 414–465. Academic Press, New York.

Devinoy, E., Houdebine, L. M., and Delouis, C. (1978). *Biochim. Biophys. Acta* **517,** 360–366.

Disorbo, D. M., and Litwack, G. (1981). *Biochem. Biophys. Res. Commun.* **99,** 1203–1208.

Elias, J. J. (1957). *Science* **126,** 842–844.

Forsyth, I. A. (1971). *J. Dairy Res.* **38,** 419–444.

Gala, R. R., and Westphal, U. (1965). *Acta Endocrinol. (Copenhagen)* **55,** 47–61.

Ganguly, R., and Banerjee, M. R. (1978). *Nucleic Acids Res.* **5,** 4463–4477.

Ganguly, R., Mehta, N. M., Ganguly, N., and Banerjee, M. R. (1979). *Proc. Natl. Acad. Sci. U.S.A.* **76,** 6466–6470.

Ganguly, R., Ganguly, N., Mehta, N. M., and Banerjee, M. R. (1980). *Proc. Natl. Acad. Sci. U.S.A.* **77,** 6003–6006.

Ganguly, N., Ganguly, R., Mehta, N. M., Crump, L. R., and Banerjee, M. R. (1981). *In Vitro* **17,** 55–60.

Ganguly, R., Majumder, P. K., Ganguly, N., and Banerjee, M. R. (1982). *J. Biol. Chem.* **257,** 2182–2187.

Gaye, P., Houdebine, L., and Denamur, R. (1973). *Biochem. Biophys. Res. Commun.* **51,** 637–644.

Groner, B., Herrlich, P., Kennedy, N., Pouta, H., Rahmsdorf, U., and Hynes, N. E. (1982). *J. Cell. Biochem.* **20**, 349–357.

Gupta, P., Rosen, J. M., D'Eustachio, P., and Ruddle, F. H. (1982). *J. Cell Biol.* **93**, 199–204.

Hall, L., Craig, R. K., and Campbell, P. N. (1979). *Nature (London)* **277**, 54–56.

Hall, L., Davies, M. S., and Craig, R. K. (1981). *Nucleic Acids Res.* **9**, 65–84.

Hall, L., Craig, R. K., Edbrooke, M. R., and Campbell, P. N. (1982). *Nucleic Acids Res.* **10**, 3503–3515.

Hennighausen, L. G., and Sippel, A. E. (1982a). *Eur. J. Biochem.* **125**, 131–141.

Hennighausen, L. G., and Sippel, A. E. (1982b). *Nucleic Acids Res.* **10**, 2677–2684.

Hennighausen, L. G., Stendle, A., and Sippel, A. E. (1982a). *Eur. J. Biol. Biochem.* **126**, 569–572.

Hennighausen, L. G., Sippel, A. E., Hobbs, A. A., and Rosen, J. M. (1982b). *Nucleic Acids Res.* **10**, 3733–3744.

Hobbs, A. A., and Rosen, J. M. (1982). *Nucleic Acids Res.* **10**, 8079–8098.

Hobbs, A., Richards, D. A., Kessler, D. J., and Rosen, J. M. (1982). *J. Biol. Chem.* **257**, 3598–3605.

Houdebine, L. M. (1980). *Horm. Cell Regul.* **4**, pp. 175–196.

Ichinose, R. R., and Nandi, S. (1964). *Science* **145**, 496–497.

Iyer, A. P., and Banerjee, M. R. (1981). *JNCI, J. Natl. Cancer Inst.* **66**, 893–905.

Jeness, R. (1974). *In* "Lactation: A Comprehensive Treatise" (B. L. Larson and V. R. Smith, eds.), Vol. 3, pp. 3–107. Academic Press, New York.

Jensen, E. V., and DeSombre, E. R. (1972). *In* "Biochemical Actions of Hormones" (G. Litwack, ed.) Vol. 2, pp. 215–255. Academic Press, New York.

Johnson, M. L., Levy, J., Supowit, S. C., Yu-Lee, L., and Rosen, J. M. (1983). *J. Biol. Chem.* **258**, 10805–10811.

Juergens, W. G., Stockdale, F. E., Topper, Y. J., and Elias, J. J. (1965). *Proc. Natl. Acad. Sci. U.S.A.* **54**, 629–634.

Karlson, P. (1963). *Perspect. Biol. Med.* **6**, 203–314.

Kulski, J. K., Topper, Y. J., Chomcaynski, P., and Qasba, P. (1983). *Biochem. Biophys. Res. Commun.* **114**, 380–387.

Leder, P., Konkel, D. A., Nishioka, Y., Leder, A., Homer, D. H., and Kashler, M. (1980). *Recent Prog. Horm. Res.* **36**, 241–260.

Lin, F. K., Banerjee, M. R., and Crump, L. R. (1976). *Cancer Res.* **36**, 1607–1614.

Litwack, G. (1979). *Trends Biochem. (Pers. Ed.) Sci.* **4**, 217–220.

Lodish, H. F. (1976). *Annu. Rev. Biochem.* **45**, 39–72.

Lyons, W. R., Li, C. H., Cole, R. D., and Johnson, R. E. (1958). *Recent Prog. Horm. Res.* **14**, 219–248.

McKnight, G. S. (1978). *Cell* **14**, 403–413.

Majumder, P. K., Joshi, J. B., and Banerjee, M. R. (1983). *J. Biol. Chem.* **258**, 6793–6798.

Maurer, R. A. (1982). *J. Biol. Chem.* **257**, 2133–2136.

Medina, D. (1978). *In* "Breast Cancer" (W. L. McGuire, ed.), Vol. 2, pp. 47–102. Plenum, New York.

Mehta, R. G., and Banerjee, M. R. (1975). *Acta Endocrinol. (Copenhagen)* **80**, 501–516.

Mehta, N. M., Ganguly, N., Ganguly, R., and Banerjee, M. R. (1980). *J. Biol. Chem.* **255**, 4430–4434.

Mehta, N. M., El-Gewely, M. R., Joshi, J., Helling, R. B., and Banerjee, M. R. (1981). *Gene* **15**, 285–288.

Mena, F., Enjalbert, L., Carbonell, M., Priam, M., and Kordan, C. (1976). *Endocrinology* **99**, 445–451.

Mukherjee, A. S., Washburn, L. L., and Banerjee, M. R. (1973). *Nature (London)* **246**, 159–160.

Mulvihill, E. R., LePennec, J.-P., and Chambon, P. (1982). *Cell* **24**, 621–632.

Nandi, S. (1958). *J. Natl. Cancer Inst. (U.S.)* **21**, 1039–1063.

Nandi, S. (1959). *Univ. Calif., Berkeley, Publ. Zool.* **65**, 1–129.

Nandi, S. (1978). *J. Environ. Pathol. Toxicol.* **2**, 13–20.

Nandi, S., and McGrath, C. S. (1973). *Adv. Cancer Res.* **17**, 353–414.

Nguyen-Huu, M. C., Sippel, A. A., Hynes, N. E., Groner, B., and Schutz, G. (1978). *Proc. Natl. Acad. Sci. U.S.A.* **75**, 686–690.

Oka, T., and Topper, Y. J. (1971). *J. Biol. Chem.* **246**, 7701–7707.

Oka, T., Perry, J. W., Toshiyuki, T., Tadashi, S., Hirada, N., and Inoue, H. (1982). *In* "Hormonal Regulation of Mammary Tumors" (B. Leung, ed.), pp. 205–228. Eden Press, Montreal.

O'Malley, B. W., and Means, A. R. (1974). *Science* **183**, 610–620.

O'Malley, B. W., Towle, H. C., and Swartz, R. J. (1977a). *Annu. Rev. Genet.* **11**, 239–275.

O'Malley, B. W., Tsai, M. J., Tsai, S. Y., and Towele, H. C. (1977b). *Cold Spring Harbor Symp. Quant. Biol.* **42**, 605–615.

Orkin, S. H., and Swerdlow, P. S. (1977). *Proc. Natl. Acad. Sci. U.S.A.* **74**, 2475–2479.

Perry, R. P. (1967). *Nucleic Acid Res. Mol. Biol.* **6**, 219–257.

Perry, R. P. (1976). *Annu. Rev. Biochem.* **45**, 605–629.

Prop, F. J. A. (1966). *Exp. Cell Res.* **42**, 386–388.

Qasba, P. K., and Chakrabartty, P. K. (1978). *J. Biol. Chem.* **253**, 1167–1173.

Richards, D. A., Rodgers, J. R., Supowit, S. C., and Rosen, J. M. (1981a). *J. Biol. Chem.* **256**, 526–532.

Richards, D. A., Blackburn, D. E., and Rosen, J. M. (1981b). *J. Biol. Chem.* **256**, 533–538.

Rigby, P. W. J., Diechmann, M., Rhodes, C., and Berg, P. (1977). *J. Mol. Biol.* **113**, 237–251.

Rilema, J. A. (1982). *In* "Hormonal Regulation of Mammary Tumors" (B. S. Leung, ed.), Vol. 2, pp. 77–87. Eden Press, Montreal.

Rivera, E. (1971). *In* "Methods in Mammalian Embryology" (J. C. Danial, ed.), pp. 442–471. Freeman, San Francisco, California.

Rivera, E. M., and Bern, H. A. (1961). *Endocrinology* **69**, 340–353.

Rosen, J. M. (1976). *Biochemistry* **15**, 5263–5271.

Rosen, J. M., Matusik, R., Richards, D. A., Gupta, P., and Rodgers, J. R. (1980). *Recent Prog. Horm. Res.* **36**, 157–193.

Schechter, I. (1974). *Biochemistry* **13**, 1875.

Scheidereit, C., Geisse, S., Westphal, H. M., and Beato, M. (1983). *Nature (London)* **304**, 749–752.

Schimke, R. T., McKnight, G. S., and Shapiro, D. J. (1975). *In* "Biochemical Actions of Hormones" (G. Litwack, ed.), Vol. 3, pp. 245–269. Academic Press, New York.

Shiu, R. P. C., and Friesen, H. G. (1976). *Science* **192**, 259–261.

Shyamala, G. (1973). *Biochemistry* **12**, 3085–3090.

Shyamala, G. (1982). *In* "Hormonal Regulation of Mammary Tumors" (B. S. Leung, ed.), Vol. 1, pp. 245–286. Eden Press, Montreal.

Shyamala, G., and Dickson, C. (1976). *Nature (London)* **262**, 107–112.

Singh, D. V., DeOme, K. B., and Bern, H. A. (1969). *J. Endocrinol.* **45**, 579–583.

Singh, D. V., DeOme, K. B., and Bern, H. A. (1970). *J. Natl. Cancer Inst. (U.S.)* **45**, 657–675.

Spindler, S. R., Mellon, S. H., and Baxter, J. D. (1982). *J. Biol. Chem.* **257**, 11627–11632.

Strobl, J. S., and Lippman, M. E. (1979). *Cancer Res.* **39**, 3319–3327.

Suard, Y. M. L., Tosi, M., and Kraehenbuhl, J. P. (1982). *Biochem. J.* **201**, 81–90.

Tata, J. R. (1966). *Prog. Nucleic Acid Res. Mol. Biol.* **5,** 191–250.
Tata, J. R. (1970). *In* "Biochemical Actions of Hormones" (G. Litwack, ed.), Vol. 1, pp. 89–133. Academic Press, New York.
Tata, J. R. (1976). *Cell* **9,** 1–14.
Tata, J. R., and Smith, D. F. (1979). *Recent Prog. Horm. Res.* **35,** 47–95.
Telang, N. T., Banerjee, M. R., Iyer, A. P., and Kundu, A. B. (1979). *Proc. Natl. Acad. Sci. U.S.A.* **76,** 5886–5890.
Terry, P. M., Ganguly, R., Ball, E. M., and Banerjee, M. R. (1975a). *Cell Differ.* **4,** 113–122.
Terry, P. M., Ball, E. M., Ganguly, R., and Banerjee, M. R. (1975b). *J. Immunol. Methods* **9,** 123–134.
Terry, P. M., Banerjee, M. R., and Lui, R. M. (1977a). *Proc. Natl. Acad. Sci. U.S.A.* **74,** 2441–2445.
Terry, P. M., Lin, F. K., and Banerjee, M. R. (1977b). *Mol. Cell. Endocrinol.* **9,** 169–182.
Teyssot, B., Houdebine, L. M., and Djiane, J. (1981). *Proc. Natl. Acad. Sci. U.S.A.* **78,** 6729–6733.
Thomas, P. (1980). *Proc. Natl. Acad. Sci. U.S.A.* **77,** 5201–5205.
Tomkins, G. M. (1974). *Harvey Lect.* **68,** 37–65.
Tonelli, Q. J., and Sorof, S. (1980). *Nature (London)* **285,** 250–252.
Topper, Y. J. (1970). *Recent Prog. Horm. Res.* **26,** 287–308.
Topper, Y. J., and Freeman, C. S. (1980). *Physiol. Rev.* **60,** 1049–1106.
Topper, Y. J., and Oka, T. (1974). *In* "Lactation: A Comprehensive Treatise" (B. L. Larson and V. R. Smith, eds.), Vol. 1, pp. 327–348. Academic Press, New York.
Topper, Y. J., Nicholas, K. R., and Sankaraw, L. (1984). *In* "Biochemical Actions of Hormones" (G. Litwack, ed.), Vol. 11, pp. 163–186. Academic Press, New York.
Tucker, H. A. (1974). *In* "Lactation: A Comprehensive Treatise" (B. L. Larson and V. R. Smith, eds.), Vol. 1, pp. 277–326. Academic Press, New York.
Turkington, R. W. (1972). *In* "Biochemical Actions of Hormones" (G. Litwack, ed.), Vol. II, pp. 55–80. Academic Press, New York.
Turkington, R. W., Mazumdar, G. C., Kadohama, N., MacIndoe, J. H., and Frantz, W. L. (1973). *Recent Prog. Horm. Res.* **29,** 417–455.
Vondehaar, B. K. (1975). *Biochem. Biophys. Res. Commun.* **67,** 1219–1225.
Weissbach, H., and Ochoa, S. (1976). *Annu. Rev. Biochem.* **45,** 191–216.
Welsch, C. W., Squires, M. D., Casseby, E., Chen, C. L., and Meites, J. (1971). *Am. J. Physiol.* **221,** 1714–1717.
Willis, I. M., Stewart, A. F., Caputo, A., Thompson, A. R., and Mackinlay, A. G. (1982). *DNA* **1,** 375–386.
Wood, B. G., Washburn, L. L., Mukherjee, A. S., and Banerjee, M. R. (1975). *J. Endocrinol.* **65,** 106.
Yamamoto, R., and Albert, B. (1976). *Annu. Rev. Biochem.* **38,** 722–746.
Yu-Lee, L., and Rosen, J. M. (1983). *J. Biol. Chem.* **258,** 10794–10804.

CHAPTER 9

Control of Prolactin Production by Estrogen

Priscilla S. Dannies

Department of Pharmacology
Yale University School of Medicine
New Haven, Connecticut

I. INTRODUCTION

The stimulation of prolactin by estrogen was first recognized almost 50 years ago (reviewed in Turner, 1977), and the means by which this stimulation occurs has been investigated by many laboratories. Estrogen affects almost every conceivable aspect of prolactin production; this chapter reviews

BIOCHEMICAL ACTIONS OF HORMONES, VOL. XII

the processes that are changed and what we know about the mechanisms by which estrogen causes these changes.

II. ESTROGEN STIMULATES THE GROWTH OF PROLACTIN-PRODUCING CELLS

A. IDENTIFICATION OF PROLACTIN-PRODUCING CELLS

Prolactin cells have been distinguished from other cell types in the pituitary gland by three different methods. The secretory granules in which prolactin is stored can be stained with acidic dyes, and this technique was the earliest used to identify prolactin cells. Later, identification depended on morphological characteristics detectable with the electron microscope; prolactin cells are the only cells in the gland that may contain granules as large as 500–900 nm in diameter (Farquhar, 1977). More recently, the ability to visualize prolactin in the cells by immunocytochemical techniques has been used to identify prolactin cells. Several laboratories found using this technique that the pituitary gland contains prolactin cells that have only small granules in addition to the cells with the large secretory granules (Baker, 1970; Nogami and Yoshimura, 1980; Sato, 1980).

Use of the first technique, staining the granules with acidic dyes, missed cells that had few granules. Chromophobe cells that did not stain with acidic or basic dyes were often classified as cells not producing hormones, but subsequent studies showed that some of them were producing large amounts of prolactin but storing little. Identification of prolactin cells by granule size alone means that only a subpopulation of prolactin cells may have been examined. Immunocytochemical techniques can stain prolactin in the rough endoplasmic reticulum and Golgi apparatus as well as prolactin in granules, which means that cells that are synthesizing but not storing prolactin may be detected (Tougard *et al.*, 1980). This method, therefore, is the most extensive way of examining prolactin cells, and the emphasis in this discussion will be on results obtained using immunostains when possible.

B. ESTROGEN INCREASES THE NUMBER OF PROLACTIN CELLS

Gersten and Baker (1970) demonstrated that estrogen pellets implanted in the anterior pituitary gland of ovariectomized rats caused hyperplasia of prolactin cells, revealed by immunological staining. Corenblum and associates (1980) did a quantitative study of the effects of daily injections of estradiol on the number of prolactin cells present in the glands of male rats with and without treatment with estradiol, detecting the cells by immunostaining. They found the percentage of cells that stained for prolactin increased from 15% in untreated male rats to 50% after 22 days of estradiol treatment. There are two experiments that indicate that the increase in the number of prolactin cells is a direct effect of estradiol on the anterior pituitary gland. The first experiment was performed in intact animals. In the study by Gersten and Baker, estrogen increased the number of prolactin cells only in the lobe in which the pellet was planted, but not in the other lobe. In addition, the estrogen effects were localized to particular parts of that lobe, only occurring in areas where the blood flow had first passed by the pellet and not occurring upstream of the pellet. The second experiment was performed in primary cell cultures of anterior pituitary glands. Lieberman *et al.* (1982) demonstrated that a 5-day incubation with estradiol increased the number of prolactin cells to 130% of the number in control cultures. Both experiments indicate that estrogen can act directly at the level of the pituitary gland to stimulate cell number, but do not indicate a direct action on the prolactin cells themselves, since the cells in the gland are heterogeneous.

The mitotic activity of the pituitary gland changes during the estrous cycle (Hunt, 1943). The changes may be caused by estrogen, because estrogen increases mitotic activity in the pituitary gland 2 days after injections in female and male rats (Hunt, 1947; Lloyd *et al.*, 1975). Treatment with estrogen also increases the ability of isolated pituitary glands or pieces of glands to incorporate [^{3}H]thymidine into DNA, which is interpreted as an increase in DNA synthesis. There may be problems with using [^{3}H]thymidine as a measure of DNA synthesis. Changes in the amount of incorporation may reflect changes in the specific activity of the precursor pools, not changes in the rate of synthesis, and incorporation may reflect repair of existing DNA, not synthesis of new DNA. One of the most thorough studies of [^{3}H]thymidine incorporation is that of Wiklund and Gorski (1982). They demonstrated that *in vivo* treatment of rats with estradiol did not change the specific activity or the size of the pool of thymidine triphosphate during a subsequent *in vitro* incubation of the glands with [^{3}H]thymidine. These workers also showed that increased incorporation occurred in isolated nuclei and that 80–90% of this activity had the characteristics expected if the enzyme involved was the DNA polymerase thought to be responsible for new DNA synthesis rather than the polymerase involved in repair. These data indicate that stimulation of [^{3}H]thymidine incorporation into the pituitary gland is a good reflection of DNA synthesis.

The cells that take up [^{3}H]thymidine in the pituitary gland include prolactin cells; 3% of the prolactin cells in male rats incorporated [^{3}H]thymidine *in vivo,* determined by a combination of immunoperoxidase staining and auto-radiography (Corenblum *et al.,* 1980). Mitotic cells that stain immuno-logically for prolactin have been seen (Sato, 1980), indicating that at least some of the new prolactin cells come from previously existing cells; whether others come from stem cells that differentiate into prolactin cells after divid-ing is not known.

III. ESTROGEN AFFECTS THE MORPHOLOGY OF PROLACTIN-PRODUCING CELLS

Estrogen increases the size of the prolactin cells in addition to increasing prolactin cell number (Gersten and Baker, 1970). Many laboratories have studied the changes in the morphology of the cell by electron microscopy. These studies are reviewed by Farquhar (1977); the changes include in-creases in the size of the Golgi apparatus and increases in the amount of rough endoplasmic reticulum, which is often found arrayed in long rows parallel to the plasma membrane or in whorled formations. A more recent study combined the techniques of immunoperoxidase staining with electron microscopy to examine the pituitary glands of mature female rats before ovariectomy, 4 weeks after ovariectomy, and after treating the ovariec-tomized rats with estrogen for 4 days (Osamura *et al.,* 1982). In normal female rats, they found staining for prolactin in the rough endoplasmic re-ticulum, in the Golgi saccules, and in membrane-bound secretory granules. The cells contained the large secretory granules (about 600 nm in diameter) commonly associated with prolactin cells. After ovariectomy, the size of the cells that stained for prolactin was markedly decreased, and both the amount of the rough endoplasmic reticulum and the size of the Golgi apparatus were reduced. The cytoplasm was filled with small secretory granules (120–190 nm) that stained for prolactin. When estrogen was given for 4 days, the most prominent feature that stained positively for prolactin was the rough endo-plasmic reticulum that was found in the characteristic large whorls or in rows parallel to and close to the plasma membrane. The cells had only a few secretory granules that did not stain heavily.

IV. ESTROGEN INDUCES PITUITARY TUMORS

A. PRIMARY TUMORS

Long-term treatment with estrogen induces pituitary adenomas that are derived from the multiplication of prolactin-producing cells and cells without granules (Clifton and Meyer, 1956). In the early weeks of treatment, the pituitary glands show the same morphological changes that occur with short-term treatment—hypertrophy; increases in the amount of rough endoplasmic reticulum, again in rows and whorls; and increases in the size of the Golgi apparatus. Cells are found in all stages of granulation, and mitoses occur in both granulated acidophil cells and chromophobe cells. At later stages, most cells have only a few small granules (Clifton and Meyer, 1956; Furth and Clifton, 1966; Olivier *et al.*, 1975; DeNicola *et al.*, 1978).

The ability of estrogen to cause these pituitary tumors varies with the strain of rat. Dunning and co-workers (1947) noticed that the Fischer 344 strain of rat was susceptible to pituitary tumor induction. Stone and associates (1979) found that estrogen did not increase pituitary weight in Sprague Dawley rats after 130 days of treatment, but increased the weight of the pituitary glands in ACI rats to 2–7 times as much as in control glands after 130 days. The uteri of the ACI rats were not larger, but those of the Sprague Dawley were, after estrogen treatment. Wiklund *et al.* (1981a) compared pituitary and uterine growth in ovariectomized rats using the Fischer 344 strain, in which tumors develop after 2 months of estrogen treatment, and in the Holtzman strain, in which there is no tumor development within this time. They found that estrogen rapidly increased uterine wet weight over threefold in both strains, and this increase reached a plateau after 2 weeks. Estrogen increased prolactin synthesis, expressed as a percentage of total protein synthesis in the gland, from 7% to about 40% in both strains. Estrogen, however, increased pituitary wet weight six- to tenfold in the Fischer rats, but caused no change in the Holtzman rats. These experiments indicate that the uterus in the Holtzman rats can respond to estrogen by growing and that the pituitary gland in the Holtzman rats can respond to estrogen in other ways, even though it does not grow, so the lesion is not just a general loss of responsiveness. Wiklund *et al.* (1981a) showed that pituitary glands transplanted under the kidney capsule of an F_1 recipient have the same tendencies to develop tumors as they do *in situ*, indicating that the lesion is actually in the pituitary gland itself. A series of crosses between Holtzman and Fischer parents and offspring indicate that a small number of loci, but more than one, are probably involved (Wiklund *et al.*, 1981b). These studies were continued by Wiklund and Gorski in 1982, when they demonstrated that estradiol and diethylstilbestrol both increase the weight of the gland and the amount of DNA synthesis, but DNA synthesis does not remain elevated in Holtzman rats. Estrogen increases DNA synthesis in both strains by 2 days, but synthesis returns to untreated levels after 1 week of treatment in the Holtzman strain and remains elevated in the Fischer strain. The increase in the weight of the gland is also maintained in the Fischer rats, but not in the Holtzman rats. The Holtzman strain, therefore, seems to have a mechanism to shut off estrogen-stimulated growth.

B. Transplantable Tumors and Cell Lines

Pituitary tumors that have been induced by estrogen can be transplanted to other animals. Exogenous estrogen is usually required at first for growth of these transplanted tumors, but the tumors will grow autonomously with continued passages (reviewed in Furth and Clifton, 1966). Clifton and Furth (1961), in one of the more thorough studies of effects of various doses of estrogen, found that in the early passages transplanted tumors appear to become progressively more sensitive to diethylstilbestrol. The response of the early passage tumors was biphasic; doses of diethylstilbestrol that maximally stimulated tumor growth had little effect on the weight of the normal gland, and higher doses that caused no stimulation of tumor growth compared to controls did stimulate the normal gland to grow. Estradiol stimulated growth of normal glands with the same dose–response pattern, whether they were in their usual position or transplanted under the kidney capsule. Because connections to the hypothalamus were not necessary to see the difference in sensitivity between normal glands and tumors, the difference could not be explained by hypothalamic factors influencing the normal gland. These data suggest that at least some tumors may no longer require exogenous estradiol, because they have become sensitive enough to respond to endogenous estrogens.

There are two autonomous prolactin-producing tumors, $MtTF_4$ and 7315a, that were each initiated by estrogen but whose growth is now strongly inhibited by high doses of estrogen (10 μg of 17β-estradiol daily) (Morel *et al.*, 1982; Lamberts *et al.*, 1982). Lamberts and co-workers found that growth of the pituitary tumor was inhibited by estradiol, but the uterus and the pituitary gland both showed a normal weight gain in response to estradiol, indicating that the inhibitory effect of estradiol is specific for the tumors. At present, the inhibitory effect has only been seen in animals and is not understood; it is of interest in part because large doses of estradiol are used to treat other tumors thought to be estrogen dependent, such as breast carcinomas (Hellman *et al.*, 1982).

Some of these autonomous hormone-producing tumors have been used to establish cell lines that grow continuously in culture. One of these, the GH cell strain, was started from a tumor induced by irradiating the head of a female rat (Tashjian *et al.*, 1968; Takemoto *et al.*, 1962). This tumor, MtTW5, grew in female rats after transplantation without needing exogenous estrogens. Two laboratories have found that injections of cell lines established from this tumor will give rise to tumors only in females and not in males (Sorrentino *et al.*, 1976; Sonnenschein *et al.*, 1973). The difference was interpreted as a requirement for estrogen, because both laboratories found that treating males with estrogen enabled the injected cells to form tumors. Sorrentino and co-workers, however, measured estradiol levels in the serum of the rats and found that females, with 25 tumors in 25 animals, had serum estradiol levels of 40 pg/ml, and males, with no tumors in 14 animals, had levels of 20 pg/ml. Treatment with exogenous estradiol raised serum levels to over 500 pg/ml. Ovariectomized females had estradiol levels of less than 12 pg/ml, but 15 of 24 animals developed tumors, although the average tumor mass was much smaller than in normal females. Therefore, although it is clear from the two papers that large doses of estrogen stimulate the growth of these tumors in both sexes, it seems unlikely, considering the tumors in the ovariectomized females, that the twofold difference in serum estradiol levels accounts for the all-or-none effect in females versus males. Other differences in males and females besides average serum estradiol levels must be important.

Sorrentino and co-workers did not see stimulation of growth of the cells in tissue culture and concluded that estrogen acts indirectly, stimulating other organs to make growth factors. Estrogen effects in tissue culture, however, have been difficult to see reproducibly. One reason for the difficulty is the presence of endogenous estrogens in the serum usually used to supplement the medium in which the cells are grown. Estradiol can stimulate cell growth in cultures at concentrations as low as 10^{-11} M (Lippman *et al.*, 1976), and the amount of estrogen present in the serum usually used to supplement medium may be higher by one to three orders of magnitude—there is wide variation among serum lots. In order to remove endogenous estrogens, serum has been treated with dextran-coated charcoal. This procedure obviously removes many factors besides estrogens that may be necessary to see all the estrogen effects. In addition, estrone sulfate, not usually measured in assays of estradiol, is not extracted from serum by charcoal treatment and can act as a precursor for more active estrogens (Vignon *et al.*, 1980). These problems may explain why charcoal-treated serum has been difficult to use to measure reproducible estrogen effects in breast or pituitary cultures.

A second approach has been to develop a serum-free medium in which all of the components are known. So far, using GH cells in serum-free medium, laboratories have seen no effect of estrogen on cell growth or a decrease in cell growth at physiological concentrations (Hayashi and Sato, 1976; Tixier-Vidal *et al.*, 1983; Brunet *et al.*, 1982). Wyche and Noteboom (1979) also reported that estradiol inhibited growth of a human pituitary cell line in defined medium, but this inhibition occurred at concentrations above 1 μM, concentrations higher than those found physiologically. A medium that is satisfactory for expressing one effect of estrogen may not be sufficient to allow expression of other effects. For example, Evans *et al.* (1981) found that induction of ovalbumin gene transcription by estrogen required a somatomedinlike activity, but induction of the conalbumin gene did not. Serum-free medium that has been developed for the expression of one effect may not allow the expression of all.

We have reduced the amount of endogenous estrogens in medium by using serum from castrated horses, or geldings. The main source of estrogen in the male is the conversion of testosterone from the testis to estrogens in the peripheral tissues, such as skin and fat. Gelding serum, therefore, has low levels of estrogen, but other compounds have not been removed. Using serum from one horse, we have found maximum stimulation occurring between 1 and 3×10^{-11} M estradiol; the doubling time was decreased from roughly 2.5 to 1.5 days (Amara and Dannies, 1983). This response was biphasic; the rate of growth decreased between 3×10^{-11} and 3×10^{-9} M. We know that these effects of estradiol depend on factors present in the serum for two reasons. First, the increase in growth was substantially less after the serum had been heat-inactivated, and, second, the effect was much smaller in a batch of commercial gelding serum that we tried. Although we have found that the estrogen stimulation of growth has been reproducible with serum from the same horse, it appears to be necessary to screen batches of serum to use gelding serum for estrogen stimulation.

It would be satisfying to be able to relate the biphasic response we see with low concentrations of estradiol on GH cell growth to the biphasic effect of diethylstilbestrol on tumor growth at concentrations too low to affect normal pituitary growth (Clifton and Furth, 1961). Both the increase and the decrease in the rate of growth in GH cells fell within concentration ranges that could be mediated by the estrogen receptor characterized in these cells (discussed in Section VIII). The dose–response relationship of estrogen concentrations to the ability of GH cells to form tumors in animals is not known, and the response may not be biphasic. Stimulation of growth in serum is different from the inhibition seen by Tixier-Vidal and co-workers in serum-free medium, and it is not clear which conditions are more relevant to growth in animals. Estrogen obviously affects many processes in prolactin-producing cells, and changes in some of these properties might enable the cells to grow differently on plastic without changing the ability to grow as a tumor in animals. Furthermore, estrogen has been shown to increase blood supply to the pituitary gland (Elias and Weiner, 1983), an effect that could be a cause of increased tumor growth that would not show up in tissue culture. One method to determine whether the estrogen response in culture is related to effects in animals is to isolate stable variants from an estrogen-sensitive population in culture and ascertain whether the response of tumor growth in animals also changes. These types of experiments have not yet been done, either for GH cells or for breast cell lines, in which the stimulatory effects of estrogen on growth in monolayer culture have been more extensively studied and such variants are available.

V. ESTROGEN STIMULATES SYNTHESIS
OF PROLACTIN

Many of the early studies, some of which have been cited here, showed that estrogen increases serum prolactin levels. Meites and his co-workers demonstrated that this increase is a direct effect on the pituitary gland by showing that incubating glands in culture for days or for 12 hours with estradiol caused more prolactin to accumulate in the medium (Nicoll and Meites, 1962; Lu *et al.*, 1971).

An increase in prolactin in the medium over a period of hours or days may reflect many processes—release of previously synthesized stores, increased synthesis of prolactin, increase in the number of prolactin-producing cells, or stabilization of intracellular prolactin. Later work showed that treating rats with estradiol *in vivo* increased the amount of [^{3}H]leucine incorporated into prolactin by the glands *in vitro* (MacLeod *et al.*, 1969; Maurer and Gorski, 1977) and that incubating dispersed cells with estradiol also caused the same increase (Lieberman *et al.*, 1978). A control to show that incorporation was linear over the time period measured seemed routine, but turned out to be important. Incorporation of leucine over a period of hours can reflect a combination of synthesis and breakdown, and changes in incorporation can reflect changes in either process. If incorporation of the radioactive amino acid is linear over the incubation period, then the rate of synthesis alone is the primary effect measured (Schimke and Doyle, 1970). More recent studies on prolactin degradation have indicated that [^{3}H]prolactin can be rapidly broken down before it is secreted from the cells, both in pituitary halves or in monolayer cultures, and that the amount of degradation may vary from one experiment to another (Shenai and Wallis, 1979; Maurer, 1980). These reports on degradation emphasize the need for caution in interpreting changes in leucine incorporation as changes in synthesis.

As techniques for quantitating mRNA were developed, these studies on prolactin synthesis were extended to show that estrogen treatment increased prolactin mRNA, measured by activity in a cell-free translational system or by quantitating the sequences by hybridization (Stone *et al.*, 1977; Ryan *et al.*, 1979; Seo *et al.*, 1979a). The studies of Gorski and co-workers showed that the increase in message activity and in messenger sequences agreed well with the increase in prolactin synthesis when male rats were treated for 3 or 6 days with estrogen (Ryan *et al.*, 1979) and that, in dispersed cell cultures from male rats, the increase in prolactin synthesis corresponded to the increase in prolactin mRNA (Lieberman *et al.*, 1982). Seo *et al.* (1979a), however, found that estrogen treatment of male rats for 1 week caused a 3-fold increase in prolactin synthesis, but an 11-fold increase in prolactin message activity; at longer times, the two parameters agreed. In a second paper, Seo *et al.* (1979b) again demonstrated discrepancies between increases in prolactin synthesis and increases in prolactin message. They found that single injections in male rats increased message activity and sequences without measurable changes in prolactin synthesis. Chronic treatment, however, resulted in equal increases in prolactin message levels and synthesis. This group had shown that [^{3}H]leucine incorporation was linear over the time period used and, therefore, they did not appear to be underestimating the amount of synthesis because of degradation. The experiments of Gorski and co-workers, who saw agreement, and Seo and co-workers, who did not, used different species of rats, and there are other technical differences that may explain why the different results occurred. It appears that estrogen, under certain conditions, can induce prolactin message in male rats faster than it can induce the capacity to translate this message. There is one reservation about this conclusion; estrogen-induced increases in prolactin synthesis and production have not been seen reproducibly in culture using medium containing charcoal-treated serum or serum-free medium (Raymond *et al.*, 1978; West and Dannies, 1980; Maurer, 1982a; Giguère *et al.*, 1982), and the reasons for this variation have not been determined. It may be that it is easier to see increases in mRNA than in prolactin synthesis *in vitro* for reasons unrelated to physiological changes.

Increases in prolactin mRNA levels may reflect stabilization of existing message or synthesis of new message. By giving estrogen to ovariectomized female rats, isolating the nuclei, and measuring incorporation of [^{32}P]UTP into prolactin messenger RNA precursors, Maurer (1982b) determined that estrogen does increase synthesis of new message. Estradiol increased incorporation within 20 minutes of injection into the animal, indicating that it has a rapid effect on induction of transcription of the prolactin gene.

A question that has been raised is whether estrogen increases the synthesis of prolactin by increasing the number of cells synthesizing prolactin. Experiments with DNA synthesis inhibitors, which have been performed, have to be subject to reservations because of the toxicity of the drugs. Lieberman *et al.* (1982) showed that the increase in prolactin synthesis is greater than the increase in prolactin cell number, which suggests that the increase in synthesis cannot be accounted for by the change in cell number. Prolactin cells, however, are heterogeneous, and different morphological populations are not affected in the same way by physiological changes that affect estradiol serum levels (Merchant, 1974; Sato, 1980). Therefore, one could postulate a preferential increase in cells highly active in synthesizing prolactin to account for the discrepancy between cell number and synthesis. The best evidence for a direct effect of estrogen on the prolactin gene itself is the rapid effect on transcription of prolactin RNA sequences; an effect occurring in 20 minutes cannot be accounted for by cell division.

Estrogen can stimulate prolactin synthesis in tumor cell lines as well as in primary cultures (Tashjian and Hoyt, 1972; Haug and Gautvik, 1976; Herbert *et al.*, 1978; Tixier-Vidal *et al.*, 1983). Under conditions where we found both an increase in growth and an increase in prolactin synthesis, we have examined a series of estrogenic compounds and found that growth of GH cells was always tenfold more sensitive to estrogen stimulation than was prolactin production (Amara and Dannies, 1983, and unpublished data). Such differences in the sensitivity of various responses to steroids have been seen with glucocorticoids in other cell lines (Mercier *et al.*, 1983). At present, it is not known whether the difference in sensitivity of the two responses is also seen at the level of mRNA transcription and accumulation or whether it is caused by posttranscriptional factors. With the techniques now available, it will be possible to determine this.

VI. ESTROGEN INCREASES PROLACTIN STORAGE

We began studies in GH cells to attempt to cause these cells to differentiate into a more normal phenotype. One of the noticeable differences between GH cells and normal cells is the amount of prolactin they contain; GH cells store a much smaller proportion of the prolactin that they secrete over a 24-hour period than normal prolactin cells do, and they lack the dense secretory granules seen in electron micrographs of normal prolactin cells (Tixier-Vidal, 1975). We found that treating the cells with insulin and estradiol caused an increase in intracellular prolactin that was larger than the increase in prolactin in the medium (Kiino and Danies, 1981, 1982). In early experiments, we found three- to sevenfold increases in intracellular prolactin after treating the cells for 6 days with 180 nM insulin and 1 nM estradiol, compared to increases of less than twofold in the amount of prolactin produced in the medium. Insulin and estrogen acted synergistically to increase intracellular prolactin, but were less than additive in increasing extracellular prolactin. In subsequent experiments, we have shown that the effect was larger when we plated cells at lower initial densities or added 10 nM epidermal growth factor. The three hormones together increased intracellular prolactin 10- to 30-fold, while increasing extracellular prolactin 2- to 4-fold. These experiments were performed in medium containing serum that had not been treated in any special way to remove exogenous steroids, so this effect was apparently less sensitive to estradiol concentrations than the stimulation of growth was.

We have shown that prolactin synthesis was specifically increased by the combination of insulin and estrogen, but that the increase was not large enough to account for the increase in intracellular prolactin (Kiino and Dannies, 1982). We have shown also that the increase in the time it takes newly synthesized, rapidly released prolactin to be discharged from the cells in large quantities (about 1 hour in GH cells) was not affected by this treatment. Although intracellular prolactin content increased as cells passed through the cell cycle, insulin and estrogen increased prolactin storage at each stage of the cycle and did not affect the cell cycle distribution (Kiino *et al.*, 1982).

There appear to be at least two components of prolactin release in the pituitary cells (reviewed in Dannies, 1982), and how these relate to the morphology has not been clearly demonstrated. The most likely form for stored prolactin, based on current knowledge, is secretory granules. Using another clonal cell strain, 2B8, McGill (1983) showed that insulin and estrogen increased the percentage of the area of the cell occupied by granules sixfold and that these granules contained prolactin, visualized by immunostaining. In 2B8 cells, as in GH cells, granules are not uniformly distributed among the cells, so this kind of study has to be reported by the quantitative examination that McGill did.

We began these experiments to see if we could cause differentiation of GH cells into more normal cells, but the ability to induce storage is not restricted to continuous cell lines. We have found more recently that insulin and estrogen also increased intracellular prolactin stores in primary cultures of normal male rat pituitary cells in gelding serum (C. M. Van Itallie and P. S. Dannies, unpublished results). There are some suggestions that such processes also occur in intact animals; estrogen increased the pituitary content of prolactin (Meites *et al.*, 1972; Lloyd *et al.*, 1973) as well as the amount of prolactin that could be released (Labrie *et al.*, 1980). In the morphological studies of Osamura *et al.* (1982), however, castration resulted in the disappearance of large secretory granules and the appearance of many small secretory granules; these disappeared after injection of estradiol, a result that does not appear to agree with the studies performed in culture. The situation in animals is complicated by interactions of estrogen with the hypothalamus as well as with the pituitary gland, interactions that may make it more difficult to distinguish effects on storage from other effects. The ability to manipulate storage conditions in cells in culture provides a way of resolving the proteins involved in creating storage. Once these are identified, the question of whether they also change in intact animals can be directly answered.

A role of estrogen in increasing the storage of prolactin by decreasing the ability of the cells to degrade prolactin has been suggested. After prolactin secretion in lactating rats is prevented by removing the suckling pups, the contents of secretory granules can be seen in the lysosomes (Smith and Farquhar, 1966). As mentioned previously, there is biochemical evidence that pituitary glands and cells will degrade newly synthesized prolactin under some conditions. Dopaminergic agents enhance this ability (Maurer, 1980; Dannies and Rudnick, 1980). Nansel *et al.* (1981a) found that dopamine increased the activity of β-glucuronidase, an enzyme found in lysosomes and microsomes of the cells. They reported that the levels of β-glucuronidase decreased as estrogen levels increased and that estradiol decreased enzyme levels in ovariectomized rats (Nansel *et al.*, 1981b). Other laboratories, however, did not see similar changes. Nagy and co-workers (1983) did not see changes in acid phosphatase, another enzyme found in the lysosomes, or in β-glucuronidase after dopamine or estrogen treatment, and Chowdhury and Sarkar (1983) found a decrease in β-glucuronidase activity, but an increase in acid phosphatase activity, with estrogen treatment. Interpretation of any experiment is obviously complicated by the heterogeneous populations of cells in the gland; it is not clear in which cells changes occur when differences are found. The only conclusion that can be reached at this time is that changes in enzyme activity sufficiently large to be detectable are not necessary for the effects on prolactin production. Estrogen regulation of prolactin degradation remains an unproven possibility. Regulation of intracellular prolactin stability, if it exists, may not occur only at the lysosomal level; evidence in several systems suggests a nonlysosomal component of the degradation of secretory proteins (Bienkowski, 1983).

VII. ESTROGEN CHANGES THE RESPONSE OF PROLACTIN CELLS TO AGENTS THAT AFFECT PROLACTIN RELEASE

In addition to causing direct increases in prolactin synthesis and storage, estrogen affects the ability of other factors to stimulate or inhibit prolactin release. This effect was first shown for thyrotropin-releasing hormone (TRH) in intact animals. DeLéan and co-workers (1977a) showed that estrogen injections increased the amount of prolactin released in response to TRH. This effect appeared to be physiologically relevant, because prolactin responses to TRH were lowest in diestrus and highest in proestrus, and TRH binding to the pituitary gland was lowest in diestrus and highest in proestrus (DeLéan *et al.*, 1977b). The ability of estrogen to increase the binding of TRH in GH cells and to directly increase TRH-induced prolactin release in normal cells and GH cells has been demonstrated (Gershengorn *et al.*, 1979; Giguère *et al.*, 1982).

At the same time that estradiol enhanced the effects of TRH, it lessened the inhibitory action of dopaminergic agents (Raymond *et al.*, 1978). We extended these studies to show that estradiol caused a shift in the half-maximally effective concentration of dihydroergocryptine, a dopaminergic agonist, that ranged from 10- to 30-fold and, in addition, reduced the maximal amount of inhibition obtained to about half the amount of inhibition in untreated cultures (West and Dannies, 1980). These effects of estradiol occurred within 2 days, a time span that could be relevant to the estrous cycle, and occurred with a maximal effect at 50 pM estradiol. Measurements of plasma estradiol concentrations during the diestrous period of the rat range from 7 to 370 pM (Butcher *et al.*, 1974; Brown-Grant *et al.*, 1970; Shaikh and Shaikh, 1975), so these effects of estradiol may have physiological relevance.

Although Heiman and Ben-Jonathan (1982) showed that dopaminergic receptors varied during the estrous cycle, DiPaolo *et al.* (1979) found no effect of estradiol on pituitary dopaminergic receptors when the steroid was injected into rats, and suggested that a postreceptor step was involved. Giguère *et al.* (1982) have found that estrogen increased the amount of release occurring in response to isobutylmethylxanthine, a phosphodiesterase inhibitor. It is difficult to interpret this result cleanly, even if the only effect of isobutylmethylxanthine is to inhibit phosphodiesterase activity, except to say that a receptor is not involved. Estrogen may have increased the activity of adenylate cyclase so that more cyclic AMP can accumulate when enzymatic breakdown is prevented, and therefore more release occurs. Alternatively, estrogen may have affected some step other than cAMP formation, such as storage, to make the release of more prolactin possible. The estrogen-induced changes in response to TRH and dopamine may be completely accounted for by changes in receptor number and increases in intracellular stores of prolactin, but further investigations may show that other mechanisms are involved as well.

In serum-free medium, almost any component that we added enhanced or inhibited the ability of estrogen to decrease the response to dopamine (B. West and P. S. Dannies, unpublished results). One problem is to determine which of these effects occur *in vivo*; effects found in culture may be different from those in the animal. For example, Maurer (1980) found that estradiol could not overcome thyroid hormone inhibition of prolactin synthesis in primary cultures, but DeLéan *et al.* (1977a) found that estrogen could overcome thyroid hormone inhibition of prolactin production in intact animals. It is possible now to determine in the animal whether the effect of estrogen observed by DeLéan *et al.* is an effect on synthesis and whether the *in vivo* results are different from the results obtained in tissue culture.

VIII. RAPID EFFECTS OF ESTROGEN

Most, if not all, of the estrogenic effects described up to this point are probably mediated through the same kinds of estrogen–receptor genomic interactions that occur in other systems. Pituitary glands and GH cells have estradiol receptors similar to those that have been characterized in other systems, with reported affinities ranging from 2×10^{-10} to 1×10^{-9} M (Eisenfeld, 1970; Leavitt *et al.*, 1969; Vreeburg *et al.*, 1975; Haug *et al.*, 1978; Roos *et al.*, 1980; Mester *et al.*, 1973). The best evidence that these binding sites mediate biological responses comes by analogy with results obtained using receptor mutants in other systems. Cells with defective steroid binding show altered responses to steroids (reviewed by Strobl and Thompson, 1984). It seems reasonable to assume that, if pituitary cells with altered estrogen receptors were examined, many or all of the responses described would be affected. There may, however, be nongenomic membrane-mediated events. Estradiol at 1-nM concentrations caused a rapid increase (within 1–2 minutes) in formation of action potentials in 30% of the cells in a clone of GH cells (Dufy *et al.*, 1979). These action potentials may have a calcium component because they could be blocked by D600, a calcium channel blocker. 17α-Estradiol was not as effective in stimulating action potentials, but blocked the action of 17β-estradiol. These effects were so rapid that it seems likely that they were not mediated by genomic interactions. Zyzek *et al.* (1981) have found that 17β-estradiol concentrations of 10^{-8} M or higher stimulated release of prolactin 10 minutes after the steroid was added to the same clone of GH cells in which the electrophysiological effects were found. At times longer than 10 minutes, the large amount of basal release obscured the stimulation. Because increasing intracellular calcium concentrations can cause prolactin release, it is possible that the rapid increase in formation of action potentials accounts for estrogen-stimulated release. There are rapid effects of steroids seen in other systems, reviewed by Baulieu (1978) and Duval *et al.* (1983). These effects include rapid changes in the firing rates of neurons at steroid concentrations that sometimes are 1 nM or less. One of the ways in which prolactin cells resemble nerve cells is in their ability to show action potentials. Both cell types apparently have the ability to respond to steroids with rapid membrane effects.

IX. EFFECTS OF ANTIESTROGENS

The reports of the effects of estrogen antagonists on prolactin levels in intact normal animals vary. Clomiphene has been found to decrease basal serum prolactin levels (Burdman *et al.*, 1979) and to cause a twofold increase (Tobias *et al.*, 1981). Tamoxifen had no effect on basal serum prolactin in studies by Nicholson and Golder (1975), Spona and co-workers (1980), and Leibl and workers (1981). On the other hand, Spona and Leibl (1981) and Prysor-Jones and co-workers (1983) found increases in serum prolactin levels after tamoxifen. Nagy *et al.* (1980) found no change in serum prolactin levels in Buffalo rats, but a threefold increase in Wistar Furth rats, although this change was evidently not statistically significant. Estrogen antagonists are known to be partial agonists, and it is therefore not necessarily surprising that there are conditions under which they show stimulatory activity. Agents that have only partial agonist activity should partially block the activity of agents with full activity. Jordan *et al.* (1975), Jordan and Koerner (1976), and Clemens *et al.* (1983) found that tamoxifen could partially block the estrogen-induced rise in serum prolactin, but Spona *et al.* (1980) and Leibl *et al.* (1981) found that tamoxifen increased the estrogen-induced rise in serum prolactin levels in the same experiments where it had no effects on its own.

Tamoxifen effects on prolactin synthesis have been measured by treating rats with the compound and then removing the pituitary glands and incubating them with [^{3}H]leucine. Several laboratories have observed decreased incorporation of leucine into prolactin, either of basal levels or of estrogen-induced increases (Spona and Leibl, 1981; Nagy *et al.*, 1980; DeQuijada *et al.*, 1980). The decrease was seen even in cases when serum prolactin levels or prolactin levels in the cultures increased or were not affected. The interpretation of these results as decreases in synthesis must be done with caution, because the incubation times were as long as 4 hours. In view of the previously described occurrence of degradation, it is probably necessary to confirm under each set of experimental conditions that changes in synthesis are being measured. Spona and Leibl (1981) found that tamoxifen had no effect on basal incorporation of [^{3}H]leucine into prolactin, but caused increases in translatable prolactin mRNA, and tamoxifen decreased estrogen stimulation by both techniques. If the leucine incorporation is a good measure of synthesis, then the discrepancy between prolactin mRNA activity and leucine incorporation may indicate control of a translational process in the gland.

The results of estrogen antagonists on tumor growth also vary. The growth of pituitary tumor 7315a was inhibited by tamoxifen and was also inhibited by estrogen as previously discussed (DeQuijada *et al.*, 1980; Nagy *et al.*, 1980; Lamberts *et al.*, 1981). Nagy *et al.* (1980) found that the growth of MtTW15 tumors was inhibited by tamoxifen, but Winneker *et al.* (1981) found that the growth of these tumors was stimulated by tamoxifen and other antiestrogens.

Many factors may account for the differences summarized here. Results in intact animals obviously can occur through indirect as well as direct effects on the gland. The variability in experiments in intact animals may be caused by the age or sex of the animal, whether the animal has been castrated or ovariectomized, the dose of antagonist administered, the times of administration, and perhaps even the strain of rat; more than one of these factors may affect the response. The studies cited above have too many differences among them to be able to determine causes. It is important to resolve eventually what conditions cause estrogen antagonists to elevate prolactin levels in the serum. Clomiphene is used clinically as a fertility drug, but hyperprolactinemia causes infertility. If clomiphene elevates prolactin levels in some patients, the effect could interfere with the desired stimulation of fertility. Estrogen antagonists are also used to treat breast cancer. Again, if prolactin is elevated in some patients by these agents, it may interfere with inhibition of growth of the cancer.

The actions of estrogen antagonists have been widely studied in other tissues; one review of this work is that by Sutherland and Murphy (1982). Estrogen antagonists compete with estrogen for binding to the estrogen receptor. Unoccupied estrogen receptors are primarily found in the cytoplasm when cells are homogenized; binding of estrogen or most estrogen antagonists causes the receptor to be retained in the nucleus. The retention of the estrogen receptor in the nucleus is longer with most estrogen antagonists than it is with estrogen. Tamoxifen appears to behave in the pituitary gland as it does in other systems, causing prolonged retention of the estrogen receptor in the nucleus (Bowman *et al.*, 1982; Kirchoff *et al.*, 1983). Sutherland and Murphy point out in their review that tamoxifen has direct effects on estrogen biosynthesis, prostaglandin synthesis, and enzymes of carbohydrate metabolism; these effects are not always reversed by estrogen. Winneker *et al.* (1983) have shown that tamoxifen can bind to a site on the serum low-density lipoprotein, an effect that may interfere with cholesterol synthesis. There is also an intracellular binding site for estrogen antagonists distinct from its binding site on the estrogen receptor. Studies with variant cell lines resistant to tamoxifen suggest that this binding site is important for the action of these compounds in inhibiting the growth of a breast cancer cell line (Faye *et al.*, 1983). Although estrogen can compete with the antiestrogens to prevent the growth inhibition, Faye and co-workers suggest that this competition may be at a physiological level, rather than at the level of the receptor. Therefore, the various results reported with estrogen antagonists in animals may not all be mediated through the estrogen receptor—in fact, it is not yet proven that any effects are.

Lieberman *et al.* (1983a) have approached this question pharmacologically by using cell cultures of normal pituitary glands, which avoids actions at sites other than the gland itself. They have measured estrogen-induced prolactin synthesis and its inhibition by antiestrogens. If an antagonist is competitive, it ought to shift the dose–response curve of the agonist without affecting the shape of the curve. Increasing concentrations of antiestrogens ideally should result in a parallel series of estrogen dose–response curves, with increases in the apparent half-maximally effective concentration of estrogen. Interactions in a whole cell are never ideal, but Lieberman *et al.* (1983a) did show at least that two concentrations of hydroxytamoxifen increased the apparent half-maximal concentrations of estradiol. Therefore, the antagonist appears to behave in a competitive manner. Lieberman *et al.* (1983b) present a second kind of pharmacological evidence that antiestrogens exert their effects through the estrogen receptor; they showed that the relative potencies of the compounds in inhibiting prolactin synthesis were similar to the relative binding affinity for the estrogen receptor. At present, pharmacological correlations are the best evidence for the action of antiestrogens. Cell lines with mutations in estrogen receptors and antiestrogen binding sites are not yet available for pituitary cell lines.

In the series of experiments using cells in culture, described above, estrogen antagonists behaved as antagonists are expected to behave, suggesting that culture systems may be simpler than intact animals. This is not always the case. In GH cells grown in normal horse serum and fetal calf serum, we showed that several estrogen antagonists stimulated prolactin production after a week or more of treatment, but estradiol did not (Dannies *et al.*, 1977). Estrogen actually prevented the increase in prolactin production. The lack of effect of estradiol may have been caused by endogenous estrogens in the serum, since in this series of experiments we made no effort to remove them, but because the estrogen effect may depend on other serum factors, this explanation is not the only one possible. If the antiestrogens were increasing prolactin production by acting as estrogens, then they appeared to be better estrogens than estradiol under those circumstances. More recently, we have used antiestrogens in medium containing gelding serum, and we found that most antiestrogens were partial agonists in stimulating both prolactin production and cell growth (J. F. Amara and P. S. Dannies, unpublished results). Whether the difference in the results in GH cells and those in normal cells is caused by trivial differences in culture conditions or by more interesting differences in gene induction in normal and GH cells is not yet known.

X. CONCLUSION

Estrogen affects prolactin cells in several ways. With the technology now available, it will be possible to use pituitary glands and cell lines to learn more about how estradiol regulates transcription. It is also now possible to isolate messages induced by estrogen in addition to prolactin. These other induced proteins must regulate growth and secretion, and by learning more about these proteins we will know more about how these processes function and are regulated, both in cell culture and in animals.

REFERENCES

Amara, J. F., and Dannies, P. S. (1983). *Endocrinology* **112**, 1141–1143.

Baker, B. L. (1970). *J. Histochem. Cytochem.* **18**, 1–8.

Baulieu, E. E. (1978). *Mol. Cell. Endocrinol.* **12**, 247–254.

Bienkowski, R. S. (1983). *Biochem. J.* **214**, 1–10.

Bowman, S. P., Leake, A., and Morris, I. D., (1982). *J. Endocrinol.* **94**, 167–175.

Brown-Grant, K., Exley, D., and Naftolin, F. (1970). *J. Endocrinol.* **48**, 295–296.

Brunet, N., Gourdji, D., Tixier-Vidal, A., and Rizzino, A. (1982). *Cold Spring Harbor Conf. Cell Proliferation* **9**, 169–177.

Burdman, J. A., Szijan, I., Jahn, G. A., Machiavelli, G., and Kalbermann, L. E. (1979). *Experientia* **35**, 1258–1259.

Butcher, R. L., Collins, W. E., and Fugo, N. W. (1974). *Endocrinology* **94**, 1704–1708.

Chowdhury, M., and Sarkar, M. (1983). *Biochem. Biophys. Res. Commun.* **116**, 230–236.

Clemens, J. A., Bennett, D. R., Black, L. J., and Jones, C. D. (1983). *Life Sci.* **32**, 2869–2875.

Clifton, K. H., and Furth, J. (1961). *Cancer Res.* **21**, 913–920.

Clifton, K. H., and Meyer, R. K. (1956). *Anat. Rec.* **125**, 65–81.

Corenblum, B., Kovacs, K., Penz, G., and Ezrin, C. (1980). *Endocr. Res. Commun.* **7**, 137–144.

Dannies, P. S. (1982). *Biochem. Pharmacol.* **31**, 2845–2849.

Dannies, P. S., and Rudnick, M. S. (1980). *J. Biol. Chem.* **255**, 2776–2781.

Dannies, P. S., Yen, P. M., and Tashjian, A. H., Jr. (1977). *Endocrinology* **101**, 1151–1156.

DeLéan, A., Ferland, L., Drouin, J., Kelly, P. A., and Labrie, F. (1977a). *Endocrinology* **100**, 1496–1503.

DeLéan, A., Garon, M., Kelly, P. A., and Labrie, F. (1977b). *Endocrinology* **100**, 1505–1510.

DeNicola, A. F., Lawzewitsch, I., Kaplan, S. E., and Libertun, C. (1978). *JNCI, J. Natl. Cancer Inst.* **61**, 753–763.

DeQuijada, M., Timmermans, H. A. T., and Lamberts, S. W. J. (1980). *J. Endocrinol.* **86**, 109–116.

DiPaolo, T., Carmichael, R., Labrie, F., and Raynaud, J. P. (1979). *Mol. Cell. Endocrinol.* **16**, 99–106.

Dufy, B., Vincent, J. D., Fleury, H., DuPasquier, P., Gourdji, D., and Tixier-Vidal, A. (1979). *Science* **204**, 509–510.

Dunning, W. F., Curtis, M. R., and Segaloff, A. (1947). *Cancer Res.* **7**, 511–521.

Duval, D., Durant, S., and Homo-Delarche, F. (1983). *Biochim. Biophys. Acta* **737**, 409–442.

Eisenfeld, A. (1970). *Endocrinology* **86**, 1313–1318.

Elias, K. A., and Weiner, R. I. (1983). *Proc. 65th Annu. Meet., Am. Endocr. Soc.,* Abstract 414, p. 184.

Evans, M. I., Hager, L. J., and McKnight, G. S. (1981). *Cell* **25**, 187–193.

Farquhar, M. G. (1977). *In* "Comparative Endocrinology of Prolactin" (H. D. Dellman, J. A. Johnson, and D. M. Klacho, eds.), pp. 37–94. Plenum, New York.

Faye, J. C., Jozan, S., Redeuilh, G., Bauleiu, E. M., and Bayard, F. (1983). *Proc. Natl. Acad. Sci. U.S.A.* **80**, 3158–3162.

Furth, J., and Clifton, K. H. (1966). *In* "The Pituitary Gland" (G. W. Harris and B. T. Donovan, eds.), Vol. 2, pp. 260–497. Univ. of California Press, Berkeley.

Gershengorn, M. C., Marcus-Samuels, B. E., and Geras, E. (1979). *Endocrinology* **105**, 171–176.

Gersten, B. E., and Baker, B. L. (1970). *Am. J. Anat.* **128**, 1–20.

Giguère, V., Meunier, H., Veilleux, R., and Labrie, F. (1982). *Endocrinology* **111**, 857–862.

Haug, E., and Gautvik, K. M. (1976). *Endocrinology* **99**, 1482–1489.

Haug, E., Naess, O., and Gautvik, K. M. (1978). *Mol. Cell. Endocrinol.* **12**, 81–95.

Hayashi, I., and Sato, G. H. (1976). *Nature (London)* **259**, 134–136.

Heiman, M. L., and Ben-Jonathan, N. (1982). *Endocrinology* **111**, 37–41.

Hellman, S., Harris, J. R., Canellos, G. P., and Fisher, B. (1982). *In* "Cancer: Principles and Practice of Oncology" (V. T. DeVita, Jr., S. Hellman, and S. A. Rosenberg, eds.), pp. 914–962. Lippincott, Philadelphia, Pennsylvania.

Herbert, D. C., Ishikawa, H., Shiino, M., and Rennels, E. G. (1978). *Proc. Soc. Exp. Biol. Med.* **157**, 605–609.

Hunt, T. E. (1943). *Endocrinology* **32**, 334–339.

Hunt, T. E. (1947). *Anat. Rec.* **97**, 127–137.

Jordan, V. C., and Koerner, S. (1976). *J. Endocrinol.* **68**, 305–311.

Jordan, V. C., Koerner, S., and Robinson, C. (1975). *J. Endocrinol.* **65**, 151–152.

Kiino, D. R., and Dannies, P. S. (1981). *Endocrinology* **109**, 1264–1269.

Kiino, D. R., and Dannies, P. S. (1982). *Yale J. Biol. Med.* **55**, 409–420.

Kiino, D. R., Burger, D. E., and Dannies, P. S. (1982). *J. Cell Biol.* **93**, 459–462.

Kirchhoff, J., Hoffman, B., and Ghraf, R. (1983). *J. Steroid Biochem.* **18**, 631–633.

Labrie, F., Ferland, L., Denizeau, F., and Beaulieu, M. (1980). *J. Steroid Biochem.* **12**, 323–330.

Lamberts, S. W. J., Uitterlinden, P., Zuiderwjk-Roest, J. M., Bonsvan Evelingen, E. G., and de Jong, F. H. (1981). *Endocrinology* **108**, 1878–1884.

Lamberts, S. W. J., Nagy, I., Uitterlinden, P., and MacLeod, R. M. (1982). *Endocrinology* **110**, 1141–1146.

Leavitt, W. W., Friend, J. P., and Robinson, J. A. (1969). *Science* **165**, 496–498.

Leibl, H., Bieglmayer, G. H., and Spona, J. (1981). *Endocrinol. Exp.* **15**, 35–44.

Lieberman, M. E., Maurer, R. A., and Gorski, J. (1978). *Proc. Natl. Acad. Sci. U.S.A.* **75**, 5946–5949.

Lieberman, M. E., Maurer, R. A., Claude, P., and Gorski, J. (1982). *Mol. Cell. Endocrinol.* **25**, 277–294.

Lieberman, M. E., Jordan, V. C., Fritsch, M., Santos, M. A., and Gorski, J. (1983a). *J. Biol. Chem.* **258**, 4734–4740.

Lieberman, M. E., Gorski, J., and Jordan, V. C. (1983b). *J. Biol. Chem.* **258**, 4741–4745.

Lippman, M., Bolan, G., and Huff, K. (1976). *Cancer Res.* **36**, 4595–4601.

Lloyd, H. M., Meares, J. D., and Jacobi, J. (1973). *J. Endocrinol.* **58**, 227–231.

Lloyd, H. M., Meares, J. D., and Jacobi, J. (1975). *Nature (London)* **255**, 497–498.

Lu, K. H., Koch, Y., and Meites, J. (1971). *Endocrinology* **89**, 229–233.

McGill, J. R. (1983). *Anat. Rec.* **206**, 43–48.

MacLeod, R. M., Abad, A., and Eidson, L. L. (1969). *Endocrinology* **84**, 1475–1483.

Maurer, R. A. (1980). *Biochemistry* **19**, 3573–3578.

Maurer, R. A. (1982a). *Endocrinology* **110**, 1515–1520.

Maurer, R. A. (1982b). *J. Biol. Chem.* **257**, 2133–2136.

Maurer, R. A., and Gorski, J. (1977). *Endocrinology* **101**, 76–84.

Meites, J., Lu, K. H., Wuttke, W., Welsch, C. W., Nagasawa, H., and Quadri, S. K. (1972). *Recent Prog. Horm. Res.* **28**, 471–526.

Merchant, F. W. (1974). *Am. J. Anat.* **139**, 245–268.

Mercier, L., Thompson, E. B., and Simons, S. S., Jr. (1983). *Endocrinology* 112, 601–609.

Mester, J., Brunelle, R., Jung, I., and Sonnenschein, C. (1973). *Exp. Cell Res.* 81, 447–452.

Morel, Y., Albaladejo, V., Bouvier, J., and Andre, J. (1982). *Cancer Res.* 42, 1492–1497.

Nagy, I., Valdenegro, C. A., and MacLeod, R. M. (1980). *Neuroendocrinology* 30, 389–395.

Nagy, I., Rappay, G., Makara, G. B., Horvath, G., Bacsy, E., and MacLeod, R. M. (1983). *Endocrinology* 112, 470–475.

Nansel, D. D., Gudelsky, G. A., Reymond, M. J., Neaves, W. B., and Porter, J. C. (1981a). *Endocrinology* 108, 896–902.

Nansel, D. D. Gudelsky, G. A., Reymond, M. J., and Porter, J. C. (1981b). *Endocrinology* 108, 903–907.

Nicholson, R. I., and Golder, M. P. (1975). *Eur. J. Cancer* 11, 571–597.

Nicoll, C. S., and Meites, J. (1962). *Endocrinology* 70, 272–277.

Nogami, H., and Yoshimura, F. (1980). *Cell Tissue Res.* 211, 1–4.

Olivier, L., Vila-Porcile, E., Racadot, O., Peillon, F., and Racadot, J. (1975). *In* "The Anterior Pituitary" (A. Tixier-Vidal and M. G. Farquhar, eds.), pp. 231–276. Academic Press, New York.

Osamura, R. Y., Komatsu, N., Izumi, S., Yoshimura, S., and Watanabe, K. (1982). *J. Histochem. Cytochem.* 30, 919–925.

Prysor-Jones, R. A., Silverlight, J. J., and Jenkins, J. S. (1983). *J. Endocrinol.* 97, 261–266.

Raymond, V., Beaulieu, M., Labrie, F., and Boissier, J. (1978). *Science* 200, 1173–1175.

Roos, W., Strittmatter, B., Fabbro, D., and Eppenberger, U. (1980). *Horm. Res.* 12, 324–332.

Ryan, R., Shupnik, M. A., and Gorski, J. (1979). *Biochemistry* 18, 2044–2048.

Sato, S. (1980). *Endocrinol. Jpn.* 27, 573–583.

Schimke, R. T., and Doyle, D. (1970). *Annu. Rev. Biochem.* 39, 929–976.

Seo, H., Refetoff, S., Martino, E., Vassart, G., and Brocas, H. (1979a). *Endocrinology* 104, 1083–1090.

Seo, H., Refetoff, S., Vassart, G., and Brocas, H. (1979b). *Proc. Natl. Acad. Sci. U.S.A.* 76, 824–828.

Shaikh, A. A., and Shaikh, S. A. (1975). *Endocrinology* 96, 37–44.

Shenai, R., and Wallis, M. (1979). *Biochem. J.* 182, 735–743.

Smith, R. E., and Farquhar, M. G. (1966). *J. Cell Biol.* 31, 319–347.

Sonnenschein, S., Posner, M., Saududdin, S., and Krasnay, M. (1973). *Exp. Cell Res.* 78, 41–46.

Sorrentino, J. M., Kirkland, W. L., and Sirbasku, D. A. (1976). *J. Natl. Cancer Inst. (U.S.)* 56, 1149–1153.

Spona, J., and Leibl, H. (1981). *Biochim. Biophys. Acta* 656, 45–54.

Spona, J., Bieglmayer, C., and Leibl, H. (1980). *Biochim. Biophys. Acta* 633, 361–375.

Stone, J. P., Holtzman, S., and Shellabarger, C. J. (1979). *Cancer Res.* 39, 773–778.

Stone, R. T., Maurer, R. A., and Gorski, J. (1977). *Biochemistry* 16, 4915–4921.

Strobl, J. S., and Thompson, E. B. (1984). *In* "Sex Steroid Receptors" (F. Auricchio, ed.) (in press).

Sutherland, R. L., and Murphy, L. C. (1982). *Mol. Cell. Endocrinol.* 25, 5–23.

Takemoto, H., Yokoro, K., Furth, J., and Cohen, A. I. (1962). *Cancer Res.* 22, 917–924.

Tashjian, A. H., Jr., and Hoyt, R. F., Jr. (1972). *In* "Molecular Genetics and Developmental Biology" (M. Sussman, ed.), pp. 353–372. Prentice-Hall, Englewood Cliffs, New Jersey.

Tashjian, A. H., Jr., Yasumura, Y., Levine, L., Sato, G. H., and Parker, M. L. (1968). *Endocrinology* 82, 342–352.

Tixier-Vidal, A. (1975). *In* "The Anterior Pituitary" (A. Tixier-Vidal, M. Farquhar, eds.), pp. 181–229. Academic Press, New York.

Tixier-Vidal, A., Brunet, N., and Gourdji, D. (1983). *In* "Prolactin and Prolactinomas" (G. Tolis, C. Stefanis, T. Mountokalakis, and F. Labrie, eds.), pp. 327–337. Raven Press, New York.

Tobias, H., Carr, L. A., and Voogt, J. L. (1981). *Life Sci.* **29,** 711–716.

Tougard, C., Picart, R., and Tixier-Vidal, A. (1980). *Am. J. Anat.* **158,** 471–490.

Turner, C. W. (1977). *In* "Comparative Endocrinology of Prolactin" (H. D. Dellman, J. A. Johnson, and D. M. Klacho, eds.), pp. 1–17. Plenum, New York.

Vignon, F., Terqui, M., Westley, B., Derocq, P., and Rochefort, H. (1980). *Endocrinology* **106,** 1079–1086.

Vreeburg, J. T. M., Schretlen, P. J. M., and Baum, M. J. (1975). *Endocrinology* **97,** 969–977.

West, B., and Dannies, P. S. (1980). *Endocrinology* **106,** 1108–1113.

Wiklund, J. A., and Gorski, J. (1982). *Endocrinology* **111,** 1140–1149.

Wiklund, J. A., Wertz, N., and Gorski, J. (1981a). *Endocrinology* **109,** 1700–1707.

Wiklund, J. A., Rutledge, J., and Gorski, J. (1981b). *Endocrinology* **109,** 1708–1714.

Winneker, R. C., Welshons, W. V., and Parsons, J. A. (1981). *Mol. Cell. Endocrinol.* **23,** 333–344.

Winneker, R. C., Guthrie, S. C., and Clark, J. H. (1983). *Endocrinology* **112,** 1823–1827.

Wyche, J. H., and Noteboom, W. D. (1979). *Endocrinology* **104,** 1765–1773.

Zyzek, E., Dufy-Barbe, L., Dufy, B., and Vincent, J. D. (1981). *Biochem. Biophys. Res. Commun.* **102,** 1151–1157.

CHAPTER 10

Genetic and Epigenetic Bases of Glucocorticoid Resistance in Lymphoid Cell Lines

Suzanne Bourgeois

Regulatory Biology Laboratory
The Salk Institute for Biological Studies
San Diego, California

Judith C. Gasson

Division of Hematology-Oncology
Department of Medicine
UCLA School of Medicine
Los Angeles, California

This chapter is dedicated to the memory of Gordon Tomkins (1926–1975) on the tenth anniversary of his death.

BIOCHEMICAL ACTIONS OF HORMONES, VOL. XII

I. INTRODUCTION

The basic distinction between genetic and epigenetic events is that genetic changes involve alterations in the primary structure of DNA, while epigenetic phenomena shift the expression of the genome in a clonally heritable manner without change in DNA sequence. Mutants resulting from base substitutions or deletions represent classic examples of genetic variations. The traditional criteria used to define mutants are that their altered phenotype

1. Occurs randomly, at a low frequency increased by mutagens,
2. Is inheritable and stable in the absence of selection,
3. Is reversible by specific mutagens,
4. Is associated with changes in the properties of a specific protein,
5. Can be mapped to a specific region of the genome, and
6. Can be transferred to other cells.

However, genetic events include not only mutations but also gene amplification, chromosome rearrangements, and segregation of genetic material. The criteria used to define mutations, therefore, do not necessarily apply to the other genetic events. Gene amplification, for example, occurs at relatively high frequency, can be unstable in the absence of selection, and does not lead to changes in the properties of a specific protein, but rather to increased synthesis of the amplified gene product (for examples, see Schimke, 1982).

Epigenetic variations involve the state of DNA methylation (for a review, see Adams and Burdon, 1982) and other structural features of chromatin, revealed, for example, by nuclease sensitivity (Weintraub and Groudine,

1976), which appear correlated with gene expression. These properties of chromatin are stably transmitted to progeny cells and play a role in the developmental activation of tissue-specific genes. Little is known about the mechanisms which, probably under the influence of hormonal signals, alter these structural features of chromatin during development. The notion that changes in DNA methylation are "epigenetic" can be confusing, since they actually involve changes in DNA sequence from cytosine to 5-methylcytosine. This postsynthetic modification does not, however, alter the sequence of the transcript and of the protein product. Further confusion can arise from the fact that a variety of mutagens and carcinogens inhibit DNA methylation *in vitro* (Wilson and Jones, 1983) and generate variants at high frequency (see Section III,D).

Clearly, a variety of criteria are needed to identify the mechanism of a heritable variation, whether genetic or epigenetic. If the mechanism has not been identified, the cautious term *variant*, rather than *mutant*, should be used to describe cells having an altered phenotype. All variants, if stable, can be analyzed by somatic cell genetic approaches involving complementation, dominance tests, and mapping. It is, however, important in interpreting the results of such tests to realize that DNA methylation, like gene amplification, can involve more than one genetic locus. In this chapter, we will review evidence that four different mechanisms can generate glucocorticoid resistance in T-lymphoid cell lines: mutations, chromosome segregation, DNA methylation, and, probably, gene amplification.

II. GENETIC DEFECTS IN GLUCOCORTICOID RECEPTOR

A. MUTATIONS

The direct lethal effect of glucocorticoids on T-lymphocytes is mediated by cytoplasmic receptors which, after binding of the hormone, undergo activation and translocation to the nucleus. Glucocorticoid-sensitive T-cell lines established in tissue culture from both mouse and human tumors have provided a genetic approach to the analysis of this response, based on the selection *in vitro* of variants resistant to glucocorticoid-induced killing. Genetic and biochemical characterizations of such variants have identified some of the determinants of glucocorticoid sensitivity and mechanisms of acquisition of resistance *in vitro*.

Extensive studies carried out with the murine T-cell lines S49 and W7 brought compelling evidence for the role of the glucocorticoid receptor in hormone-induced lymphocytolysis and demonstrated that glucocorticoid resistance can result from mutations affecting either the quality or the quantity of receptors. These studies have recently been reviewed (Stevens *et al.*, 1983) and will only be briefly summarized in this chapter. It should be emphasized that *all* variants derived from the S49 and W7 cell lines by selection at high concentrations of dexamethasone (0.1–10 μM) result either from alterations in glucocorticoid receptor properties or reduction in receptor amount. Early work by Sibley and Tomkins (1974b) described two S49 variants, designated as "deathless," having receptor indistinguishable from the wild type. Subsequent studies (Bourgeois and Newby, 1977, 1979; Pfahl and Bourgeois, 1980) strongly suggest that these variants, which were both derived from pseudotetraploid S49 cells, arose by chromosome segregation resulting in a reduced intracellular receptor concentration (for discussion, see Section II,D).

Comparison of the S49 and W7 cell lines revealed important differences: the W7 line is sensitive to lower dexamethasone concentrations than the S49 line, and W7 cells contain 30,000 glucocorticoid binding sites, which represents twice as many receptors as in S49 cells (Bourgeois and Newby, 1977). Moreover, dexamethasone-resistant variants arise spontaneously from S49 cells at frequencies on the order of 10^{-6} to 10^{-5} (Sibley and Tomkins, 1974a; Bourgeois and Newby, 1977), while this frequency is $<1.2 \times 10^{-10}$ in the case of W7 cells (Huet-Minkowski *et al.*, 1981). These results led to the conclusion that S49 cells are functionally hemizygous for a gene encoding the glucocorticoid receptor (r^+/r^-), while W7 cells contain two functional copies of that gene (r^+/r^+) (Bourgeois and Newby, 1977). This accounted for the higher frequency at which S49 resistant variants were obtained and for the presence of twice as much receptor in W7 cells as the result of a gene dosage effect. This conclusion was supported by the fact that W7 variants were isolated that were resistant to low dexamethasone concentrations (10^{-9} to 10^{-8} M) and which, like S49 cells, contained only 15,000 dexamethasone binding sites per cell and gave rise to fully resistant derivatives at increased frequency. These results also provided the first evidence that a reduction in the amount of normal receptors resulted in partial resistance to dexamethasone (Bourgeois and Newby, 1977, 1979). The functional hemizygosity of S49 cells for the gene encoding receptor was later confirmed by karyotypic analysis of hybrids, which assigned this gene to chromosome 18 of the mouse (Francke and Gehring, 1980). Recent results suggest that the amount of receptor in S49 cells can be further reduced by a mechanism as yet unidentified but that must be different from gene dosage (Gehring *et al.*, 1982).

The observations that receptor inactivation occurs at low frequencies, which can be increased by mutagens (Sibley and Tomkins, 1974a; Bourgeois and Newby, 1977; Pfahl *et al.*, 1978b; Bourgeois *et al.*, 1978; Huet-Minkowski *et al.*, 1981) and which depend on the ploidy of the cells for the gene encoding receptor, strongly indicate that these events result from mutations. The evidence for mutational events becomes overwhelming when one considers the finding in some of the dexamethasone-resistant S49 and W7 variants of receptor proteins with altered properties. In both cell lines, variant receptors with decreased nuclear transfer capacity (nt^-) have been described, and rare S49-receptor variants that display increased nuclear transfer capacity (nt^i) have been found (Sibley and Tomkins, 1974b; Yamamoto *et al.*, 1976; Pfahl *et al.*, 1978a,b). The properties of these altered receptors have been extensively reviewed (Stevens *et al.*, 1983). Therefore, this information will only be updated in this chapter by reviewing recent results obtained with nt^- and nt^i receptors (Sections II,B and C). Extensive complementation analysis of hybrids obtained by fusions of a variety of S49 and W7 receptor-defective variants was carried out (Pfahl and Bourgeois, 1980). These did not provide evidence for the existence of more than one genetic locus determining receptor activity. The absence of complementation between receptor-defective variants does not, however, rule out the possibility that a locus, distinct from the receptor structural gene *r*, might exist that plays a role in receptor activity. If the function encoded by that locus is vital to the cell, mutations inactivating that function would be lethal and, therefore, would not be found.

Similar studies were carried out using the glucocorticoid-sensitive human leukemic line CEM-C7 (Norman and Thompson, 1977; Schmidt *et al.*, 1980; Harmon and Thompson, 1981). Resistant variants, selected in the presence of 1 μM dexamethasone, occurred at frequencies on the order of 10^{-5}, increased by mutagens. It appears, therefore, that resistance in the CEM-C7 line is acquired in a single step by mutation in a functionally hemizygous locus. As in the case of S49 cells, this haploid locus encodes the glucocorticoid receptor since all CEM-C7 variants obtain result from receptor defects. One glucocorticoid-resistant CEM-C7 clone, containing approximately 30% of the parental level of receptor, had a phenotype not previously observed among the murine cell line variants, namely a complete absence (rather than reduction) of nuclear translocation. This receptor defect was designated "activation labile" because this variant receptor cannot form stable activated receptor–steroid complexes. The stability of the altered receptors of nt^- variants of S49 or W7 lines has not been examined. It is likely that some of the murine nt^- receptors also have increased lability, either in their activated or nonactivated form. This would account for the observation that most of these variants contain a reduced amount of glucocorticoid-binding activity.

B. DNA BINDING OF nt⁻ VARIANT RECEPTOR

A collection of nt⁻ variant receptors has been examined for its capacity to bind nuclei or calf-thymus DNA cellulose *in vitro* (reviewed by Stevens *et al.*, 1983). Reduced binding and altered sensitivity of DNA and nuclear binding to ionic strength have been observed. These tests monitor the general affinity of receptor–steroid complexes for DNA and/or other nuclear components. Recent evidence shows that activated glucocorticoid–receptor complexes recognize specific sequences in mouse mammary tumor virus (MMTV) DNA (Payvar *et al.*, 1981; Geisse *et al.*, 1982; Govindan *et al.*, 1982; Pfahl, 1982; Scheidereit *et al.*, 1983). The fact that some of the DNA sites having high affinity for glucocorticoid receptor are located in the region of the MMTV genome necessary for glucocorticoid-regulated transcription suggests that these sites play a biological role in hormonal control (Chandler *et al.*, 1983; Hynes *et al.*, 1983; Majors and Varmus, 1983; Pfahl *et al.*, 1983). Pfahl (1982) used a DNA–cellulose competition assay to compare the DNA-binding properties of glucocorticoid receptors from nt⁻ variants with those of receptor from the glucocorticoid-sensitive W7 line and from rat liver receptor. This assay, which does not require purified glucocorticoid receptor, measures the ability of free DNA to compete in the binding of receptor–steroid complexes to calf thymus DNA immobilized on cellulose. The receptor–steroid complexes were labeled by binding of [³H]triamcinolone acetonide, and various MMTV DNA fragments were used as competitors. A 0.55-kilobase (kb) restriction fragment that contains the promoter region of the MMTV proviral DNA was found to be the strongest competitor and, therefore, to have the highest affinity for the receptor–hormone complex. Further analysis (Pfahl *et al.*, 1983) revealed the existence of at least two high-affinity receptor binding sites in that region, one located between −202 and −137 and another between −135 and −50 base pairs (bp) from the site of initiation of transcription.

This assay was used to examine MMTV site-specific and unspecific DNA binding of two S49 glucocorticoid-resistant variants, nt⁻ 81 and 78, and of one W7 variant, nt⁻ 378. The nuclear transfer capacities of these variant receptors have been found to be 38% (nt⁻ 81), 44% (nt⁻ 78), and 51% (nt⁻ 378) in assay conditions in which 70% of wild-type S49 or W7 receptors were associated with the nucleus (Pfahl *et al.*, 1978b). The results obtained are illustrated in Fig. 1. Panel A shows that the variant receptor–hormone complexes have a reduced capacity to bind calf thymus DNA as compared to wild-type receptors. Panels B and C demonstrate that, in the case of the nt⁻ 378 and nt⁻ 78 variant receptors, the 0.55-kb DNA fragment containing the MMTV promoter region is a better competitor than 0.9-kb (Panel B) or 0.7-kb (Panel C) fragments, which do not include that region. Therefore, it

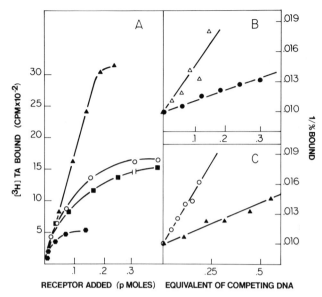

FIG. 1. DNA binding of nuclear transfer-deficient glucocorticoid receptors. Cytosolic extracts were prepared, and the activated receptor–steroid complexes were formed by incubation with 1, 2, 4 N [^{3}H] triamcinolone acetonide (TA) as described by Pfahl (1982). The amount of receptor present in the extract was calculated from the specifically bound [^{3}H] TA. (A) Binding of increasing amounts of extract to a constant amount of calf thymus DNA–cellulose. Receptor extracts were obtained from wild-type W7 cells (▲), variant 78 (○), variant 378 (■), or variant 81 (●). (B) Competition experiment using variant 378 receptor and 0.55 kb DNA fragment containing high-affinity receptor binding sites (△) or 0.9 kb nonspecific DNA fragment (●). (C) Competition experiment using variant 78 receptor and 0.55 kb DNA fragment (○) or 0.7 kb nonspecific DNA fragment (▲). [Reproduced from Pfahl (1982). Copyright 1982 M.I.T.]

appears that the nt$^-$ variant receptors are still to some extent capable of recognizing the high-affinity binding sites of MMTV DNA. However, since in the DNA–cellulose competition assay one compares relative affinities and these receptors have a reduced affinity for calf thymus DNA, the nt$^-$ receptors must have reduced affinity for the specific MMTV promoter sites as well. Therefore, the nt$^-$ phenotype appears to be due to a decreased affinity of their receptor–steroid complexes for both specific and unspecific DNA sites.

The same assay was used to show that binding of the steroid antagonist RU-486 to wild-type glucocorticoid receptors from W7 cells or rat liver mimicks pharmacologically the properties of nt$^-$ variant receptors (Bourgeois *et al.*, 1984). RU-486 is an antifertility steroid (Herrmann *et al.*, 1982) that also has antiglucocorticoid effects and was shown to be a strong antagonist of the glucocorticoid-induced cytolytic response of W7 cells and of the induction of MMTV mRNA in the T_1M_1b lymphoid cell line. The receptor–RU-486 complex was found to have only 40% nuclear transfer capacity in W7 cells, compared to the 70% nuclear transfer observed with receptor–dexamethasone complexes. Moreover, like nt⁻ receptors, wild-type receptor–RU-486 complexes have decreased affinity for DNA in general and a reduced specific recognition of the MMTV promoter region when compared to receptor–triamcinolone acetonide complexes. In the case of the RU-486 complex formed with rat liver receptor, it was shown that only a fraction of these complexes are activated by temperature and that these form highly salt-sensitive interactions with DNA. The capacity of nt⁻ receptor–hormone complexes to be activated has not yet been examined, but one can expect that at least some nt⁻ receptors will probably have defects in activation.

C. Reevaluation of the Size and Properties of nt^i Variant Receptor

Several of the glucocorticoid-resistant variants isolated from the S49 cell line were shown to contain receptors with increased nuclear transfer capacity (Sibley and Tomkins, 1974b; Yamamoto *et al.*, 1976). These nt^i variants are rare and have not been observed in W7 cells (Pfahl *et al.*, 1978a). Early studies (Yamamoto *et al.*, 1976) using sucrose gradient sedimentation and gel permeation chromatography indicated that nt^i receptors are considerably smaller than wild-type receptor, with a molecular weight of approximately 50,000, compared to 90,000 for the receptor of parental S49 cells. Recent size determinations using photoaffinity labeling confirmed the reduced size of nt^i receptors and gave a more precise estimate of molecular weight of 39,000 to 42,000 (Nordeen *et al.*, 1981; Dellweg *et al.*, 1982). Higher ionic strength was found to be required to elute nt^i than wild-type receptor–hormone complexes from DNA–cellulose columns, indicating an increased affinity of nt^i receptors for DNA. This behavior led Yamamoto *et al.* (1976) to interpret the resistant phenotype of nt^i variants as resulting from an increased general affinity of these receptors for DNA. This interpretation needs, however, to be reexamined in the light of recent results.

All the studies mentioned above were carried out with cytosolic extracts of nt^i variants. Therefore, the size and properties of nuclear nt^i receptors had not been assessed. Recently Gruol *et al.* (1984b) used radiation inactivation and target analysis to compare the sizes of nt^i and wild-type receptors both in cytosol and nuclei. This technique (Lea, 1955) has been successfully used to measure the size of a large number of enzymes (for a review, see Kempner and Schlegel, 1979) and a variety of hormone receptors (Houslay *et al.*, 1977; Harmon *et al.*, 1980; Gruol and Kempner, 1982). It involves the exposure of frozen samples to a beam of high-energy electrons and the subsequent determination of a residual activity. An exponential decay of activity is observed as a function of the dose of radiation received, with the rate of inactivation being related to the mass of the functional unit measured. In this case, the activity measured was the ability of receptors to retain prebound ^{3}H-labeled triamcinolone acetonide, and the analysis measured the size of the hormone-binding unit of glucocorticoid receptors. This approach allows measurements of the size of receptor as it exists inside nuclei by labeling receptors in intact cells at 37°C, to allow nuclear translocation, and subsequently submitting the isolated nuclei to target analysis. This method, then, avoids the potential problem of receptor degradation, which could be introduced by extracting receptors from nuclei for analysis. For comparison, the same measurements were performed on cytosolic extracts prepared from cells labeled with hormone in the cold (4°C).

The results of this analysis are illustrated in Fig. 2. The rate of radiation inactivation of cytosolic nt^i receptors is considerably slower than that of wild-type cytosolic receptors, confirming the reduced size of cytosolic nt^i receptors. However, the rate of inactivation of nuclear nt^i receptors is not significantly different from that of wild-type receptors, indicating that nuclear nt^i receptors have the same target size as wild-type receptors. The values obtained for the size of these receptors, based on several determinations, are summarized in Table I. The size of wild-type receptors, whether nuclear or cytosolic, was calculated to be 75,000–79,000, a value that is in good agreement with estimates on the order of 90,000 (reviewed by Stevens *et al.*, 1983), the difference being most likely due to the dissimilar methodologies. In contrast, the size of the nt^i receptor was found to be very different depending on whether it was measured in cytosol or nuclei: while cytosolic nt^i receptors have a molecular weight of only 40,000, the nuclear nt^i receptors have a size of 72,000, which is, within experimental errors, indistinguishable from wild-type receptors. These results strongly indicate that the small form of nt^i receptors found in cytosol by us and by others results from proteolytic attack, while the native nt^i receptor has the same size as wild-type receptor and is protected from proteolysis after nuclear translocation. This suggests that the nt^i mutation has probably increased the receptor's susceptibility to proteolytic attack, rather than creating a deletion or nonsense mutation that would result in a truncated protein.

So far, all DNA and nuclear binding studies of nt^i receptors have been carried out with the small cytosolic form of these receptors, probably representing a proteolytic fragment. Therefore, these properties need to be investigated with the nuclear, presumably intact, form of nt^i receptors. Gruol *et al.* (1984a,b) compared some properties of translocated wild-type and nt^i receptors using preparations of isolated nuclei similar to those described

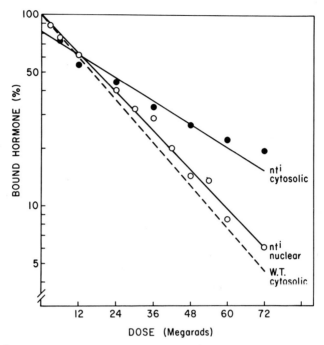

Fig. 2. Radiation inactivation of glucocorticoid receptors from wild-type cells and nt[i] variant. In all cases, binding of 1, 2, 4 N [³H] triamcinolone acetonide (TA) was carried out with intact cells: cytosolic extracts were prepared from cells labeled with [³H] TA in the cold (4°C), while nuclei were obtained from cells incubated with labeled hormone as 37°C, as described by Gruol *et al.* (1984b). After irradiation, the bound hormone retained was measured using hydroxyapatite in the case of cytosolic extracts and a filter binding assay in the case of nuclei. Each point represents the average of several measurements with nt[i] cytosol (●———●) or nt[i] nuclei (○———○). The dotted line represents the average slope obtained in several independent experiments with wild-type (W.T.) cytosol. [Adapted and redrawn from Gruol *et al.* (1984b).]

above, which contained the large form of nt[i] receptors. Significant differences were found in the release of wild-type and nt[i] receptors from nuclei by nuclease digestion, spermidine, and salt. A greater proportion of nt[i] receptors than of wild-type receptors can be released by nucleases and spermidine. Moreover, in contrast with studies showing that higher ionic strengths are required to release the (small form of) nt[i] receptors from DNA–cellulose, the translocated (intact) nt[i] receptors are *more sensitive* to release by salt than wild-type receptors. These studies suggest that at least a portion of the wild-type receptors are retained within the nucleus through a type of interaction that cannot be sustained by nt[i] receptors. Moreover, the interpretation of the nt[i] phenotype as resulting from increased DNA-binding affinity of the nt[i] receptors may not be valid, especially since Dellweg *et al.*

TABLE I

SIZE OF WILD-TYPE AND nt[i] VARIANT RECEPTOR ESTIMATED
BY RADIATION INACTIVATION[a]

Receptor		
Type	Localization	Molecular weight[b]
Wild type	Nuclear	75,000 ± 3,500 (4)
Wild type	Cytosolic	79,000 ± 3,200 (3)
nt[i]	Nuclear	72,000 ± 5,200 (3)
nt[i]	Cytosolic	40,000 ± 5,600 (2)

[a] Summarized from Gruol *et al.* (1984b).

[b] Mean ± standard deviation calculated from the number of determinations shown in parentheses.

(1982) showed that limited proteolysis of wild-type receptor also yields a
39,000-dalton steroid-binding fragment that has an increased affinity for
DNA indistinguishable from that of nt[i] receptor. Therefore, the increased
affinity for DNA observed *in vitro* for the small cytosolic form of nt[i] receptor
is not a characteristic resulting from the nt[i] mutation and cannot be imputed
as the cause of the observed phenotype. DNA binding studies of intact nt[i]
receptors remain to be done.

D. CHROMOSOME SEGREGATION

The amount of gene product present in a cell can be the consequence of
gene dosage resulting from events such as functional hemizygosity, gene
amplification, or chromosome loss. In the case of glucocorticoid receptors,
the functional hemizygosity of S49 cells for the structural gene encoding this
receptor (r^+/r^-) has been convincingly established (Section II,A). An
important consequence of the reduced amount of receptor in S49 cells is the
fact that these cells are less sensitive to dexamethasone-induced killing than
homozygous (r^+/r^+) W7 cells (Bourgeois and Newby, 1977). This indication
that intracellular glucocorticoid receptor concentration could limit the biological response was further investigated in cell hybrids (Bourgeois and
Newby, 1979). Hybrid clones carrying one, two, three, or four functional
copies of the receptor allele (r^+) were obtained by fusion between thymoma
lines that were either homozygous $(r^+/r^+$ or $r^-/r^-)$ or hemizygous
(r^+/r^-) for that gene. The receptor content of these hybrids reflected the
r^+ gene dosage, and a tight correlation was found between receptor concentration and level of sensitivity to dexamethasone. Remarkably, pseudo-

tetraploid hybrids containing a single copy of the r^+ allele $(1r^+/4n)$, and therefore 15,000 receptor sites per cell, were considerably more resistant to dexamethasone than pseudodiploid S49 cells $(1r^+/2n)$ that contain the same number of receptors (Bourgeois and Newby, 1979).

Another important observation made in these studies was that glucocorticoid-sensitive hybrids generated glucocorticoid-resistant variants at frequencies that were orders of magnitude higher than expected on the basis of the number of r^+ genes present in those cells (Bourgeois and Newby, 1979, 1980; Pfahl and Bourgeois, 1980). For example, glucocorticoid-resistant clones arose at frequencies of 10^{-6} to 10^{-5} from hybrids containing two functional receptor alleles $(2r^+/2r^-)$, while a frequency of $<1.2 \times 10^{-10}$ was observed in the case of the diploid W7 cell line, which also contains two copies of that allele (r^+/r^+) (Huet-Minkowski *et al.*, 1981). Moreover, hybrids containing a single copy of the r^+ allele generated resistant clones at very high frequencies, on the order of 10^{-3} to 10^{-2}. This suggested that different mechanisms give rise to the dexamethasone-resistant phenotype in pseudodiploid lymphoid cell lines and in pseudotetraploid hybrids of these cell lines. Segregation of chromosome(s) carrying the r^+ allele was demonstrated to be the major mechanism responsible for generating glucocorticoid resistance in pseudotetraploid lymphoid cells. Glucocorticoid-resistant segregants were shown to have lost functional receptors, and karyotypic analysis demonstrated that loss of receptors from hybrids containing two r^+ alleles was accompanied by a reduction in the modal number of chromosomes from 80 to 78. A similar phenomenon was later observed in the case of hybrids containing four copies of the r^+ allele but only two functional copies of a gene (l^+) encoding another function essential for glucocorticoid induced lysis (Gasson and Bourgeois, 1983b). In that case, the dexamethasone-resistant segregants retained all four copies of the r^+ gene, while losing two chromosomes presumably carrying the "lysis" loci (Section III,C).

These observations provide a reasonable explanation for the early observation by Sibley and Tomkins (1974b) of S49 variants that were called "deathless" because they appear to contain normal receptor with high nuclear transfer capacity. While several of the variants originally classified as deathless were later found to belong to the nt^i class (e.g., clone 55R), two clones (61.4R and 61.10R) remained in the so-called deathless class because their receptor was indistinguishable from wild-type receptor by all tests used (Yamamoto *et al.*, 1976). In view of the functional hemizygosity of the r^+ gene in the S49 line, it appears improbable that this line would yield variants having a defect in a function other than the receptor, and a more likely explanation for the nature of these two deathless variants is required. It should be emphasized that these two clones were both derived from a pseudotetraploid (S49.1A.61) parental line (Sibley and Tomkins, 1974b). The

S49 cell line established in culture by Horibata and Harris (1970) is pseudo-diploid, with a modal number of 40 chromosomes. However, as is commonly observed in tissue cultures, pseudotetraploid cells spontaneously appear in the population after prolonged growth without cloning and eventually supplant diploid cells. The pseudotetraploid parental line S49.1A.61, having a modal number of 80 chromosomes, resulted from subcloning of such a population (Sibley and Tomkins, 1974a). In view of the functional hemizygosity of the diploid S49 cell line at the receptor locus (Bourgeois and Newby, 1977), the tetraploid S49.1A.61 clone must have contained only two functional r^+ alleles. As discussed above, such tetraploid cell lines are unstable and segregate chromosomes at high frequency. Since the loss of one r^+ allele from a tetraploid line occurs at frequencies on the order of 10^{-3} to 10^{-2}, the two deathless variants are most likely segregants, having lost one r^+ allele and retained a single copy of the r^+ gene. The presence of a single gene dose of receptors in a tetraploid cell $(1r^+/4n)$ is known to result in considerable resistance to dexamethasone (Bourgeois and Newby, 1979). Therefore, it appears likely that $1r^+/4n$ segregants would yield colonies in the presence of 0.1 μM dexamethasone, the hormone concentration used in the selection of the deathless variants, although these colonies may be smaller and appear at lower plating efficiency than fully resistant variants. The interpretation of the two deathless variants in terms of $1r^+/4n$ segregants predicts that these clones should be only partially resistant to dexamethasone and contain 15,000 receptors/cell, which would, obviously, be wild type. Unfortunately, no data have been reported in the literature about the level of resistance of these clones, and their receptor content has not been measured quantitatively, since the two putative deathless clones in which Sibley and Tomkins (1974b) measured dexamethasone binding turned out later to belong to the nt^i class (Yamamoto *et al.*, 1976). Furthermore, complementation analysis was not carried out with these clones because of their tetraploidy. As stated by Sibley and Tomkins (1974b): "Thus, the phenotype originally designated 'deathless' (where binding and transfer were normal) has not been isolated."

E. FUTURE DIRECTIONS

One can foresee that, in the near future, molecular cloning of genes encoding the glucocorticoid receptor as well as the other steroid receptors will be achieved. Moreover, an increasing number of cloned hormone-responsive genes will become available. The isolation of somatic cell variants defective in receptor or in hormonal response will, then, be replaced by *in vitro* mutagenesis of cloned genes. Specific base substitutions in genes encoding receptor will be used to introduce amino acid substitutions in various regions of the protein. This approach, combined with hormone and DNA binding studies, will establish the correlation between receptor structure and function. Transfection of receptor or hormone-responsive genes into heterologous species or cell types will provide an additional tool to examine the specificity and mechanism of hormone-induced responses.

III. EPIGENETIC CONTROL OF "LYSIS" FUNCTION

A. T-CELL MATURATION AND GLUCOCORTICOID RESISTANCE

The differentiation of T-lymphocytes in the thymus involves a coordinated series of events during which large, immature cortical thymocytes appear to give rise to smaller, more mature medullary cells, which are thought to be the precursors of immunocompetent T-cells in the periphery. Changes in the pattern of expression of several cell surface antigens are seen during thymocyte maturation; in general, immature cortical cells express higher levels of Thy-1, TL, and ThB than more mature medullary cells, which themselves express higher levels of H2 antigens (Cantor and Weissman, 1976; Chen *et al.*, 1983). In addition, some enzymes, such as terminal deoxynucleotidyl transferase (TdT), appear to be preferentially expressed in immature thymocytes (Rothenberg, 1980). Among the many changes involved in T-cell differentiation is the apparent transition from glucocorticoid sensitivity to resistance; immature cortical cells are glucocorticoid sensitive, whereas those in the medulla are glucocorticoid resistant, as are circulating peripheral T-lymphocytes (Claman, 1972).

Genetic analyses of glucocorticoid-resistant variants, derived from sensitive cell lines either spontaneously or by mutagenic treatments, have revealed many important aspects of the receptor–hormone interaction. However, no defects in functions other than the glucocorticoid receptor have been proven, by complementation analysis, to exist in glucocorticoid-resistant cell lines generated *in vitro* (discussed in Sections II and V). For this reason, it is important to examine and characterize the types of glucocorticoid resistance that arise *in vivo*. By screening thymocyte cell lines, it is possible to study the mechanisms by which the cells, from which the cell line arose, have attained hormone resistance. Since the more mature immunocompetent thymocytes are resistant to glucocorticoid hormones *in vivo*, at least some cell lines should display this phenotype, which probably does not involve a genetic alteration, but more likely an epigenetic change(s).

B. Glucocorticoid-Induced Responses in SAK Cells

The SAK8 cell line was derived from a spontaneous T-lymphoma in an AKR/J mouse (Gasson and Bourgeois, 1983b). Figure 3 shows a comparison of the effect of dexamethasone on the growth of the SAK8 line and on the growth of W7 wild-type cells and a receptor-deficient W7 variant. SAK8 cells are not lysed by glucocorticoid hormones, but, intriguingly, an effect of the hormone is seen on the growth rate as well as the final cell density (Panel C), suggesting that these cells contain functional glucocorticoid receptors. The growth characteristics of SAK8 cells are not due to a mixed population of sensitive and resistant cells, because the original cloned cell line, SAK, was

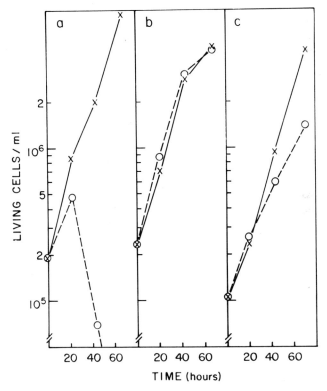

FIG. 3. Effect of dexamethasone on the growth of three murine T-lymphoid cell lines. Cells were grown in Dulbecco's modified Eagle's medium containing 10% fetal calf serum in the absence of hormone (X———X) or in the presence of 10 μM dexamethasone (O- - -O). Living cells were monitored by Trypan blue exclusion and counted. (a) W7 wild-type line. (b) Receptor-deficient W7 variant. (c) SAK line. [From Gasson and Bourgeois (1983a).]

subcloned, and all of the clones (of which SAK8 is one) displayed identical growth properties in the presence of the steroid.

Scatchard analyses of glucocorticoid binding data showed that the SAK8 cells contain approximately 30,000 binding sites per cell with a K_a of 1×10^8 M^{-1}. In addition, approximately 65% of the receptor–hormone complexes are translocated into the nucleus (Gasson and Bourgeois, 1983b). These values are strikingly similar to those obtained for the glucocorticoid-sensitive W7 cell line (Bourgeois and Newby, 1977); thus, no gross receptor defects could be detected in SAK8 cells that would account for the resistance to cytolysis.

In addition to the effects of dexamethasone on the growth properties of

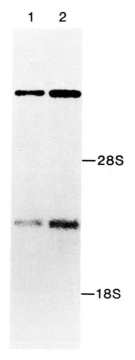

FIG. 4. Induction of leukemia virus mRNA by dexamethasone in SAK8 cells. Cells were incubated in medium in the absence of hormone (lane 1) or in the presence of 0.1 μM dexamethasone for 6 hours (lane 2). RNA was prepared, and mRNA was selected using oligo(dT) cellulose as described elsewhere (Wahl *et al.*, 1979). RNA samples were denatured in glyoxal, fractionated in a 1% agarose gel, transferred to nitrocellulose paper, and probed with cDNA made to Moloney leukemia virus RNA (generously provided by Dr. Inder Verma, Salk Institute). The transfer was washed, and exposed film was used to quantitate the enhancement in viral mRNA accumulation. The positions of the 18 S and 28 S ribosomal RNA markers are indicated.

SAK8 cells, other responses could be detected at the molecular level. Work by Palmiter and collaborators has shown that expression of the metallothionein gene is regulated in a number of cell types by glucocorticoids as well as metal ions (Mayo and Palmiter, 1981). Following incubation of SAK8 cells with 10^{-6} *M* dexamethasone for 20 hours, metallothionein mRNA levels increase from approximately 90 to 220 molecules/cell (Gasson and Bourgeois, 1983b). This effect is similar to that seen with W7 cells after demethylation of the metallothionein gene by 5-azacytidine (Compere and Palmiter, 1981); no metallothionein expression is seen in W7 cells prior to demethylation.

A number of investigators have reported that glucocorticoids enhance the synthesis of type C retroviruses (Ihle *et al.*, 1975; Paran *et al.*, 1973; Dunn *et al.*, 1975). AKR/J mice have stably integrated copies of murine leukemia virus (a type C retrovirus) in their genome, and the SAK8 cell line constitutively expresses viral proteins and mRNA (Fig. 4, lane 1). The upper band in Fig. 4 consists of genomic viral mRNA (approximately 9 kbp in length), and the lower band is a processed form of the mRNA, which encodes the envelope glycoprotein (Gielkens, 1976). Incubation of SAK8 cell with 0.1 μM dexamethasone for 6 hours results in a threefold increase in both genomic and processed viral mRNAs (Fig. 4, lane 2).

The increases in metallothionein and murine leukemia virus mRNA induced by dexamethasone, together with the hormone binding data and effects on cell growth, provide strong evidence that the glucocorticoid receptors in SAK8 cells are functional and that these cells are dexamethasone resistant due to a defect in another function which we have designated the "lysis" function. A genetic analysis has been used to demonstrate the existence of this function.

C. Genetic Analysis of Glucocorticoid Resistance in SAK Cells

To determine whether the glucocorticoid resistance of SAK cells is dominant or recessive, SAK cells were fused with dexamethasone-sensitive W7 cells and the resulting hybrids were tested for their hormone responsiveness. Figure 5A shows the growth of the SAK (dex^r) and W7 (dex^s) parent cell lines and one of the hybrid clones in 10 μM dexamethasone. Analysis of several hybrid clones showed that the glucocorticoid resistance in SAK cells is recessive, since the hybrids are dexamethasone sensitive. As shown in Figure 5A, the kinetics of cell killing is not as rapid in the hybrid as in the dexamethasone-sensitive W7 parent. One possible explanation for this observation is that both parental cell lines contribute functional glucocorticoid

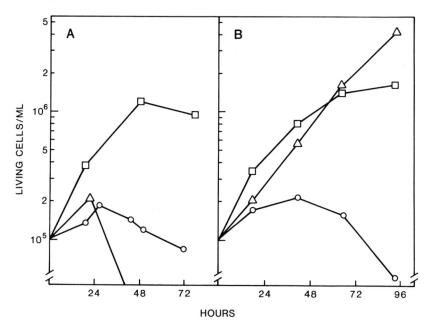

FIG. 5. Dominance and complementation analysis of the glucocorticoid resistance of the SAK cell line. Growth was monitored as described in Fig. 3 in medium containing 10 μM dexamethasone. Hybrids were obtained as described elsewhere (Gasson and Bourgeois, 1983b). (A) The parental cell lines SAK (□) and wild-type W7 (r^+/r^+) (△) were used to generate the hybrid (○). (B) The parental cell lines SAK (□) and a receptor-deficient W7 variant (r^-/r^-) (△) were used to generate the hybrid (○). [Panel B from Gasson and Bourgeois (1983b). Redrawn from *The Journal of Cell Biology*, 1983, Volume 96, p. 412 by copyright permission of the Rockefeller University Press.)

receptor, but only the W7 parent contributes functional lysis loci. Indeed, 60,000 glucocorticoid binding sites were found per hybrid cell, the sum of the number of binding sites contributed by SAK and W7. This fusion can be summarized as follows, where r^+ represents functional glucocorticoid receptor loci and l^+ represents functional lysis loci.

$$\text{SAK}(2r^+/2l^-) \times \text{W7}(2r^+/2l^+) \rightarrow (4r^+/2l^+2l^-)$$
$$\langle\text{dex}^r\rangle \qquad \langle\text{dex}^s\rangle \qquad \langle\text{dex}^s\rangle$$

The observation that glucocorticoid resistance in SAK is recessive supports the idea that these cells are resistant to lysis due to a defect or absence of a function in the lytic pathway, rather than the generation of some "protective substance" that inhibits cytolysis. In order to prove that this defect exists in a function distinct from the glucocorticoid receptor, complementation analysis was performed. Dexamethasone-resistant SAK cells were fused with a variant of the W7 cell line that is resistant due to the absence of measurable glucocorticoid receptor. The resulting hybrids were tested for their response to dexamethasone. Figure 5B shows that, while both parental cell lines grow in the presence of 1 μM dexamethasone, the hybrid is lysed. This positive complementation phenomenon was seen with all of the hybrid clones tested from this fusion. Analyses of the receptor content of the hybrids showed that they contain approximately 30,000 binding sites per cell—the number of binding sites contributed by the SAK parent. Since the variant W7 parent has no detectable hormone binding and no new receptor sites are activated in the hybrid, this parent must be contributing the lysis function, absent in the SAK cells, to regenerate dexamethasone sensitivity in the hybrid.

$$\text{SAK}(2r^+/2l^-) \times \text{W7}(2r^-/2l^+) \rightarrow (2r^+2r^-/2l^+2l^-)$$
$$\langle\text{dex}^r\rangle \qquad\qquad \langle\text{dex}^r\rangle \qquad\qquad \langle\text{dex}^s\rangle$$

In order to obtain further genetic proof for the existence of the lysis function, it should be possible to obtain dex^r derivatives of the dex^s hybrids by segregation of chromosomes bearing the "lysis loci" with no loss of glucocorticoid receptor (assuming that the lysis locus is not linked to the receptor locus). The hybrid between the dex^r variant W7 and SAK would not be a good choice, because it contains only two copies of functional receptor genes; thus, the likelihood of achieving hormone resistance through the loss of receptor would be as great as through the loss of lysis loci, making the results difficult to interpret. However, the hybrid between the dex^s W7 and SAK contains four copies of the receptor locus (approximately 60,000 binding sites/cell) and only 2 copies of the lysis locus: therefore segregation of l should be favored.

Dex^r derivatives of dex^s hybrids containing four copies of the glucocorticoid receptor locus were selected at a frequency of approximately 2.5×10^{-5}; the growth of one such derivative in 1 μM dexamethasone is shown in Fig. 6A. Scatchard analysis of the glucocorticoid binding data showed that this resistant derivative retained all four copies of the receptor gene. The modal number of chromosomes in the dex^s hybrid is 80 (Fig. 6B). In the dex^r derivative (Fig. 6C), the modal number of chromosomes has shifted to 78, consistent with the idea that two chromosomes carrying the lysis loci (originating from the W7 parent) have been segregated, giving rise to a dex^r derivative.

$$(4r^+/2l^+2l^-) \rightarrow (4r^+/2l^-)$$
$$\langle\text{dex}^s\rangle \qquad\quad \langle\text{dex}^r\rangle$$

In summary, these genetic analyses of glucocorticoid resistance in SAK cells show that this type of glucocorticoid resistance is recessive (Fig. 5A)

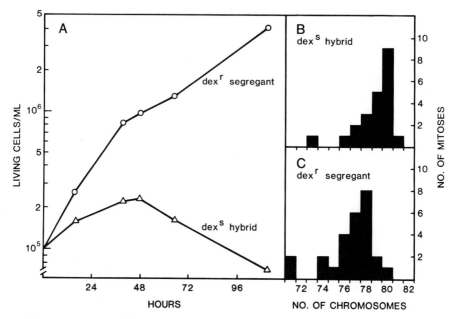

FIG. 6. Segregation of the "lysis" function. The dex^s hybrid was constructed by fusion of SAK cells with wild-type W7 cells, as described elsewhere (Gasson and Bourgeois, 1983b). The dex^r segregant was obtained by cloning in the presence of 10 μM dexamethasone. (A) Growth in medium containing 10 μM dexamethasone. (B, C) Metaphase spreads were prepared as described elsewhere (Bourgeois and Newby, 1977), and the chromosomes were counted. [From Gasson and Bourgeois (1983b). Adapted and redrawn from *The Journal of Cell Biology*, 1983, Volume 96, p. 413 by copyright permission of The Rockefeller University Press.]

and that SAK cells are not dexamethasone resistant due to a receptor defect (Fig. 5B). The defect must therefore be in another step, designated the lysis function. While genetic complementation demonstrates the existence of that function, this analysis does not distinguish whether it is encoded by one or several genetic loci. These results, then, raised the question of the mechanism by which the lysis function was inactivated. The next series of experiments was designed to determine whether SAK8 cells became dex^r through a mutation or through an epigenetic process.

D. ROLE OF DNA METHYLATION IN GLUCOCORTICOID RESISTANCE

The most common DNA base modification found in higher eukaryotes is methylation of the 5-position of cytosine residues. Approximately 2–5% of cytosine residues in vertebrate DNA are methylated; the vast majority of 5-methylcytosines exist in the 5'-M^{5}C-G-3' dinucleotide (reviewed by Ehrlich and Wang, 1981). No methylcytosines have been found in insects or yeast; thus, the role of this modified base cannot be universal in eukaryotes.

The pattern of DNA methylation in an organism is tissue specific. Individual patterns are preserved during cell division by a "maintenance" methylase, which methylates the newly synthesized DNA strand at sites that are methylated in the template strand (hemimethylated regions). The observation that the pattern of DNA methylation is tissue specific suggests a role for DNA methylation in differentiation and gene expression. Although the correlation is not perfect, numerous studies on viral and cellular genes have demonstrated a correlation between DNA hypomethylation and gene expression (reviewed by Doerfler, 1981; Razin and Riggs, 1980). Possible mechanisms for the effects of DNA methylation on gene expression could involve conformational changes (transition from B to Z DNA) and/or changes in the affinity of DNA-binding proteins. An attractive model for steroid hormone–induced differentiation involves heritable changes in methylation patterns of specific genes resulting from the interaction of the receptor–hormone complex with DNA. This hypothesis is supported by changes observed in the methylation pattern of hormone-responsive genes following steroid treatment (Wilks *et al.*, 1982; Mermod *et al.*, 1983; Burch and Weintraub, 1983).

The analogs 5-azacytidine and 5-azadeoxycytidine cause clonally heritable undermethylation of DNA, which often results in changes in gene expression. These compounds have been used in a number of systems to activate previously unexpressed genes (Taylor and Jones, 1979; Groudine *et al.*, 1981; Harris, 1982; Compere and Palmiter, 1981). Data from numerous investigators suggest that DNA hypomethylation may be necessary for expression of specific genes in certain tissues, but not sufficient for expression of those genes in other tissues.

Since DNA methylation may play a role in gene expression and differentiation, and since mature T-lymphocytes become glucocorticoid resistant, it is possible that DNA methylation could inactivate genes involved in the cytolytic response in mature T-cells, leaving receptor genes functional and capable of mediating other hormone responses. The SAK cells that may have arisen from a tumor that was glucocorticoid resistant *in vivo* were an obvious system in which to test this hypothesis.

SAK8 cells were treated overnight with a concentration of 5-azacytidine that only slightly affected cell growth, washed, and allowed to recover until the normal growth rate resumed (usually in about 48 hours). Cells from the recovered population were cloned by limiting dilution, and subclones were picked at about 10 days. Individual subclones were tested for their responsiveness to dexamethasone, and in several experiments 10% or more of the subclones had become glucocorticoid sensitive (see Fig. 7A, 1 week). Control experiments showed that dex[s] derivatives did not preexist at this frequency among the SAK8 cells, but were a result of the treatment with 5-azacytidine. This result suggests that genes involved in the lysis function are intact in SAK8 cells but are inactivated by DNA methylation. Thus, in these cells the lysis function appears to be under epigenetic control–DNA methylation.

The dex[s] clones derived from treatment of SAK8 cells with 5-azacytidine were maintained in the absence of dexamethasone but were tested frequently for continued hormone sensitivity to ascertain the stability of the

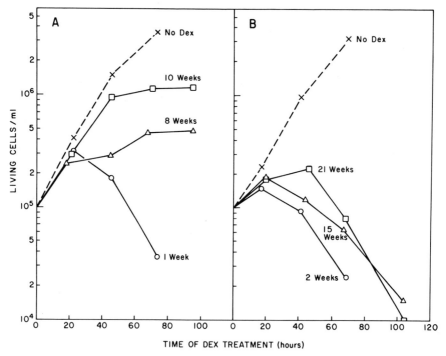

FIG. 7. Reversion of SAK8 clones after 5-azacytidine treatment. SAK8 cells were treated for 13 hours with 3 μM 5-azacytidine, allowed to recover, and subcloned, as described elsewhere (Gasson *et al.*, 1983). Dexamethasone-sensitive subclones were maintained in culture in the absence of hormone, and aliquots of the cultures were tested for growth in the presence of 1 μM dexamethasone at weekly or longer intervals. The growth in the absence of hormone (dotted line) did not change with time. (A) Unstable subclone A2. (B) Stable subclone A95. [Panel A from Gasson *et al.* (1983). Reprinted by permission from *Nature*, Volume 302, p. 621. Copyright © 1983 Macmillan Journals Limited.]

newly acquired dex^s phenotype. Figure 7A shows one clone, which, over a period of 2–3 months, reverted back to dex^r. One possible mechanism for reversion to dex^r would be remethylation of genes involved in the lysis function that were demethylated as a result of treatment with 5-azacytidine. This would require *de novo* methylation of regions of DNA containing genes involved in the lysis response rather than the mere maintenance of the methylation pattern that occurs during cell division. It was possible to determine whether a large amount of *de novo* methylation had occurred by using HPLC to measure total levels of 5-methylcytosine in cellular DNA during the reversion process (Gasson *et al.*, 1983). The results showed that, in untreated SAK8 cells, approximately 4.5% of the cytosine residues are methylated (a typical result for mammalian DNA), but after 5-azacytidine treatment, massive demethylation occurs. One week after growing up the dex^s clone shown in Fig. 7A, only 2.5% of the cytosine residues were methylated, a 50% decrease from untreated cells. However, after 9 weeks in culture (well into the reversion process), 3.8% of cytosine residues existed as 5-methylcytosine. These results clearly demonstrate striking demethylation by 5-azacytidine, which correlates with dexamethasone sensitivity, followed by *de novo* methylation, which correlates with reversion to dexamethasone resistance. If spontaneous remethylation causes the reversion from dexamethasone sensitivity to resistance, it should be possible to again make the dex^r revertants dex^s by treatment with 5-azacytidine. Such is the case; treatment of revertant cells with dexamethasone in the presence of 5-azacytidine results in a reappearance of the sensitive phenotype (Gasson *et al.*, 1983).

Reversion of dex^s derivatives of SAK8 to the dex^r phenotype is a frequent event. Four of five dex^s clones tested, generated in three different experiments, reverted to dex^r over periods of 1–2 months; the clone shown in Fig. 7A was thawed three times, and on all three occasions it reverted to dex^r within 4–10 weeks. Direct microscopic observations have shown that many dex^s clones revert to dex^r within the first week of culture. Of all the dex^s derivatives of SAK8 characterized, only one has been found that does not revert to dex^r within a short period of time. Figure 7B shows a clone that remains dex^s for over 5 months after 5-azacytidine treatment. Several hypotheses are being examined to explain this phenotype. Possible explanations include that perhaps these cells are incapable of *de novo* remethylation, or that a change in sequence or conformation of the control region of the lysis gene prevents its methylation.

It is tempting to speculate that DNA methylation plays a role in the acquisition of glucocorticoid resistance during T-cell maturation *in vivo* and that SAK8 cells were derived from a tumor that was glucocorticoid resistant in the animal. However, recent results by MacLeod *et al.* (1984) using a different AKR T-lymphoma cell line provide another possible explanation for the dex^r phenotype of SAK8 cells. The SL12 tumor displayed heterogeneity with regard to glucocorticoid sensitivity, giving rise to dexamethasone-sensitive and dexamethasone-resistant subclones. Cloned dexamethasone-sensitive SL12 cells generate *in vitro* spontaneous dexamethasone-resistant subclones, which, as is the case with SAK8 cells, can be converted to dexamethasone sensitivity by treatment with 5-azacytidine. Furthermore, these dexamethasone-resistant clones display coordinate changes in cell surface antigens, specifically reduced Thy-1 and ThB expression. Thus, the SL12 tumor provides evidence for a role of DNA methylation in tumor heterogeneity, and this system may well provide insights into T-cell differentiation. In addition, these data raise the possibility that SAK8 cells may have become glucocorticoid resistant *in vitro* before the tumor was subcloned and assayed for hormone sensitivity.

Genetic complementation studies will determine whether lysis-defective SAK8 cells and SL12 cells share precisely the same defect or whether these lines have become dex^r through methylation of different genes in the cytolytic pathway. The nature of the lysis function remains unknown; however, the existence of these dex^r cell lines strongly suggests that it cannot be a vital function and that it must be induced or activated by glucocorticoids. Recent work in two laboratories has suggested that an endonuclease activity may be involved in programmed cell death (Wyllie, 1980; Duke *et al.*, 1983; Cohen and Duke, 1984). The possible role of this nuclease in the dexamethasone-induced cytolytic response of T-cell lines remains to be investigated.

IV. MEMBRANE PERMEABILITY AND DEXAMETHASONE RESISTANCE

Entry of glucocorticoids into cells is, obviously, required for binding of cytoplasmic receptors. It has generally been assumed that steroids enter cells by passive diffusion through the cell membrane by virtue of their small size and lipophilic properties. The role of passive diffusion has, however, not been demonstrated. Some steroid-transport systems have been postulated, but these have remained ill-defined (for reviews, see Ballard, 1979; Duval *et al.*, 1983). The steroid entry process has received relatively little attention, since it was not thought to be a rate-limiting step in steroid hormone action. None of the glucocorticoid-resistant variant selected from the S49 and W7 cell lines at high concentrations of dexamethasone (0.1–10 μM) resulted from impaired hormone entry. However, recent evidence demonstrates that W7 variants with reduced permeability to dexamethasone can be obtained by selection for resistance to low concentrations of the hormone (Johnson *et al.*, 1984).

As mentioned in Section II,A, selection at dexamethasone concentrations between 1 and 10 nM yielded W7 variants having half the parental amount of receptors as the result of the inactivation of one allele (r^+/r^-) encoding receptor (Bourgeois and Newby, 1977). However, several of the partially resistant W7 variants obtained appeared to have more than half the parental amount of receptors. One such variant, MS23, was recently characterized and found to have acquired a permeability barrier preventing dexamethasone from accumulating inside cells at the same concentration as that of the incubation medium. As a result, the MS23 variant was found, in whole-cell hormone-binding assays, to contain the parental amount of receptors (30,000 binding sites per cell) with a reduced *apparent* affinity for dexamethasone, but unchanged affinity for triamcinolone acetonide. However, when measured in cytosolic extracts, the affinities of the MS23 receptor for both dexamethasone and triamcinolone acetonide were indistinguishable from those of the wild-type W7 receptor. These results were in agreement with the phenotype of the MS23 variant, which had acquired partial resistance to dexamethasone but had retained unchanged sensitivity to triamcinolone acetonide.

The hypothesis that the MS23 variant had acquired a permeability barrier predicted that this variant should have increased resistance to drugs unrelated to dexamethasone but known to enter cells by passive diffusion. This prediction was fulfilled, since MS23 cells have increased resistance to puromycin and colchicine. These results are summarized in Table II, which shows that inhibition of growth of an MS23 population by 50% required an approximately 2-fold higher concentration of dexamethasone, a 12-fold higher concentration of puromycin, and a 5-fold higher concentration of colchicine than required for a similar effect on wild-type W7 cells.

Cross-resistance to unrelated drugs resulting from altered membrane permeability has been observed in a number of cell types, including Chinese hamster ovary cells (Bech-Hansen *et al.*, 1976) and lung cells (Garman and

TABLE II

CROSS-RESISTANCE OF W7 VARIANTS TO DEXAMETHASONE AND OTHER DRUGS[a]

Cell line	Dexamethasone (nM)	Puromycin (μM)	Colchicine (ng/ml)	Triamcinolone acetonide (nM)
W7TB	2.1	1.0	8.8	0.85
MS23	3.9	12.5	44	0.74
S7CD-5	140	180	450	1.3

[a] Summarized from Johnson *et al.* (1984). The results are expressed as the concentration of drug required to inhibit growth by 50%.

Center, 1982), neuroblastoma cells (Baskin *et al.*, 1981), L-cells (Debenham *et al.*, 1982), CCRF-CEM human leukemic cells (Beck *et al.*, 1979), and murine L5178Y lymphoblasts (Kessel and Bosmann, 1970; Hill and Whelan, 1982). However, resistance to dexamethasone could not be investigated in nonlymphoid cells, which are not killed by glucocorticoids. As for the CCRF-CEM and L5178Y lymphoid cells used in previous studies, their sensitivity to dexamethasone was not assessed. Since both these lines give rise spontaneously to dexamethasone-resistant variants (Harmon and Thompson, 1981; Lampkin and Potter, 1958), the parental cells used in multidrug resistance studies could have been resistant to dexamethasone because of receptor or other defects. In a number of systems, drug resistance could be increased by stepwise selection in progressively higher drug concentrations, and the multidrug resistance phenotype associated with altered membrane permeability was found to be correlated with increased expression of a 170K-dalton plasma membrane glycoprotein (P-glycoprotein) (Kartner *et al.*, 1983). These results are consistent with a mechanism involving gene amplification leading to overproduction of the P-glycoprotein.

To examine the possibility that a similar mechanism could confer dexamethasone resistance and cross-resistance to the MS23 variant, these cells were submitted to seven rounds of selection in increasing concentrations of dexamethasone and colchicine. This combination of two drugs was used to avoid glucocorticoid receptor mutants that would arise by selection in dexamethasone alone and possible microtubule mutants that could result from selection in colchicine alone. Clones isolated at several stages of this selection were found to have acquired increased resistance to dexamethasone and cross-resistance to unrelated drugs. Table II shows that clone S7CD-5, isolated from the MS23 variant after seven stages of selection in dexamethasone and colchicine, had considerably increased resistance to puromycin and colchicine. This clone was found to have also acquired increased resistance to daunomycin, gramicidin, and vincristine (data not shown). Strikingly, resistance to triamcinolone acetonide did not develop (Table II). In whole-cell assays, binding of [^{3}H]dexamethasone to S7CD-5 cells was undetectable, while binding of [^{3}H]triamcinolone acetonide was normal. In cytosolic extracts of these cells, receptors with normal affinity for both dexamethasone and triamcinolone acetonide were found. The observation that permeability and sensitivity to triamcinolone acetonide are not affected in these variant cells was unexpected, since this glucocorticoid is structurally related to dexamethasone. Perhaps some physicochemical properties of these two steroids are sufficiently dissimilar to result in differential effects of membrane changes, although the possibility that these two glucocorticoids enter these cells by distinct mechanisms has not been eliminated. However, Chinese hamster ovary cell variants can also display considerable differences in resistance to two closely related drugs, colchicine and colcemid, which have a similar mode of action (Bech-Hansen *et al.*, 1976).

The rate of uptake of [³H]puromycin was greatly reduced compared to the parental W7 line in MS23 cells and was further decreased in the S7CD-5 derivatives resulting from seven stages of selection. Procaine, a membrane-active anesthetic, potentiates uptake of dexamethasone and puromycin in S7CD-5 cells. These results support the view that dexamethasone enters these cells by passive diffusion and demonstrate that membrane permeability can be a rate-limiting step in steroid hormone action. Alterations in permeability are the basis for a new type of glucocorticoid resistance in lymphoid cells, namely resistance to dexamethasone and unrelated drugs, but not to triamcinolone acetonide. The level of resistance of these variants to other glucocorticoids remains to be assessed. Although the observation of stepwise increase in resistance is suggestive of a gene amplification event, this mechanism has not been established in this case, and the nature of the membrane change involved remains to be elucidated.

V. UNIDENTIFIED DETERMINANTS OF GLUCOCORTICOID SENSITIVITY

Since all variants derived so far by selection for full resistance to dexamethasone *in vitro* result from receptor defects (see Section II,A), other approaches have been taken to search for new types of murine (Mermod *et al.*, 1981; Danielson *et al.*, 1983) and human T-cell (Zawydiwski *et al.*, 1983) variants. In the three systems described below, selection for glucocorticoid resistance *in vitro* was either avoided or combined with a procedure aimed at retaining functional receptor. Although the nature of the variants obtained is still uncertain, these recent results will be briefly reviewed as they illustrate alternative approaches, which could be applicable to other systems, and their limitations.

A. SUPERSENSITIVE VARIANTS

The rationale for the selection of variants that are supersensitive rather than resistant to dexamethasone is that defects in a nonreceptor function involved in the lytic response would be lethal if that function is vital to the cell. Therefore, hormone-resistant variants in which such a function has been inactivated would not be found, while variants in which the activity of that function has been amplified might be obtained and could display increased hormone sensitivity. The selection used (J.-J. Mermod and S. Bourgeois, unpublished results) was based on the finding that dexamethasone delays murine T-cell lines in the G-1 phase of the cell cycle and that the delayed cells are viable and can be rescued. Moreover, dexamethasone-resistant cells are not delayed, while increased sensitivity to the hormone can be expected to cause longer arrest in G-1. After release of the G-1 block, cells entering S phase were killed by cytosine arabinoside, whereas cells delayed in G-1 by dexamethasone survived this suicide selection.

This procedure was applied to two glucocorticoid-sensitive cell lines, W7 and T_1M_1b, using several rounds of selection. Among the surviving populations, supersensitive clones were found that are killed faster and are sensitive to lower hormone concentrations than wild-type cells (Mermod $et\ al.$, 1981). Figure 8 illustrates the phenotype of two supersensitive clones obtained, one from each cell line. Their glucocorticoid receptor was found to be indistinguishable from that of the parental lines in terms of dexamethasone receptor sites per cell, affinity for dexamethasone, and nuclear transfer capacity. No significant changes were observed in nuclear fragility, glucose uptake, or metabolism. No increase in membrane permeability could be detected in the supersensitive W7 variant using the procedure of Lalande $et\ al.$ (1981), which measures the kinetics of uptake of the dye Hoescht 33342. However, cross-sensitivity to the drugs tested in the case of the MS23 variant (Section IV) was not assessed, and this biological test could conceivably be more sensitive than the dye uptake assay. Therefore, the possibility that supersensitive variants result from a subtle increase in membrane permeability has not been eliminated.

It is not known whether the basis for the supersensitive phenotype is genetic or epigenetic. Since these variants resulted from several rounds of enrichment rather than a one-step selection, the frequency at which they arise cannot be accurately estimated. The facts that they were derived without mutagenic treatment of the cells and that they were obtained repeatedly suggest that their frequency is considerably higher than expected for mutational events. Gene amplification or DNA demethylation are possible mechanisms that could have led to overproduction of a determinant of the lytic response. While binding assays demonstrate that receptor is not overproduced, the possibility exists that increased expression of the lysis gene, demonstrated to be active in W7 cells and inactivated by DNA methylation in SAK8 cells (see Section III,C), could be responsible for the supersensitive phenotype. Conversely, spontaneous $de\ novo$ DNA methylation could have taken place, as has been observed $in\ vitro$ in SL12 cells (Section III,D). In that instance, a reduction in the expression of a gene encoding a membrane glycoprotein affecting permeability could have taken place, resulting in increased permeability to dexamethasone (Section IV). At any rate, the supersensitive phenotype appears stable, and our knowledge of the role of a lysis

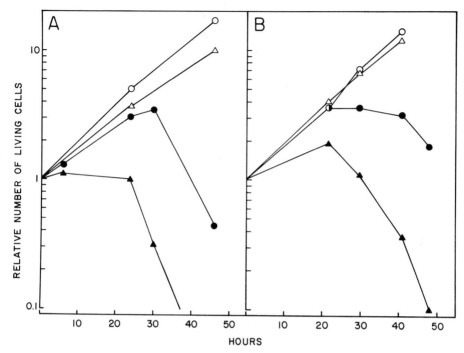

FIG. 8. Phenotype of supersensitive variants. The growth conditions and counting of living cells were as described in Fig. 3. Cells were plated at approximately 10^5 cells/ml, and the results are expressed as number of living cells per milliliter relative to the inoculum. Open symbols indicate growth in the absence of dexamethasone; closed symbols indicate growth in the presence of 0.1 μM dexamethasone. (A) Parent W7 cell line ($\bigcirc$, $\bullet$); supersensitive derivative W7 Dex^{ss} ($\triangle$, $\blacktriangle$). (B) Parent T_1M_1 cell line ($\bigcirc$, $\bullet$); supersensitive derivative T_1M_1 Dex^{ss} ($\triangle$, $\blacktriangle$). (Reprinted with permission from *Journal of Steroid Biochemistry*, Volume 15, by J. J. Mermod, L. Intriere, C. MacLeod, and S. Bourgeois, "Characterization of a new type of thymoma variants supersensitive to dexamethasone," 1981, Pergamon Press Ltd.)

function, of permeability, and of DNA methylation in the cytolytic response suggests testable hypotheses.

B. Variants Expressing Glucocorticoid-Induced MMTV Gene Products

The procedure described by Danielsen *et al.* (1983) combines selection for dexamethasone resistance with immunological selection for expression of glucocorticoid-induced MMTV cell surface proteins. The immunological "panning" procedure, designed to select for variants having retained functional receptor, involves binding of the cells to dishes coated with specific monoclonal antibodies against the MMTV p27 protein. Although the parental W7 cell line contains three endogenous copies of MMTV provirus, these are not expressed. Therefore, W7 cells had to be infected with MMTV either before or after selection for dexamethasone resistance. An MMTV-infected parental line, W7MG1, containing 10 additional copies of the provirus was used in the selection following mutagenic treatment with ethyl methane sulfonate. Approximately 90% of these cells were found to bind to MMTV antibody–coated dishes after 8 hours of dexamethasone treatment, while only 0.1% of the untreated cells were bound. The principle of the selection is simple in that it consists of four successive rounds of alternating selection for dexamethasone resistance and for hormone-induced expression of MMTV p27 protein. However, this approach is seriously complicated by the fact that, through an unknown mechanism, MMTV-infected cells grown in dexamethasone for extended periods accumulate very large numbers of integrated MMTV proviral sequences. In an attempt to circumvent that problem, only relatively brief periods (36 hours) of dexamethasone treatment were used in the selection for resistant cells. This treatment was followed by long periods (10 generations) of hormone-free growth and immunological elimination of the cells having elevated basal levels of MMTV expression indicative of large numbers of provirus copies. These precautions did not, however, entirely eliminate the problem, since a number of the variants obtained still had acquired additional copies of the viral genome. Moreover, the majority of the variants that had retained MMTV inducibility had only acquired partial resistance to dexamethasone, probably because the selection for resistance had to be limited to a relatively brief period.

Of the 164 clones resulting from the final selection, 22 represented parental cells that had escaped selection and 91 appeared receptor-deficient, having lost both MMTV inducibility and dexamethasone sensitivity. Another 27 clones that remained MMTV inducible had acquired only partial resistance to dexamethasone and, most likely, had reduced levels of receptors. Only 24 clones had the desired phenotype, namely MMTV inducibility and full resistance to dexamethasone. However, one of these clones, which was further characterized, was found to contain additional copies of MMTV sequences. As a result, the basal level of MMTV expression was greatly elevated, and induction of MMTV expression by hormone was drastically reduced compared to the parental line. This behavior can, again, be most simply explained by a qualitative defect in receptor, resulting in reduced MMTV induction, and/or by a decrease in the number of free receptors as a result of the presence of multiple copies of MMTV sequences known to bind receptor with high affinity (Section II,B). No fully resistant clone having retained full MMTV inducibility and the parental number of MMTV provirus copies has been described. Moreover, no data on glucocorticoid receptor levels and properties in these clones are available, and their complementation analysis by fusion with receptor-defective mutants has not been carried out.

As in other multistep enrichment methods, the frequency of the events selected cannot be accurately estimated. However, the scheme used by Danielsen *et al.* (1983) is consistent with the idea that the variants obtained resulted from mutational events in the receptor structural gene. Mutagenesis of W7 cells with ethyl methane sulfonate was shown to generate receptor-defective mutants at frequencies on the order of 2.5×10^{-7} (Bourgeois *et al.*, 1978). Considering that initial populations of 10^8 mutagenized cells were used and that selected cells were allowed to grow for 10 generations between each of the enrichment steps, the accumulation of receptor-defective mutants and their siblings can be expected. From these considerations and the fact that the only variant described having the desired phenotype had also acquired a large number of additional MMTV sequences, it appears that this approach has failed to produce new types of variants.

A similar approach was previously used by Grove *et al.* (1980) to select for hepatoma cell variants unable to produce the MMTV glycoprotein gp52 in response to dexamethasone. In that system, variants expressing decreased amounts of gp52 were selected in a fluorescence-activated cell sorter that can effectively discriminate lower levels of antigen than the panning method. That approach, which is applicable to cells having a single provirus copy, yielded hepatoma cell variants that had a defective or reduced level of glucocorticoid receptor (Grove *et al.*, 1980) as well as some variants in which the changes in production of MMTV RNA were subtle and which appeared to have normal receptor (Grove and Ringold, 1981). Immunological selection is certainly an attractive approach that could be successfully applied to other systems, not complicated by the selection for multiple copies of proviral sequences.

C. Human CEM Variant Expressing Dexamethasone-Induced Glutamine Synthetase

The uncloned human acute lymphoblastic leukemic cell line CCRF-CEM is only slightly sensitive to dexamethasone. This phenotype was shown to be due to a mixture of resistant and sensitive cells (Norman and Thompson, 1977). This result was recently confirmed using a different stock of CCRF-CEM cells, which was found to contain subclones of intermediate sensitivity as well (J. Smith and S. Bourgeois, unpublished results). The glucocorticoid-sensitive CEM subclone C7 was extensively used to derive a collection of receptor-deficient resistant variants *in vitro* (Section II,A). Another subclone, CEM-Cl, which preexisted in the original cell population and is fully resistant to dexamethasone, was recently characterized (Zawydiwski *et al.*, 1983). Using a variety of biochemical criteria, the glucocorticoid receptor of the CEM-Cl clone was indistinguishable from that of the sensitive CEM-C7 clone. However, comparison of the receptors from these two cell lines may not be entirely valid, since the CEM-Cl clone was not derived from the CEM-C7 line *in vitro*, but, rather, both lines preexisted in this original population. The observation that dexamethasone induces glutamine synthetase in CEM-Cl cells provides evidence that this receptor is functional in that response. Complementation analysis in hybrids between CEM-Cl cells and receptor-defective CEM variants has, however, not been carried out to demonstrate that CEM-Cl receptors are capable of mediating the cytolytic response.

The origin of the CEM-Cl clone is unclear: since these hormone-resistant cells preexisted together with sensitive cells in the tumor line, it is unknown whether this heterogeneity resulted from independent transformation events *in vivo* or, alternatively, occurred *in vitro* after the CEM tumor had been established in culture. However, the demonstration (Section III,D) in the murine cell line SAK8 that expression of a lysis function can be inactivated by DNA methylation while glucocorticoid receptors remain normal, suggested that a similar event could have taken place in CEM-Cl cells. Furthermore, the CEM tumor presents striking analogies with the SL12 murine T-lymphoma cell line, which was also found, upon subcloning, to contain a mixture of glucocorticoid-sensitive cells and of resistant cells containing apparently normal receptor (Section III,D). In that case, DNA methylation was shown to be responsible for this tumor heterogeneity, and spontaneous DNA methylation was observed *in vitro*, generating glucocorticoid-resistant cells from sensitive SL12 clones.

These findings in murine systems suggested the possibility that DNA methylation may be responsible for the inactivation of a function other than the receptor in CEM-Cl cells. Evidence for the role of DNA methylation in the glucocorticoid resistance of SAK8 was obtained by showing that these cells can be converted to glucocorticoid sensitivity by treatment with 5-azacytidine (Gasson and Bourgeois, 1983b; Gasson *et al.*, 1983). The same observation was made with glucocorticoid-resistant SL12 cells, which, like CEM-Cl cells, preexisted in the heterogeneous tumor or with SL12 clones that were generated from sensitive SL12 cells *in vitro* (MacLeod *et al.*, 1984). Therefore, the effect of treatment by DNA-demethylating drugs on CEM-Cl cells is being investigated, and preliminary results indicate that glucocorticoid-sensitive clones can be generated from CEM-Cl cells by DNA demethylation (J. Smith and S. Bourgeois, unpublished results). Pending further characterization of the sensitive clones obtained, these preliminary results encourage the view that a function analogous to the lysis function demonstrated in SAK8 murine cells may mediate the dexamethasone-induced cytolysis of human T-lymphoid cells. Furthermore, the expression of the lysis gene(s) determining that function would also be sensitive to DNA methylation. This view implies that the mechanism of glucocorticoid-induced lymphocytolysis and the modes of acquisition of resistance would be similar in human and mouse T-cell lines.

VI. ROLE OF GROWTH FACTORS IN GLUCOCORTICOID SENSITIVITY

A. T-CELL GROWTH REQUIREMENTS FOR INTERLEUKIN-2

Interleukin-2 (IL-2, T-cell growth factor) is a lymphokine that mediates the clonal expansion of T-cells in response to lectin or antigen. IL-2 is produced by activated Lyt-1$^+$, 2$^-$/Thy-1$^+$ cells in the mouse and the OKT-4$^+$ "helper-inducer" subset of human T-cells. In addition, the existence of IL-2–dependent cell lines has made it possible to identify continuous cell lines, of both murine and human origin, that produce IL-2. Purified murine IL-2 has an apparent molecular weight of 23,000, and material purified from human sources has an apparent molecular weight of 15,000 (Gillis *et al.*, 1982). Specific binding of metabolically labeled IL-2 has revealed receptors with dissociation constants of about 10 pM on activated T-lymphocytes of human and mouse origin, but not on B-cells or unstimulated lymphocytes (Robb *et al.*, 1981).

T-lymphocyte proliferation is inhibited by glucocorticoids when administered early after mitogen. This suppressive effect could be on the production of IL-2 or on the ability of cells to respond to the lymphokine. Experiments demonstrating that the inhibitory effects of glucocorticoids can be overcome by the addition of exogenous IL-2 prove that the inhibition is at the level of IL-2 production (Gillis *et al.*, 1979a,b). Inhibitory effects of glucocorticoids on lymphokine and monokine (IL-1) production (Snyder and Unanue, 1982) are probably an important component of immunosuppressive effects of glucocorticoids.

These results raise the question of whether the glucocorticoid-induced lysis observed with T-cell lines, such as W7, may be due to the inhibition of IL-2 production. The W7 cell line has been shown to produce IL-2 in response to ConA stimulation (Smith *et al.*, 1980); therefore, it was of interest to determine what effect, if any, exogenous IL-2 would have on the cytolytic response of W7 cells to glucocorticoids. The murine cell line LBRM

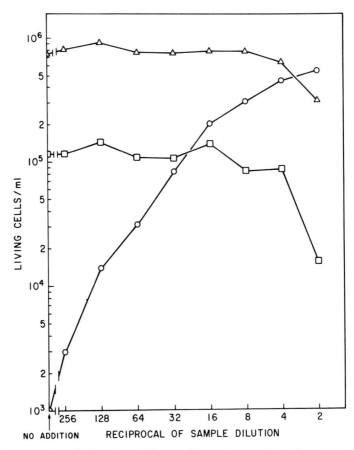

Fig. 9. Assay of interleukin-2 (IL-2) effect on dexamethasone-induced lysis. Culture supernatant containing IL-2 was obtained by growing the LBRM-33 (clone 4A2) cell line, described
by Gillis *et al.* (1980), in Dulbecco modified Eagle's medium supplemented with 1% fetal calf
serum, 1% phytohemaglutinin-M, 1% nonessential amino acids, and 5 μM β-mercaptoethanol.
After 18 to 24 hours of growth, the culture was centrifuged, and the phytohemaglutinin-M was
removed as described by Fagnani and Braatz (1980). After sterilization by filtering, samples
were diluted in fresh medium containing 10% fetal calf serum; reciprocals of the dilutions tested
are indicated on the abcissa. In the case of the W7 line, the effect of this IL-2–containing
supernatant was tested in the presence of 10 nM dexamethasone (□) as well as in the absence of
hormone (△). The IL-2–dependent CTLL-2 line, described by Gillis and Smith (1977), was
used as a control for the presence of IL-2 in the supernatant (○). All three cultures were
inoculated with 2 × 10⁴ cells/ml and living cells were counted after growth for 3 days.

33 was stimulated with PHA, and the supernatant was used as a source of IL-2. The IL-2-dependent cell line CTLL was used to monitor the amount of IL-2 in LBRM33-conditioned medium (Fig. 9). The results in Fig. 9 show that exogenous IL-2 has no effect on the inhibition of W7 cells even at low concentrations $(10^{-8} M)$ of dexamethasone. The possibility exists that these cells lack IL-2 receptors and that exogenous IL-2 cannot replace the IL-2 produced inside the cells. More likely the growth of W7 cells is independent of IL-2, and the lethal effect of glucocorticoids on these cells involves a direct cytolytic mechanism not attributable to reduced IL-2 production. These findings support the idea that not all of the immunosuppressive effects of glucocorticoids on T-cells are mediated through decreased IL-2 production.

B. Effect of Growth Factors on the Cloning Efficiency of SAK Cells

As mentioned in Section III,B, SAK cells are not lysed by glucocorticoids, but effects are seen on growth rate and final cell density. In addition, dexamethasone was found to reduce the cloning efficiency of these cells. In the absence of glucocorticoids, 100% of SAK cells plated at 1 cell/well will form colonies; 1 μM dexamethasone reduces the cloning efficiency to between 20 and 50% (Table III), and the clones that do grow up are much smaller. Based on the results of Gillis *et al.* (1979a,b), it seemed possible that this effect could be due to a decreased production of growth factors by SAK cells in the presence of glucocorticoids. A variety of supernatants were tested to determine whether the cloning efficiency could be increased by adding exogenous sources of growth factors. The results in Table III show that increased fetal calf serum (Experiments I and II), as well as EL4.E1 and ConA-stimulated mouse spleen cell supernatants (Experiment III) increase the cloning efficiency in a dose-dependent way. Based on these results, it appears that the effect of glucocorticoids on SAK8 cloning efficiency may be mediated by a decreased production of one or more growth factors; the identification of these growth factor(s) is under investigation.

The effects of glucocorticoids on the cloning efficiency of SAK cells may have important implications in terms of isolating new types of glucocorticoid-resistant variants from glucocorticoid-sensitive cell lines. In particular, this observation might account for the fact that no mutant defective in the lysis function has ever been isolated *in vitro* (Section II,A). In such mutant selection experiments, a population of sensitive cells is mutagenized and then plated in the presence of the selective agent, in this case dexamethasone. Resistant cells then form clones, which are picked and characterized to analyze the defect. If a lysis-defective mutant were generated, it is possible

TABLE III

CLONING EFFICIENCY OF SAK8 IN 1 μM DEXAMETHASONE[a]

			Cloning conditions		
				Supernatant	Cloning
		FCS[b]			efficiency[c]
Experiment	Medium	(%)	%	Source	(%)
I	DME[d]	10			50
	DME	20			70
	DME + HAMS[e]	10			60
II	DME	10			30
	DME	20			100
III	DME	10			20
	DME	10	23	EL4.E1[f]	86
	DME	10	8	EL4.E1	44
	DME	10	23	Spleen[g]	57
	DME	10	8	Spleen	22

[a] From Gasson and Bourgeois (1983a).

[b] Fetal calf serum.

[c] Expressed as percentage of a control without dexamethasone in which the cloning efficiency is 100% in all culture conditions tested.

[d] Dulbecco's modified Eagle's medium.

[e] 50% DME + 50% HAMS F-12 medium.

[f] Culture supernatant from EL4.E1 cells, prepared as described by Farrar *et al.* (1980).

[g] Culture supernatant from ConA-stimulated mouse spleen cells, prepared as described by Dennert *et al.* (1981).

that such a cell would not be able to form a clone in the presence of glucocorticoids, because of effects of dexamethasone on cloning efficiency unrelated to the lytic response. Such effects cannot be detected in cells such as W7, because they are lysed by glucocorticoids. It appears, then, that glucocorticoids can induce two distinct potentially lethal pathways in T-cells: the lytic response, which is unaffected by the addition of IL-2 (Fig. 9), and a reduction in cloning efficiency, which can be overcome by the addition of growth factors (Table III). Only receptor mutations would block both pathways; the cells would not lyse nor would effects on cloning efficiency be seen in the absence of functional receptor to mediate these responses. This could explain the fact that, by selection at high concentrations of dexamethasone (0.1 to 10 μM), only receptor-defective mutants have been generated to date from sensitive cell lines. It is possible that mutagenized populations selected in media enriched with exogenous growth factors will yield new types of variants.

VII. CONCLUSIONS

Studies of glucocorticoid-induced lysis of murine T-cell lines have established the role of three determinants in the response: the glucocorticoid receptor, a lysis function, and the permeability of the plasma membrane. Alterations in these elements can arise by four different mechanisms, which all result in glucocorticoid resistance: mutation, chromosome segregation, DNA methylation, and, possibly, gene amplification. Receptor quality can be altered by mutations, and receptor quantity can be affected both by mutations and by chromosome segregation. DNA methylation appears to modulate expression of the lysis function, and this mechanism appears responsible for generating lymphoid tumor heterogeneity. However, the lysis function can be lost by chromosome segregation as well. As for the changes in permeability that limit dexamethasone entry into cells, their basis will likely turn out to be gene amplification. While the receptor has been extensively characterized, the lysis function and the membrane element(s) affecting hormone entry remain unidentified. However, the availability of variants in which those elements are not expressed or are overproduced provides tools to approach the question of their nature.

In the human T-lymphoid system studied so far, receptor is the only determinant of the response for which a role has been definitely demonstrated. However, there is no compelling reason to believe that the elements of the response and mechanisms of acquisition of resistance are fundamentally different in human and in mouse cells. On the contrary, the recent analogies found between the human CEM leukemic tumor and murine T-lymphomas encourage the view that the cytolytic response may involve similar mechanisms in both species.

Receptor defects are, so far, the only bases for glucocorticoid resistance generated by mutations. These have been extensively characterized and are the subject of numerous reviews. We have, therefore, limited our discussion to a critical reappraisal of early results and to bringing the characterization of receptor-defective variants up to date. It is remarkable that most of the conclusions derived from the pioneer work of Gordon Tomkins and his colleagues have received support and confirmation over the past 10 years. However, two of their conclusions need to be revised in view of more recent information: (1) the fact that the S49 variants classified as "deathless" now appear most likely to be segregants having a reduced amount of normal receptor (Section II,D), and (2) the interpretation of the phenotype of nt^i receptor variants as resulting from an increased general affinity of a small form of these receptors for DNA (Section II,C).

Finally, one should raise the question regarding what contribution the direct cytolytic response of T-lymphoid cells to glucocorticoids makes to the immunosuppressive effects of these hormones. The discovery in recent years of glucocorticoid regulation of various lymphokines, and in particular of T-cell growth factor (IL-2), has shifted the attention away from possible direct cytotoxic effects of glucocorticoids on T-cells. However, recent results show that glucocorticoid-sensitive T-cells are not protected from dexamethasone-induced lysis by exogenous IL-2 (Section VI,A). This suggests that not all the cytotoxic effects of glucocorticoids on T-cells result from inhibition of IL-2 production. The effect of growth factors on the cloning efficiency of SAK cells in the presence of dexamethasone (Section VI,B) raises the possibility that glucocorticoids induce two distinct and potentially lethal pathways in T-cells. These two pathways may account for the fact that no variants resulting from mutational alterations in the "lysis" function have been obtained so far. The recognition of the existence of this dual mechanism and the availability of an increasing number of lymphokines may open the way to the isolation of lysis-defective mutants, which would be invaluable for the identification of that function.

ACKNOWLEDGMENTS

The work by the authors is supported by PHS Grant No. CA36146 awarded by the National Cancer Institute, DHHS, and by a Grant from the Elsa U. Pardee Foundation to Suzanne Bourgeois; Judy Gasson is supported by a Grant from the University of California Cancer Research Coordinating Committee and was the recipient of Fellowship AM06179 from the National Institute of Arthritis, Metabolic, and Digestive Diseases. We wish to thank all our collaborators who, over the years, have contributed much to this work. We are especially grateful to Ronald F. Newby, Jean-Jacques Mermod, and Jennifer Smith for allowing us to quote some of their unpublished results, and to Magnus Pfahl, Donald J. Gruol, and Ronald F. Newby for their critical reading of sections of our manuscript. We greatly appreciate the help of Connie Meloan, not only her expert typing of this manuscript but also her good-spirited secretarial assistance that makes every task easier.

REFERENCES

Adams, R. L. P., and Burdon, R. H. (1982). *Crit. Rev. Biochem.* **14**, 349–384.
Ballard, P. L. (1979). *Monogr. Endocrinol.* **12**, 25–48.
Baskin, F., Rosenberg, R. N., and Dev, V. (1981). *Proc. Natl. Acad. Sci. U.S.A.* **78**, 3654–3658.
Bech-Hansen, N. T., Till, J. E., and Ling, V. (1976). *J. Cell. Physiol.* **88**, 23–32.
Beck, W. T., Mueller, T. J., and Tanzer, L. R. (1979). *Cancer Res.* **39**, 2070–2076.
Bourgeois, S., and Newby, R. F. (1977). *Cell* **11**, 423–430.
Bourgeois, S., and Newby, R. F. (1979). *Cancer Res.* **39**, 4749–4751.
Bourgeois, S., and Newby, R. F. (1980). *Prog. Cancer Res. Ther.* **14**, 67–77.
Bourgeois, S., Newby, R. F., and Huet, M. (1978). *Cancer Res.* **38**, 4279–4284.

Bourgeois, S., Pfahl, M., and Baulieu, E. E. (1984). *EMBO J.* **3**, 751–755.
Burch, J. B. E., and Weintraub, H. (1983). *Cell* **33**, 65–76.
Cantor, H., and Weissman, I. (1976). *Prog. Allergy* **20**, 1–64.
Chandler, V. L., Maler, B. A., and Yamamoto, K. R. (1983). *Cell* **33**, 489–499.
Chen, S. S., Tung, J. S., Gillis, S., Good, R. A., and Hadden, J. W. (1983). *Proc. Natl. Acad. Sci. U.S.A.* **80**, 5980–5984.
Claman, H. N. (1972). *N. Engl. J. Med.* **287**, 388–397.
Cohen, J. J., and Duke, R. C. (1984). *J. Immunol.* **132**, 38–42.
Compere, S. J., and Palmiter, R. D. (1981). *Cell* **25**, 233–240.
Danielsen, M., Peterson, D. O., and Stallcup, M. R. (1983). *Mol. Cell. Biol.* **3**, 1310–1316.
Debenham, P. G., Kartner, N., Siminovitch, L., Riordan, J. R., and Ling, V. (1982). *Mol. Cell. Biol.* **2**, 881–889.
Dellweg, H.-G., Hotz, A., Mugele, K., and Gehring, U. (1982). *EMBO J.* **1**, 285–289.
Dennert, G., Yoguswaran, G., and Yamagata, S. (1981). *J. Exp. Med.* **153**, 545–556.
Doerfler, W. (1981). *J. Gen. Virol.* **57**, 1–20.
Duke, R. C., Chervenak, R., and Cohen, J. J. (1983). *Proc. Natl. Acad. Sci. U.S.A.* **80**, 6361–6365.
Dunn, C. Y., Aaronson, S. A., and Stephenson, J. R. (1975). *Virology* **66**, 579–588.
Duval, D., Durant, S., and Homo-Delarche, F. (1983). *Biochim. Biophys. Acta* **737**, 409–442.
Ehrlich, M., and Wang, R. Y. H. (1981). *Science* **212**, 1350–1357.
Fagnani, R., and Braatz, J. A. (1980). *J. Immunol. Methods* **33**, 313–322.
Farrar, W. L., Mizel, J. G., and Farrar, J. J. (1980). *J. Immunol.* **124**, 1371–1374.
Francke, U., and Gehring, U. (1980). *Cell* **22**, 657–664.
Garman, D., and Center, M. S. (1982). *Biochem. Biophys. Res. Commun.* **105**, 157–163.
Gasson, J. C., and Bourgeois, S. (1983a). *In* "UCLA Symposia on Molecular and Cellular Biology: Rational Basis for Chemotherapy" (B. A. Chabner, ed.), pp. 153–176. Alan R. Liss, Inc., New York.
Gasson, J. C., and Bourgeois, S. (1983b). *J. Cell Biol.* **96**, 409–415.
Gasson, J. C., Ryden, T., and Bourgeois, S. (1983). *Nature (London)* **302**, 621–623.
Gehring, U., Ulrich, J., and Segnitz, B. (1982). *Mol. Cell. Endocrinol.* **28**, 605–611.
Geisse, S., Scheidereit, C., Westphal, H. M., Hynes, N. E., Groner, B., and Beato, M. (1982). *EMBO J.* **1**, 1613–1619.
Gielkens, A. L. J., Van Zaane, D., Bloemers, H. P. J., and Bloemendahl, H. (1976). *Proc. Natl. Acad. Sci. U.S.A.* **73**, 356–360.
Gillis, S., and Smith, K. A. (1977). *Nature (London)* **268**, 154–156.
Gillis, S., Crabtree, G. R., and Smith, K. A. (1979a). *J. Immunol.* **123**, 1624–1631.
Gillis, S., Crabtree, G. R., and Smith, K. A. (1979b). *J. Immunol.* **123**, 1632–1638.
Gillis, S., Scheid, M., and Watson, J. (1980). *J. Immunol.* **125**, 2570–2578.
Gillis, S., Mochizuki, D. Y., Conlon, P. J., Hefeneider, S. H., Ramthun, C. A., Gillis, A. E., Frank, M. B., Henney, C. S., and Watson, J. D. (1982). *Immunol. Rev.* **63**, 167–209.
Govindan, M. V., Spiess, E., and Majors, J. (1982). *Proc. Natl. Acad. Sci. U.S.A.* **79**, 5157–5161.
Groudine, M., Eisenman, R., and Weintraub, H. (1981). *Nature (London)* **292**, 311–317.
Grove, J. R., and Ringold, G. M. (1981). *Proc. Natl. Acad. Sci. U.S.A.* **78**, 4349–4353.
Grove, J. R., Dieckmann, B. S., Schroer, T. A., and Ringold, G. M. (1980). *Cell* **21**, 47–56.
Gruol, D. J., and Kempner, E. S. (1982). *J. Biol. Chem.* **257**, 708–713.
Gruol, D. J., Dalton, D. K., and Bourgeois, S. (1984a). *J. Steroid Biochem.* **20**, 255–257.
Gruol, D. J., Kempner, E. S., and Bourgeois, S. (1984b). *J. Biol. Chem.* **259**, 4833–4839.
Harmon, J. M., and Thompson, E. B. (1981). *Mol. Cell. Biol.* **1**, 512–521.

Harmon, J. T., Kahn, C. R., Kempner, E. S., and Schlegel, W. (1980). *J. Biol. Chem.* **255**, 3412–3419.

Harris, M. (1982). *Cell* **29**, 483–492.

Herrmann, W., Wyss, R., Riondel, A., Philibert, D., Teutsch, G., Sakiz, E., and Baulieu, E.-E. (1982). *C. R. Hebd. Seances Acad. Sci., Ser. III* **294**, 933–938.

Hill, B. T., and Whelan, D. H. (1982). *Cancer Chemother. Pharmacol.* **8**, 163–169.

Horibata, K., and Harris, A. W. (1970). *Exp. Cell Res.* **60**, 61–77.

Houslay, M. D., Ellory, J. C., Smith, G. A., Hesketh, T. R., Stein, J. M., Warren, G. B., and Metcalfe, J. C. (1977). *Biochim. Biophy. Acta* **467**, 208–219.

Huet-Minkowski, M., Gasson, J. C., and Bourgeois, S. (1981). *Cancer Res.* **41**, 4540–4546.

Hynes, N., Van Doyen, A. J. J., Kennedy, N., Herrlich, P., Ponta, H., and Groner, B. (1983). *Proc. Natl. Acad. Sci. U.S.A.* **80**, 3637–3641.

Ihle, J. N., Lane, S. E., Kenney, F. T., and Farrelly, J. G. (1975). *Cancer Res.* **35**, 442–446.

Johnson, D. M., Newby, R. F., and Bourgeois, S. (1984). *Cancer Res.* **44**, 2435–2440.

Kartner, N., Riordan, J. R., and Ling, V. (1983). *Science* **221**, 1285–1288.

Kempner, E. S., and Schlegel, W. (1979). *Anal. Biochem.* **92**, 2–10.

Kessel, D., and Bosmann, H. B. (1970). *Cancer Res.* **30**, 2695–2701.

Lalande, M. E., Ling, V., and Miller, R. G. (1981). *Proc. Natl. Acad. Sci. U.S.A.* **78**, 363–367.

Lampkin, J. M., and Potter, M. (1958). *J. Natl. Cancer Inst. (U.S.)* **20**, 1091–1108.

Lea, D. E. (1955). "Actions of Radiation in Living Cells." Cambridge Univ. Press, London and New York.

MacLeod, C. L., Hays, E. F., Hyman, R., and Bourgeois, S. (1984). *Cancer Res.* **44**, 1784–1790.

Majors, J., and Varmus, H. E. (1983). *Proc. Natl. Acad. Sci. U.S.A.* **80**, 5866–5870.

Mayo, K. E., and Palmiter, R. D. (1981). *J. Biol. Chem.* **256**, 2621–2624.

Mermod, J. J., Intrière, L., MacLeod, C., and Bourgeois, S. (1981). *J. Steroid Biochem.* **15**, 25–34.

Mermod, J. J., Bourgeois, S., Defer, N., and Crépin, M. (1983). *Proc. Natl. Acad. Sci. U.S.A.* **80**, 110–114.

Nordeen, S. K., Lan, N. C., Showers, M. O., and Baxter, J. D. (1981). *J. Biol. Chem.* **256**, 10503–10508.

Norman, M. R., and Thompson, E. B. (1977). *Cancer Res.* **37**, 3785–3791.

Paran, M., Gallo, R. C., Richardson, L. S., and Wu, A. M. (1973). *Proc. Natl. Acad. Sci. U.S.A.* **70**, 2391–2395.

Payvar, F., Wrange, Ö., Carlstredt-Duke, J., Okret, S., Gustafsson, J. A., and Yamamoto, K. (1981). *Proc. Natl. Acad. Sci. U.S.A.* **78**, 6628–6632.

Pfahl, M. (1982). *Cell* **31**, 475–482.

Pfahl, M., and Bourgeois, S. (1980). *Somat. Cell Genet.* **6**, 63–74.

Pfahl, M., Sandros, T., and Bourgeois, S. (1978a). *Mol. Cell. Endocrinol.* **10**, 175–191.

Pfahl, M., Kelleher, R. J., and Bourgeois, S. (1978b). *Mol. Cell. Endocrinol.* **10**, 193–207.

Pfahl, M., McGinnis, D., Hendricks, M., Groner, B., and Hynes, N. (1983). *Science* **222**, 1341–1343.

Razin, A., and Riggs, A. D. (1980). *Science* **210**, 604–610.

Robb, R. J., Munck, A., and Smith, K. A. (1981). *J. Exp. Med.* **154**, 1455–1474.

Rothenberg, E. (1980). *Cell* **20**, 1–9.

Scheidereit, C., Geisse, S., Westphal, H. M., and Beato, M. (1983). *Nature (London)* **304**, 749–752.

Schimke, R. T. (1982). "Gene Amplification." Cold Spring Harbor Lab., Cold Spring Harbor, New York.

Schmidt, T. J., Harmon, J. M., and Thompson, E. B. (1980). *Nature (London)* **286**, 507–510.

Sibley, C. H., and Tomkins, G. M. (1974a). *Cell* **2**, 213–220.

Sibley, C. H., and Tomkins, G. M. (1974b). *Cell* **2**, 221–227.

Smith, K. A., Gilbride, K. J., and Favata, M. F. (1980). *Nature (London)* **287**, 853–855.

Snyder, D. S., and Unanue, E. R. (1982). *J. Immunol.* **129**, 1803–1805.

Stevens, J., Stevens, Y.-W., and Haubenstock, H. (1983). *In* "Biochemical Actions of Hormones" (G. Litwack, ed.), Vol. 10, pp. 383–446. Academic Press, New York.

Taylor, S. M., and Jones, P. A. (1979). *Cell* **17**, 771–779.

Wahl, G. M., Padgett, R. A., and Stark, G. R. (1979). *J. Biol. Chem.* **254**, 8679–8689.

Weintraub, H., and Groudine, M. (1976). *Science* **193**, 848–856.

Wilks, A. F., Cozens, P. J., Mattaj, I. W., and Jost, J.-P. (1982). *Proc. Natl. Acad. Sci. U.S.A.* **79**, 4252–4255.

Wilson, V. L., and Jones, P. (1983). *Cell* **32**, 239–246.

Wyllie, A. H. (1980). *Nature (London)* **284**, 555–556.

Yamamoto, K. R., Gehring, U., Stampfer, M. R., and Sibley, C. H. (1976). *Recent Prog. Horm. Res.* **32**, 3–32.

Zawydiwski, R., Harmon, J. M., and Thompson, E. B. (1983). *Cancer Res.* **43**, 3865–3873.

CHAPTER 11

Estrogen and Antiestrogen Binding Sites: Relation to the Estrogen Receptor and Biological Response

J. H. Clark, R. C. Winneker, and B. M. Markaverich

Department of Cell Biology
Baylor College of Medicine
Houston, Texas

BIOCHEMICAL ACTIONS OF HORMONES, VOL. XII

I. INTRODUCTION

Estrogenic hormones are thought to act via receptor-binding interactions that stimulate target cells to respond. We have been interested in the relationship between estrogen receptor binding and biological response for some time. These studies entailed the careful examination of estrogen receptor–binding parameters as a function of hormone dose, time after exposure to hormone, and physiological state. In the course of these experiments, we discovered a secondary binding site for estrogens that we called the type II estradiol binding site. At first these sites were considered to be a nuisance because they interfered with the accurate determination of estrogen receptor–binding parameters; however, their potential biological importance was realized when we discovered that estrogen administration influenced the level of these sites.

In addition to our studies of the involvement of type II sites in estrogen action, we have been examining the role of antiestrogen binding sites in the mechanism of action of estrogen antagonists. Both of these lines of research have led to the discovery of two different endogenous ligands that are probably involved in the mechanisms by which estrogen and antiestrogens function. The purpose of this chapter is to review these findings.

II. TYPE II ESTROGEN BINDING SITES
AND AN ENDOGENOUS LIGAND

Type II estrogen binding sites are found in both the cytosol and nuclear fractions of various target organs for estrogen (Eriksson *et al.*, 1978; Clark *et al.*, 1978). The characteristics of these sites and their relevance to a possible role in hormone action will be reviewed in this section.

A. CYTOSOL TYPE II ESTRADIOL BINDING SITES

The cytosol from immature rat uteri contains, in addition to the estrogen receptor (type I sites), a proteinaceous macromolecule, which we have named the cytosol type II estradiol binding site. These sites are observed when saturation analysis by [³H]estradiol exchange is performed on uterine cytosol obtained from immature rats. Unlike the estrogen receptor, type II sites do not appear to undergo translocation to the nucleus (Eriksson *et al.*, 1978; Clark *et al.*, 1978). That is, an injection of estradiol that causes cytoplasmic depletion and concomitant nuclear accumulation of the estrogen receptor does not deplete type II sites from the cytosol. Type II sites have a somewhat lower affinity ($K_d \sim 20$ nM) than the receptor ($K_d \sim 1$ nM), but the number of sites may greatly exceed that of type I sites. Type II sites display stereospecificity for estrogenic compounds and are present in other estrogen target tissues such as the vagina (Clark *et al.*, 1978), mouse (Watson and Clark, 1980) and human mammary tumors (Panko *et al.*, 1981), MCF-7 cells (Mercer *et al.*, 1981), rabbit endometrial cells (Murai *et al.*, 1979), and Mullerian ducts of the chick embryo (MacLaughlin *et al.*, 1983). Similar secondary binding sites have been observed in the prostate (Swaneck *et al.*, 1982; Ekman *et al.*, 1983), the chick oviduct (Smith *et al.*, 1979), and the rabbit corpus luteum (Yuh and Keyes, 1979). In addition, multiple binding sites have been described for glucocorticoids and progesterone in a number of tissues (Barlow *et al.*, 1979; Do *et al.*, 1979; Giannopoulos and Munowitz, 1980). Thus, the presence of secondary binding sites for steroid hormones appears to be a general phenomenon and is not restricted to estrogens.

Although the function of cytosol type II sites is not known, their presence complicates the interpretation of receptor assays. The quantity of these sites varies with many factors and may range from 2 to 10 times the quantity of estrogen receptor. The influence of these kinds of variation on the determination of the type I receptor can be significant. As the quantity of type II sites increases, the error introduced in the estimation of the K_d and the number of type I sites progressively increases. This only becomes apparent when saturation analysis is run over a wide range of hormone concentrations. Consequently, assays that are limited to a single concentration of hormone (1–10 nM) will measure both sites and may lead to overestimates of the K_d and numbers of type I sites. These points have been discussed in detail in Clark and Peck (1979).

B. Nuclear Type II Estradiol Binding Sites

As discussed previously, an injection of estradiol will cause the depletion of type I sites from uterine cytosol. This depletion is accompanied by the accumulation of these sites in the nucleus and represents the well-known cytoplasmic-to-nuclear translocation phenomenon. Analysis of nuclear fractions for estrogen binding sites by the [³H]estradiol exchange assay reveals a complex picture that also involves at least two sites (Eriksson *et al.*, 1978; Markaverich and Clark, 1979). One conforms to the type I site, which was depleted from the cytosol and is undoubtedly identical to the classically described estrogen receptor. As shown in Fig. 1A, type I sites display the usual saturation curve, which has the shape of a rectangular hyperbola and can be analyzed by a Scatchard plot to yield a linear component. Nuclear type II sites, however, have a more complex binding function, which is

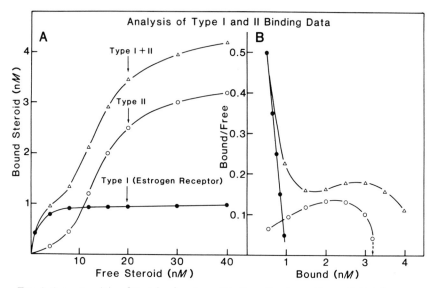

FIG. 1. Saturation (A) and Scatchard analyses (B) of type I and type II estradiol binding sites. The total amount of specific binding (△) is the sum of type I (●) (estrogen receptor) and type II sites (○).

sigmoidal and curvilinear by saturation and Scatchard analysis, respectively (Fig. 1A, B). Complex curves such as these are difficult to resolve into their components; however, we have observed that dithiothreitol (DTT) exposure causes the disappearance of type II sites and permits the independent measurement of the estrogen receptor (Markaverich *et al.*, 1981a).

Nuclear type II sites do not appear to be identical to cytosol type II sites, and we have no evidence of a precursor–product relationship. However, the quantity of these nuclear type II sites is elevated by treatment with estrogen and is modulated by other steroids. These points are considered in the following sections.

C. Effects of Estradiol and Estriol on Nuclear Type II Sites

We have examined the relationship between the stimulation of nuclear type II sites and uterotropic responses by comparing the effects of estradiol and estriol (Markaverich and Clark, 1979). Maximal levels of type I and type II sites are reached by 1 hour after an injection of estradiol in mature castrate rats (Fig. 2). The quantity of type I sites then declines gradually to control levels by 72 hours. The quantity of type II sites also declines gradually but is maintained two- to threefold above controls at 24, 48, and 72 hours. Estriol treatment also elevates the quantity of type I sites after 1 hour after the injection and causes a corresponding increase in uterine wet weight at 4 hours. However, only estradiol induced long-term nuclear retention of the type I site (4–6 hours), sustained elevated levels of nuclear type II sites (1–48 hours), and stimulated true uterine growth (uterine wet weight at 24–48 hours). Failure of an injection of estriol to stimulate true uterine growth is correlated with the inability of this hormone to induce long-term (4–6 hours)

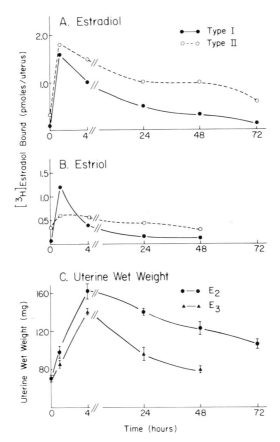

FIG. 2. Effects of an injection of estradiol or estriol on nuclear type I and II sites and uterine weight. Mature ovariectomized rats were injected with 10 μg of estradiol or estriol and sacrificed at various times after treatment. The quantity of specifically bound [³H]estradiol was determined by saturation and Scatchard analyses of uterine nuclear fractions. [From Markaverich and Clark (1979). © 1979, The Endocrine Society.]

nuclear retention of type I sites or increase the levels of nuclear type II estrogen binding sites above control levels.

To further examine the relationship between nuclear type II sites and estrogen stimulation of true uterine growth, mature ovariectomized rats were treated with paraffin pellets containing either estradiol or estriol and sacrificed 48 hours following hormone administration (Fig. 3B) (Markaverich and Clark, 1979). As we have shown in previous work, under these conditions estriol treatment results in the sustained elevation of nuclear type I sites and the stimulation of true uterine growth in the immature rat (Clark *et al.*, 1977; Martucci and Fishman, 1977). If elevated levels of nuclear type II

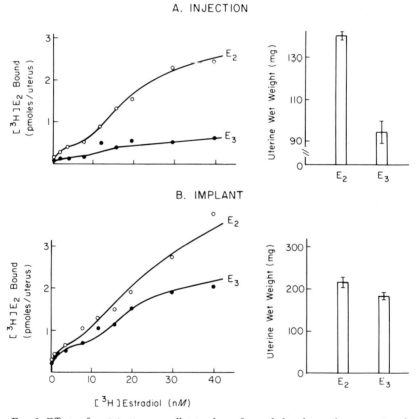

FIG. 3. Effects of an injection or pellet implant of estradiol and estriol on type I and II nuclear binding and uterine growth. Mature ovariectomized rats were either injected with estradiol or estriol (10 μg) or implanted with paraffin pellets containing 2 mg of either hormone. Animals were sacrificed at 24 hours following the injection or 48 hours after the implant. Saturation analysis was performed on the uterine nuclear fraction by [³H]estradiol exchange assays (left panel), and uterine weights were determined (right panel).

sites are related to estrogen stimulation of true uterine growth (either causally or as a secondary response), then increased quantities of this second nuclear estrogen–binding component should be observed in animals treated with an estriol implant. Saturation analysis of nuclear fractions by the [^{3}H]estradiol exchange assay demonstrated that, while not as effective as estradiol, administration of estriol by paraffin implant resulted in the sustained elevation of occupied type I sites (0.4 pmoles/uterus) and a six- to eightfold increase in the numbers of nuclear type II sites compared to the paraffin controls. Under these conditions, estriol stimulated a full uterine growth response, which is identical to that observed with estradiol.

In contrast to these observations with pellet implants, it can be seen from the data in Fig. 3A that a single injection of estradiol has no effect on the elevation of type II sites or the stimulation of uterine growth.

These results demonstrate that a positive correlation exists between elevated levels of nuclear type II sites and the stimulation of true uterine growth. This correlation is better than that observed for the classic estrogen receptor (type I site). Type I sites accumulate rapidly in the nucleus after an injection of estradiol; however, they decline to low levels by 24 hours. In contrast, the level of type II remains elevated for 24–48 hours, and true growth of the uterus is observed during this time. An injection of estriol also causes nuclear accumulation of type I, but these sites rapidly disappear from the nucleus, and, additionally, neither stimulation of type II sites nor true uterine growth occurs. We have previously demonstrated that a single injection of estradiol stimulated sustained RNA polymerase activity, increased chromatin template activity over long periods of time, and elevated DNA synthesis. A single injection of estriol, in contrast, failed to cause these long-term uterotropic responses (Fig. 3A) (Hardin *et al.*, 1976; Markaverich *et al.*, 1978). We have suggested that these events relate to the ability of estradiol to maintain receptor occupancy in the nucleus for a period of time that is sufficient to stimulate the nuclear-mediated events that are obligatory for the production of true growth. One of these obligatory events may be the elevation of type II sites. The failure of an estriol injection to cause true growth results from its inability to maintain type I sites in the nucleus for a sufficient period of time. That type II sites at least attend, if not cause, true growth appears to be the case, since implants of estriol, which sustain occupancy of type I sites, cause the elevation of type II sites and true uterine growth. Thus, estrogen stimulation of true uterine growth correlates with nuclear retention of type I sites and sustained elevation of the level of the nuclear type II estrogen binding sites.

The precise requirements for estrogenic stimulation of the nuclear type II site remain to be resolved. The ability of estriol, when administered by paraffin implant, to increase nuclear type II sites and to stimulate true uterine growth suggests that one requirement for the elevation of nuclear type II sites may be sustained nuclear occupancy by receptor–hormone complexes. In addition, the specificity of the interaction between receptor–hormone complexes and nuclear sites that results in the increase in type II sites may also be considered. This conclusion is supported by the observation that, while a single injection of either estradiol or estriol resulted in an equivalent accumulation of receptor–hormone complexes at 1–4 hours postinjection, only the receptor–estradiol complexes were associated with rapid and sustained elevations of nuclear type II sites between 1 and 48 hours after treatment. Whether the increase in nuclear type II sites in estriol-implanted animals was due to long-term nuclear occupancy by receptor–estriol complexes or to saturation of specific nuclear binding sites through a lower affinity interaction with receptor–estriol complexes remains to be established.

In conclusion, these data indicate that two estrogen binding sites may be involved in the response of the rat uterus to estrogenic hormones. Whereas responses may be mediated through the interaction of estrogen with type I sites (Anderson *et al.*, 1975; Gorski and Gannon, 1976; O'Malley and Means, 1974), nuclear events associated with true uterine growth (Hardin *et al.*, 1976; Markaverich *et al.*, 1978; Stormshak *et al.*, 1976) may require not only long-term nuclear retention of type I sites, but the sustained elevation of the level of nuclear type II sites.

D. Progesterone and Dexamethasone Antagonism of Type II Sites and Uterine Growth

As discussed earlier, the elevation of nuclear type II sites is closely correlated with the stimulation of true uterine growth, and therefore it is conceivable that these sites might be involved in the mechanism by which estrogens cause uterotropic stimulation. One way to test this hypothesis is to block the stimulation of nuclear type II sites and examine the uterotropic response pattern. Since progesterone and glucocorticoids have been used to block uterotropic responses in various ways (Szego and Roberts, 1953; Huggins and Jensen, 1955; Lerner, 1964), it seemed possible that these hormones could be used for this purpose (Markaverich *et al.*, 1981a).

Mature, ovariectomized rats were given two daily injections of estradiol or a single injection of estradiol on day 1 and an injection of either estradiol plus dexamethasone or estradiol plus progesterone on day 2. All animals were sacrificed 24 hours following the second injection. Pretreatment with estradiol (day 1) was to increase the uterine response to progesterone, presumably by increasing the level of progesterone receptor (Milgrom *et al.*, 1973;

Leavitt *et al.*, 1974; Walters and Clark, 1978). Saturation analysis of specific nuclear binding sites by the [^{3}H]estradiol exchange assay revealed that uterine nuclei from estradiol-treated controls contained approximately 0.2 and 6.0 pmoles/uterus of type I and type II sites, respectively (Fig. 4).

Dexamethasone treatment completely blocked the estrogen-stimulated increase in the nuclear type II site and in the uterine wet weight ($p < .01$) normally observed 24 hours following a second injection of estradiol (Fig. 4) (Markaverich *et al.*, 1981b). Nuclear levels of the type I site were very similar (0.2 pmoles/uterus) in the estradiol and estradiol plus dexamethasone treatment groups, suggesting that this antagonist failed to alter nuclear estrogen receptor levels at 24 hours. While not as effective as dexamethasone, administration of progesterone to mature ovariectomized rats reduced levels of the nuclear type II site and decreased ($p < .05$) the uterine wet-weight response to estradiol but failed to influence nuclear levels of the type I site.

These results suggest that the antagonistic properties of dexamethasone and progesterone on estradiol-induced uterine growth reside in the ability of these compounds to reduce the numbers of nuclear type II sites while not altering nuclear levels of type I estrogen binding sites. However, these compounds could interfere with nuclear translocation and "processing" of type I sites, thereby reducing the availability of estrogen receptor at 1, 4, and 24 hours following dexamethasone or progesterone administration to mature ovariectomized rats (Markaverich *et al.*, 1981b). As shown in Fig. 5, the levels of cytoplasmic type I sites were identical in animals treated with estradiol, estradiol plus dexamethasone, or estradiol plus progesterone at 1 and 4 hours postinjection. By 24 hours, the level of cytoplasmic type I was increased above control (2.0 pmoles/uterus) in estradiol-treated (3.6 pmoles/uterus) and estradiol plus dexamethasone-treated (3.0 pmoles/uterus) animals. The lower level of type I sites in the cytosol of progesterone-treated rats (2.0 pmoles/uterus) compared to the estradiol treatment groups (3.6 pmoles/uterus) is consistent with previous reports from this laboratory demonstrating that progesterone blocks the estrogen-induced synthesis of cytoplasmic estrogen receptors 8–24 hours postinjection (Hseuh *et al.*, 1976). Apparently, dexamethasone treatment does not inhibit this phase of cytoplasmic receptor synthesis. Similarly, the antagonistic effects of dexamethasone and progesterone on nuclear type II sites and uterine growth do not appear to be the result of alterations in nuclear retention patterns of type I sites, since nuclear levels of estrogen receptor were identical at 1, 4, and 24 hours following injection of estradiol, estradiol plus dexamethasone, or estradiol plus progesterone.

These data suggest that the nature of dexamethasone and progesterone antagonism of uterotropic responses to estradiol is due to an inhibition of the expression of nuclear type II sites rather than in impedance of receptor–

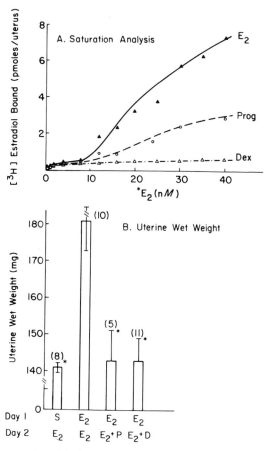

FIG. 4. Saturation analysis (A) of nuclear estrogen binding sites in rat uterine fractions. The quantity of specifically bound [³H]estradiol (pmoles/uterus) for each estradiol concentration was determined by subtracting the nonspecific binding ([³H]estradiol bound in the presence of 100-fold excess diethylstilbestrol) from the total quantity of [³H]estradiol bound. Mature ovariectomized rats were primed with an injection of estradiol (10 µg) 24 hours prior to receiving a second injection of estradiol (▲———▲), estradiol + progesterone (○- - -○), or estradiol + dexamethasone (△-·-··-△). Animals were sacrificed 24 hours following the second injection. Estradiol (10 µg), progesterone (2.5 mg), and dexamethasone (5 mg) were injected subcutaneously in 30% ethanol/0.9% NaCl (v/v). Effects of progesterone and dexamethasone on uterine wet weight (B). Animals received a priming injection of vehicle (S) [30% ethanol/0.9% NaCl (v/v)] or estradiol (E₂) (10 µg) on day 1 and a second injection of estradiol, estradiol + progesterone (E₂ + P), or estradiol + dexamethasone (E₂ + D) on day 2 and were sacrificed 24 hours later. Hormones were injected exactly as described in the legend to Fig. 1A. Values represent the mean ± SEM for the number of observations per experiment, indicated in parenthesis. * indicates significant difference from animals receiving two daily injections of estradiol ($p < 0.01$). (Reprinted with permission from *Journal of Steroid Biochemistry*, Volume 14, by B. M. Markaverich, S. Upchurch, and J. H. Clark, An endogenous ligand for the triphenylethylene antiestrogen binding site. Copyright 1981, Pergamon Press, Ltd.)

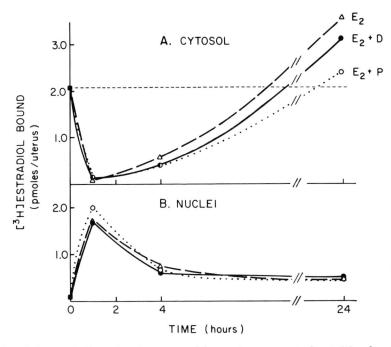

FIG. 5. Temporal effects of progesterone and dexamethasone on cytoplasmic (A) and nuclear (B) levels of nuclear type I sites. Mature ovariectomized rats were treated exactly as described in Fig. 1 and were sacrificed 1, 4, and 24 hours following the second injection of estradiol ($\triangle$- - -$\triangle$), estradiol + progesterone ($\bigcirc\cdots\bigcirc$), or estradiol + dexamethasone ($\bullet$——$\bullet$). Cytoplasmic and nuclear levels of type I sites were estimated at the indicated times following injection by saturation analysis utilizing the [³H]estradiol exchange assay or hydroxylapatite adsorption assay. The values (pmoles/uterus) represent the quantities of type I sites in the cytosol and nuclear fractions corrected for the influence of type II sites by graphic analysis. (Reprinted with permission from *Journal of Steroid Biochemistry,* Volume 14, by B. M. Markaverich, S. Upchurch, and J. H. Clark, An endogenous ligand for the triphenylethylene antiestrogen binding site. Copyright 1981, Pergamon Press, Ltd.)

nuclear interactions, "processing," and/or cytoplasmic receptor replenishment. This concept is supported by the observation that a single injection of dexamethasone 24 hours prior to estradiol administration inhibited estrogen stimulation of uterine growth and nuclear type II sites, even though effects on type I sites do not appear to be involved in this inhibition (Markaverich *et al.,* 1981b). Apparently, antagonistic effects of progesterone on nuclear type II sites and uterine growth are dependent on estrogen pretreatment, since progesterone failed to antagonize either of these parameters in the unprimed rat uterus.

In summary, these data demonstrate that dexamethasone and progesterone inhibit the ability of estradiol to elevate nuclear type II estrogen binding sites in the rat uterus, and this is correlated with an antagonism of uterine growth. Since the nuclear binding and cytoplasmic replenishment of type I receptors are normal under these circumstances, we propose that the estrogen-induced elevation of nuclear type II sites may be involved in the mechanism by which estrogen causes uterine growth.

E. Differential Uterine Cell Stimulation and Nuclear Levels of Nuclear Type I and II Sites

Triphenylethylene drugs, such as nafoxidine and clomiphene, stimulate epithelial cells of the uterus while having little effect on the stromal or myometrial components (Clark and Peck, 1979). This finding plus the discovery of type II sites prompted us to examine the relationships between these two phenomena.

Mature castrate rats were implanted with estradiol, nafoxidine, or clomiphene, and epithelial, stromal, and myometrial cells were prepared as described in McCormack and Glasser (1980). Saturation analysis demonstrated that these cells contain both type I and type II estrogen binding sites and that sustained nuclear occupancy by type I sites and the elevation in nuclear type II sites are correlated to a certain degree with the growth of the epithelium that we observed histologically (Fig. 6) (Markaverich *et al.*, 1981c). Surprisingly, estradiol stimulation of nuclear type II sites in the uterine epithelium was approximately twofold greater than that obtained with nafoxidine and clomiphene, even though histologically the triphenylethylenes were more active in this regard. Thus, whether or not elevations in this second nuclear binding site for estradiol are directly proportional to the epithelial growth response remains to be established. Likewise, nuclear levels of the type I site were not directly correlated with luminal epithelial growth. Both estradiol and clomiphene treatment stimulated uterine growth to the greatest extent, both histologically and on a wet-weight basis. Yet these compounds elevated nuclear type I sites only slightly above controls. Conversely, nafoxidine caused maximal accumulation of type I sites and was equally effective in stimulating epithelial growth, but was the least effective of the three compounds in increasing uterine wet weight. The elevated levels of type I sites in the control group appear to be due to a redistribution artifact resulting from the cell separation technique (McCormack and Glasser, 1980). As shown in Fig. 4, these sites are unoccupied by hormone in control animals, whereas those from the hormone-treated groups are occupied and assumed to be physiologically active receptor–hormone complexes.

Nuclear levels of both estrogen binding sites in uterine stromal cells corre-

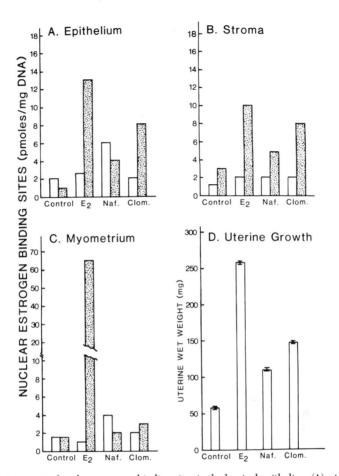

FIG. 6. Summary of nuclear estrogen binding sites in the luminal epithelium (A), stroma (B), myometrium (C), and uterine wet weight response (D) in beeswax controls and in rats treated with estradiol (E_2), nafoxidine (Naf.), and clomiphene (Clom.). Nuclear levels of type I (open bars) and type II (stippled bars) estrogen binding sites were determined by graphic analysis of the saturation curves and are expressed as specific binding (pmoles/mg DNA).

lated more closely with the uterotropic responses to estradiol and the tri-phenylethylene derivatives (Fig. 6). Similar but more pronounced effects were observed in cellular preparations of myometrium. In this tissue, estradiol elevated the level of type II sites 30-fold above controls, while nafoxidine and clomiphene had little effect on type II sites in the myometrium. This ability of estradiol and the failure of nafoxidine and clomiphene to cause elevations in type II sites is highly correlated with their differential capacities to stimulate growth in the myometrium (Clark and Peck, 1979; Markaverich *et al.*, 1981c). Nuclear levels of type I sites in estradiol-, clomiphene-, and nafoxidine-treated rats were not significantly elevated above controls; however, as noted earlier, these sites in the control animals are not occupied by hormone.

From these studies we conclude that estradiol, clomiphene, and nafoxidine cause accumulation of type I sites in the epithelium, stroma, and myometrium of the rat uterus. Likewise, nuclear type II sites are elevated to some degree in all three tissues; however, the ability of estradiol to stimulate these sites in the myometrium greatly exceeds that of nafoxidine and clomiphene. This stimulation of nuclear type II sites is correlated with the agonistic properties of estradiol, while the reduced responses observed with clomiphene and nafoxidine are correlated with their antagonistic properties.

The differential cellular response to nafoxidine and clomiphene has important implications with respect to their proposed activity as "antiestrogens." Compounds such as clomiphene, tamoxifen, and nafoxidine are used clinically to induce ovulation in anovulatory women and in the treatment of breast cancer. The rationale for their use is based on their definition as antiestrogens. However, the differential cellular response to the triphenylethylene derivatives requires that their activity as estrogen antagonists be re-evaluated. Since these compounds have mixed agonist–antagonist activities that are related to target cell response, their definition as antiestrogens requires careful reassessment.

F. NUCLEAR TYPE II SITES AND THE NUCLEAR MATRIX

Nuclear type II sites are resistant to salt extraction procedures, which suggests that they are bound very tightly to nuclear components. Salt-insoluble or salt-resistant receptor sites for androgens and estrogens in the uterus, liver, and ventral prostate have been reported to be associated with the nuclear matrix. Since the nuclear matrix is thought to be involved in the structure–function components that control DNA and RNA synthesis, it was of interest to examine binding of type II sites to these structures.

The data presented in Fig. 7 suggest that type II sites in the rat uterus are also associated with the nuclear matrix of this tissue (Clark and Markaverich, 1982b). In these experiments, nuclear matrix was prepared from uterine nuclei obtained from estradiol-implanted rats (2 mg for 96 hours) essentially as described by Barrack *et al.* (1977). Briefly, uteri were homogenized in high magnesium buffer (10 mM Tris; 5 mM MgCl$_2$, pH 7.4) and the homogenate was centrifuged at 800 g to obtain the crude nuclear pellet. The pellet was washed three times by resuspension and centrifugation (800 g for 20 minutes) in high magnesium buffer and split into two equal aliquots. One

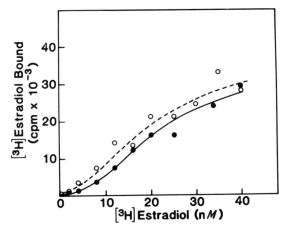

Fɪɢ. 7. Saturation analysis of the specific binding of [³H]estradiol to crude uterine nuclei (O- - -O) and nuclear matrix (●———●).

aliquot was assayed directly for nuclear type II sites by [³H]estradiol exchange (Fig. 7) under conditions that are optimum (4°C for 60 minutes) for the measurement of this site. The remaining nuclei (Fig. 3) were extracted three times with 2 *M* NaCl, washed with 1% Triton X-100, and also assayed for nuclear type II sites by [³H]estradiol exchange. Analysis of these data revealed that 95–98% of the nuclear type II sites were resistant to these extraction procedures and are presumably associated with nuclear matrix, even though this matrix preparation was devoid of 90–95% of the total nuclear DNA. Preliminary data also suggest that these sites are resistant to DNase digestion and are dramatically reduced by trypsin (data not shown), further supporting their association with nuclear matrix.

G. An Endogenous Ligand for Type II Sites

As explained earlier, the presence of type II sites in nuclear preparations complicates the measurement of the estrogen receptor. In addition, we observed that the quantity of nuclear type II sites varied with the homogenization conditions used in the assay. In order to establish the quantitative and qualitative relationships between type I and type II binding and to optimize the assay conditions for measurement of both binding sites, we performed estrogen binding assays at various dilutions of homogenate. The results of such experiments are shown in Fig. 8, which demonstrates that, as uterine homogenates are diluted, more nuclear type II sites are measured (Markaverich *et al.*, 1983). Note that this is not true for the estrogen recep-

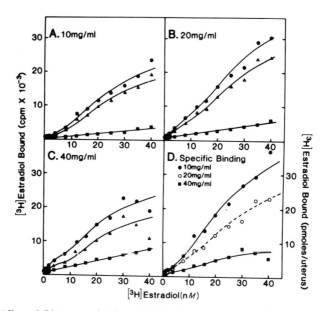

FIG. 8. Effect of dilution on [3H]estradiol binding in uterine nuclear fractions from 17β-estradiol-implanted (4 mg × 96 hours) adult ovariectomized rats. Uterine nuclei were prepared, diluted in TE (10 mM Tris, 1.5 mM EDTA) buffer in final volumes equivalent to 10 (A), 20 (B), or 40 (C) mg fresh uterine equivalent per milliliter and assayed for estrogen binding sites by [3H]estradiol exchange (37° × 30 minutes). Specific binding (▲ in panels A–C) was determined by subtraction of nonspecific binding (■ in panels A–C, noncompetable with 300-fold excess diethylstibestrol) from the total quantity (● in panels A–C) of [3H]estradiol bound. Panel D represents the specific binding measured at 10, 20, or 40 mg nuclear equivalents per milliliter (panels A–C) corrected for the dilution effect (pmoles/uterus). Identical results are obtained when these data are expressed per μg DNA or as numbers of estrogen binding sites per cell (data not shown). [From Markaverich *et al.* (1983).]

tor. These findings suggested the possibility that an endogenous inhibitor (ligand) was dissociating from type II sites upon dilution, which then permitted a greater number of sites to be measured.

The presence of an endogenous ligand for type II sites was confirmed by demonstrating that cytosol preparations contained substance that inhibited the binding of [3H]estradiol to nuclear type II sites (Fig. 9). Note in this figure that there was no effect of the addition of cytosol preparation on the binding of [3H]estradiol of either the cytosol or the nuclear estrogen receptor. Thus, the inhibiting effect appears to be specific for type II sites.

Preliminary characterization of this inhibitor in rat uterine cytosol demonstrates that this molecule(s) is stable to heat (100° × 60 minutes) and 0.1 N HCl, and, therefore, it is unlikely to be protein in nature. In addition, trypsin and proteinase K do not destroy its activity, and the inhibitor activity

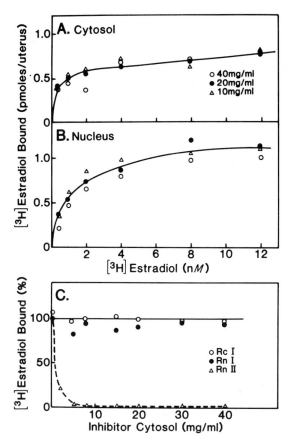

FIG. 9. Effects of dilution and cytosol inhibitor preparations on [3H]estradiol binding to cytoplasmic and nuclear estrogen receptor (type I sites). Uterine cytosol (ovariectomized controls) (A) and nuclei (10 μg estradiol injection, 30 minutes prior to sacrifice) (B) were prepared from appropriately treated animals, diluted to the indicated concentrations (△, 10 mg/ml; ●, 20 mg/ml; ○, 40 mg/ml) and assayed for estrogen receptor by [3H]estradiol exchange. Results are expressed as specific binding corrected for the dilution effect (pmoles/uterus). (C) Uterine cytosol (○, Rc I) or nuclei (●, Rn I) from above were diluted to 10 μg fresh uterine equivalents per milliliter and incubated (cytosol, 30° × 30 minutes; nuclei, 37° × 30 minutes) in the presence of increasing concentrations of a uterine cytosol (2.5–40 mg/ml) inhibitor preparation and 10 nM [3H]estradiol ± 300-fold excess DES. Specific binding of [3H]estradiol in cytosol (○) was determined by the hydroxylapatite adsorption assay, and measurement of nuclear type I sites (●) was as routinely performed in nuclear exchange assays. As a control, uterine nuclei (estradiol-implanted rats) containing nuclear type II sites were diluted to 10 mg/ml (△, Rn II) and incubated (4° × 60 minutes); 40 nM [3H]estradiol bound where 100% (~5000 cpm, type I; ~35,000 cpm, type II) represents binding to cytosol or nuclear sites in the absence of the inhibitor preparation. [From Markaverich *et al.* (1983).]

chromatographs on Sephadex G-25 or LH-20 as two major peaks with an estimated molecular weight of ~350 (Fig. 10). We have purified the β-peak material from rat liver (which appears identical to that seen in the uterus) by thin layer chromatography and HPLC, and it appears to consist of two nearly identical phenanthrene-like compounds with molecular weights on the basis of mass spectrometry of 302 and 304. Proof that these are in fact the inhibitor molecules awaits purification to homogeneity, structural identification, and

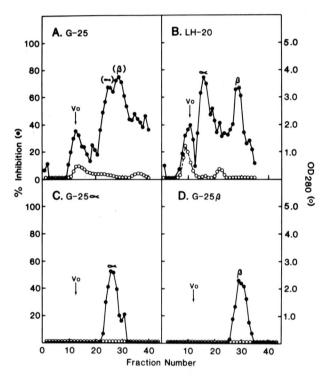

FIG. 10. Chromatography of rat uterine cytosol inhibitor preparations on Sephadex G-25 (A, C, D) or LH-20 (B) columns. Acid-precipitated boiled cytosol (100 mg fresh tissue equivalents per milliliter) was loaded (1 ml) on these columns and eluted (0.5 ml/fraction) with TE (10 mM Tris, 1.5 mM EDTA) buffer. Each fraction was assayed (125 μl) for inhibitor activity, and binding data are expressed as percent inhibition, which represents the relative quantity of [3H]estradiol specifically bound to nuclear type II sites in the presence of the column fractions, as compared to control (nuclei + buffer; ~35,000 cpm). Panels C and D represent rechromatography and assay of inhibitor activity from pooled lyophilized LH-20 α and β peak fractions (resuspended in 1 ml TE and rechromatographed) on Sephadex G-25. Identical results are obtained with "native" cytosol from rat uterus, and therefore the α and β inhibitor forms are not generated by the boiling or acid-precipitation steps. [From Markaverich *et al.* (1983).]

demonstration that the "identified" material has equivalent biological activity. At the present time, we feel that these phenanthrene derivatives are good candidates for the inhibitor activity since the only other measurable compounds in the sample preparation (free fatty acids) did not inhibit [^{3}H]estradiol binding to nuclear type II sites.

We do not know the cellular origin of the inhibitor activity. Excluding the possibility that the inhibitor activity has an extremely long biological half-life (>7–10 days), it is unlikely to be of adrenal or ovarian origin. Ablation of these endocrine glands (7–10 days prior to analysis) did not change the measurable quantities of this activity in uterine cytosol. Likewise, estrogen, progesterone, or dexamethasone administration to adult-ovariectomized rats does not alter detectable levels of this material. We currently feel that this material may be a steroid metabolite of liver origin, since the liver contains high quantities of the activity. Perhaps chronic hormone (estrogen, glucocorticoid, etc.) administration will regulate the synthesis of this compound in the liver.

Another possibility for regulation is that ovarian steroids do not directly regulate the synthesis of this inhibitor activity, but instead regulate the concentration of the compound that is available for binding to nuclear type II sites. Preliminary experiments suggest that estrogen may modulate the levels of an inhibitor binding protein, and we are currently investigating this possibility. We speculate at this time that when the inhibitor is bound to this protein it may be "inactive", and consequently nuclear type II sites are activated or expressed.

On the basis of the above observations we can only conclude that this inhibitor very effectively blocks estradiol binding to nuclear type II sites. Since nuclear type II sites display very complex [^{3}H]estradiol-binding behavior, we could not definitively determine the nature of this interaction. Competition experiments with the inhibitor suggest that the inhibition occurs by a competitive inhibition mechanism; however, noncompetitive allosteric effects cannot be ruled out. It appears that the "dissociation" of the inhibitor from nuclear type II sites as suggested by the dilution experiments (Fig. 8) is estrogen dependent, since this dilution effect is not observed with uterine nuclear fractions from untreated ovariectomized control animals.

Since we have not been able to directly assess the effects of this inhibitor activity *in vivo*, it is very difficult at this early time to ascribe any direct role for this compound in estrogen action. These experiments await chemical identification of the inhibitor, as mentioned earlier, and we are currently attempting to purify this material to homogeneity and to structurally identify the molecule from rat liver. Once a positive identification has been made, determination of its biological significance *in vivo* should be straightforward. Preliminary *in vitro* experiments, however, are very promising. It appears that there is a deficiency in the β-inhibitor component in rat mammary tumor cytosol compared to normal uterus and in lactating mammary gland (Fig. 11). In experiments to be presented elsewhere, we have observed that inhibitor preparations from rat mammary tumors that were deficient in the β-peak material did not inhibit growth of uterine stromal and myometrial cells or of rat mammary tumor cells in culture. In contrast, inhibitor preparations from uterus or liver, which contain the β material, reduced cell numbers by approximately 80% following 4–7 days of treatment. Whether or not this inhibition of cell growth in culture resulted from an acceleration of cell death or an inhibition of cell division or both remains to be resolved. We are currently initiating more definitive experiments with the HPLC-purified β-peak material to answer these questions.

Although the physiological significance of this inhibitor remains to be resolved, we speculate at this time that the inhibitor may act to modify or regulate uterotropic responses to estrogen or perhaps to act in a "protective" capacity in cases of hyperestrogenization. Such hypotheses are consistent with our current knowledge concerning a possible role for nuclear type II sites in estrogen action. As described previously, we have shown that these secondary nuclear estrogen binding sites are only activated or stimulated in the nucleus under conditions that cause uterine hypertrophy, hyperplasia,

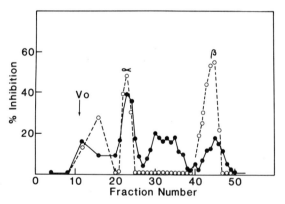

FIG. 11. Comparison of LH-20 elution profiles from acid-precipitated boiled cytosol preparations (100 mg fresh tissue equivalents per milliliter) from rat uterus (O- - -O) or from an estrogen-induced rat mammary tumor (●———●). The column (1.0 × 30 cm; 20 ml bed volume) was eluted (0.5 ml/minute) in TE buffer, and 0.5 ml fractions were collected and assayed as described (Fig. 7). Data are expressed as percent inhibition (see Fig. 7) and represent one of three separate experiments. Analysis of cytosol inhibitor preparations from three separate mammary tumors provided essentially identical results to those shown above except that the β-peak material was nonmeasurable in one mammary tumor preparation. [From Markaverich *et al.* (1983).]

and DNA synthesis (Markaverich and Clark, 1979; Markaverich *et al.*, 1981b,c). Furthermore, dexamethasone and progesterone antagonism of uterine growth in the rat are associated with an inhibition of estrogen stimulation of nuclear type II sites, and these antagonists do not affect the normal functions of the estrogen receptor. On the basis of these experiments, we have suggested that nuclear type II sites may be involved in estrogen action. Since nuclear type II estrogen binding sites may be localized on the nuclear matrix that has been implicated in DNA replication (Pardoll *et al.*, 1980), we feel that this inhibitor activity may modulate or block estrogen-induced DNA synthesis by inhibiting estrogen stimulation of these secondary nuclear estrogen binding sites. Structural identification of the inhibitor molecule will aid in the determination of the precise function of type II sites in estrogen action. Hopefully these studies will lead to an understanding of the intracellular mechanisms by which endogenous substances may modulate estrogenic responses in estrogen target tissues. Perhaps the failure of estrogen to stimulate cell growth (hyperplasia, DNA synthesis) in estrogen target tissues such as the pituitary and hypothalamus (Kelner and Peck, 1981) is related to the inability of estrogen to modulate the activity of this inhibitor in these tissues. Certainly, the failure of estrogen to stimulate nuclear type II sites in these estrogen target organs makes this a tenable hypothesis. Our findings that rat and mouse mammary tumors and human breast cancer (Markaverich *et al.*, 1984) contain significantly lower levels ($\sim$15- to 20-fold) of this inhibitor activity, which is correlated with a deficiency in the β-peak component, are consistent with this hypothesis. Likewise, nuclear type II sites appear to be permanently activated in ovarian-dependent (Watson and Clark, 1980) or ovarian-independent (Watson *et al.*, 1980) mouse mammary tumors and human breast cancer (Syne *et al.*, 1982a,b), regardless of the endocrine status. Therefore, these higher levels of nuclear type II sites in malignant tissues are correlated with this inhibitor deficiency. Likewise, we have measured basal levels of nuclear type II sites in a variety of tissues that do not normally respond to estrogen via hypertrophy and hyperplasia (diaphragm, spleen, liver). These tissues do contain significant quantities of inhibitor activity. Therefore, our hypothesis is that this inhibitor may be component of all tissues, as are nuclear type II sites. In tissues that do not normally respond to estrogen in a proliferative manner, type II sites are complexed with this inhibitor, and consequently the functions of these sites are not expressed. Conversely, in tissues that do respond to estrogens, the association of the receptor–estrogen complex with target cell nuclei may result in a dissociation of the inhibitor from nuclear type II sites. Under these conditions, cellular hypertrophy and hyperplasia are observed. Consistent with this hypothesis is our observation that in estrogen-treated nuclei additional nuclear type II sites are observed following dilution. Since this effect is not observed in uterine nuclei from ovariectomized animals, we feel that this dissociation of the inhibitor from nuclear type II sites is estrogen dependent. Obviously, the lower levels of inhibitor activity in neoplastic tissues are consistent with the elevated levels of type II sites measured in tumors and the rapid proliferation rate in these cell populations. Although only tentative at this point in time, we feel that this is a reasonable model for potential regulation of cell proliferation by this type II binding inhibitor.

In addition to the potential role for this inhibitor in uterine physiology, its presence in a variety of rat tissues has important implications with respect to the measurement of nuclear estrogen receptor and nuclear type II sites. Although we have shown that the inhibitor does not directly interfere with [^{3}H]estradiol binding to cytoplasmic or nuclear type I sites (Fig. 9), indirect effects on these sites cannot be ruled out. We have previously demonstrated that the quantity of nuclear type II estrogen binding sites in the rat uterus will have variable, but profound, effects on receptor measurement (Markaverich *et al.*, 1981a). Consequently, an endogenous inhibitor that interferes with estradiol binding to nuclear type II sites in [^{3}H]estradiol exchange assays will also indirectly influence estimates of estrogen receptor. As discussed previously, the degree of interference is dependent upon the dilution of nuclei used in these exchange assays. Furthermore, we have previously shown that 0.4 M KCl extraction of uterine nuclei can have profound effects on the measurement of salt-extractable and salt-resistant nuclear type I sites (Markaverich *et al.*, 1981d). Since exposure of uterine nuclei to 0.4 M KCl increases the numbers of type II estrogen binding sites in these nuclear fractions, the error introduced into receptor measurement under these experimental conditions is substantial and varies with hormone administered and duration of exposure. On the basis of the present studies, it is quite possible that removal and/or dilution of this endogenous inhibitor with 0.4 M KCl extraction procedures was, at least in part, responsible for the "opening up" of nuclear type II sites in these salt extracts of nuclei.

III. ANTIESTROGEN BINDING SITES AND AN ENDOGENOUS LIGAND

Antiestrogens, such as clomiphene and tamoxifen, are triphenylethylene derivatives that are used to induce ovulation and to treat hormone-dependent breast cancer. Although they have been used effectively for years, their mechanism of action remains unknown. Most investigators believe antiestrogens interfere with the action of estrogen at the receptor level; however, as we describe below, the picture must be more complex than this.

A. The Agonistic–Antagonistic
Actions of Antiestrogens

Antiestrogens are thought to interfere with estrogen action by competing for estrogen receptor sites and thereby reducing the number of active receptor–estrogen complexes. The receptor antiestrogen complexes are thought to be inactive or partially active. Indeed, this explanation does appear to have validity in experiments that are done with cells *in vitro* (Lieberman *et al.*, 1983). However, this concept fails when it is applied to the *in vivo* situation. Triphenylethylene drugs are mixed agonist–antagonists when injected in the animal, and this agonist–antagonist activity expresses itself as a function of time. During the first 24 hours after an injection of estradiol or nafoxidine, early uterotropic events, such as the stimulation of RNA polymerase I and II activities, are equally elevated, and no suggestion of antagonism can be observed (Hardin *et al.*, 1976). This is also true for the amount of receptor–hormone complex found in the nuclear fraction. However, antiestrogens not only cause equivalent nuclear binding of the receptor, but also cause occupancy of these sites for much longer time periods than estradiol (Clark *et al.*, 1973). It is only after 24 hours that antiestrogens begin to exert their antagonistic effects, even though they maintain a significant level of estrogenic stimulation. Thus, by 3–4 days after the beginning of such an experiment, both antagonistic and agonistic effects of these compounds can be observed (Clark and Peck, 1979).

It can be concluded from the above discussion that triphenylethylene antiestrogens are estrogenic during the first 24 hours after exposure *in vivo* and that antiestrogenicity is expressed after this time. Therefore, it appears that the concept of direct receptor blocking is not valid *in vivo* and that indirect actions of these compounds are likely. Such indirect actions may result from the binding of these compounds to the specific antiestrogen binding sites that have been described by Sutherland *et al.* (1980).

B. Specific Binding Sites for Triphenylethylene
Antiestrogens

Sutherland *et al.* (1980) showed that there are antiestrogen-specific binding sites in various tissues and suggested that these sites might be receptors for antiestrogens. The presence of these sites has been confirmed by several investigators (Gulino and Pasqualini, 1980; Faye *et al.*, 1980; Sudo *et al.*, 1983; Kon, 1983). Our interest in these sites arose from the possibility that there might be an endogenous ligand for these sites, which might represent an endogenous antiestrogen.

In order to test the possibility of an endogenous ligand, we first examined the characteristics of the triphenylethylene antiestrogen binding site (TABS). These sites are found in the low-speed cytosol of several different tissues. They appear to be associated with the particulate components of the homogenate, since they can be cleared from the cytosol by high-speed centrifugation (Sudo *et al.*, 1983).

TABS have some properties in common with receptors and some unique properties. There are a limited number of sites per cell that have a high affinity (K_d, = 2 nM) for the binding of triphenylethylene drugs (Fig. 12). These sites are very specific for the binding of triphenylethylenes and do not recognize estrogens or any of the other steroids. They are found in several tissues of the body and are not restricted to estrogen target tissues (Sudo *et al.*, 1983; Kon, 1983). This distribution makes it unlikely that TABS are antiestrogen receptors per se, but does not rule out an indirect role in estrogen antagonism.

The possible involvement of TABS in the mechanism of action of antiestrogens is suggested by the observation that estrogen administration and the physiological state of the ovary have effects on the level of TABS in both liver and uterus (Winneker *et al.*, 1983). At the time of puberty, the liver TABS concentration increased significantly in the female when compared to both mature males and immature females. TABS levels in the rat uterine cytosol increased significantly in mature females when compared to either castrated or younger animals. In addition, both uterine and liver TABS levels fluctuated throughout the estrous cycle and reached a peak approx-

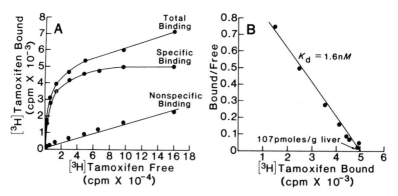

FIG. 12. Saturation (A) and Scatchard (B) analysis of [³H]tamoxifen binding to mature, intact rat liver cytosol. Samples of liver cytosol were exposed to different concentrations of [³H]-tamoxifen for 1 hour at 30°C followed by dextran charcoal separation. A 200-fold excess of DES was added to all assay tubes to inhibit [³H]tamoxifen estrogen receptor interactions. Only specific binding data were used for Scatchard plots. [From Winneker and Clark (1983). © 1983, The Endocrine Society.]

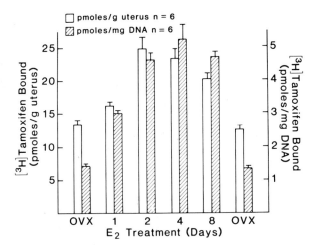

FIG. 13. The effect of estradiol treatment on rat uterine cytosol TABS. Ovariectomized rats implanted with beeswax pellets containing 20 μg of estradiol were sacrificed 1, 2, 4, and 8 days later. Control animals were sacrificed on days 1 and 8 only. The concentration of TABS normalized per gram of uterus and per milligram of DNA are shown. [From Winneker and Clark (1983). © 1983, The Endocrine Society.]

imately on the day of estrus. Treatment of ovariectomized rats with physiological amounts of estradiol causes a twofold increase in TABS levels in the uterus, thus mimicking the midcycle peak of TABS (Fig. 13). A similar elevation in TABS occurs in the liver following estrogen treatment. Gulino and Pasqualini (1983) have shown that the levels of TABS are modulated in the guinea pig uterus by estradiol and progesterone.

These results indicate that TABS are being regulated by ovarian steroids, primarily estrogens. If TABS were involved in antiestrogen action, it might be expected that estrogens would regulate or modify the level of these sites. That is, one can speculate that one of the estrogenic responses of target tissues is to produce TABS, which may in some way modify the ability of the tissue to respond to estrogen.

C. TRIPHENYLETHYLENE BINDING SITES AND LOW-DENSITY LIPOPROTEINS

During the course of studies discussed above, we also examined rat serum for the presence of TABS and were surprised to find substantial quantities of sites that resemble but are not identical to the sites found in the liver and uterus (Winneker *et al.*, 1983). The serum TABS has less affinity for triphenylethylene drugs ($K_d = 28$ nM), but the hormonal specificity is similar.

Since there were high concentrations of this site present in serum, we decided to characterize this site. Preliminary studies using 1.5 *M* agarose columns indicated that the molecular weight of TABS was greater than 10^6. Since serum lipoproteins are found in these large-molecular-weight classes, we examined the possibility that these lipoproteins contained the TABS.

When serum is separated into its lipoprotein fractions by flotation sucrose density gradient centrifugation, specific binding of [^{3}H]tamoxifen can be found in the gradient fraction containing low-density lipoproteins (LDL) (Fig. 14). These LDL TABS have the same binding characteristics and hormone specificity as the serum TABS. They are destroyed by exposure to protease enzymes and not by DNase or RNase. Therefore, these sites are probably associated with the protein component of the LDL.

The physiological significance of our findings is not known; however, it has been recognized for some time that triphenylethylene drugs inhibit cholesterol synthesis (for a review of this topic, see Clark and Markaverich, 1982a). In addition, since cellular cholesterol synthesis is thought to be controlled by LDL cholesterol (Goldstein and Brown, 1979), it is possible that triphenylethylene drugs are involved in this process. Also, it has been demonstrated that treatment with hyperphysiological levels of estrogen decreases serum LDL levels in the rat (Hay *et al.*, 1971) and increases the uptake of LDL by the rat liver (Kovanen *et al.*, 1979). We have recently observed that

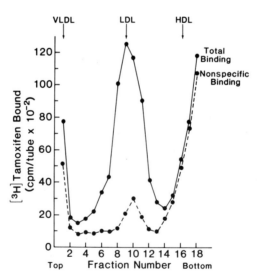

Fig. 14. Potassium bromide density gradient centrifugation profile illustrating the fractionation of rat serum lipoproteins (VLDL, LDL, and HDL) and the binding of [^{3}H]tamoxifen to these fractions. Note that the TABS resides under the LDL marker. [From Winneker *et al.* (1983). © 1983, The Endocrine Society.]

physiological levels of estradiol will also decrease LDL TABS in ovariec-tomized rats (Winneker and Clark, 1983). These effects of estrogen may be related to the observations discussed in the previous section, that estradiol treatment increases the number of intracellular TABS in the liver and uterus.

D. An Endogenous Ligand for the Triphenylethylene Antiestrogen Binding Site

The presence of specific binding sites for triphenylethylene in various tissues and in the LDL fraction of rat serum opens the possibility that the activity of these sites is regulated by an endogenous ligand. We examined this possibility by extracting liver tissue in boiling ethanol and fractionating the extract by silica gel column chromatography. Each fraction was assayed for its ability to inhibit the binding of [3H]tamoxifen to liver TABS, and these were collected and used in a competitive binding assay (Fig. 15) (Clark *et al.*, 1983). These data show that various dilutions of the endogenous ligand inhibit the binding of [3H]tamoxifen to TABS in a fashion similar to that of nonlabeled tamoxifen.

The ability of the endogenous ligand to inhibit the binding of [3H]tamoxifen to serum LDL fractions was also tested. The data in Fig. 16

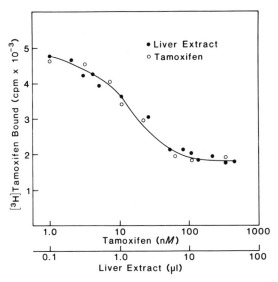

Fig. 15. Inhibition of the binding of [3H]tamoxifen to liver TABS by nonlabeled tamoxifen and endogenous ligand. [From Clark *et al.* (1983). © 1983, The Endocrine Society.]

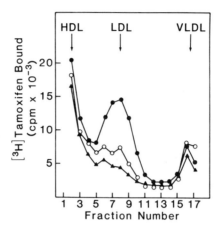

F‍ɪɢ. 16. Density gradient profiles of serum lipoproteins labeled with [³H]tamoxifen alone (●), with [³H]tamoxifen plus 100-fold excess of nonlabeled tamoxifen (▲), or with [³H]tamoxifen plus 100 µl of endogenous ligand (○). [From Clark *et al.* (1983). © 1983, The Endocrine Society.]

show that [³H]tamoxifen binds to HDL (high-density lipoprotein), LDL, and VLDL (very low-density lipoprotein) fractions; however, inhibition of binding by 100-fold excess of nonlabeled tamoxifen or 100 µl of endogenous ligand is observed only in the fractions containing LDL.

These data suggest that an endogenous ligand is present in the ethanol extracts of rat liver that acts as a competitive inhibitor of the binding of [³H]tamoxifen to TABS in liver cytosol and serum LDL. The presence of such a ligand implies that it may be an endogenous antiestrogen; however, the binding of triphenylethylene antiestrogens to TABS has not been shown to be involved in antiestrogen action. Therefore, the term *endogenous antiestrogen* is used with reservation and is an operational term rather than a functional one.

The significance of TABS associated with LDL is not known; however, as mentioned previously, LDL is known to be involved in the control of cholesterol metabolism (Goldstein and Brown, 1979), and triphenylethylene drugs are known to inhibit these pathways (for review of this topic, see Clark and Markaverich, 1982a). Therefore, it seems possible that LDL TABS and the endogenous ligand may be involved in the control of cholesterol metabolism. If such were the case, it is possible to suggest a mechanism of indirect estrogen antagonism by triphenylethylene drugs. The binding interactions of estrogens with target tissues stimulate the biosynthetic processes that culminate in cell growth and proliferation. This occurs between 24 and 72 hours after exposure to estrogens. Triphenylethylene antiestrogens may interfere with the uptake or proper utilization of cholesterol during this 24- to 72-hour period and thus block the ability of cells to synthesize new membranes, which are necessary for growth. It is well known, as explained earlier, that antiestrogens act as agonists during the period prior to 24 hours and act as antagonists after this time. Thus, it is possible that these compounds block the full expression of estrogen action by interfering with the delivery or utilization of cholesterol by target tissue cells. In nontarget tissues, which also contain TABS, estrogens are not active as stimulators of cell growth, and, hence, no dramatic effect would be expected. However, triphenylethylene drugs are known to have effects on many tissues other than those of the reproductive tract, and it is possible that these effects occur via the TABS system.

ACKNOWLEDGMENTS

This work was supported by NIH grants HD-08436 and HD-35480. We thank Lee Graham for secretarial assistance and David Scarff for the artwork.

REFERENCES

Anderson, J. N., Peck, E. J., Jr., and Clark, J. H. (1975). *Endocrinology* **96**, 160–167.

Barlow, J. W., Kraft, N., Stockigt, J. R., and Funder, J. W. (1979). *Endocrinology* **105**, 1055–1063.

Barrack, E. R., and Coffey, D. S. (1980). *J. Biol. Chem.* **255**, 7265–7275.

Barrack, E. R., Hawkins, E. F., Allen, S. L., Hicks, L. L., and Coffey, D. S. (1977). *Biochem. Biophys. Res. Commun.* **79**, 829–836.

Clark, J. H., and Markaverich, B. M. (1982a). *Pharmacol. Ther.* **15**, 467.

Clark, J. H., and Markaverich, B. M. (1982b). *In* "The Nuclear Envelope and the Nuclear Matrix" (G. Maul, ed.), pp. 259–269. Alan R. Liss, Inc., New York.

Clark, J. H., and Peck, E. J., Jr. (1979). "Female Sex Steroids: Receptors and Function." Springer-Verlag, Berlin and New York.

Clark, J. H., Anderson, J. N., and Peck, E. J., Jr. (1973). *Steroids* **22**, 707–718.

Clark, J. H., Paszko, Z., and Peck, E. J., Jr. (1977). *Endocrinology* **100**, 91–96.

Clark, J. H., Hardin, J. W., Upchurch, S., and Eriksson, H. (1978). *J. Biol. Chem.* **253**, 7630–7634.

Clark, J. H., Markaverich, B., Upchurch, S., Eriksson, H., and Hardin, J. W. (1979). *In* "Steroid Hormone Receptor Systems" (W. W. Leavitt and J. H. Clark, eds.), pp. 17–46. Plenum, New York.

Clark, J. H., Winneker, R. C., Gutherie, S. C., and Markaverich, B. M. (1983). *Endocrinology* **113**, 1167–1169.

Do, Y. S., Loose, D. S., and Feldman, D. (1979). *Endocrinology* **105**, 1055–1063.

Ekman, P., Barrack, E. R., Greene, G. L., Jensen, E. V., and Walsh, P. C. (1983). *J. Clin. Endocrinol. Metab.* **57**, 166–176.

Eriksson, H., Upchurch, S., Hardin, J. W., Peck, E. J., Jr., and Clark, J. H. (1978). *Biochem. Biophys. Res. Commun.* **81**, 1–7.

Faye, J.-C., Lasserre, B., and Bayard, F. (1980). *Biochem. Biophys. Res. Commun.* **93**, 1225.

Giannopoulos, G., and Munowitz, P. (1980). *Proc. 62nd Annu. Meet., Am. Endocr. Soc.,* Abstract No. 7.

Goldstein, J. L., and Brown, M. S. (1979). *Annu. Rev. Genet.* **13**, 259–291.

Gorski, J., and Gannon, F. (1976). *Annu. Rev. Physiol.* **38**, 425–450.

Gulino, A., and Pasqualini, J. R. (1980). *Cancer Res.* **40**, 3821.

Gulino, A., and Pasqualini, J. R. (1983). *Endocrinology* **112**, 1871–1873.

Hardin, J. W. H., Clark, J. H., Glasser, S. R., and Peck, E. J., Jr. (1976). *Biochemistry* **17**, 3146–3152.

Hay, R. V., Potenger, L. A., Reingold, A. L., Getz, G. S., and Wissler, R. W. (1971). *Biochem. Biophys. Res. Commun.* **44**, 1471–1476.

Hseuh, A. J. W., Peck, E. J., Jr., and Clark, J. H. (1976). *Endocrinology* **98**, 438–444.

Huggins, C., and Jensen, E. V. (1955). *J. Exp. Med.* **102**, 335–346.

Kelner, K. L., and Peck, E. J., Jr. (1981). *J. Recept. Res.* **2**, 47–62.

Kon, O. L. (1983). *J. Biol. Chem.* **258**, 3173–3177.

Kovanen, P. T., Brown, M. S., and Goldstein, J. L. (1979). *J. Biol. Chem.* **254**, 1137.

Leavitt, W. W., Toft, D. O., Strott, C. A., and O'Malley, B. W. (1974). *Endocrinology* **94**, 1041–1053.

Lerner, J. L. (1964). *Recent Prog. Horm. Res.* **20**, 435–490

Lieberman, M. E., Jordan, V. C., Fritsch, M., Santos, M. A., and Gorski, J. (1983). *J. Biol. Chem.* **258**, 4734–4740.

McCormack, S. A., and Glasser, S. R. (1980). *Endocrinology* **106**, 1634–1649.

MacLaughlin, D. T., Hutson, J. M., and Donoahue, P. K. (1983). *Endocrinology* **113**, 141–145.

Markaverich, B. M., and Clark, J. H. (1979). *Endocrinology* **105**, 1458–1462.

Markaverich, B. M., Clark, J. H., and Hardin, J. W. (1978). *Biochemistry* **17**, 3146–3152.

Markaverich, B. M., Upchurch, S., and Clark, J. H. (1980). *In* "Perspectives in Steroid Receptor Research" (F. Bresciani, ed.), pp. 143–164. Raven Press, New York.

Markaverich, B. M., Williams, M., Upchurch, S., and Clark, J. H. (1981a). *Endocrinology* **109**, 62–69.

Markaverich, B. M., Upchurch, S., and Clark, J. H. (1981b). *J. Steroid Biochem.* **14**, 125–132.

Markaverich, B. M., Upchurch, S., McCormack, S. A., Glasser, S. R., and Clark, J. H. (1981c). *Biol. Reprod.* **24**, 171–181.

Markaverich, B. M., Upchurch, S., and Clark, J. H. (1981d). *J. Recept. Res.* **1**, 415–438.

Markaverich, B. M., Roberts, R. R., Finney, R. W., and Clark, J. H. (1983). *J. Biol. Chem.* **258**, 11663–11671.

Markaverich, B. M., Roberts, R. R., Alejandro, M. A., and Clark, J. H. (1984). *Cancer Res.* **44**, 1575–1579.

Martucci, C., and Fishman, J. (1977). *Endocrinology* **101**, 1709–1715.

Mercer, W. D., Edwards, D. P., Chamness, G. C., and McGuire, W. L. (1981). *Cancer Res.* **41**, 4644–4652.

Milgrom, E., Thi, L., Atgers, M., and Baulieu, E. E. (1973). *J. Biol. Chem.* **248**, 6366–6377.

Murai, J. T., Lieberman, R. C., Yang, J. J., and Gerschenson, L. E. (1979). *Endocr. Res. Commun.* **6**, 235–247.

O'Malley, B. W., and Means, A. R. (1974). *Science* **183**, 610–620.

Panko, W. B., Watson, C. S., and Clark, J. H. (1981). *J. Steroid Biochem.* **14**, 1311–1316.

Pardoll, D. M., Vogelstein, B., and Coffey, D. S. (1980). *Cell* **19**, 527–536.

Smith, R. G., Clarke, S. G., Zalta, E., and Taylor, R. N. (1979). *J. Steroid Biochem.* **10**, 31–38.

Stormshak, F., Leake, R., Wertz, N., and Gorski, J. (1976). *Endocrinology* **99**, 1501–1511.

Sudo, K., Monsma, F. J., Jr., and Katzenellenbogen, B. S. (1983). *Endocrinology* **112**, 425–434.

Sutherland, R. L., Murphy, L. C., Foo, M. S., Green, M. D., and Whybourne, A. M. (1980). *Nature (London)* **228**, 273.

Swaneck, G. E., Alvarez, J. M., and Sufrin, G. (1982). *Biochem. Biophys. Res. Commun.* **106**, 1441–1445.

Syne, J. S., Markaverich, B. M., Clark, J. H., and Panko, W. B. (1982a). *Cancer Res.* **42**, 4443–4448.

Syne, J. S., Markaverich, B. M., Clark, J. H., and Panko, W. B. (1982b). *Cancer Res.* **42**, 4449–4454.

Szego, C. M., and Roberts, S. (1953). *Recent Prog. Horm. Res.* **8**, 419–464.

Walters, M. R., and Clark, J. H. (1978). *Endocrinology* **98**, 601–609.

Watson, C. S., and Clark, J. H. (1980). *J. Recept. Res.* **1**, 91–111.

Watson, C. S., Medina, D., and Clark, J. H. (1980). *Endocrinology* **107**, 1432–1437.

Winneker, R. C., and Clark, J. H. (1983). *Endocrinology* **112**, 1910–1915.

Winneker, R. C., Guthrie, S. C., and Clark, J. H. (1983). *Endocrinology* **112**, 1823–1827.

Yuh, K.-C., and Keyes, P. L. (1979). *Endocrinology* **105**, 690–696.

CHAPTER 12

The Mineralocorticoid Receptor

Diana Marver

Departments of Internal Medicine and Biochemistry
University of Texas Health Science Center
Southwestern Medical School
Dallas, Texas

BIOCHEMICAL ACTIONS OF HORMONES, VOL. XII

I. INTRODUCTION

Aldosterone influences the transepithelial transport of Na, K, and H ions in specific target tissues. The initiation of the physiological response requires 1–1.5 hours, or the period of time required for receptor binding, translocation of receptor complexes to the nucleus, synthesis of RNA and mineralocorticoid-specific proteins, and insertion of these proteins into their active sites within the cell (Fimognari *et al.*, 1967). If urinary Na/K ratios are used as an index of mineralocorticoid action, an intravenous injection of aldosterone, with a biological half-life of about 30 minutes, results in a maximal fall in urinary Na/K ratios at 4 hours in adrenalectomized rats, with a marked recovery in the ratio by 12 hours (Fimognari *et al.*, 1967; Kirsten and Kirsten, 1972). Recent experiments have shown that there is no difference in the time course of the change in urinary Na or K concentrations, although documentation of increases in urinary K following aldosterone may be compromised by both dietary K intake and factors that determine K recycling in the renal medulla (Horisberger and Diezi, 1983; Fimognari *et al.*, 1967; Stokes, 1982). Prolonged administration of aldosterone leads to renal "escape" from the Na-retaining actions of this hormone. The exact factors that result in escape are controversial, but may include prostaglandins and the activation of the kallekrein–kinin system. Notably, escape is a renal phenomenon, since other target tissues are not similarly affected following chronic mineralocorticoid therapy (Mulrow and Forman, 1972).

Well-recognized target organs for mineralocorticoids are the mammalian kidney, colon, and salt glands, the toad/turtle urinary bladder, and frog skin. Current data would suggest that at least two functionally distinct types of cells respond to mineralocorticoids in both kidney and amphibian bladder; one is responsible for steroid-dependent Na reabsorption (and K secretion), and the other, for H secretion. These two cell types are depicted in Fig. 1. It is assumed that both of these cells contain mineralocorticoid receptors, although a rigorous argument has not been presented for the presence of receptors in acid-secreting cells. In the kidney, these cells are typified by the cortical (Na-reabsorbing, K-secreting) and medullary collecting tubule (H-secreting). In the toad bladder, they are equivalent to the granular and mitochondrial-rich cells, respectively (Gross *et al.*, 1975; Schwartz and Burg, 1978; Marver and Lombard, 1981; Stokes *et al.*, 1981; Stone *et al.*, 1983; Marver, 1980a).

As a clarification of the schema shown in Fig. 1, aldosterone freely enters all cells, but is fixed within target cells by the presence of mineralocorticoid receptors. Antagonists compete with aldosterone for these sites, but, once bound, cannot induce that conformation of the receptor required for subsequent nuclear attachment (Fanestil and Edelman, 1966; Ausiello and Sharp,

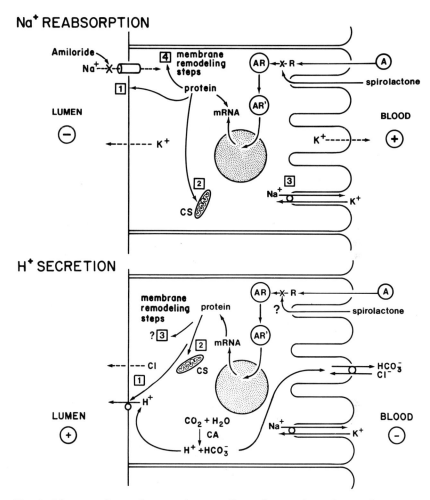

FIG. 1. Schematic of mineralocorticoid target cells regulating either sodium reabsorption or acid secretion. Aldosterone (A) freely enters these cells and binds to a mineralocorticoid-specific receptor (R). AR complexes then undergo an activation step (AR'), which enhances their affinity for key chromatin binding sites; both RNA and protein synthesis ensue. Regulatory changes in Na-reabsorbing cells include an increase in (a) luminal membrane Na permeability, (b) TCA cycle enzyme levels, and (c) Na,K-ATPase activity, while peculiar to acid-secreting cells may be the induction or activation of a luminal membrane proton ATPase.

1968; Alberti and Sharp, 1970; Marver *et al.*, 1974). On the other hand, agonists bound to receptors result in increased mRNA, rRNA, and protein synthesis (Rossier *et al.*, 1974). Posited synthesized or activated proteins in the Na-reabsorbing cells include a Na channel on the apical membrane, various mitochondrial enzymes involved in ATP synthesis, Na, K-ATPase, and as yet unidentified factors that may alter fatty acid and phospholipid metabolism (Sharp *et al.*, 1966; Kirsten *et al.*, 1970; Petty *et al.*, 1981; Geering *et al.*, 1982; Goodman, 1981; Yorio and Bentley, 1976, 1978). Available data support the concept that the rate-limiting step in the action of aldosterone on Na transport is an increase in the luminal membrane Na permeability and thus the induction or activation of Na channels, sometimes referred to in the literature as "sodium permeases." Potassium secretion increases secondarily to a rise in the electrochemical gradient for K entry into the lumen. The gradient is enhanced as a result of the increased turnover of Na, K-ATPase, of pumping more K into the cell, and of the increased lumen negativity, which favors the translocation of cations such as K into the lumen. Whether or not aldosterone also increases luminal membrane K conductance in some tissues has not been resolved. Less is known about the action of aldosterone on H transport, although the rate-limiting step in this process is thought to be the induction or activation of a H ATPase embedded within the luminal membrane (Dixon and Al-Awqati, 1979).

Given this brief introduction on the physiological action of aldosterone [for further details, see Marver (1980a) and Marver and Kokko (1983)], the intent of this chapter is to focus on the initial step in this process, namely the receptor. We will examine its physical characteristics and steroid specificity and determine to the best of our ability how the number of receptors and receptor occupancy relate to the various physiological actions of aldosterone. From the outset, it is important to realize that there is a paucity of data on the mineralocorticoid receptor compared to other steroid hormones due to the lability of isolated complexes. Nonetheless, the studies outlined herein may serve as a basis from which to plan for future experiments on the purification and further characterization of this interesting protein.

II. METHODS

A. RECEPTOR ASSAYS

The three most commonly used analyses to examine aldosterone–receptor interactions include binding assays, which evaluate the equilibrium dissociation constant (K_d) and the maximal number of binding sites (N_{max}), competition analyses with a fixed dose of [³H]aldosterone to determine the relative affinity of a series of unlabeled steroids for the mineralocorticoid binding site, and density gradient analyses to determine the influence of a particular steroid or milieu on the sedimentation coefficients (S values) of labeled complexes. The lability of the mineralocorticoid receptor (termed type I corticosteroid binding site) combined with the awareness that corticosteroids have significant affinity for three closely related receptors or binding proteins, termed type I→III sites (Feldman *et al.*, 1972), makes it important that the reader become aware of the problems encountered in assaying the mineralocorticoid receptor and how to limit these problems. The problems include (a) metabolism or inadvertent sequestration of labeled and unlabeled steroids during assay, (b) an inappropriately high ratio of binding site–steroid concentration, and (c) inactivation of receptor.

The question of metabolism has been addressed in several tissues and under a variety of conditions. The mammalian and amphibian kidney and the rabbit aorta have been found to metabolize steroids such as progesterone, corticosterone, cortisol, and aldosterone (Winkel *et al.*, 1980; Watlington *et al.*, 1982; Hierholzer *et al.*, 1982; McDermott *et al.*, 1983; Kornel *et al.*, 1982). The relative rate varies. For instance, Kornel *et al.* (1982) found that if rabbit aorta cytosolic fractions were incubated for 6 hours at 4°C, 98% of [³H]corticosterone (B), 94% of [³H]aldosterone, 88% of [³H]dexamethasone (DM), 86% of [³H]deoxycorticosterone (DOC), and 28% of [³H] cortisol (F) remained unmetabolized. Obviously, if competition assays were carried out using [³H]aldosterone and varying concentrations of either unlabeled aldosterone or F in this tissue, the relative affinity of F for [³H]aldosterone sites would be underestimated by threefold if metabolism data were not available. Renal data is sparse. Rat renal slices incubated at 37°C with [³H]aldosterone produce primarily 5α reduced metabolites, with no major difference between cortical and medullary activity. This is an interesting contrast to the findings of Winkel *et al.* (1980), which showed that the activity responsible for metabolism of progesterone to DOC in rabbit kidney was localized in the cortex, suggesting site-specific localization of steroid hydroxylase versus hydrogenase activity along the nephron. In the McDermott *et al.* (1983) studies, the total amount of aldosterone metabolites formed was equivalent to 10 fmoles/mg dry weight/hour at 37°C. Thus, given conditions of 21.5 nM [³H]aldosterone, 100-mg (dry weight) slices/ml, and a 30-minute incubation period (typical conditions for a receptor assay), only 2.5% of the aldosterone would be metabolized. However, since neither the kinetics nor the capacity of the reducing enzymes is known, we cannot predict how metabolism may influence determination of the K_d by Scatchard analyses where concentrations may range from 0.1 to 10 nM, that is, if the percentage error in evaluating the true concentration of unmetabolized aldosterone may increase with decreasing amounts of added steroid. Furthermore, the suggestion that the renal type III corticosteroid binding site might represent a metabolizing enzyme with high affinity for B and DOC would require a careful analysis of metabolism in receptor assays including these steroids (Marver, 1984a).

Equally important is the question of inadvertant sequestration of available steroid due to adsorption on assay tubes or dishes or to binding to high capacity, contaminating serum-binding proteins such as CBG (corticosteroid binding globulin). Meyer and Nichols (1981) found that triamcinolone acetonide was an unsuitable tag for glucocorticoid receptors since 30% of the label was bound to the assay tube. Furthermore, recent experiments using renal cytosolic samples cleared of contaminating plasma CBG either by ammonium sulfate precipitation of the sample (Beaumont and Fanestil, 1983) or by hydroxylapatite treatment (Stephenson *et al.*, 1984) have suggested that the relative affinities of B, DOC, and F for the mineralocorticoid receptor are higher than heretofore appreciated due to sequestration of unlabeled steroids in competition assays by resident CBG. Beaumont and Fanestil (1983) found that as little as 2 μl rat serum/ml assay bound >60% of 1 nM [³H]corticosterone at 4°C. This problem can be minimized by perfusing kidneys before use, by increasing the ratio of assay volume per milligram of tissue, or by selectively removing CBG; it can be evaluated in competition assays by adding [³H]corticosterone, [³H]deoxycorticosterone, or [³H]cortisol to control incubations and determining bound versus free levels.

As for the concentration of receptor sites in *in vitro* assays, Chang *et al.* (1975) demonstrated that, if the concentration of the receptor or the binding protein is not 10 times lower than the true K_d, then the apparent K_d will vary as a linear function of the receptor concentration. Thus, high-affinity systems (10^{-11}, 10^{-10} M) require the use of very low concentrations of receptor. Given that the affinity of aldosterone for the mineralocorticoid receptor is in this range, this admonition must be taken into consideration. In the example obtained from Warnock and Edelman (1978) and listed in Table I, diluting the sample by a factor of two (13–6 mg/ml protein, approximately equal to a concentration of type I sites of 50 and 32 × 10^{-11} M, respectively) increased the apparent affinity of aldosterone for type I sites by a factor of 10 (90 to 9 × 10^{-11} M), with only a modest increase in the affinity for the type II, or glucocorticoid receptor (62–41 nM). It is probable, therefore, that 9 × 10^{-11} M is a better representation of the true K_d of aldosterone for the mineralocorticoid receptor in kidney. Receptor concentration may be in part responsible for the variability in the dissociation constants obtained for the type I relative to the type II site shown in the examples listed in Table I.

TABLE I

Results of Scatchard Analyses of Rat and Rabbit Renal Receptors Using [3H]Aldosterone

		Assay conditions			Incubation		K_d (nM)		N_{max} (× 10^{-14} mol/mg protein)		
Source	Incubation	Homogenizing buffer	Centrifugation speed (g)	Separation B vs. F	Temperature (°C)	Time (hours)	Type I	Type II	Type I	Type II	Reference[c]
Rat	Cell-free	Tris/Ca^{2+}/Mg^{2+}	100,000	Charcoal	4	1.5	5	65	13	41	1
	Cell-free	Tris/EDTA/glycerol/DTT	30,000	Charcoal-dextran	4	2.5	1.7	60	3.2	38	2
	Cell-free	Tris/EDTA/glycerol/DTT	105,000	Charcoal-dextran	4	2.5	3.9	53	9.0	39	3
	Slice	Sucrose/Tris EDTA/glycerol	100,000	DE-81 filters		2	0.9[a] 0.09[b]	62[a] 41[b]	4.0[a] 0.4[b]	68[a] 34[b]	4
	Cell-free	Sucrose/Tris	100,000	Charcoal-dextran	22	0.66	3.0 0.5	25	3.5 4.6		5
	Slice	Sucrose/Tris/Mo^{2+}	105,000	Charcoal-dextran	20	0.33	3.5	47			3
	Slice	Sucrose/Mg^{2+}	30,000	G.50	25	0.5	2.3				6
	Slice	Sucrose/Ca^{2+}	30,000	G.50	37	0.33	0.5	25	~1.0	~4.0	7
Rabbit	CCTs[d]	—		Millipore filters	25	1	2.0		10.5		8
	Slice	Sucrose/TES/EDTA	34,000	DE-52/Mo^{2+}	37	0.33	3.0	25	1.5	3.4	9

[a] Cytosol concentration = 13 mg/ml.
[b] Cytosol concentration = 6 mg/ml.
[c] (1) Rousseau et al., 1972a; (2) Claire et al., 1978; (3) Rafestin-Oblin et al., 1977; (4) Warnock and Edelman, 1978; (5) Grekin and Sider, 1980; (6) Genard and Palem-Vliers, 1980; (7) Funder et al., 1973a; (8) Doucet and Katz, 1981; (9) Marver, 1980b.
[d] CCTs, cortical collecting tubules.

Inactivation of receptor during processing probably accounts for the next most serious problem in binding assays. The unlabeled receptor in a cell-free state is labile and can be protected to some degree by the presence of steroid, glycerol, or sodium molybdate and by reducing assay temperature. Thus, the time required to prepare a 100,000-g supernatant for cell-free incubations may be critical, as shown by Rafestin-Oblin *et al.* (1977). These investigators examined the K_d of [^{3}H]aldosterone for high-affinity sites (20°C) in rat renal slices and in two cell-free preparations. In the first cell-free assay, steroid was added immediately following a short 700-g centrifugation step; then the usual prolonged high-speed centrifugation step followed. In the second assay, steroid was added only after the 100,000-g for 1 hour step. In the slice and the 700-g assay, high-affinity sites were demonstrable (K_d = 3.5 and 3.9 nM), but they were not so in the delayed assay, suggesting a loss of binding activity in the absence of protective steroid. The presence of [^{3}H]aldosterone alone, however, does not eliminate loss of binding with time. Incubation times at 37°C >30 minutes or at 0°C in excess of 4 hours have been shown to decrease labeled receptor recovery (Doucet and Katz, 1981; Beaumont and Fanestil, 1983). The addition of Ca^{2+} to the homogenization buffer and determination of type I sites using cell-free extracts incubated at 25°C have resulted in an apparent 95% loss of these sites (Warnock and Edelman, 1978). On the other hand, receptor complexes are stabilized to some degree by the addition of 15–30% glycerol in the homogenization buffer (Herman *et al.*, 1968; Alberti and Sharp, 1969; Marver *et al.*, 1972; Rafestin-Oblin *et al.*, 1977). In fact, substitution of glycerol for sucrose in density gradients and addition of labeled aldosterone to density gradient media have markedly improved the recovery of labeled species with [^{3}H]-aldosterone or [^{3}H]spirolactone (Marver *et al.*, 1972).

Maximal protection can be obtained, however, with the addition of 15–20 mM sodium molybdate to homogenizing buffers and to solutions used for column chromatography (Marver, 1980b; Grekin and Sider, 1980). Figure 2 illustrates this property of molybdate. In these experiments, unlabeled rabbit renal cortical and medullary cell-free extracts were incubated for various periods of time in the presence or absence of MoO_4 and then challenged with [^{3}H]aldosterone for binding analyses. Without molybdate there was a 40–50% fall in binding activity in 1 hour at 20°C, with no fall in activity plus molybdate. Grekin and Sider (1980) also found that the presence of 100 mM molybdate decreased the apparent K_d for type I sites by sixfold at 22°C (3 nM → 0.5 nM) with a 31% increase in the moles [^{3}H]aldosterone-bound/mg protein (Table I). The molybdate effect is common to all steroid receptor complexes and is thought to be due to its role as a phosphatase inhibitor (Neilson *et al.*, 1977; Sherman *et al.*, 1982). This compound, however, pre-

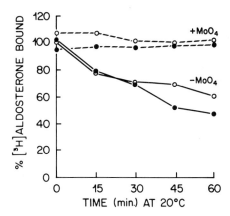

FIG. 2. The influence of molybdate on the stability of the mineralocorticoid receptor. Un-labeled cytoplasmic fractions were prepared from rabbit renal cortex (○) or red medulla (●) and incubated with (broken lines) or without (solid lines) 20 mM sodium molybdate for various periods of time at 20°C. At the times indicated, samples were withdrawn and added to 5 nM [^{3}H]aldosterone ± unlabeled steroid (to determine nonspecific binding) and incubated for 2 hours at 4°C. Values indicate the percentage of specific binding relative to controls maintained at 4°C. [From Marver (1980b).]

vents binding of receptor complexes to chromatin or nuclei, so it cannot be used in transfer assays in which the investigator wishes to estimate the capacity of labeled cytosolic receptors to bind to isolated nuclei or chromatin (Lan *et al.*, 1981).

The last point to be made regarding the receptor assay is the choice of a means to separate bound versus free steroid. Here several methods have been used, such as G-50, DE-52, and hydroxylapatite column or batch chromatography, DE-81 filters, and charcoal-dextran (Marver *et al.*, 1972; Marver, 1980b; Stephenson *et al.*, 1984; Warnock and Edelman, 1978; Rafestin-Oblin *et al.*, 1977). All of these appear to be acceptable, although both DE-52 and hydroxylapatite fractionations allow a degree of separation of classes of binding proteins. In summary of this section, it would appear that mineralocorticoid receptors would be best monitored in slices with [^{3}H]steroid followed by homogenization in molybdate EDTA-containing buffers. An alternate method would be cell-free extracts containing sodium molybdate, although it is not clear yet if this compound alters the K_d independent of its effects on inactivation. In such studies, both metabolism and the influence of contaminating CBG (if DOC, B, or F are included) on the binding reaction should be evaluated.

B. Companion Bioassays

It is desirable to relate *in vitro* binding assays with *in vivo* mineralocorticoid potency. The ability of a steroid to enhance Na reabsorption *in vivo* relative to its potency determined in *in vitro* binding assays depends on its biological half-life, its agonist versus antagonist properties, its affinity for plasma-binding proteins, and the suitability of the bioassay. This section will evaluate the influence of plasma protein and the bioassay used. Table II lists the affinity of several endogenous steroids (aldosterone, B, F, and DOC) for human CBG and plasma-free versus total concentrations of these steroids. Spironolactone and dexamethasone are also added to show that these steroids have negligible affinity for CBG. It is to be expected, therefore, that, although B has about half the affinity of dexamethasone for glucocorticoid or type II sites *in vitro*, 0.2 nM plasma dexamethasone should approximate the glucocorticoid response to 12 nM plasma B *in vivo*, allowing that the free concentration of B is 0.4 nM.

In addition to the contribution of plasma-binding proteins to apparent *in vivo* versus *in vitro* mineralocorticoid activity, there has been recent controversy regarding the best way to bioassay this activity in mammals. The difficulty has to do with the variety of renal mechanisms which influence K excretion. For instance, aldosterone can increase K secretion as a reciprocal act of its effect on Na reabsorption. Glucocorticoids, on the other hand, can increase K secretion as a consequence of their action on glomerular filtration rate. Furthermore, K secreted into the lumen of the renal cortical collecting tubule in response to aldosterone can be either excreted into the urine or can be recycled into the interstitium surrounding the medullary collecting tubule before it enters the renal pelvis (Stokes, 1982). There is also the

TABLE II

AFFINITY OF VARIOUS STEROIDS FOR HUMAN PLASMA CORTICOSTEROID BINDING GLOBULIN (CBG) AT 37°C[a]

Steroid	K_d CBG (μM)	Plasma concentration steroid (nM)	% Free	Free concentration (nM)
Aldosterone	0.53	0.35	37.0	0.13
B	0.013	12	3.3	0.40
F	0.013	400	3.9	16
DOC	0.022	0.2	2.7	0.005
DM	>10		~100	
Spironolactone	>10		~100	

[a] Data from Dunn *et al.*, 1981 and Pugeat *et al.*, 1981.

suggestion that the actions of aldosterone on K transport may be more complicated than the model presented in Fig. 1, since mineralocorticoid effects on Na and K are apparently uncoupled under certain circumstances; ergo, actinomycin D reportedly blocks the effect of aldosterone on Na, but not on K transport (Fimognari *et al.*, 1967).

Parameters that have been used to bioassay activity include urinary Na/K ratios, $U_{Na}V$ and $U_{Na} \div U_{Cr}$, measured 3–5 hours after steroid or diluent. Campen *et al.* (1983) have suggested that urinary Na/K ratios alone are an inappropriate index since dexamethasone, with some apparent mineralocorticoid activity as indexed by Na/K values (dexamethasone activity is equal to one-fiftieth that of aldosterone), is actually less potent than this ratio suggests, because dexamethasone primarily increases K secretion as opposed to Na reabsorption. In examination of this data in Table III, example A shows that it is important to evaluate both $U_{Na} \div U_{Cr}$ and $U_K \div U_{Cr}$ independently of urinary Na/K ratios. As reported by Fimognari *et al.* (1967), animals should also be placed on low-K diet the night before assay to reduce the dietary K component of U_KV. While the absolute change in K secretion seen with mineralocorticoids does not change with this maneuver, the fractional change is magnified and is thus easier to detect and quantify (Horisberger and Diezi, 1983).

Two variants of the usual mineralocorticoid-induced decrease in urinary Na and increase in urinary K are found in examples B and C in Table III. In the first example, 19-OH androstenedione enhanced the mineralocorticoid activity of submaximal doses of aldosterone, although it was devoid of mineralocorticoid activity when given alone (Sekihara *et al.*, 1979; Sekihara, 1983). In the second example, Thomas *et al.* (1983) found that although 50 μg of 19-oxo DOC provided about the same decrease in Na excretion as 3 μg of aldosterone, aldosterone, but not 19-oxo DOC, enhanced K secretion. Since these particular animals received both K and Na supplements before bioassay, these findings need to be supported by similar clearance studies using low-K diet overnight. While it is possible to explain the findings in examples B and C using several models, the 19-OH androstenedione and 19-oxo DOC results may point to (a) a class of steroids that amplifies the mineralocorticoid response by an as yet unknown mechanism, or (b) a class of steroids that differentially affects specific segments along the nephron monitoring either Na or K transport.

Two final points should be made concerning clearance studies. First, the dose–response curves for male rats exceed those for females, and thus, a single sex should be used for bioassay (Morris *et al.*, 1973). Second, it may be preferable to give small doses of dexamethasone to all adrenalectomized animals, thereby maintaining adequate urinary volumes during the course of the experiment.

TABLE III

COMPARISON OF URINARY INDICES USED TO DETERMINE MINERALOCORTICOID ACTIVITY OF VARIOUS STEROIDS IN ADX RATS

Steroid	Dose required to decrease Na/K by one-half (μg)	Relative mineralo-corticoid activity (Na/K)	Dose of steroid (μg)	$U_{Cr}V$ (μg/hour)	$U_{Na}V$ (μEq/hour)	U_{KV} (μEq/hour)	$U_{Na} \div U_{Cr}$	$U_K \div U_{Cr}$	Na/K
Example A[a]									
Control	—	—	—	172	73	1.0	0.424	0.006	73
Aldosterone	0.2	100	1[b]	171	12	2.1	0.070	0.012	5.7
DOC	3.3	6	1[b]	168	35	1.5	0.208	0.009	23
DM	10	2	10[b]	206	116	1.3	0.563	0.006	89
Example B[c]									
Control			—		57	15			3.3
Aldosterone			0.05		57	18			3.3
19-OH androstenedione			300		56	16			3.2
19-OH androstenedione + aldosterone			0.05 + 300		20	17			1.8
Example C[d]									
Control			—		254	171			1.5
Aldosterone			3		147	208			0.7
19-Oxo DOC			50		152	152			1.0
Aldosterone + 19-Oxo DOC			3 + 50		106	216			0.5

[a] Data from Campen and Fanestil, 1982. Details of protocol: Low-K+ diet overnight + 2 ml/100 g saline IP just before assay.

[b] Per 100 g body weight, given at 0 and 2.5 hours.

[c] Data from Sekihara et al., 1979. Details of protocol: Fasted overnight, 3 ml saline per rat.

[d] Data from Thomas et al., 1983. Details of protocol: 3 ml/100 g 0.45% NaCl–0.25% KCl SQ.

III. CHARACTERISTICS OF THE
MINERALOCORTICOID RECEPTOR

A. GENERAL PROPERTIES AND KINETICS

Mineralocorticoids bind to three classes of receptors or binding sites. The first, type I, is the mineralocorticoid receptor; the second, type II, is the glucocorticoid receptor; while the third, type III, is corticosterone-specific, and may be either a true receptor, a CBG-like binding protein, or an enzyme (Feldman *et al.*, 1973; Marver, 1984a). The sites are indeed proteins, since [^{3}H]aldosterone-specific binding is sensitive to pronase and chymotrypsin treatment of target cytosol, but not to lipase or DNase and RNase action (Herman *et al.*, 1968). The proteins can usually be precipitated by 30–50% ammonium sulfate fractionation (Herman *et al.*, 1968; Beaumount and Fanestil, 1983).

Table I lists the K_d's determined for [^{3}H]aldosterone binding to type I and type II receptors in rat and rabbit. Due to the problems outlined in the previous section, neither the K_d nor the N_{max} for type I sites predictably varies with assay temperature or degree of purification of the sample. However, averaging all data, the K_d of aldosterone for the renal type I site is 2.2 ± 0.4 nM (range 0.09–5 nM) and the N_{max} is $5 \pm 1 \times 10^{-14}$ mol/mg protein; the K_d of aldosterone for the type II site is 45 ± 5 nM (range 25–65 nM), and the maximum number of binding sites is about six times that of type I sites. Similar parameters have been found in human kidney (Fuller and Funder, 1976). Fewer data are available on type III site interactions. The K_d for [^{3}H]corticosterone binding to rat renal type III sites (25°C) was 3 nM in one study (Feldman *et al.*, 1973) and 25 nM in another (Lee *et al.*, 1983). The steroid specificities also differ somewhat between these two analyses in that in the former, the relative affinities are B > F > DOC > progesterone > aldosterone > dexamethasone, while in the latter, B > progesterone > DOC > aldosterone > dexamethasone or F. The K_d of aldosterone for type III sites (Feldman *et al.*, 1973) is 1.2 μM, similar to that noted in Table II for aldosterone binding to plasma CBG, thus the suggestion that these are CBG-like sites. The maximal number of type III renal sites is 50–60 times that of type I sites.

The relative affinities of a series of steroids for corticosteroid-binding proteins are approximated in Table IV. The data are not directly comparable since there are species, temperature, and procedural differences among the values listed. They, however, give a rough index of the fractional occupancy of these proteins by each steroid. As noted in Table IV, the relative receptor potency of A ≧ DOC > B > DM > F for type I sites, and DM > B > F >

TABLE IV
RELATIVE K_d's AND BINDING HIERARCHIES OF CORTICOSTEROIDS
FOR VARIOUS BINDING PROTEINS[a]

A. Relative K_d

Steroid	Type I (nM)	Type II (nM)	Type III (μM)	CBG (μM)	Ratio type I/type II
Aldosterone	2	45	1.2	0.5	23
DOC	2.4	30	0.020	0.022	13
B	27	7	0.003	0.013	0.26
F	102	18	0.005	0.013	0.18
DM	56	3	5.6	>10	0.05

B. Apparent binding hierarchy

Type I:	A ≧ DOC > B > DM > F
Type II:	DM > B > DOC > A > F
Type III:	B > F > DOC > A > DM[b]
	B > DOC > A > DM, F[c]

[a] Data compiled from Tables I and II and the following references: Feldman *et al.*, 1972, 1973; Rousseau *et al.*, 1972b; Lan *et al.*, 1982; Lee *et al.*, 1983.

[b] Data from Feldman *et al.*, 1973.

[c] Data from Lee *et al.*, 1983.

DOC > A for Type II sites. Those investigators who treat receptor fractions to remove CBG-like protein report a relatively higher affinity for B and F (Beaumont and Fanestil, 1983; Krozowski and Funder, 1984). Although the endogenous compound DOC has been listed in this table, it is noteworthy that DOCA, commonly used in the laboratory, has one-half the affinity of DOC for the type I site (Palem-Vliers *et al.*, 1982).

B. SEDIMENTATION VALUES

Sedimentation values for all cytoplasmic steroid hormone agonist–receptor complexes vary between 7–9 S in low salt (≦0.1 *M*) and 4–5 S in high salt (0.3–0.4 *M*) (Marver, 1980a). Therefore, it is not surprising that the aldosterone–type I receptor complex has a major 8.5 or 4.5 S peak depending on the ionic conditions (Table V). The presence of millimolar calcium results in the appearance of a 3.5 S as well as 4.5 S species, probably due to a Ca-dependent cleavage of the protein to a basic steroid-binding subunit, termed a meroreceptor (Marver *et al.*, 1972; Sherman *et al.*, 1978). If antagonists are bound to these sites, the protein no longer sediments as a 7–9 S aggregate on low-salt gradients, but as a 3 S complex. The formation of the 8 S species does not require receptor activation, since the aggregate forms even if samples are incubated at 4°C, or below the activation temperature (Marver *et al.*, 1972). Molybdate, which blocks binding of receptor complexes to chromatin, does not alter the sedimentation profile in low salt (Grekin and Sider, 1980; Lan *et al.*, 1981). Thus, the 8 S complex can be assumed to be composed of preactive complexes, while those bound to spirolactones in low salt (3 S) can be considered inactive complexes. Furthermore, molybdate does not inhibit interaction of receptors with nuclear binding sites by inducing the 3 S antagonist form of the receptor. Antagonists also result in a minor modification of the sedimentation value of the type I and type II receptors in high salt relative to agonist complexes, decreasing the values by approximately 0.5 S.

If renal slice binding assays are performed with [³H]aldosterone at either 4 or 25°C, nuclei isolated following incubation contain a significant amount of bound [³H] complexes at 25°C but not at 4°C (Marver *et al.*, 1972). Early studies isolated two separate [³H] steroid-binding proteins from nuclei; one easily extracted with 0.1 M Tris-HCl and 3 mM CaCl$_2$ and usually concentrated by ammonium sulfate precipitation, and a second more tightly bound and extracted with 0.4 M KCl. The former has a 3 S and the latter a 4 S sedimentation coefficient (Marver *et al.*, 1972; Swaneck *et al.*, 1970). Figure

TABLE V

SEDIMENTATION (S) VALUES OF MINERALOCORTICOID AND GLUCOCORTICOID RECEPTOR COMPLEXES

Fraction	Ca²⁺	Sedimentation value		Agonist/antagonist	[³H] Steroid	Reference[a]
		Low salt	High salt			
Cytosolic	−	8.5 S (4 S)[b]	4.5 S	Agonist	Aldosterone	1
Cytosolic	+		4.5 S + 3.5 S	Agonist	Aldosterone	1
Nuclear	+	3 S		Agonist	Aldosterone	1
Nuclear	−		4 S	Agonist	Aldosterone	2
Cytosolic	−	3 S	4 S	Antagonist	Spirolactone (SC-26304)	3
Cytosolic	−	7.5 (3.5 S)	4 S	Agonist	Triamcinolone	4
Cytosolic	−	3.5 S	3.5 S	Antagonist	Cortexolone	4

[a] (1) Marver *et al.*, 1972; (2) Marver *et al.*, 1974; (3) Swaneck *et al.*, 1970; (4) Kaiser *et al.*, 1972.

[b] Values in parentheses indicate minor labeled species which may or may not appear.

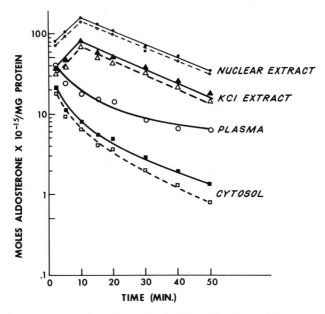

FIG. 3. The time course of renal receptor labeling following an intravenous injection of [³H]aldosterone. Adrenalectomized rats were injected with 0.3 nmoles of [³H]aldosterone ± 100-fold unlabeled steroid and sacrificed 2–50 minutes thereafter. The total concentration of [³H]aldosterone in plasma is shown (O————O), as well as the total (————) and specific (- - -) binding to cytosolic receptors (■,□) and to low (●,○) and high (▲,△) salt-extracted nuclear complexes. [From Marver *et al.* (1972). Reprinted from *Kidney International* (Vol. 1: pp. 210–223, 1972) with permission.]

3 indicates the time course of formation of cytoplasmic, Tris-soluble, and KCl-soluble nuclear complexes following an intravenous injection of [³H]aldosterone into adrenalectomized rats. The loss of [³H]aldosterone binding activity from the cytosolic receptor pool mimicked the biological half-life of aldosterone in plasma. In contrast, the activity in the two nuclear extracts rose simultaneously following injection, reaching a peak in 10 minutes, followed by a steady decline. While earlier models suggested that the Tris-soluble form was a nuclear precursor of the KCl extracted form, the presence of Ca^{2+} in the Tris extracts in these studies may have resulted in modification of a susceptible fraction of the nuclear complexes. Thus, the relationship between the nuclear 3 and 4 S–labeled species still needs to be clarified. Indeed, Kalimi *et al.* (1983) reported that Ca can influence loss of apparent binding activity, receptor activation, as well as processing.

Finally, Palem-Vliers *et al.* (1982) reported that the mobility of unactivated (4°C) and activated (25°C) [³H]aldosterone-bound cytosolic complexes differed on nondenaturing disc gels (R_f = 0.02 at 4°C and 0.36 at 25°C). The fact that the R_f of KCl-extracted nuclear complexes was 0.35 supports the concept that this nuclear complex is closely related to the activated cytoplasmic receptor.

IV. MINERALOCORTICOID ANTAGONISTS

A. PHYSICAL PROPERTIES

The spirolactones are a class of compounds with a C-17 γ lactone ring with variable agonist–antagonist properties (Porter and Edelman, 1964; Porter, 1968; Marver *et al.*, 1974; Knauf, 1976). Table VI lists a series of seven spirolactones that were assayed in toad bladder for relative agonist–antagonist activity; also shown are their approximate affinities for the mineralocorticoid receptor. Unfortunately, only a single dose of each compound was used (10^{-5} M), so that with low-affinity compounds, insufficient steroid was present to completely occupy the receptor. Nonetheless, the data demonstrate not only that several compounds are pure antagonists, but also that some are suboptimal inducers, that is, they have mixed agonist–antagonist actions (Rousseau *et al.*, 1972b). Examples are SC-26304, SC-23133, SC-8109, and SC-5233. The ratio of agonist–antagonist varies. The numbers in columns (A) and (C) of Table VI give the percentage decrease in current if compounds are given with aldosterone (relative to current with aldosterone alone) and the percentage increase in current if compounds are given alone. Correcting for the average basal current at 5 hours in these studies [column (B)] and the average rise in current following aldosterone [column (D)] allows a better estimate of the actual antagonist and agonist activities of the spirolactones. Theoretically, the antagonist and agonist activities should equal 100%. The fact that they actually range from 67–89% probably indicates the degree of error in the assumptions made to derive columns (B) and (D). As evidenced in Table VI, the ratio of antagonist–agonist activity ranges from 2.0 (SC-26304) to >90 (SC-9420, SC-9376).

The action of individual spirolactones varies with species, since SC-26304, with appreciable agonist activity in toad bladder (~17% that of aldosterone), behaves as a pure antagonist in rat and rabbit (Marver *et al.*, 1974; Marver and Schwartz, 1980; Petty *et al.*, 1981). The compounds may also have variable activities on Na reabsorption versus H secretion. Mueller and Steinmetz (1978) reported that SC-9240 enhanced acid secretion while decreasing Na reabsorption in turtle bladder. This concept, however, needs rigorous testing since it does not comply with our current concept of receptor action

TABLE VI

RELATIVE K_d, ANTAGONIST, AND AGONIST ACTIVITIES OF VARIOUS SPIROLACTONES IN TOAD BLADDER[a,b]

Steroid	Approximate K_d (nM)	Assay concentration (nM)	(A) % Decrease in SCC SC + A vs. A alone	(B) % Decrease corrected for average basal SCC	(C) % Increase in SCC + SC or A alone	(D) % Increase relative to aldosterone	Approximate antagonist/agonist activity
Aldosterone	14	50	—	—	235 (avg.)	100	—
SC-26304	37	10,000	37	50	51	17	2
SC-23133	90	10,000	51	63	23	8	6
SC-8109	140	10,000	59	75	39	13	4
SC-9420	190	10,000	72	89	0	0	>90
SC-5233	380	10,000	53	65	21	7	9
SC-9376	480	10,000	58	70	0	0	>70
SC-14266	4800	10,000	9	11	0	0	?

[a] Numbers derived from Kusch et al., 1978; Sakauye and Feldman, 1976.

[b] Relative antagonist and agonist activities determined 5 hours after addition of aldosterone ± spirolactones [antagonist activity, columns (A) and (B)] and aldosterone or spirolactones alone [agonist activity, columns (C) and (D)].

in target epithelia. It is also clear that spirolactones and progesterone, an endogenous antagonist, bind to type II sites if sufficient compound is added and, once bound, block the physiological action of glucocorticoids (Campen and Fanestil, 1982; Rousseau *et al.*, 1972b; Claire *et al.*, 1979). Nonetheless, their effects favor the mineralocorticoid receptor; the apparent K_d of spironolactone for type I sites is approximately seven times less than that for type II sites, while progesterone has about a twofold higher affinity for type I: type II sites in rat assays (Table VII).

In addition to mineralocorticoid agonists, antagonists, and suboptimal inducers, there of course exists a class of inactive steroids. These include isoaldosterone, estradiol, and dihydrotestosterone (DHT) (Herman *et al.*, 1968; Grekin and Sider, 1980; Butkus *et al.*, 1976). The latter steroid is an interesting inclusion since spirolactones have significant affinity for the DHT receptor and manifest this clinically by causing gynecomastia in male recipients (Corvol *et al.*, 1975). In rat prostate, spironolactone has one-sixth the affinity of unlabeled DHT for [^{3}H]DHT binding (Claire *et al.*, 1979), while aldosterone and dexamethasone are inactive (Mainwaring *et al.*, 1972; Bullock and Bardin, 1974); the K_d for [^{3}H]DHT binding to androgen receptors, like aldosterone for type I sites, is about 2 nM (Bullock and Bardin, 1974), and, thus, circulating therapeutic concentrations of spironolactone in man ($\sim 10^{-6}$ M) would appreciably occupy both mineralocorticoid and androgen receptors (Cutler *et al.*, 1978).

TABLE VII

RELATIVE K_d'S OF MINERALOCORTICOID ANTAGONISTS FOR TYPE I AND TYPE II RECEPTORS IN RAT RENAL CYTOPLASMIC FRACTIONS[a]

Steroid	Common name	Type I (nM)	Type II (nM)
Aldosterone		2	
DM			3
Progesterone		64	128
SC-26304		2	
SC-9420	Spironolactone	22	150
SC-9376	Canrenone	92	—
SC-16266	K$^+$ Canrenoate	50	1280
SC-23233	Prorenone	14	300
SC-23992	K$^+$ Prorenoate	59	>>300

[a] Calculated from Table IV and Funder *et al.*, 1974; Wambach and Casals-Stenzel, 1983; Funder *et al.*, 1973b; Claire *et al.*, 1979.

B. MODEL OF MINERALOCORTICOID
AGONIST–ANTAGONIST ACTIONS

We have reviewed the physical properties of mineralocorticoid agonists and antagonists and have shown that they compete with each other for type I receptors. We have also found that cytoplasmic Type I sites labeled with spirolactone (SC-26304) or type II sites labeled with cortexolone sediment at S values that differ from complexes labeled with either aldosterone or triamcinolone acetonide respectively; i.e., neither forms the characteristic 7–9 S complexes on low-salt gradients. The number of type I sites titrated by [³H]aldosterone has also been shown to be equivalent to the number of type I sites titrated by [³H]SC-26304 using rat renal receptors (Warnock and Edelman, 1978). [³H]SC-26304 was further used to determine the mechanism by which spirolactone blocked the physiological action of aldosterone. Thus, if either slices or cell-free extracts mixed with purified nuclei/chromatin were incubated with [³H]SC-26304, neither specific Tris-soluble nor KCl-soluble labeled complexes could be isolated from the nuclei or chromatin, a finding in marked contrast to that seen with [³H]aldosterone (Marver *et al.*, 1974). A lack of apparent nuclear binding following the addition of sufficient corticosteroid antagonist to labeled cytoplasmic receptor was also reported by Claire *et al.* (1979) and Lan *et al.* (1981) using [³H]prorenone-labeled type I sites and by Kaiser *et al.* (1972) using [³H]cortexolone-labeled type II sites. Thus, the model was proposed that antagonist–receptor complexes existed in a conformational state different from agonist–receptor complexes. This basic difference prevented activation, a process necessary to uncover or create a second action site necessary for complex attachment to chromatin. This is schematically presented in Fig. 4. By shifting the equilibrium to the 3 S form of the receptor (low salt), endogenous steroids such as progesterone, which may rise and wane in activity, exclude to some degree the mineralocorticoid receptor pool from a path that would otherwise undergo activation and result in excess salt and water retention.

Suboptimal inducers can be explained by steroids having appreciable affinity for both conformational states of the receptor. The relative agonist–antagonist activities in a group of compounds such as those presented in Table VI (toad bladder studies) should then be equivalent to the relative affinity of each compound for the active and inactive site. This might be tested by showing that the equilibrium formed between 3 S and 8 S peaks on a low-salt gradient of suboptimal inducers mimicked their relative antagonist–agonist actions, but such data have not been accumulated. In Tables VI and VII, the single K_d's approximated for each compound do not discriminate between these sites, but either blend the values for both sites or are equal to the K_d's for the dominant species.

While the agonist–antagonist model shown in Fig. 4 is equivalent to that initially proposed by Monod *et al.* (1965) for allosteric proteins, another equally plausible concept, based on the formulation of Koshland *et al.* (1966), has been proposed for corticosteroid effects mediated via type II receptors. [For a detailed discussion and comparison of the kinetics of steric–allosteric reactions, the reader is referred to the monograph of Hammes and Wu (1974)]. As a basis for this alternate induced-fit model, Suthers *et al.* (1976) found it remarkable that the addition of a 1000-fold excess of progesterone to cell-free extracts accelerated the dissociation of [³H] steroid from type II sites prelabeled with 25nM [³H]dexamethasone relative to that produced by dexamethasone itself. After 30 minutes at 25°C, 60% of the label remained upon dexamethasone addition and 30% remained with progesterone addition. To explain this finding, the induced-fit model would present a receptor containing two nonequivalent, but interacting binding sites. Thus, if [³H]dexamethasone were bound to the active site, the addition of the antagonist, progesterone, and its subsequent attachment to the second modulator site would induce a conformational change in the receptor such that release of label from the active site was augmented; dexamethasone would have a low affinity for the second regulatory site. This argument is incomplete, however, since a second antagonist, cortexolone, promoted [³H]dexamethasone dissociation to about 55%, while a type II agonist,

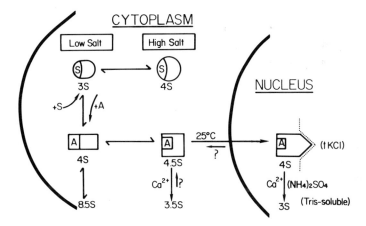

FIG. 4. A model for the interaction of agonists and antagonists with the mineralocorticoid receptor. The binding of an agonist [aldosterone (+A)] or an antagonist [spirolactone (+S)] shifts the equilibrium between an inactive (oval–round) and active (rectangle–square–pentagon) form of the receptor. Also shown are the various sedimentation coefficients obtained for cytoplasmic complexes in high- and low-salt media, as well as nuclear low-salt (Tris-soluble) and high-salt (↑KCl) extractable [³H]aldosterone-bound proteins.

deoxycorticosterone (Rousseau *et al.*, 1972b), reduced binding to about 50% that of controls in the same time frame. Thus, both an agonist and an antagonist were more potent than dexamethasone in these dissociation assays. While the results might also be explained by variations in the receptor on versus off rates of the steroids employed, the details of the experimental protocol do not offer this explanation; thus, the progesterone findings and this model need to be further explored.

The steric–allosteric model suggested by the accelerated dissociation in the presence of progesterone provided some evidence toward binding-site heterogeneity of corticosteroid cytoplasmic receptors. There is also evidence to suggest subunit heterogeneity, as well as the presence of a form of the receptor that is unable to bind either agonists or antagonists but can be recruited to do so. While these studies have been carried out with progesterone and glucocorticoid receptors, the similarity of the induction process for all steroid hormones dictates that these results be considered as possible additions to the simple scheme shown in Fig. 4. While subunit heterogeneity has been suggested for the type II receptor (Mayer *et al.*, 1983), this concept has been best defined for the progesterone receptor in chick oviduct. Here an A and a B subunit have a common core protein that contains a binding site for progesterone. The subunits differ, however, in molecular weight (79,000 and 108,000) and in their preference for DNA versus chromatin. They associate to form an approximately 7 S species similar to the aggregated form of the mineralocorticoid receptor. All tests thus far have shown that the A subunit is not a degradative product of the B subunit (Birnbaumer *et al.*, 1983).

Another important contribution involves an inactive form of the receptor, i.e., one that does not bind steroid, not to be confused with the physiologically inactive complexes formed by steroid antagonists. Studies have also shown that both glucocorticoid and progesterone receptors have phosphorylation–dephosphorylation site(s) (Weigel *et al.*, 1981; Housley and Pratt, 1983). Investigators found that glucocorticoid receptors lost steroid binding capacity if exogeneous phosphatases were added. However, if molybdate was present during this process, the activity could be reactivated with dithiothreitol (DTT) (Housley *et al.*, 1983). This combined information led investigators to conclude that dephosphorylation of the receptor leads to oxidation of a critical SH group that is required for receptor binding (Leach *et al.*, 1983). DTT can reverse this process if molybdate is present to preserve the receptor in a form that allows subsequent reduction of the receptor back to a steroid-binding state. Leach *et al.* (1983) proposed that molybdate ions complex with sulfur groups on the molecule and thus protect the receptor from sustained inactivation. Certain cytoplasmic co-factors may carry out the reduction reaction provided by the added DTT. While resident glutathione may be of some benefit, Grippo *et al.* (1983) judged that this process was accomplished by NADPH and thioredoxin using rat liver. The preservation of unlabeled cytoplasmic type I binding sites by molybdate dictates that the mineralocorticoid as well as the glucocorticoid receptor steroid-binding capacity may be influenced by a critical sulfhydryl and protected by a phosphorylation reaction.

Having considered the cytoplasmic receptor, what of the nature of transformation and of nuclear-bound receptor complexes? Little is known about the molecular basis for transformation. Vedeckis (1983b) reported that sulfhydryl groups may be important to the transformation of the receptor, as Housley *et al.* (1983) suggested for preservation of the steroid binding site. It may also involve an enzymatic clipping of the receptor, which exposes a portion of the protein with heightened affinity for chromatin–DNA (Vedeckis, 1983a,b). Certainly both nuclear forms of the type I receptor shown in Figure 4 appear to be of a lower molecular weight as judged by equilibrium density gradient analyses (3 S and 4 S as opposed to 4 S and 4.5 S). When nondenaturating polyacrylamide gel electrophoresis was used to compare the physical characteristics of the cytoplasmic receptor incubated at 4 or 25°C with the nuclear low-salt extract, both warmed cytosol (transformed?) and the low-salt nuclear extract had a coincident R_f of 0.35–0.36, while cytosol labeled at 4°C barely penetrated the origin of the gel (Palem-Vliers *et al.*, 1982). Thus, either enzymatic clipping of the receptor may occur or transformation may diminish the interaction of receptor with another constituent of the cytoplasm, a constituent that results in aggregation of receptors.

Some characterization of the nuclear acceptor site has been carried out. The number of transformed renal type I cytosolic complexes bound to nuclei isolated from various species and tissues was highly dependent on the transcriptional activity of the nuclear preparation. DNA intercalators such as ethidium bromide and proflavin sulfate inhibited 100% of the attachment of activated aldosterone complexes to chromatin. Using DNA probes with base:pair specificity, netropsin (A:T) was a more potent inhibitor than actinomycin D (G:C) (Edelman and Marver, 1980). This suggested that DNA, as opposed to chromosomal proteins, was a major template for transformed receptor complexes and that there was some base–pair selectivity in this interaction. Compton *et al.* (1983) also showed preference of binding of the A subunit of the progesterone receptor (DNA-preferring) to A:T-rich sequences. The attraction of mineralocorticoid receptor complexes for DNA does not preclude interaction with specific chromosomal proteins at key sites along the template, although the nature of such interactions has not been described.

The relationship between nuclear binding and the physiological action of aldosterone has been best studied in the toad bladder. In this tissue, two nuclear sites were characterized by computer analyses of binding data—one with an apparent K_d of 3 nM, and a second with a K_d of 460 nM. As with cytoplasmic receptor data, these two nuclear sites have been coined type I and type II. The nuclear type I site appeared to be important to the physiological action of aldosterone, since saturation of this site at 40 nM aldosterone was coincident with achieving a maximal rise in short circuit current (SCC) during the course of the experiments. The maximal number of nuclear type I sites (measured as total nuclear-associated activity, corrected for binding in the presence of ~200-fold excess of unlabeled aldosterone) was equivalent to 15 fmoles/mg nuclear protein or about 1400 high-affinity sites per nucleus. The type II sites (10-fold more than type I) were presumed to be related to glucocorticoid activity, but this has not been proven (Farman *et al.*, 1978; Kusch *et al.*, 1978). When these data were analyzed further to relate the fractional increase in SCC with the fractional increase in binding to nuclear Type I sites, a concave nonlinear association was found, such that 50% occupancy of these sites was coincident with only a 10% of maximum rise in SCC, and indeed it required more than 80% saturation of sites to bring about a 50% of maximum rise in SCC (Edelman, 1981). Whether this unusual relationship came about because of the limitations of accurately describing each part of the puzzle or whether it indeed represents the stoichiometry required of receptor–acceptor site interactions remains to be seen.

V. TARGET TISSUE EVALUATION BY RECEPTOR ANALYSES

A. KIDNEY, COLON, SWEAT GLANDS

The ability to dissect discrete segments from both rat and rabbit kidney has aided in the localization of corticosteroid receptors along the nephron. The availability of ultramicro biochemical assays and the technique of microperfusion of individual nephron segments has further allowed investigators to initiate a detailed analysis of the mechanism of action of corticosteroids at their respective target sites. We will examine both corticosterone receptor data and companion biochemical–physiological studies. Both autoradiography and segmental binding assays have been used to detect receptors. Each has its own limitations; thus, the conclusions are most defensible when both are available. Using these analyses, the cortical collecting tubule (CCT), the connecting segment (CNT), and the medullary collecting tubule (MCT) appear to be prime targets for aldosterone (for spatial relationship of these segments, see Fig. 5). The relative labeling of these segments, in terms of either specific binding per millimeter of tubule length or nuclear grains/100 μm^2 (autoradiographic analyses), is given in Table VIII. The steroid specificity of these mineralocorticoid sites was aldosterone > DOCA > DM (Doucet and Katz, 1981; Farman *et al.*, 1982). Although rabbit data are shown to define mineralocorticoid receptors in Table VIII, similar autoradiographic localization patterns were obtained for rat (Farman and Bonvalet, 1983). Binding was saturable and the equilibrium dissociation constants determined by both assays (0.5–2.2 n*M*) were within the range of those noted in Table I for renal slice and cell-free determinations.

While autoradiographic and binding analyses agreed with respect to CNT, CCT, and MCT type I site localization, these same two assays differed with respect to their evaluation of mineralocorticoid receptors in thick ascending limb and distal convoluted tubule (DCT). The binding assay performed at

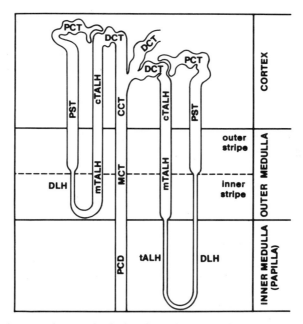

FIG. 5. A schematic of a superficial (short loop of Henle) and juxtamedullary (long loop of Henle) renal nephron. Segments are marked to indicate the position of the proximal convoluted and straight tubules (PCT, PST), thin descending and ascending limbs of Henle (DLH, tALH), medullary and cortical thick ascending limbs of Henle (mTALH, cTALH), distal convoluted tubules (DCT), and cortical and medullary and collecting tubules and papillary collecting ducts (CCT, MCT, PCD). Not shown is the connecting segment (CNT), which joins the DCT and CCT portions of the nephron. In the rabbit, approximately six nephrons empty their luminal contents into a single collecting duct system.

TABLE VIII

LOCALIZATION OF CORTICOSTEROID BINDING SITES[a]

Species	Site	Assay	Temp. (°C)	K_d (nM)	Concentration used (nM)	Relative binding								Reference[b]
						PCT	PST	mTALH	cTALH	DCT	CNT	CCT	MCT	
Rabbit	Type I	[³H]aldosterone[c]	25	2.2	6	0.07	0.01	0.03	0.04	0.04	0.92	1.00	0.96	1
Rabbit	Type I	[³H]aldosterone[d]	30	0.5	0.3	0.04	0.17	0.26	0.45	0.13	1.47	1.00	0.39	2
					1.5	<0.01	0.04	0.14	0.23	0.82	0.91	1.00	0.45	
Rabbit	Type I	CS				0	0	0.78	0.17	0		1.00	0.43	3
Rabbit	Type I	Na,K-ATPase				0.22[e]	0	0	0.04	0.74	1.07	1.00	0.14	4
						1.16[f]	0	0.20	0.20	0.65	1.24	1.00	0	
Rabbit	Type II	[³H]DM[d]	30	30	53	1.14	1.77	0.06	0.14	0.34	0.63	1.00	0.11	5
Rat	Type III	[³H]B	25	25	80	0.11	0.06	0.03	0.03	0.28	—	1.00	0.27	6

[a] In vitro receptor assays using whole, tubule segments or autoradiographic analyses of nuclear grain densities were corrected for nonspecific binding. Citrate synthase (CS) assays were performed at 25°C following in vivo administration of 10 µg/kg BW of aldosterone to adrenalectomized rabbits and sacrificed at 90 minutes. Steroid-sensitive Na,K-ATPase are expressed as the difference between normals and rabbits given chronic DOCA or low-Na diet.

[b] (1) Doucet and Katz, 1981; (2) Farman et al., 1982; (3) Marver and Schwartz, 1980; Marver and Lombard, 1981; (4) Garg et al., 1981; (5) Farman et al., 1983; (6) Lee et al., 1983.

[c] Whole tubule segment.

[d] Autoradiographic analysis.

[e] Chronic DOCA.

[f] Low-Na diet.

25°C shows no other significant binding along the nephron, while the autoradiographic study at 30°C shows significant nuclear binding in DCT at moderate concentrations of steroid (1.5 nM). There was also a significant degree of nuclear-specific [^{3}H]aldosterone in cortical thick ascending limbs of Henle (cTALH) and medullary thick ascending limbs of Henle (mTALH).

Two biochemical assays have been used to map type I sites in the rabbit, namely, citrate synthase and Na,K-ATPase activities, since both have been implicated as possible mineralocorticoid-induced proteins. Table VIII indicates that steroid increased the levels of one or both of these enzymes in the CNT, CCT, and MCT. There is again some disagreement in DCT and TALH, since citrate synthase assays document no significant change in this enzyme in DCT, with a pronounced dependence in mTALH, while Na,K-ATPase was increased in DCT from rabbits given either chronic DOCA or low-Na diet, with little or no steroid-dependent difference in activity in TALH. Surprisingly, Na,K-ATPase is increased in proximal convoluted tubules (PCT) with either chronic regimen, but the changes in activity are not significant due to a high basal Na,K-ATPase and the variability of that activity in this particular segment (Marver and Schwartz, 1980; Marver and Lombard, 1981; Garg *et al.*, 1981). The physiological role of aldosterone in the CCT is to influence both Na reabsorption and K secretion, and that of the MCT is to enhance H secretion as noted earlier (Gross *et al.*, 1975; Schwartz and Burg, 1978; Stone *et al.*, 1983). The role of aldosterone in the CNT is unclear, since chronic DOCA therapy does not alter the potential difference across this segment, as it does in the CCT (Imai, 1979). It may, however, be important to aldosterone-dependent changes in K secretion. The possible role of aldosterone at other potential sites of action (DCT, TALH) is unknown, and it may well be that putative action at these sites is related to secondary actions of the steroid or to crossover binding to Type II sites. It is also conceivable that the DCT may play a role in kallikrein–kinen stimulation following chronic steroid therapy.

The autoradiographic (nuclear) labeling pattern for the glucocorticoid type II receptor varies from that for the type I receptor in that the proximal tubule in addition to the distal tubule is well labeled. Since glucocorticoid receptors are found in all tissues (Ballard *et al.*, 1974), its general presence along the nephron is unquestioned. The only surprise is the low level of receptor in mTALH by this technique, since this is thought to be a major renal target for this steroid (Rayson and Edelman, 1982). The steroid specificity of this site is DM $\geq$ B $>>$ aldosterone (Farman *et al.*, 1983). The physiological roles of glucocorticoids in the segments other than the PCT are still unclear. In the PCT, glucocorticoids influence both gluconeogenesis and ammoniagenesis (Vandewalle *et al.*, 1981).

Finally, the results of Lee *et al.* (1983) using the endogenous glucocor-

TABLE IX
A Comparison of the Binding Parameters of [³H]Aldosterone Receptors in Well-Characterized Target Tissues with Those of Several Putative Target Sources

Species	Tissue	Temperature (°C)	Assay	Type I K_d (nM)	Type I N_{max} (×10⁻¹⁴/mg protein)	Type II K_d (nM)	Type II N_{max} (×10⁻¹⁴/mg protein)	Steroid preference Type I	Steroid preference Type II	Reference[a]
Well-characterized										
Rat & Rabbit	Kidney	4–37	Slice and cell-free	2.2 ± 0.4	5 ± 1	45 ± 5	32 ± 9	A ≧ DOC > B > DM > F	DM > B > F > DOC > A	1
Rabbit	Colon	37	Mince	6	14	60	30	A > DM	DM > A	2
Rat	Parotid	37	Mince	2	4	NA[b]	NA			3
Candidates										
Rat	Lung	37	Mince	0.7	0.2	80	12	A > DOC > DM,B		4
Rabbit/Rat	Mammary gland	4	Cell-free	3[c]	2	12	8[c]	DOC > A ≧ B > DM		5,6
				2[d]	0.4	12	4[d]			
Rabbit	Ocular lens	NA	Cell-free	0.15	0.6	NA	NA			7
Rabbit	Aorta	4	Cell-free	0.7		13	25	B ≧ DCC ≧ A > F ≧ DM	DM > B > DOC,A	8
Rat	Aorta	37	Cells		10[e]	11	242[e]	DOC > B > A > F > DM	B = DOC = F = DM >> A	9
Rabbits	Aorta	4	Cell-free	0.4	3.4	5	66		DM > F > B > DOC > A	10
Rat	Pituitary tumor	37	Cells	1	8	90	73	A ≧ DOC ≧ B ≧ F > DM		11
Rat	Pituitary	4	Cell-free	3	10	NA	NA	DOC > A		12
Rat	Pituitary	37	Cells	2	0.3[f]	80	3[f]	A > D	D > A	13
Rat	Brain	4	Cell-free	0.3	3	18	22	DOC > B > A > F > DM		14
Rat	Hippocampus	4	Cell-free	3	8	5	50	DOC > B > A > DM	DOC = B > DM > A	15
Rat	Hippocampus	4	Cell-free	3	20	NA	NA	DOC > A		12
Rat	Hippocampus	4	Cell-free	~1	7	0.6	10	DOC = A = B > F > DM		16

[a] (1) Tables I and IV; (2) Marver, 1984b; (3) Funder *et al.*, 1972; (4) Krozowski and Funder, 1972; (5) Quirk *et al.*, 1983; (6) Kelly *et al.*, 1983; (7) Hampl *et al.*, 1981; (8) Duval *et al.*, 1977; (9) Meyer and Nichols, 1981; (10) Kornel *et al.*, 1983; (11) Lan *et al.*, 1981; (12) Moguilewsky and Raynaud, 1980; (13) Krozowski and Funder, 1981a; (14) Beaumont and Fanestil, 1983; (15) Veldhuis *et al.*, 1982; (16) Krozowski and Funder, 1984.

[b] Not available.

[c] Pregnant.

[d] Lactating.

[e] Per milligram of DNA.

[f] Per pituitary.

ticoid, corticosterone, are also shown in Table VIII. In these studies, both the proximal tubule and TALH were minimally labeled. Indeed, the labeling pattern nearly reproduced that for aldosterone, although the number of specific binding sites per millimeter of segment length was two orders of magnitude higher with corticosterone. The two sites also differed in their steroid specificity. In contrast to type I sites, DOCA was more potent than aldosterone for type III site binding, and in contrast to the type II sites, B was far more potent than DM. Furthermore, in contrast to CBG (Table I), F does not compete for labeling in the presence of [^{3}H]corticosterone when given in 100-fold excess concentrations. The role of this type III binding site and its relationship to the mineralocorticoid and glucocorticoid receptor is still under evaluation (for discussion, see Marver, 1984a). The binding studies might be summarized by saying that, using modest doses of steroid, both aldosterone and type III binding sites were localized to the CNT, CCT, and MCT. Type II sites, indexed by dexamethasone, were highest in the proximal tubule (PCT, PST) and CCT, with modest to moderate labeling in all other tested segments.

Similar segmental analyses are currently being carried out for steroid control of transport along the gastrointestinal tract. To date glucocorticoid activity has been documented in the jejunum, ileum, and colon, and mineralocorticoid activity in the colon (for review of corticosteroid actions in the gut, see Bastl and Marver, 1984). Only recently, mineralocorticoid receptors have been documented in the distal colon (Marver, 1984b). Earlier attempts may have again been impeded by the instability of mineralocorticoid complexes *in vitro* (Marusic *et al.*, 1981). Table IX gives the K_d and N_{max} determined for rabbit colonic type I and type II receptors as well as values for another classic target tissue, parotid. Figure 6, on the other hand, shows competition analyses in rabbit distal colon for both type I and type II site binding and indicates that they can be distinguished by their relative steroid specificity for aldosterone and DM. Furthermore, the affinity of aldosterone and DM for type I sites in rabbit colon mimics their affinity for rabbit renal type I sites. As with the kidney and toad bladder, aldosterone was found to enhance citrate synthase activity in colon within 2 hours after administration to adrenalectomized rabbits, and it increased the potential difference and Na transport, as measured by SCC, across isolated colon tissue (Marver, 1984b). Thus, it appears that colon is a target for aldosterone and that glucocorticoids also influence transport and/or metabolism in this segment of the gastrointestinal tract.

B. Possible Targets: Brain, Aorta

Table IX also lists a series of other tissues that may be possible targets for aldosterone. They include lung, mammary gland, ocular lens, aorta, and

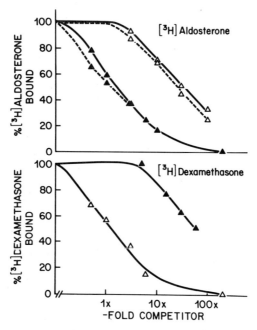

FIG. 6. Steroid competition analyses for [³H]aldosterone binding sites in rabbit colon and kidney. Either colon (———) or kidney (- - -) whole-cell preparations were incubated at 37°C for 30 minutes with 5 nM [³H]aldosterone + 10x dexamethasone or 50 nM [³H]dexamethasone + 1x aldosterone ± various concentrations of either aldosterone (▲) or dexamethasone (△). Values have been corrected for nonspecific labeling and represent the percentage of [³H] steroid specifically bound in each sample relative to controls. [From Marver (1984b).]

brain. The role of mineralocorticoids in such tissues is unclear. For instance, glucocorticoids have been found to accelerate morphological development and the appearance of surfactant in fetal lung, but no such action is known for mineralocorticoids (Kikkawa *et al.*, 1971). Even such diverse tissues as spleen have been shown to have apparent aldosterone-specific binding sites by receptor assay, again with no known physiological role of aldosterone in this organ (Swaneck *et al.*, 1969). Within this list of tissues, however, two bear special attention since the action of aldosterone on these sites could have important physiological consequences. The implication has been that the aortic site may be physiologically important in hypertension and that the brain site(s) may influence pathways such as salt–water appetite or stimulation of steroid biosynthesis. These sites have been evaluated using receptor assays, and available numbers appear in Table IX.

It is clear from Table IX that aorta, pituitary, hippocampus, and even mammary glands contain a high affinity (~2 nM) and low capacity (~6 ×

10^{-14} moles/mg protein) binding site for aldosterone. In each case, the affinity of aldosterone clearly exceeds that of DM. It is distinct from the renal type I site, however, in that the potencies of DOC and B are either equivalent to or exceed the affinity of aldosterone for this site. The binding hierarchy is in fact more reminiscent of type III sites in general, and specifically of the [^{3}H]corticosterone-specific site found in isolated renal CCTs by Lee *et al.* (1983) (B > DOC > A > DM, F). The brain and aorta receptor analyses substantiated the conclusions of studies by Ermische and Rühle (1978) and Hollander *et al.* (1965), using autoradiographic localization techniques.

Two concepts have been evoked to explain the altered hierarchy of steroid affinity seen in aorta and brain. One is that this may represent a different receptor than the classic mineralocorticoid receptor, i.e., it may be equivalent to or similar to the Type III site, or it is the mineralocorticoid receptor. In the latter case, Krozowski and Funder (1984) have suggested that earlier competition assays did not take into account the effect that small amounts of contaminating CBG might have on the apparent binding hierarchy. When these authors removed CBG-like material from renal cell-free extracts with hydroxylapatite [or $(NH_4)_2SO_4$, as per Beaumont and Fanestil, 1983], the binding affinities were such that DOC $\geq$ A > B > F > DM, or similar to that seen with brain and aorta samples. They argued that in earlier studies contaminating CBG removed sufficient unlabeled DOC/B/F such that their apparent affinity was decreased due to the unperceived decrease in free steroid. Stephenson *et al.* (1984) further argued that CBG or CBG-like protein in the renal interstitium may act as a local "sink" for the corticosteroids to enable aldosterone rather than B to occupy renal type I sites, akin to the model presented by De Kloet *et al.* (1975, 1977) to explain the role of CBG-like protein in anterior pituitary. In favor of a similarity between the brain and renal high-affinity aldosterone binding site is that the isoelectric focusing patterns of these two labeled species were identical before and after limited trypsin fragmentation, while the pattern of type II sites completely differed (Wrange and Yu, 1983).

Characteristically, this DOC- or B-preferring brain and aorta site has a very high or equivalent affinity for progesterone (Lan *et al.*, 1981; Veldhuis *et al.*, 1982; Moguilewsky and Raynaud, 1980; Lee *et al.*, 1983), which is in contrast to the average relative affinity of 3% for type I sites in kidney (Table VII; Doucet and Katz, 1981). Since progesterone has about one-half the affinity of B for CBG (Westphal, 1983), the argument could still be made that CBG may have also reduced free progesterone levels. This places emphasis on a study by Doucet and Katz (1981) using isolated single nephron segments labeled with [^{3}H]aldosterone and "free" of interstitial CBG; in this series, A > DOCA > DM > progesterone (25°C). Such findings suggest that two rather than one set of receptors are involved, i.e., that the DOC-preferring and aldosterone-preferring sites are not equivalent. Furthermore, sheep that have low-to-absent CBG levels have a renal binding hierarchy similar to that determined in Table IV for type I receptors, or A : DOC : F : prog $\cong 1 : 0.1 : 0.01 : 0.001$ (Butkus *et al.*, 1976, 1982). However, until competition assays are done so that not only free concentrations of unlabeled steroids are known, but also the contributions of metabolism during assay, the equivalence or nonequivalence of these sites cannot be settled. Interestingly, Wambach and Higgins (1979) reported that progesterone was an antihypertensive in DOCA-hypertensive rats but that progesterone did not reduce the amount of saline consumed by these rats, which speaks against either the equivalence of the brain and renal site or the purported action of mineralocorticoids in the brain.

Careful analyses of nuclear transfer studies in brain and aorta may also be revealing. When Kornel *et al.* (1983) attempted this with aortic cytosol, nuclear uptake of [^{3}H]progesterone was not evident, as with antagonists [^{3}H]SC-26304 or [^{3}H]prorenone in kidney (Marver *et al.*, 1974; Claire *et al.*, 1979). However, [^{3}H]aldosterone, [^{3}H]cortisol, [^{3}H]deoxycorticosterone, and [^{3}H]corticosterone were ≤ 0.5 as effective as [^{3}H]dexamethasone in transferring labeled complexes to nuclei, suggesting that perhaps these steroids are suboptimal inducers or that the predominant binding species is not a true receptor.

Last, liver, heart, and veins have served as nontarget tissues for mineralocorticoids in binding and physiological studies (Funder *et al.*, 1973b; Marver *et al.*, 1980; Marver, 1984c; Kornel *et al.*, 1982, 1983).

VI. RELATIONSHIP OF STEROID–RECEPTOR INTERACTIONS TO THE PHYSIOLOGICAL ROLE OF ALDOSTERONE

A. AGONIST–ANTAGONIST ACTIONS WHICH MAY OR MAY NOT BE RECEPTOR MEDIATED

Licorice and carbenoxolone (used in the treatment of peptic ulcer) contain or are derivatives of glycyrrhetinic acid, a compound with significant affinity for the mineralocorticoid receptor and clear Na-retaining properties. The affinities are low (<0.0001 that of aldosterone); nonetheless, licorice addicts can develop significant hypokalemia (Ulmann *et al.*, 1975; Armanini *et al.*, 1982). In addition, a number of nonsteroidal anti-inflammatory drugs (NSAID) promote salt and water retention in the rat. They do so as a result of their inhibition of prostaglandin synthesis or in some instances due to a modest affinity for the mineralocorticoid receptor. For instance, indomethacin, mefenamic acid, meclofenamic acid, phenylbutazone, and ibuprofen reduce [³H]aldosterone binding to receptor sites by 30–40% when added at a 10^5 molar ratio. Eicosatetraynoic acid (ETYA) also reduces binding by 30% at 100 μg/ml in the presence of 5 nM [³H]aldosterone. On the other hand, NSAIDs such as naproxen do not compete with aldosterone for binding sites, and thus their action on salt and water retention must be solely due to their role as inhibitors of prostaglandin biosynthesis (Feldman and Couropmitree, 1976; Feldman *et al.*, 1978). Corticosteroids may also alter prostaglandin biosynthesis in the CCT, since both aldosterone and DM at 50 pM concentrations have permissive action on ADH-mediated water flow. It has been suggested, but not proven, that this may be a consequence of corticosteroid inhibition of either cAMP phosphodiesterase activity, prostaglandin biosynthesis, or both (Schwartz and Kokko, 1980). The effect on prostaglandin synthesis is of import since PGE_2 inhibits electrolyte and water flux across this segment (Stokes and Kokko, 1977; Grantham and Orloff, 1968).

Steroid action on the inhibition of PGE biosynthesis can be reversed by appropriate concentrations of spirolactones (Zusman *et al.*, 1978). Current opinion would be, however, that type II sites rather than type I sites mediate this response and that glucocorticoids induce a protein responsible for this inhibition (Russo-Marie and Duval, 1982). Since steroids (Zusman *et al.*, 1978; Russo-Marie and Duval, 1982) can block prostaglandin synthesis, the amplification mechanism of 19-OH androstenedione (Sekihara *et al.*, 1979), 5α dihydro F (DHF) (Adam *et al.*, 1978), and carbenoxolone (Armanini *et al.*, 1982) are likely due to the ability of these molecules to diminish prostaglandin levels.

It also remains a strong possibility that the type I or type II binding site in aorta is linked to the effects of corticosteroids on prostaglandin biosynthesis. In this tissue, aldosterone and DOCA have been shown to increase the pressor response (Gross and Sulser, 1957; Rondell and Gross, 1960; Raab *et al.*, 1950), and prostaglandins have been shown to decrease the pressor response to catecholamines. While some have argued that the increased electrolyte content of aortic cells from DOCA-hypertensive animals simply reflects alterations in plasma electrolyte concentrations (Garwitz and Jones, 1982), the finding that DOC increases the intracellular Na concentration in aortic strips grown in culture, a process antagonized by progesterone, leaves open the possibility that steroid directly inhibits transport in this tissue (Kornel and Rafelson, 1983). This could be a classic response of aldosterone (i.e., increase in Na permeability, etc.) or could reflect an action on prostaglandin synthesis. While the search goes on for steroid-sensitive tissue sites that might aggravate hypertension, the search also goes on for novel steroids that might aggravate that hypertensive state coincident with nor-mal-to-low plasma aldosterone levels. A partial list is given in Table X. To date, only the 19 nor-derivatives of compounds such as DOC appear note-worthy, and investigators are currently trying to localize peripheral tissue sites that might carry out this demethylation reaction.

Finally, both progesterone and spirolactones have been shown to have rapid inhibitory actions in transport epithelia (Rossier and Claire, 1978; Marver, 1980a; Tomlinson, 1971). It is unclear whether these actions are receptor mediated. Results using SC-9376 are shown in Fig. 7. When SC-9376 was added to bladders pretreated with aldosterone, SCC fell rapidly, the fall following a biphasic curve. These results have been in-terpreted two ways. First, the type I receptor may function to initiate the induction process, and it may also stabilize some short-lived rate-limiting product activated or induced by steroid. Alternately, spironolactone, and by inference, aldosterone, may influence a site within the cell other than the receptor, with the stipulation that this site also modulates Na transport across the cell. Progesterone and several spirolactones have been shown to have an immediate (Tomlinson, 1971; Nutbourne *et al.*, 1970) or a more chronic effect (inhibition) on Na transport (Clarkson and Luck, 1970) in a variety of tissues, unrelated to an antagonism of aldosterone action. In each of the studies noted, the mechanism of inhibition was not defined, although the effect of progesterone was shown to be reversible in one case (Tomlin-

TABLE X

MINERALOCORTICOID ACTIVITY OF VARIOUS STEROIDS POSTULATED TO PLAY A ROLE IN ESSENTIAL HYPERTENSION

| | Activity relative to aldosterone | | |
Compound	Receptor assays	Bioassays	Reference[a]
16β-OH DHEA	<<0.001	0.025	1–3
16-oxoandrostenediol	<<0.001	0.025	1,3
18-oxo-F	0.02	0.01	4
17α-OH progesterone	0.003		5
17α,20α(OH)$_2$ progesterone	0.001		5
17α,20β(OH)$_2$ progesterone	0.0007		5
19-norprogesterone	0.4	0.01	6,7
19-nor-DOC	2.5		6
19-nor-B	0.25		6
19-nor-F	0.08		6
19-noraldosterone	0.002		6

[a] (1) Baxter *et al.*, 1976; (2) Higgins *et al.*, 1977; (3) Liddle and Sennett, 1975; (4) Ulick *et al.*, 1983; (5) Butkus *et al.*, 1982; (6) Wynne *et al.*, 1980; (7) Funder and Adam, 1981.

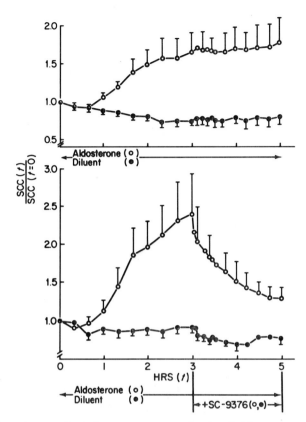

FIG. 7. The influence of spirolactone SC-9376 on basal and aldosterone-stimulated short circuit current (SCC). In the upper and lower panels, either 50 nM aldosterone (○) or diluent (●) was added to paired toad hemibladders at 0 hours. The experiments differ in that in the lower panel, 2×10^{-5} M SC-9376 was added to hemibladders 3 hours after the addition of steroid or diluent, while in the upper panel, bladders were not subjected to further additions. The normalized values shown (±SEM) represent the SCC at any time = t, divided by the SCC at time = 0 hours. [From Marver (1980a).]

son, 1971). Whether these actions are in any way related to arachidonic acid metabolism is unknown.

B. Structure–Function Analyses

Structure–function analyses (Table XI) are of interest when we wish to know how to enhance steroid binding affinity for type I sites, to enhance type I site binding relative to type II sites, or to understand the molecular

TABLE XI
STRUCTURE–FUNCTION ANALYSES[a]

A. Alterations in affinity for type I and type II sites

Parent compound	Modification	Receptor affinity relative to parent compound		
		Type I	Type II	I/II
Progesterone (P)	21-OH	29	12	2.4
17α OH P	20α-OH	0.3	0.6	0.5
	20β-OH	0.25	0.50	0.5
F	20α-dihydro	Inactive[b]		
P	19-nor	3	3	1
DOC	19-nor	3	1.5	2
F	19-nor	1.5	0.1	15
B	19-nor	1.0	0.3	3.3
SC-5233	19-nor	2.0		
Aldosterone	19-nor	0.002	<0.002	>1.0
DOC	19-oxo	0.3	0.12	2.5
F	18-oxo	0.1	0.07	1.4
F	18-OH	0.0005	0.008	0.06
DOC	18-OH	0.01		
B	18-OH	0.01		
Aldosterone	18-deoxy	0.3	0.05	6
P	17α-OH	0.4	0.6	0.7
B	17α-OH	0.6	1.1	0.5
F	11-deoxy	1.4		
B	11-deoxy	3.6	0.9	4.0
F	9α-fluoro	62		
Prednisolone	9α-fluoro	33		
SC-5233	7-carboxyl (isopropyl ester)	5		
DOCA	6-dehydro	1.0		
SC-5233	6-dehydro	0.25		
F	5α-dihydro	0.45	0.05	9
F	5β-dihydro	0.22	0.01	22
5α DHF	3α-dihydro	Inactive		

B. Alterations in agonist–antagonist activity

Increasing agonist activity	Increasing antagonist activity
DOC	21-deoxy DOC
Aldosterone	18-deoxyaldosterone
DOCA	6-dehydro DOCA
SC-5233	6-dehydro SC-5233
19-norprogesterone	Progesterone

[a] References: Butkus *et al.*, 1982; Feldman and Funder, 1973; Funder and Adam, 1981; Funder *et al.*, 1974, 1978; Genard and Palem-Vliers, 1980; Lan *et al.*, 1982; Marver and Edelman, 1978; Sakauye and Feldman, 1976; Thomas *et al.*, 1983; Ulick *et al.*, 1979, 1983; Wambach and Casals-Stenzel, 1983; Wynne *et al.*, 1980.

[b] Inactive = No displacement of [³H] steroid within the range of concentrations tested.

requirements for agonist versus antagonist activity. Considering first structural modifications that influence affinity, reduction of the C-4,5 double bond, the C-3 or C-20 keto function on C-21 steroid hormones is met with a fall in both binding and bioassayable mineralocorticoid activity. Thus, 5α and 5β DHF have about one-half the activity of F in a rat bioassay monitoring urinary Na and K ratios, while tetrahydro F (THF) and 20α DHF are inactive in renal binding assays against [³H]aldosterone (Marver and Edelman, 1978). Similar findings were obtained with reduction of aldosterone to dihydroaldosterone (DHA) and tetrahydroaldosterone (THA) (Kenyon *et al.*, 1983). The C-20 α or β OH derivative of 17-OH progesterone shows a 70–80% fall in affinity for the mineralocorticoid binding site. Loss of the 11,18 hemiacetal function on aldosterone also diminishes activity. 18-Deoxyaldosterone, which maintains the 11,18 epoxy structure, has about one-third the binding activity of aldosterone, while 18-OH corticosterone, which cannot form the epoxide or a hemiacetal, has about 1% the binding activity of corticosterone (Ulick *et al.*, 1979; Feldman and Funder, 1973). On the other hand, 19 noraldosterone has less than 1% type I binding activity, despite the fact that the 11,18 hemiacetal remains intact, and the 19 nor-derivative of DOC, F, and the spirolactone SC-5233 show a 1.5- to 3-fold enhancement of binding activity (Wynne *et al.*, 1980). Since a structural analysis was not provided to show authenticity of the 19 noraldosterone derivative, this provocative finding awaits further clarification. Modification of the C-19 methyl on DOC to an oxo group detracts from, rather than stimulates, binding activity.

The ability of a 19 nor- modification to enhance receptor binding is dependent on the status of the B ring. The C-19 methyl group projects onto the β face of the steroid from C-10, a carbon shared by the unsaturated A and saturated B rings of the steroid molecule. Thus, if the C-19-CH₃ is removed from SC-5233, a compound without B-ring substitutions in the 6,7 positions, binding activity is increased twofold. In contrast, if the same maneuver (C-19 demethylation) is carried out with SC-9376 or SC-9420, with either a C-6,7 double bond or a C-7 thioacetate function, the C-19 nor derivative does not have an increased affinity relative to the parent compound (Funder *et al.*, 1974). In fact, the 6,7 modifications in themselves enhance affinity two- to threefold. Thus, it is probably not the steric hindrance of the C-19 methyl or oxo group that influences binding, but the influence of C-10 substitution on ring-inductive effects, an influence which can be countermanded by *para* substitution at C-7.

The removal of the 18-hydroxy function of aldosterone, leaving the epoxy intact, has minimal influence on binding activity, while addition of an oxo or hydroxyl function at C-18 (to B, DOC, and F as noted in Table XI) reduces activity to a greater degree. The 18-hydroxy function is especially detrimental, resulting in an activity only $\leq 1\%$ of the parent compound. On the other hand, the most striking increase in type I binding is that following 9α fluoro substitution of F or prednisolone (30- to 60-fold rise in affinity), leading some to conclude that the alpha surface of steroid has intimate contact with the receptor site and that the fluorine at the C-9 position binds, by van der Waals forces, to the receptor (Genard and Palem-Vliers, 1980).

We might also ask about the effect of substitution on binding of steroid to type I versus type II receptors. Obviously, the 17- and 11-OH function increases glucocorticoid relative to mineralocorticoid-specific binding, while C-19 demethylation has the opposite effect. Finally, the 5α or β reduced derivatives of F maintain more mineralocorticoid than glucocorticoid affinity.

Examining antagonist structural requirements, it is readily apparent that antagonist versus agonist activity is not related to binding affinity. First, both a pure agonist such as aldosterone and a pure antagonist such as SC-26304 can have equivalent affinities for the rat type I receptor (Funder *et al.*, 1974). Second, there is some species difference in the degree of antagonism of a given molecule. SC-26304, which is an apparent "pure" antagonist in rat and rabbit, has some agonist activity in toad bladder (Marver *et al.*, 1974; Marver and Schwartz, 1980; Sakauye and Feldman, 1976). Third, the γ lactone ring emanating from C-17 is the sine qua non of the spirolactone group. Opening of the lactone ring results in a decrease in receptor affinity such that K^+ canrenoate (SC-14266) has one-tenth the affinity of canrenone (SC-9376), but without a concomitant decrease in antagonist activity. Unsaturation of the lactone ring reduces the affinity for type I sites some 10–50%, with an unreported change in the degree of antagonism of parent and product compounds. Modifications at the C on the 7 position change both affinity and degree of antagonism. The introduction of a C-6,7 double bond (SC-9376) (or a C-6,7 cyclopropane ring) decreases the affinity of the parent compound SC-5233 for the receptor while increasing antagonist properties (Chinn *et al.*, 1981). Both 6-dehydro DOCA and 6-dehydro SC-5233 have improved antagonist properties, while C-7 thioacetylation (SC-9420) increases both the affinity and the degree of antagonism of the parent compound SC-5233 (Funder *et al.*, 1978; Sakauye and Feldman, 1976). In this series, the final modification of interest is 18-deoxyaldosterone, a suboptimal inducer with the 11,18 epoxide intact, and a C-21–OH group (Ulick *et al.*, 1979). C-21 deoxyaldosterone, on the other hand, unlike C-21–deoxy,11-deoxycorticosterone, is an agonist, not an antagonist (Wynne *et al.*, 1981); thus, the spatial relationships between these oxygens (C-11, C-18, C-21) and/or the presence of these oxygens can influence agonism versus antagonism of these compounds. As with the agonists listed in Table XI, substitutions on C-10 and on the *para* carbon, C-7, influence the affinity and, at times (C-7), the degree of antagonism of resultant compounds. Finally, a major goal of chemists in this field is to produce a spirolactone with reduced affinity for the DHT receptor, which maintains significant antimineralocorticoid action. Such a derivative is SC-25152, with a C-7 carboxymethyl substitution. SC-25152 has about a 20% reduction in affinity to type I sites and an 80% reduction in affinity to DHT receptors compared to spironolactone (Cutler *et al.*, 1978).

C. Up- and Down-Regulation

With the suggestion that renal mineralocorticoid receptors may undergo up- and down-regulation, investigators have attempted to determine whether up-regulation aggravates hypertension or down-regulation results in the condition known as pseudohypoaldosteronism. The latter is a congenital salt-losing syndrome in infancy, which persists in the face of high circulating renin and aldosterone levels. This suggests a renal defect, and both proximal and distal sites have been posited (Proesmans *et al.*, 1978; Oberfield *et al.*, 1979). Since it is conceivable that the end-organ defect could be a down-regulation of receptor, Postel-Vinay *et al.* (1974) evaluated [³H]aldosterone binding to colonic mucosal cells of both normal volunteers and of a patient with pseudohypoaldosteronism. As shown in Table XII, no significant difference in receptor labeling was found, nor was there any indication that translocation of receptor to nuclei was defective in this patient. An alternate explanation for the syndrome was demonstrated by Bierich and Schmidt (1976), who found that both basal and hormone-stimulated Na,K-ATPase activity in cells all along the nephron were markedly depressed in patients relative to controls. Also shown in Table XII, hypertensive rats did not show up-regulation of [³H]aldosterone binding sites, nor was there a change in the K_d or nuclear translocation of bound receptors to nuclei in aortas from hypertensive versus normotensive rats (Nichols *et al.*, 1982). Renal hypertrophy increased the number of receptors per kidney, but not when normalized per gram tissue (Rafestin-Oblin *et al.*, 1981). Thus, to date only adrenalectomy has led to an increase in receptor number (about 3.5-fold). Still to be determined is whether this is due to an increase in synthesis, a decrease in degradation, or a shift in inactive plus nuclear-bound receptors to preactive cytoplasmic sites (Claire *et al.*, 1981). Earlier studies suggested however, that receptor was not rapidly degraded and synthesized under normal conditions, since the presence of cycloheximide over a 4-hour incubation period did not perceptibly alter receptor levels (Funder *et al.*, 1972). The apparent up-regulation following adrenalectomy is most likely related to steroid absence rather than Na depletion and volume contraction,

TABLE XII

Evaluation of Possible Up- and Down-Regulation of Type I Receptors

Species	Tissue	Basal condition	Experimental condition	N_{max} (± SEM)		Units (moles)	Significant?	Reference[a]
				Basal	Experimental			
Rat	Kidney	Normal	Adx	0.83 ± 0.01	3.05 ± 0.04	$\times 10^{-14}$/mg protein	Yes	1
Sheep	Kidney	Na deplete (adx; steroid replaced)	Na replete (adx; steroid replaced)	~14	~14	$\times 10^{-14}$/mg protein	No	2
Rat	Kidney	Normal	Renal hypertrophy	10.6 ± 3.2	10.5 ± 2.2	$\times 10^{-13}$/g tissue	No	3
Human	Colon	Normal	Pseudohypo-aldosteronism	15.8 ± 6	9.5	$\times 10^{-14}$/mg DNA	No	4
Rat	Aorta	Normal (WKY)	Hypertensive (SHR)	7.7 ± 4.0	11.5 ± 13.3	$\times 10^{-14}$/mg DNA	No	5

[a] (1) Claire et al., 1981; (2) Butkus et al., 1976; (3) Rafestin-Oblin et al., 1981; (4) Postel-Vinay et al., 1974; (5) Nichols et al., 1982.

since adrenalectomized animals maintained on exogenous steroids had no significant change in receptor number despite marked alterations in Na status (Butkus *et al.*, 1976).

VII. NEW CONCEPTS AND UNRESOLVED ISSUES

A number of questions regarding the mineralocorticoid receptor remain unresolved. Certainly it will be important to extend the simplistic model presented in Fig. 4 to include the molecular requirements that determine the ability of the receptor to (a) bind aldosterone, (b) bind to chromatin or DNA, and (c) alter its normal path of induction if progesterone rather than aldosterone occupies the receptor. Purification of the receptor and the issue of subunit homogeneity or heterogeneity remain, as well as the biochemical explanation for the apparent up-regulation in adrenalectomized animals. However, two immediate and more basic issues seem critical to our understanding of type I site actions. The first has to do with the physiological role of type III or CBG-like binding sites, which appear at times to be intracellular constituents as opposed to extracellular contaminants in binding assays of mineralocorticoid target tissues. More puzzling is that, when investigators have attempted to remove this CBG-like material by chromatography or ammonium sulfate precipitation, the renal mineralocorticoid receptor loses its discrimination between a series of precursor products, namely progesterone, DOC, B, and aldosterone. The second and related issue is that there may be four rather than three corticosteroid receptors or binding sites. They may be represented as having a high affinity for DOC/progesterone and a low affinity for F (type Ia), a high affinity for aldosterone/DOC with a lower affinity for progesterone/F (type I), a high affinity for DM/B/F with a lower affinity for aldosterone (type II), and a high affinity for F/B/DOC/progesterone with a lower affinity for aldosterone/DM (type III, CBG, CBG-like?). The distinguishing steroids are F, DM, and progesterone. Type Ia sites are characteristic of those determined by Lee *et al.* (1983) in the isolated CCT and those found in aorta by Kornel *et al.* (1982, 1983). Notably aorta also contains an F-preferring site with the characteristics of a type III binding protein—receptor. New technology and perspective should allow us to address these questions in the near future.

ACKNOWLEDGMENTS

The author wishes to thank Dr. Stanley Ulick for a critical reading of the section on structure—function, as well as L. Thyrza and D. Copeland for their help with the preparation of this manuscript. A number of the studies presented in this text were funded by a National Institutes of Health Grant, AM 25176.

REFERENCES

Adam, W. R., Funder, J. W., Mercer, J., and Ulick, S. (1978). *Endocrinology* **103,** 465–471.
Alberti, K. G. M. M., and Sharp, G. W. G. (1969). *Biochim. Biophys. Acta* **192,** 335–346.
Alberti, K. G. M. M., and Sharp, G. W. G. (1970). *J. Endocrinol.* **48,** 563–574.
Armanini, D., Karbowiak, I., Krozowski, Z., Funder, J. W., and Adam, W. R. (1982). *Endocrinology* **111,** 1683–1686.
Ausiello, D. A., and Sharp, G. W. G. (1968). *Endocrinology* **82,** 1163–1169.
Ballard, P. L., Baxter, J. D., Higgins, S. J., Rousseau, G. G., and Tomkins, G. M. (1974). *Endocrinology* **94,** 998–1002.
Bastl, C. P., and Marver, D. (1984). *In* "Controversies in Nephrology and Hypertension" (R. G. Narins, ed.), pp. 579–605. Churchill-Livingston, Edinburgh and London.
Baxter, J. D., Schambelan, M., Matulich, D. T., Spindler, J. J., Taylor, A. A., and Bartter, F. C. (1976). *J. Clin. Invest.* **58,** 579–589.
Beaumont, K., and Fanestil, D. D. (1983). *Endocrinology* **113,** 2043–2051.
Bierich, J. R., and Schmidt, U. (1976). *Eur. J. Pediatr.* **121,** 81–87.
Birnbaumer, M., Schrader, W. T., and O'Malley, B. W. (1983). *J. Biol. Chem.* **258,** 7331–7337.
Bullock, L. P., and Barden, C. W. (1974). *Endocrinology* **94,** 746–756.
Butkus, A., Coghlan, J. P., Paterson, R. A., Scoggins, B. A., Robinson, J. A., and Funder, J. W. (1976). *Clin. Exp. Pharmacol. Physiol.* **3,** 557–565.
Butkus, A., Congiu, M., Scoggins, B. A., and Coghlan, J. P. (1982). *Clin. Exp. Pharmacol. Physiol.* **9,** 157–163.
Campen, T. J., and Fanestil, D. D. (1982). *Clin. Exp. Hypertens., Part A* **A4**(9&10), 1627–1636.
Campen, T. J., Vaughn, D. A., and Fanestil, D. D. (1983). *Pfluegers Arch.* **399,** 93–101.
Chang, K.-J., Jacobs, S., and Cuatrecasas, P. (1975). *Biochim. Biophys. Acta* **406,** 294–303.
Chinn, L. J., Salamon, K. W., and Desai, B. N. (1981). *J. Med. Chem.* **24,** 1103–1107.
Claire, M., Rafestin-Oblin, M. E., Michaud, A., and Corvol, P. (1978). *FEBS Lett.* **88,** 295–299.
Claire, M., Rafestin-Oblin, M. E., Michaud, A., Roth-Meyer, C., and Corvol, P. (1979). *Endocrinology* **104,** 1194–1200.
Claire, M., Oblin, M.-E., Steimer, J.-L., Nakane, H., Misumi, J., Michaud, A., and Corvol, P. (1981). *J. Biol. Chem.* **256,** 142–147.
Clarkson, E. M., and Luck, V. A. (1970). *Clin. Sci.* **39,** 16P.
Compton, J. G., Schrader, W. T., and O'Malley, B. W. (1983). *Proc. Natl. Acad. Sci. U.S.A.* **80,** 16–20.
Corvol, P., Michaud, A., Menard, J., Friefeld, M., and Mahoudeau, J. (1975). *Endocrinology* **97,** 52–58.
Cutler, G. B., Pita, J. C., Rifka, S. M., Menard, R. H., Sauer, M. A., and Loriaux, D. L. (1978). *Endocrinology* **47,** 171–175.
De Kloet, R., Burbach, P., and Mulder, G. H. (1977). *Mol. Cell. Endocrinol.* **7,** 261–273.
De Kloet, R., Wallach, G., and McEwen, B. S. (1975). *Endocrinology* **96,** 598–609.
Dixon, T. E., and Al-Awqati, Q. (1979). *Proc. Natl. Acad. Sci. U.S.A.* **76,** 3135–3138.

Doucet, A., and Katz, A. I. (1981). *Am. J. Physiol.* **241** (*Renal Fluid Electrolyte Physiol.* **10**), F605–F611.

Dunn, J. F., Nisula, B. C., and Robard, D. (1981). *J. Clin. Endocrinol. Metab.* **53**, 58–68.

Duval, D., Funder, J. W., Devynck, M.-A., and Meyer, P. (1977). *Cardiovasc. Res.* **11**, 529–535.

Edelman, I. S. (1981). *Am. J. Physiol.* **241** (*Renal Fluid Electrolyte Physiol.* **10**), F333–F339.

Edelman, I. S., and Marver, D. (1980). *J. Steroid Biochem.* **12**, 219–224.

Ermisch, A., and Rühle, H.-J. (1978). *Brain Res.* **147**, 154–158.

Fanestil, D. D., and Edelman, I. S. (1966). *Proc. Natl. Acad. Sci. U.S.A.* **56**, 872–879.

Farman, N., and Bonvalet, J. P. (1983). *Am. J. Physiol.* **245**, (*Renal Fluid and Electrolyte Physiol.* **14**), F606–F614.

Farman, N., Kusch, M., and Edelman, I. S. (1978). *Am. J. Physiol.* **235**, C90–C96.

Farman, N., Vanderwalle, A., and Bonvalet, J. P. (1982). *Am. J. Physiol.* **242** (*Renal Fluid Electrolyte Physiol.* **11**), F69–F77.

Farman, N., Vanderwalle, A., and Bonvalet, J. P. (1983). *Am. J. Physiol.* **244** (*Renal Fluid Electrolyte Physiol.* **13**), F325–F334.

Feldman, D., and Couropmitree, C. (1976). *J. Clin. Invest.* **57**, 1–7.

Feldman, D., and Funder, J. W. (1973). *Endocrinology* **92**, 1389–1396.

Feldman, D., Funder, J. W., and Edelman, I. S. (1972). *Am. J. Med.* **53**, 545–560.

Feldman, D., Funder, J. W., and Edelman, I. S. (1973). *Endocrinology* **92**, 1429–1441.

Feldman, D., Loose, D. S., and Tan, S. Y. (1978). *Am. J. Physiol.* **234**(6), F490–F496.

Fimognari, G. M., Fanestil, D. D., and Edelman, I. S. (1967). *Am. J. Physiol.* **213**, 954–962.

Fuller, P. J., and Funder, J. W. (1976). *Kidney Int.* **10**, 154–157.

Funder, J. W., and Adam, W. R. (1981). *Endocrinology* **109**, 313–315.

Funder, J. W., Feldman, D., and Edelman, I. S. (1972). *J. Steroid Biochem.* **3**, 209–218.

Funder, J. W., Feldman, D., and Edelman, I. S. (1973a). *Endocrinology* **92**, 994–1004.

Funder, J. W., Feldman, D., and Edelman, I. S. (1973b). *Endocrinology* **92**, 1005–1013.

Funder, J. W., Feldman, D., Highland, E., and Edelman, I. S. (1974). *Biochem. Pharmacol.* **23**, 1493–1501.

Funder, J. W., Mercer, J., Ingram, B., Feldman, D., Wynne, K., and Adam, W. E. (1978). *Endocrinology* **103**, 1514–1517.

Garg, L. C., Knepper, M. A., and Burg, M. B. (1981). *Am. J. Physiol.* **240** (*Renal Fluid Electrolyte Physiol.* **9**), F536–F544.

Garwitz, E. T., and Jones, A. W. (1982). *Am. J. Physiol.* **243** (*Heart Circ. Physiol.* **12**), H927–H933.

Geering, K., Girardet, M., Bron, C., Kraehenbuhl, J.-P., and Rossier, B. C. (1982). *J. Biol. Chem.* **257**, 10338–10343.

Genard, P., and Palem-Vliers, M. (1980). *J. Steroid Biochem.* **13**, 1299–1305.

Goodman, D. B. P. (1981). *Ann N.Y. Acad. Sci.* **372**, 30–38.

Grantham, J. J., and Orloff, J. (1968). *J. Clin. Invest.* **47**, 1154–1161.

Grekin, R. J., and Sider, R. S. (1980). *J. Steroid Biochem.* **13**, 835–837.

Grippo, J. F., Tienrungraj, W., Dahmer, M. K., Housley, P. R., and Pratt, W. B. (1983). *J. Biol. Chem.* **258**, 13658–13664.

Gross, F., and Sulser, F. (1957). *Arch. Exp. Pathol. Pharmakol.* **230**, 274–283.

Gross, J. B., Imai, M., and Kokko, J. P. (1975). *J. Clin. Invest.* **55**, 1284–1294.

Hammes, G. G., and Wu, C.-W. (1974). *Annu. Rev. Biophys. Bioeng.* **3**, 1–33.

Hampl, R., Stárka, L., and Obenberger, J. (1981). *Exp. Eye Res.* **33**, 581–583.

Herman, T. S., Fimognari, G. M., and Edelman, I. S. (1968). *J. Biol. Chem.* **243**, 3849–3856.

Hierholzer, K., Lichtenstein, I., Siebe, H., Tsiakiris, D., and Witt, I. (1982). *In* "Biochemistry of Kidney Functions" (F. Morel, ed.), pp. 233–240. Elsevier, Amsterdam.

Higgins, J. R., Wambach, G., Kem, D. C., Gomez-Sanchez, C., Holland, O. B., and Kaplan, N. M. (1977). *J. Lab. Clin. Med.* **89**, 250–256.

Hollander, W., Kramsch, D. M., Yogi, S., and Madoff, I. M. (1965). *In* "International Club on Arterial Hypertension" (P. Milliez and P. Tcherdakoff, eds.), pp. 305–326. L'expansion Scientifique française, Paris.

Horisberger, J.-D., and Diezi, J. (1983). *Am. J. Physiol.* **245** (*Renal Fluid Electrolyte Physiol.* **14**), F89–F99.

Housley, P. R., and Pratt, W. B. (1983). *J. Biol. Chem.* **258**, 4630–4635.

Housley, P. R., Dahmer, M. K., and Pratt, W. B. (1983). *J. Biol. Chem.* **257**, 8615–8618.

Imai, M. (1979). Kidney Int. **15**, 346–356.

Kaiser, N., Milholland, R. J., Turnell, R. W., and Rosen, F. (1972). *Biochem. Biophys. Res. Commun.* **49**, 516–521.

Kalimi, M., Hubbard, J., and Ray, A. (1983). *J. Steroid Biochem.* **18**, 665–671.

Kelly, P. A., Djiane, J., and Malancon, R. (1983). *J. Steroid Biochem.* **18**, 215–221.

Kenyon, C. J., Brem, A. S., McDermott, M. J., Decouti, G. A., Latif, S. A., and Morris, D. J. (1983). *Endocrinology* **112**, 1852–1856.

Kikkawa, Y., Kaibara, M., Motoyama, E. K., Orzalesi, M. M., and Cook, C. D. (1971). *Am. J. Pathol.* **64**, 423–442.

Kirsten, E., Kirsten, R., and Sharp, G. W. G. (1970). *Pfluegers Arch.* **316**, 26–33.

Kirsten, R., and Kirsten, E. (1972). *Am. J. Physiol.* **223**, 229–235.

Knauf, H. (1976). *Eur. J. Clin. Invest.* **6**, 17–20.

Kornel, L., and Rafelson, M. E., Jr. (1983). *Endocr. Soc. Program*, Abstracts, p. 273.

Kornel, L., Kanamarlapudi, N., Travers, T., Taff, D. J., Patel, N., Chen, C., Baum, R. M., and Raynor, W. J. (1982). *J. Steroid Biochem.* **16**, 245–264.

Kornel, L., Kanamarlapudi, N., Ramsay, C., Travers, T., Kamath, S., Taff, D. J., Patel, N., Packer, W., and Raynor, W. J. (1983). *J. Steroid Biochem.* **19**, 333–344.

Koshland, D. E., Némethy, G., and Filmer, D. (1966). *Biochemistry* **5**, 365–385.

Krozowski, Z., and Funder, J. W. (1981a). *Endocrinology* **109**, 1221–1224.

Krozowski, Z., and Funder, J. W. (1981b). *Endocrinology* **109**, 1811–1813.

Krozowski, Z., and Funder, J. W. (1983). *Proc. Natl. Acad. Sci. U.S.A.* **80**, 6056–6060.

Kusch, M., Farman, N., and Edelman, I. S. (1978). *Am. J. Physiol.* **235**(3), C82–C89.

Lan, N. C., Matulich, D. T., Morris, J. A., and Baxter, J. D. (1981). *Endocrinology* **109**, 1963–1970.

Lan, N. C., Graham, B., Bartter, F. C., and Baxter, J. D. (1982). *J. Clin. Endocrinol. Metab.* **54**, 332–342.

Leach, K. L., Dahmer, M. K., and Pratt, W. B. (1983). *J. Steroid Biochem.* **18**, 105–107.

Lee, S.-M. K., Chekal, M. A., and Katz, A. I. (1983). *Am. J. Physiol.* **244** (*Renal Fluid Electrolyte Physiol.* **13**), F504–F509.

Liddle, G. W., and Sennett, J. A. (1975). *J. Steroid Biochem.* **6**, 751–753.

McDermott, M., Latif, S., and Morris, D. J. (1983). *J. Steroid Biochem.* **19**, 1205–1211.

Mainwaring, W. I. P., Mangan, F. R., Wilce, P. A., and Milroy, E. G. P. (1972). *In* "Receptors for Reproductive Hormones" (B. W. O'Malley and A. R. Means, eds.), pp. 197–231. Plenum, New York.

Marusic, E. T., Hayslett, J. P., and Binder, H. J. (1981). *Am. J. Physiol.* **240** (*Gastrointest. Liver Physiol.* **3**), G417–G423.

Marver, D. (1980a). *Vitam. Horm. (N.Y.)* **38**, 55–117.

Marver, D. (1980b). *Endocrinology* **106**, 611–618.

Marver, D. (1984a). *Am. J. Physiol.* **246** (*Renal Fluid Electrolyte Physiol.* **15**) F111–F123.

Marver, D. (1984b). *Am. J. Physiol.* **246** (*Renal Fluid Electrolyte Physiol.* **15**) F437–F446.

Marver, D. (1984c). *Am. J. Physiol.* **246** (*Endocrinol. Metab.* **9**) E452–E457.

Marver, D., and Edelman, I. S. (1978). *J. Steroid. Biochem.* **9**, 1–7.

Marver, D., and Kokko, J. P. (1983). *Miner. Electrolyte Metab.* **9**, 1–18.

Marver, D., and Lombard, W. B. (1981). *Kidney Int.* **19**, 248.

Marver, D., and Schwartz, M. J. (1980). *Proc. Natl. Acad. Sci. U.S.A.* **77**, 3672–3676.

Marver, D., Goodman, D., and Edelman, I. S. (1972). *Kidney Int.* **1**, 210–223.

Marver, D., Stewart, J., Funder, J. W., Feldman, D., and Edelman, I. S. (1974). *Proc. Natl. Acad. Sci. U.S.A.* **71**, 1431–1435.

Marver, D., Schwartz, M. J., Petty, K., and Lombard, W. E. (1980). *In* "Hormonal Regulation of Sodium Excretion" (B. Lichardus, R. W. Schrier, and J. Ponec, eds.), pp. 229–236. Elsevier/North-Holland, Amsterdam.

Mayer, M., Schmidt, T. J., Barnett, C. A., Miller, A., and Litwack, G. (1983). *J. Steroid Biochem.* **18**, 111–120.

Meyer, W. J., III, and Nichols, N. R. (1981). *J. Steroid Biochem.* **14**, 1157–1168.

Moguilewsky, M., and Raynaud, J. P. (1980). *J. Steroid Biochem.* **12**, 309–314.

Monod, J., Wyman, J., and Changeux, J.-P. (1965). *J. Mol. Biol.* **12**, 88–118.

Morris, D. J., Berck, J. S., and Davis, R. P. (1973). *Endocrinology* **92**, 989–993.

Mueller, A., and Steinmetz, P. R. (1978). *J. Clin. Invest.* **61**, 1666–1670.

Mulrow, P. J., and Forman, B. H. (1972). *Am. J. Med.* **53**, 561–572.

Neilson, C. J., Sando, J. J., Vogel, W. M., and Pratt, W. B. (1977). *J. Biol. Chem.* **252**, 7568–7578.

Nichols, N. R., Hall, C. E., and Meyer, W. J., III (1982). *Hypertension* **4**, 646–651.

Nutbourne, D. M., Ferguson, N. E., and Howse, J. D. (1970). *Clin. Sci.* **39**, 16P.

Oberfield, S. E., Levine, L. S., Carey, R. M., Bejar, R., and New, M. I. (1979). *J. Clin. Endocrinol. Metab.* **48**, 228–234.

Palem-Vliers, M., Hacha, R., Saint-Remy, A., Fredericq, E., and Genard, P. (1982). *J. Steroid Biochem.* **16**, 457–461.

Petty, K. J., Kokko, J. P., and Marver, D. (1981). *J. Clin. Invest.* **68**, 1514–1521.

Porter, G. A. (1968). *Mol. Pharmacol.* **4**, 224–237.

Porter, G. A., and Edelman, I. S. (1964). *J. Clin. Invest.* **43**, 611–620.

Postel-Vinay, M.-C., Alberti, G. M., Ricour, C., Limal, J.-M., Rappaport, R., and Royer, P. (1974). *J. Clin. Endocrinol. Metab.* **39**, 1038–1044.

Proesmans, W., Muaka, B. K., Corbeel, L., and Eeckels, R. (1978). *J. Pediatr.* **92**, 678–679.

Pugeat, M. M., Dunn, J. F., and Nisula, B. C. (1981). *J. Clin. Endocrinol. Metab.* **53**, 69–75.

Quirk, S. J., Gannell, J. B., and Funder, J. W. (1983). *Endocrinology* **113**, 1812–1817.

Raab, W., Humphreys, R. J., and Lepeschkin, E. (1950). *J. Clin. Invest.* **29**, 1397–1404.

Rafestin-Oblin, M.-E., Michaud, A., Claire, M., and Corvol, P. (1977). *J. Steroid Biochem.* **8**, 19–23.

Rafestin-Oblin, M.-E., Claire, M., Michaud, A., and Corvol, P. (1981). *J. Steroid Biochem.* **14**, 337–340.

Rayson, B. M., and Edelman, I. S. (1982). *Am. J. Physiol.* **243** (*Renal Fluid Electrolyte Physiol.* **12**), F463–F470.

Rondell, P., and Gross, F. (1960). *Helv. Physiol. Pharmacol. Acta* **18**, 366–375.

Rossier, B. C., and Claire, M. (1978). *In* "Aldosterone Antagonists in Clinical Medicine" (G. M. Addison, N. W. Asmussen, and P. Corvol, eds.), pp. 10–16. Excerpta Medica, Amsterdam.

Rossier, B. C., Wilce, P. A., and Edelman, I. S. (1974). *Proc. Natl. Acad. Sci.* **71**, 3101–3105.

Rousseau, G. G., Baxter, J. D., Funder, J. W., Edelman, I. S., and Tomkins, G. M. (1972a). *J. Steroid Biochem.* **3**, 219–227.

Rousseau, G. G., Baxter, J. D., and Tomkins, G. M. (1972b). *J. Mol. Biol.* **67**, 99–115.

Russo-Marie, F., and Duval, D. (1982). *Biochim. Biophys. Acta* **712**, 177–188.

Sakauye, C., and Feldman, D. (1976). *Am. J. Physiol.* **231**, 93–97.

Schwartz, G. J., and Burg, M. B. (1978). *Am. J. Physiol.* **235**(6), F576–F585.

Schwartz, M. J., and Kokko, J. P. (1980). *J. Clin. Invest.* **66**, 234–242.

Sekihara, H. (1983). *Endocrinology* **113**, 1141–1148.

Sekihara, H., Ohsawa, N., and Kosaka, K. (1979). *Biochem. Biophys. Res. Commun.* **87**, 827–835.

Sharp, G. W. G., Coggins, C. H., Lichtenstein, N. S., and Leaf, A. (1966). *J. Clin. Invest.* **45**, 1640–1647.

Sherman, M. R., Pickering, L. A., Rollwagen, F. M., and Miller, L. K. (1978). *Fed. Proc., Fed. Am. Soc. Exp. Biol.* **37**, 167–173.

Sherman, M. R., Moran, M. C., Neal, R. M., Nice, E.-M., and Tuazon, F. B. (1982). *In* "Progress in Research and Clinical Applications of Corticosteroids" (H. J. Lee and T. J. Fitzgerald, eds.), pp. 45–65. Heyden Press, Philadephia, Pennsylvania.

Stephenson, G., Krozowski, Z., and Funder, J. W. (1984). *Am. J. Physiol.* **246** (*Renal Fluid Electrolyte Physiol.* **15**) F227–F233.

Stokes, J. B. (1982). *J. Clin. Invest.* **70**, 219–229.

Stokes, J. B., and Kokko, J. P. (1977). *J. Clin. Invest.* **59**, 1099–1104.

Stokes, J. B., Ingram, M. J., Williams, A. D., and Ingram, D. (1981). *Kidney Int.* **20**, 340–347.

Stone, D. K., Seldin, D. W., Kokko, J. P., and Jacobson, H. R. (1983). *J. Clin. Invest.* **72**, 77–83.

Suthers, M. B., Pressley, L. A., and Funder, J. W. (1976). *Endocrinology* **99**, 250–269.

Swaneck, G. G., Highland, E., and Edelman, I. S. (1969). *Nephron* **6**, 297–316.

Swaneck, G. E., Chu, L. L. H., and Edelman, I. S. (1970). *J. Biol. Chem.* **245**, 5382–5389.

Thomas, C. J., Gomez-Sanchez, C. E., Marver, D., and Gomez-Sanchez, E. P. (1983). *Endocrinology* **113**, 517–522.

Tomlinson, R. W. S. (1971). *Acta Physiol. Scand.* **83**, 463–472.

Ulick, S., Marver, D., Adam, W. R., and Funder, J. W. (1979). *Endocrinology* **104**, 1352–1356.

Ulick, S., Land, M., and Chu, M. D. (1983). *Endocrinology* **113**, 2320–2322.

Ulmann, A., Menard, J., and Corvol, P. (1975). *Endocrinology* **97**, 46–51.

Vandewalle, A., Wirthensohn, G., Heidrich, H.-G., and Guder, W. G. (1981). *Am. J. Physiol.* **240** (*Renal Fluid Electrolyte Physiol.* **9**), F492–F500.

Vedeckis, W. V. (1983a). *Biochemistry* **22**, 1975–1983.

Vedeckis, W. V. (1983b). *Biochemistry* **22**, 1983–1989.

Veldhuis, H. D., Van Koppen, C., Van Ittersum, M., and De Kloet, E. R. (1982). *Endocrinology* **110**, 2044–2051.

Wambach, G., and Casals-Stenzel, J. (1983). *Biochem. Pharmacol.* **32**, 1479–1485.

Wambach, G., and Higgins, J. R. (1979). *Am. J. Physiol.* **236** (*Endocrinol. Metab. Gastrointest. Physiol.* **5**), E366–E370.

Warnock, D. G., and Edelman, I. S. (1978). *Mol. Cell. Encrinol.* **12**, 221–233.

Watlington, C. O., Perkins, F. M., Munson, P. J., and Handler, J. S. (1982). *Am. J. Physiol.* **242** (*Renal Fluid Electrolyte Physiol.* **11**), F610–F619.

•Weigel, N. L., Tash, J. S., Means, A. R., Schrader, W. T., and O'Malley, B. W. (1981). *Biochem. Biophys. Res. Commun.* **102**, 513–519.

Westphal, U. (1983). *J. Steroid Biochem.* **19**, 1–15.

Winkel, C. A., Milewich, L., Parker, C. R., Gant, N. F., Simpson, E. R., and MacDonald, P. C. (1980). *Proc. Natl. Acad. Sci. U.S.A.* **77**, 7069–7073.

Wrange, N., and Yu, Z.-Y. (1983). *Endocrinology* **113**, 243–250.

Wynne, K. N., Mercer, J., Stockigt, J. R., and Funder, J. W. (1980). *Endocrinology* **107**, 1278–1280.

Wynne, K. N., Rae, I. D., O'Keefe, D. F., Adams, W. R., Pearce, P., Stockigt, J. R., and Funder, J. W. (1981). *J. Steroid Biochem.* **14**, 1041–1044.

Yorio, T., and Bentley, P. J. (1976). *Nature (London)* **261**, 722–723.

Yorio, T., and Bentley, P. J. (1978). *Nature (London)* **271**, 79–81.

Zusman, R. M., Keiser, H. R., and Handler, J. S. (1978). *Am. J. Physiol.* **234** (*Renal Fluid Electrolyte Physiol.* 3), F532–F540.

CHAPTER 13

Purification and Properties of the Nerve Growth Factor Receptor*

Stephen E. Buxser,[†] Patricia Puma,[††] and Gary L. Johnson

Department of Biochemistry
University of Massachusetts Medical Center
Worcester, Massachusetts

*Abbreviations: NGF, nerve growth factor; NGF receptor, receptor protein for nerve growth factor; NGF–receptor, complex of NGF bound to the NGF receptor; ConA, Concanavalin A; HGH, human growth hormone; HSAB, hydroxysuccinimydyl-azidobenzoate; K_d, equilibrium affinity binding constant; PC, phosphatidylcholine; TCA, trichloroacetic acid; SDS–PAGE, sodium dodecylsulfate polyacrylamide gel electrophoresis; WGA, wheat germ agglutinin.

†Present address: Pharmaceutical Research and Development, Cell Biology Research Group, The Upjohn Company, Kalamazoo, Michigan 49001.

††Present address: Collaborative Research, Inc., 128 Spring Street, Lexington, Massachusetts 02173.

BIOCHEMICAL ACTIONS OF HORMONES, VOL. XII

I. INTRODUCTION

How does nerve growth factor (NGF) produce the diverse morphological and biochemical alterations observed during the development of sympathetic and some sensory neurons? After nearly three decades of research, the answer is still unclear. Recent advances in the development of model systems to study NGF action have led to rapid progress in unraveling many of the cellular functions that are regulated by NGF. Specific receptors for NGF have been described on cells from primary explants of embryonic sensory ganglia, dorsal root ganglia, and superior cervical ganglia (Sutter *et al.*, 1979; Banerjee *et al.*, 1976; Frazier *et al.*, 1974a). These culture systems have provided the initial descriptions of NGF action and characterization of the cell-surface NGF receptor. One of the greatest advances in recent years in defining NGF action and its receptor has been the development of clonal cultured cell lines that grow in the absence of NGF. The cell line PC12 pheochromocytoma, developed by Greene and Tischler (1976), has been the most valuable culture system to study NGF action (for review, see Greene and Tischler, 1982). When NGF is added to the culture medium for these cells, specific responses are stimulated, such as neurite outgrowth, neurotransmitter synthesis, phosphorylation of proteins, and the induction of specific proteins such as ornithine decarboxylase. In addition to PC12 pheochromocytoma cells, our laboratory has used another cell line, human A875 melanoma, to study the cell-surface receptor for NGF. A875 melanoma cells were originally characterized by Todaro and co-workers (Fabricant *et al.*, 1977; Sherwin *et al.*, 1979) and were shown to have large numbers of NGF receptors on their surface. They responded to NGF with increased survival in serum-depleted medium, similar to the survival effect of NGF on primary cultures of sympathetic neurons (for review, see Yankner and Shooter, 1982) and on PC12 cells in serum-free medium (Greene, 1978).

Cells that express receptors and respond to NGF have a common embryological origin in that they are neural crest–derived. Table I briefly outlines the properties of the NGF receptor from the cells previously described. Kinetic and structural data available at this time suggest a great deal of phylogenetic conservation in the properties of the NGF receptor. Definitive analysis of NGF-receptor homology will require detailed characterization using antireceptor antibodies and molecular cloning of receptor genes. Although many details remain to be worked out, we have succeeded in purifying the NGF receptor and are elucidating many of its properties.

II. NGF-RECEPTOR PROPERTIES ON INTACT CELLS

The affinity of [^{125}I]NGF for its cell surface receptor on sympathetic ganglia has been examined in several laboratories (Herrup and Shooter, 1973;

TABLE I

KINETIC AND EQUILIBRIUM BINDING PROPERTIES OF NGF RECEPTOR IN INTACT CELLS

Cell type	K_d (nM)	Association rate	Dissociation rate	Comments	References
Chicken embryo sympathetic and sensory ganglia	0.1 100	$7.5 \times 10^6 \ M^{-1} \ sec^{-1}$	$3.8 \times 10^{-4} \ sec^{-1}$	One high-affinity class of sites and one very low-affinity class of sites	Frazier et al., 1974a
Chicken embryo sensory ganglia	0.023 1.7	$4.8 \times 10^7 \ M^{-1} \ sec^{-1}$ 10^7–$10^8 \ M^{-1} \ sec^{-1}$	$10^{-3} \ sec^{-1}$ $2 \times 10^{-1} \ sec^{-1}$	Two apparent binding sites	Sutter et al., 1979
Chicken embryo dorsal root ganglia	n.d.[a]	n.d.	$1.6 \times 10^{-4} \ sec^{-1}$ $3.7 \times 10^{-4} \ sec^{-1}$ $1.8 \times 10^{-4} \ sec^{-1}$ $3.5 \times 10^{-4} \ sec^{-1}$	Two classes of binding sites: dilution $\}$ without removal of dilution + unlabeled $\}$ unbound [125I]NGF dilution $\}$ with removal of dilution + unlabeled $\}$ unbound [125I]NGF	Tait et al., 1981
Paravertebral sympathetic ganglia	0.011 0.5	$2.1 \times 10^7 \ M^{-1} \ sec^{-1}$	$1.1 \times 10^{-3} \ sec^{-1}$ $1.6 \times 10^{-2} \ sec^{-1}$	Two classes of binding sites	Olender and Stach, 1980
PC12 pheochromocytoma	0.2	0°C: 1/2 max = 2 minutes 1/2 max = 60 minutes 37°C: 1/2 max = 1 minute 1/2 max = 4 minutes	$t_{1/2}$ = 5 minutes $t_{1/2}$ = n.d. $t_{1/2}$ = 30 seconds $t_{1/2}$ = 20 minutes	Proposed two independent sites with distinguishable kinetic parameters, but equivalent equilibrium parameters; association and dissociation rates are temperature sensitive	Schechter and Bothwell, 1981
PC12 pheochromocytoma	3.0	n.d.	n.d.	Detected only one class of binding sites; binding performed at low temperature	Herrup and Thoenen, 1979
PC12 pheochromocytoma	0.3 5.2	n.d.	n.d.	Two classes of binding sites	Buxser et al., 1983a
A875 melanoma	1.0	n.d.	n.d.	One class of binding site	Fabricant et al., 1977
A875 melanoma	1.0	n.d.	n.d.	One class of binding site	Buxser et al., 1983a

[a] n.d., not done.

Banerjee *et al.*, 1973, 1976; Frazier *et al.*, 1974a,b). General agreement among these early studies suggested a K_d of approximately 0.2 nM for [^{125}I]NGF. Binding properties of PC12 NGF receptors, initially reported by Herrup and Thoenen (1979), suggested a single class of binding sites having a K_d = 2.9 nM by Scatchard analysis. More thorough analysis of binding to PC12 cells using a wider range of NGF concentrations has subsequently detected a second, higher-affinity class of receptors having a K_d = 0.2 nM (Yankner and Shooter, 1979; Schechter and Bothwell, 1981; Buxser *et al.*, 1983a). Similar results were reported for disrupted neural ganglia that exhibit NGF receptors present in both high- and low-affinity states (Sutter *et al.*, 1979; Frazier *et al.*, 1974a,b). The similarity in equilibrium binding studies betweeen PC12 cells and neural ganglia preparations in strong evidence that the NGF receptor in the different cell types is highly conserved.

The two classes of specific NGF receptors on PC12 and ganglia cells may also be distinguished on the basis of dissociation kinetics and by their sensitivity to tryptic digestion. The NGF receptor is highly susceptible to tryptic digestion prior to the binding of NGF, and binding of [^{125}I]NGF is completely inhibited in the presence of 10 μg/ml unlabeled NGF. Within minutes after association of NGF, 20–30% of the NGF–receptor complexes become resistant to tryptic digestion (Landreth and Shooter, 1980). Likewise, 20–30% of [^{125}I]NGF initially bound to receptor in the absence of unlabeled NGF is not dissociated by subsequent addition of 10 μg/ml unlabeled NGF. The high concentration of unlabeled NGF added after equilibration of [^{125}I]NGF binding results in rapid dissociation of the low-affinity (K_d = 2 nM) binding, and the trypsin digests [^{125}I]NGF–receptor complexes that are not in the slowly dissociating, high-affinity form (Landreth and Shooter, 1980; Buxser *et al.*, 1983a). High affinity (as a consequence of slow dissociation) and trypsin resistance temporally increase in parallel, and, thus, two independent assays appear to measure different properties of the same subpopulation of receptors.

Two interpretations of these findings have been presented by different laboratories. Landreth and Shooter (1980) suggested that a portion of low-affinity, trypsin-sensitive NGF receptors are converted to a high-affinity, trypsin-resistant state when NGF binds to PC12 cells. The hypothesis of receptor conversion is based primarily on an apparent 2-minute lag in appearance of high-affinity receptor, whereas no lag in binding to the low-affinity receptor was detected. This interpretation relies on the ability to accurately quantitate binding of [^{125}I]NGF to the high-affinity state of the receptor during a short incubation period in the presence of a three- to tenfold excess of low-affinity receptors to which [^{125}I]NGF is also binding simultaneously. Schechter and Bothwell (1981) used a very similar technique to distinguish between high- and low-affinity receptor and reported differences in both the association and dissociation rates for the two forms of the receptor. This observation further complicates interpretation of experiments employed to simultaneously assess high- and low-affinity receptors. However, Schechter and Bothwell (1981) also reported that the high-affinity, trypsin-resistant receptor was associated with the Triton-insoluble cytoskeletal matrix. Removing the Triton-soluble receptor before analysis of binding resulted in [^{125}I]NGF specifically bound to trypsin-resistant binding sites that apparently exist associated with the cytoskeleton before addition of NGF. This was interpreted as evidence that high-affinity binding sites exist associated with the cytoskeleton before contact with NGF, and, therefore, conversion to the high-affinity state after binding of NGF is not a necessary step.

The concept of negative cooperativity has also been considered in an attempt to explain the binding properties of the NGF receptor. Support for this idea was based on the observation that the presence of unlabeled NGF during the dissociation of prebound [^{125}I]NGF accelerates the rate of dissociation compared to the dissociation rate induced by dilution alone (Frazier *et al.*, 1974a). The involvement of negative cooperativity in NGF-receptor interactions was refuted by Sutter *et al.* (1979), who demonstrated that increased dissociation of bound [^{125}I]NGF took place even when the unlabeled NGF concentrations used resulted in decreased receptor occupancy. Riopelle *et al.* (1980) presented further evidence against negative cooperativity by demonstrating monoexponential dissociation of [^{125}I]NGF that was apparently bound only to the high-affinity form of the receptor. Both of these observations are at odds with the concept of negative cooperativity. However, Tait *et al.* (1981) reported that [^{125}I]NGF dissociation from its receptor on intact chicken embryo ganglia cells is not monoexponential and concluded that the data from this type of approach was insufficient to allow discrimination between models of multiple noninteracting states of the receptor and negative cooperativity.

To further complicate the analysis of NGF-receptor properties on intact cells, it is clear that several cell types demonstrate receptor-mediated endocytosis of NGF. Levi *et al.* (1980) used a biologically active rhodamine derivative of NGF to study the fate of NGF bound to either immature sensory neurons or PC12 cells. Initially, the rhodamine NGF bound to diffusely distributed receptors on the surface of the cells. At 37°C the rhodamine NGF complexed with receptors and rapidly formed clusters and immobile patches. The clustered patches required energy for internalization and underwent retrograde transport along neuronlike processes. Other techniques used to measure the internalization of NGF have demonstrated receptor-mediated endocytosis. However, the fate of internalized NGF and its receptor remains in question. Yankner and Shooter (1979) observed accumulation of label in a time-dependent manner in nuclear fractions of PC12 cells after incubation of [^{125}I]NGF with intact PC12 cells. A fraction of the nuclear-associated label was insoluble in Triton, not unlike what Schechter and Bothwell (1981) reported as evidence for cytoskeletal association of NGF–receptor complexes. Andres *et al.* (1977) analyzed the binding of [^{125}I]NGF to chick embryonic dorsal root ganglia plasma membrane and nuclear-enriched fractions and reported a class of pre-existing high-affinity binding sites associated with the nuclear preparation. The nuclear receptors were insoluble in Triton, and evidence was presented suggesting that binding was to chromatin. The chromatin association of binding is in contrast to the findings of Yankner and Shooter (1979).

Recently, Bernd and Greene (1983) used electron microscopy and radio-autography and found that [^{125}I]NGF specifically associated with plasma membranes, lysosomes, and nuclear membranes in PC12 cells. No specific association of [^{125}I]NGF with euchromatin or heterochromatin was observed. The results suggest that at least part of the receptor-internalized [^{125}I]NGF can associate with the nuclear membrane. The technique used only analyzed for the presence of [^{125}I]NGF. Evidence for the presence of receptor on the nuclear membranes, other than the apparent binding of [^{125}I]NGF, was not presented. Thus, [^{125}I]NGF associated with the nuclear membrane was demonstrated, but whether this is associated with the same receptor as is observed on the plasma membrane is not clear.

In contrast to this study, Rohrer *et al.* (1982) found association of [^{125}I]-NGF with the plasma membrane and cytoplasmic compartments, but no accumulation of [^{125}I]NGF in a nuclear pellet after cell fractionation. Using rat sympathetic neurons, Claude *et al.* (1982) observed binding, internalization, and retrograde transport of [^{125}I]NGF. The membrane binding appeared more dense on neurites than on cell bodies. After a 1-hour exposure to [^{125}I]NGF, localization was predominantly in lysosomes and multivesicular bodies. Even after 8 hours, when steady state transport was achieved, [^{125}I]NGF was primarily localized in lysosomes and multivesicular bodies. No label was detected associated with the nuclear membrane, nucleolus, or chromatin. Hogue-Angeletti *et al.* (1982) also used quantitative radioautography of [^{125}I]NGF associated with PC12 cells to localize the NGF–receptor complex within cells. Significant labeling of lysosomes was observed, as was labeling of other cytoplasmic components, including cytoskeletal elements. However, nuclei did not appear to be labeled. The same study (Hogue-Angeletti *et al.*, 1982) indicated that [^{125}I]NGF internalization is relatively slow and does not begin immediately after binding. In agreement with this interpretation, Buxser *et al.* (1983a) observed [^{125}I]-NGF bound to PC12 cells at 0°C, where approximately 20–30% of the bound [^{125}I]NGF was trypsin resistant. Because the trypsin-resistant binding occurs at 0°C, it does not appear to be due to internalization of [^{125}I]NGF. After stepping up the temperature to 37°C, an increase in trypsin-resistant binding was observed, which reached a steady state after approximately 2 hours. Degradation of [^{125}I]NGF, as assessed by trichloroacetic acid (TCA)-soluble label, was delayed by 60–120 minutes after step-up to 37°C, suggesting that lysosomal degradation of [^{125}I]NGF internalized by receptor-mediated endocytosis is significantly delayed compared to formation of the high-affinity, trypsin-resistant state of bound [^{125}I]NGF.

The experiments characterizing the interaction of [^{125}I]NGF with its receptor in intact cells are obviously important and complex. There is general agreement among workers in the field that multiple affinity states of the NGF receptor exist. Furthermore, there is general agreement that, in responsive neurons and PC12 cells, NGF is internalized by a receptor-mediated mechanism. The functional significance of each of these receptor states relative to the developmental and functional roles of NGF is not clear. The failure of NGF microinjected into the cytoplasm or nucleus of PC12 cells to induce neurite outgrowth of PC12 cells may indicate that NGF receptors on the cell surface are necessary for NGF action (Seeley *et al.*, 1983). Which of the kinetic states and properties of the receptor are important in initiating biological activity after NGF is bound is not clear. In order to gain insight into the specific signaling mechanisms that occur at NGF-receptor sites, we chose to purify the receptor and characterize its properties. Use of purified receptor should enable us to reconstitute receptor into defined systems and thereby determine how NGF receptors interact with other cellular components involved in both receptor signaling and regulation.

III. PURIFICATION OF THE NGF RECEPTOR

A. Comparison of the NGF Receptor on PC12 and A875 Melanoma Cells

Purification of cell surface hormone and growth factor receptors has been generally hampered by the low abundance of receptor protein in responsive cells and tissues. Recent isolation of cell lines expressing large numbers of specific hormone or growth factor receptors has been a major advance in purifying and characterizing these proteins. Our initial approach to purifying the NGF receptor was to identify a cell line that expressed large numbers of specific NGF receptors and could be grown in large quantity. Unfortunately, PC12 cells, although particularly useful in elucidating NGF action, do not grow to high densities and have only about 50,000–80,000 NGF receptors per cell. Several years ago, Todaro and his co-workers described human melanoma cell lines that expressed NGF receptors (Fabricant *et al.*, 1977; Sherwin *et al.*, 1979). One of these clonal cell lines, termed A875, expresses 6 to 8 × 10^5 receptors per cell. A875 human melanoma cells advantageously grow to high densities in culture and were chosen to begin purification and initial characterization of the NGF receptor.

Before attempts were made to purify the NGF receptor, the binding properties of receptor on A875 cells and PC12 cells were compared (Buxser *et al.*, 1983a). Scatchard analyses, summarized in Table I, indicated that PC12 cells express both a high-affinity form and a low-affinity form of the NGF receptor. As described in detail previously, the high-affinity form of receptor is also trypsin resistant. A875 melanoma cells, on the other hand, express a single-affinity form of receptor with $K_d = 1$ nM. All NGF receptors on A875 cells are trypsin sensitive and kinetically indistinguishable from low-affinity receptors on PC12 cells. Additionally, lysis of PC12 cells resulted in loss of the high-affinity state of NGF receptor concomitant with loss of trypsin-resistant receptor sites. High-affinity receptor sites were not preserved by inclusion of protease inhibitors in the lysis buffer. Microsomal membrane preparations from both PC12 and A875 cells contained only low-affinity, trypsin-sensitive receptor sites. The lack of high-affinity receptor in PC12 microsomal membrane fractions was not due to localization of NGF receptor to other cell fractions. Careful analysis of soluble and particulate cell fractions failed to detect high-affinity NGF receptors (Buxser *et al.*, 1983a). Block and Bothwell (1983) also observed that PC12 microsomal membranes contain only low-affinity, trypsin-sensitive receptors. However, when PC12 membranes were fused to 3T3 cells, which do not express any NGF receptor, transferred receptors were all present in the high-affinity, trypsin-resistant state. The data from these studies strongly imply that differences in receptor binding properties are related to cell factors other than the NGF-binding component of the receptor. Upon breakage of cells, these cell factors are rapidly dissociated from the NGF receptor, but can be reconstituted by fusing NGF receptor–containing membranes with appropriate intact cells. The nature of this modification is unclear. Unlike receptors that influence adenylate cyclase activity, the nucleotide triphosphates ATP and GTP do not affect NGF-receptor affinity (S. E. Buxser and G. L. Johnson, unpublished observation). However, association of NGF receptor with the cytoskeleton does appear to influence the binding properties of NGF receptor (Schechter and Bothwell, 1981). The interaction of NGF-receptor with the cytoskeleton is an important area for further investigation.

The structural relationship between NGF receptors on A875 and PC12 cells was directly assessed by photoaffinity covalent cross-linking of [^{125}I]NGF to specific receptor. Figure 1 shows that the major protein specif-

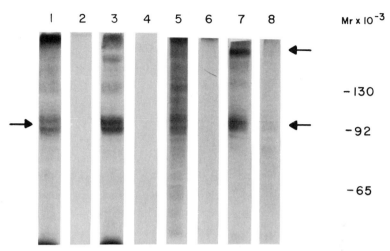

FIG. 1. Autoradiograph of SDS–polyacrylamide gel showing covalent cross-linking of [^{125}I]NGF to PC12 and A875 cells and membranes. [^{125}I]NGF was bound and covalently cross-linked to PC12 cells (lanes 1 and 2), A875 cells (lanes 3 and 4), and the plasma membrane–enriched fractions from PC12 (lanes 5 and 6) or A875 cells (lanes 7 and 8). Control incubations contained 10 μg/ml unlabeled NGF (lanes 2, 4, 6, and 8). [^{125}I]NGF was photoaffinity cross-linked to NGF-binding proteins using hydroxysuccinimydyl-azidobenzoate (HSAB) (Buxser *et al.*, 1983a). Molecular weight standards are indicated on the right. The major cross-linked peptides (indicated by arrows) are at 106 kd and 200 kd. The ratio of specific cpm's in the A875 bands to specific cpm's in the PC12 bands was 4 : 1, which is indicative of the greater amount of NGF receptor in A875 cells and membranes. Time of exposure to X-ray film for each pair of lanes was adjusted to optimize resolution in the preparations. The detection of the 200-kd band in PC12 preparations was somewhat variable, in part due to the lower abundance of the receptor compared to A875 cells and membranes. An increased background was also observed in PC12 membrane preparations, reducing the resolution of the 200-kd band (lane 5). In these and other preparations there was also a 135-kd band of relatively low abundance that appears to be specifically cross-linked to [^{125}I]NGF (lanes 1, 3, 5, and 7). This band corresponds to the M_r of the major band labeled in rabbit superior cervical ganglia described by Massague *et al.* (1981). [From Buxser *et al.* (1983a).]

ically cross-linked to [^{125}I]NGF migrates with M_r = 106 kd (Buxser *et al.*, 1983a). If the monomer size of 13 kd for β-NGF monomer is subtracted, a molecular size of 90 kd is obtained for NGF receptor on both A875 and PC12 cells. A second protein was specifically cross-linked at M_r = 200 kd. This 200-kd protein was less prominent than the 90-kd band and was particularly evident in A875 cells. A third cross-linked protein of M_r = 135 kd was occasionally observed. Two important conclusions were drawn from this analysis. (A) Proteins of equivalent size are specifically photoaffinity cross-linked to [^{125}I]NGF on both A875 and PC12 cell or membrane preparations. This supports the hypothesis that there is significant structural homology between NGF receptor on A875 and PC12 cells. (B) No detectable shift in M_r for receptor in membranes relative to receptor in cells was detected. Therefore, the lack of high-affinity receptor sites in PC12 microsomal membranes was probably not due to proteolytic lysis of receptor during membrane preparation.

In general, these studies support the hypothesis that NGF receptor present in A875 cells is closely related to NGF receptor in PC12 cells. The hypothesis is supported by both structural data and similar binding properties of receptor in both types of cells. This was an important relationship to demonstrate since the NGF receptor on PC12 cells mediates a profound biological response, but the activity of NGF on A875 cells is limited. Therefore, the studies described previously confirm the value of isolating NGF receptor from A875 cells.

B. Affinity Chromatography of the NGF Binding Protein

The NGF receptor maintains its binding activity when solubilized in the presence of several different detergents, including Triton X-100, octyl glucoside, and cholate. Among these detergents, octyl glucoside is the most useful for maintaining stability of the receptor during purification and for ease of removal during liposome reconstitution procedures. The octyl glucoside–solubilized NGF receptor from A875 membranes may be purified by sequential affinity chromatography on NGF–sepharose (Puma *et al.*, 1983). Two proteins of approximately 85 kd and 200 kd are specifically enriched on sequential rounds of NGF–sepharose affinity chromatography. Figure 2 shows the enrichment of these proteins during affinity purification starting from octyl glucoside extracts of membranes previously iodinated using a lactoperoxidase–glucose oxidase radiolabeling procedure. Similar results are also observed when the proteins are iodinated after elution from affinity columns. Table II summarizes the NGF-receptor purification from detergent extracts of A875 membranes. Receptor fractions are enriched 1500-fold after two rounds of NGF–sepharose chromatography (Puma *et al.*, 1983). The purification procedure has been repeated 15–20 times with similar results. The NGF–sepharose columns may be regenerated by high- and low-pH washes and reused at least two times. On the basis of binding studies, we calculate that the NGF receptor, present in A875 membrane preparations used as the starting material, is about 0.1% of the total membrane protein. On the basis of this estimate, a 1000- to 2000-fold purification is necessary to purify the NGF receptor. The 1500-fold purification of the

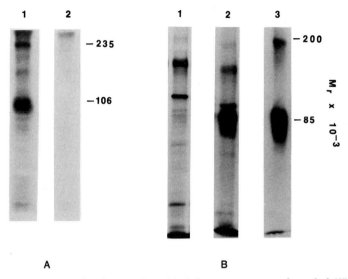

FIG. 2. Comparison of [^{125}I]NGF affinity-labeled NGF receptor and purified ^{125}I-labeled NGF receptor by SDS–PAGE. (A) Intact A875 cells were incubated with 1 nM [^{125}I]NGF in the absence (lane 1) or presence (lane 2) of 10 μg/ml unlabeled βNGF. NGF–receptor complexes were covalently linked using HSAB. (B) NGF receptors were purified by two sequential rounds of NGF–sepharose affinity chromatography. The starting material was octyl glucoside extracts of A875 membranes, which had been previously labeled with ^{125}I using lactoperoxidase-catalyzed iodination. Samples containing 10,000 cpm each were analyzed by SDS gel electrophoresis and autoradiography. Lanes represent (1) octyl glucoside extracts; (2) NGF receptor purified on one passage through an NGF–sepharose column; (3) NGF receptor passaged through two NGF–sepharose columns. The NGF-binding protein corresponds to an average size of 85 kd with a less abundant 200-kd band apparent in the preparation eluted from two NGF–sepharose columns. The 85- and 200-kd proteins correspond closely to the major cross-linked bands observed in intact cells (A) when the monomer size of βNGF is substracted from the cross-linked products. [From Puma *et al.* (1983).]

NGF receptor described previously results in receptor preparations that are purified to near homogeneity.

To verify that the 85-kd and 200-kd peptides were indeed NGF receptor–binding proteins, Puma *et al.* (1983) performed affinity labeling experiments with [^{125}I]NGF. A major band of 106 kd was specifically identified in intact A875 cells, crude octyl glucoside extracts of A875 membranes, and purified NGF receptor reconstituted into phosphatidylcholine (PC) vesicles. Subtraction of the monomer size of β-NGF gives a size on SDS gels for the NGF-binding protein similar to that observed with the iodinated proteins specifically purified by NGF–sepharose affinity chromatography. A less

TABLE II

SUMMARY OF THE PURIFICATION FOR THE NGF RECEPTOR FROM A875 MELANOMA AND PC12 PHEOCHROMOCYTOMA[a]

Sample	[^{125}I]NGF specific binding (pmoles/mg protein)	Total yield of protein (μg)	Total yield of binding activity (pmoles)	Purification (-fold)
Octyl glucoside extracts	A875 2.0 PC12 0.6	10,000 (100%) 30,000 (100%)	20 (100%) 18 .9 (100%)	— —
Extracts with treatment with NGF–sepharose (A875) or WCA sepharose (PC12)	A875 0.5 PC12 0.2	9,600 (96%) 29,700 (99%)	4.8 (24%) 5.6 (30%)	— —
NGF receptor eluted from first affinity column (A875) or WGA–sepharose (PC12)	A875 130 PC12 24	80 (0.8%) 150 (0.5%)	10 .0 (50%) 3 .7 (20%)	60 40
NGF receptor eluted from second (A 875) or first (PC12) NGF affinity column	A875 3330 PC12 2700	0.5 (.005%) 0.1 (0.0003%)	1.7 (9%) 0.28 (1.5%)	1500 4500

[a] From Puma *et al.* (1983).

prominent band at about 235 kd is also observed in the cross-linking experiments, corresponding to the 200-kd peptide purified on NGF–sepharose. Compared to intact cell cross-linking, this band was more diffuse and labeled to a lesser extent in crude solubilized and purified reconstituted preparations of the NGF receptor.

The NGF receptor from PC12 cells has also recently been purified to 20–

30% homogeneity using a modification of the procedure described for the A875 receptor (Puma and Johnson, 1984). Rather than being purified by two sequential rounds of NGF–sepharose chromatography, the NGF receptor solubilized from PC12 cell membranes in octyl glucoside was first bound to a wheat germ agglutinin (WGA)–sepharose column. Studies from several laboratories (Costrini and Kogan, 1981a; Vale and Shooter, 1982; Buxser *et al.*, 1983b) have demonstrated that the NGF receptor is a glycoprotein that binds to WGA. The column was washed extensively, and the proteins specifically bound to WGA–sepharose were eluted using N-acetylglucosamine. The fraction eluted from the WGA–sepharose column containing the NGF receptor was then adsorbed to an NGF–sepharose column and eluted as described for the receptor from A875 cells. Iodination of the final eluate showed a major band at 90 kd corresponding to the NGF-binding peptide measured in intact cells. A 200-kd peptide was also apparent, but was of much less abundance than the 90-kd peptide. Recovery of total NGF receptor was about 20% of the receptor binding activity in the octyl glucoside extract, with a final purification ranging from 500- to 6000-fold in various fractions collected from the NGF–sepharose column.

Table III summarizes the binding properties of the highly enriched NGF-receptor preparations from A875 and PC12 cells. The K_d values of purified and crude soluble receptor are in close agreement, and total binding increased several thousand fold. Calculations based on the protein recoveries and a receptor size of 90 kd indicate that greater than 50% of the purified

TABLE III

COMPARISON OF THE NGF-RECEPTOR PROPERTIES DURING PURIFICATION FROM A875 MELANOMA OR PC12 PHEOCHROMOCYTOMA CELLS

Cell type	K_d (nM)	Capacity
A875		
Intact cells	1.0	8×10^5 molecules/cell
Membranes	3.9	7.2 pmoles/mg
Octyl glucoside extract	2	
Reconstituted partially purified receptor	0.2	—
	1.7	
Purified receptor	3	28 nmoles/mg
PC12		
Intact cells	0.3	1.5×10^4 molecules/cell
	5.2	5.7×10^4 molecules/cell
Membranes	3.4	1.5 pmoles/mg
Octyl glucoside extract	1.5	1.6 pmoles/mg
Reconstituted partially purified receptor	—	—
Purified receptor	2.6	10 nmoles/mg

receptor from both A875 and PC12 cells is capable of binding [^{125}I]NGF to give specific activities approaching 30 nmoles of NGF/mg protein, compared to 1.5–8 pmoles NGF/mg protein in the octyl glucoside membrane extract.

C. Characteristics of the Purified NGF Receptor

The peptides purified from octyl glucoside extracts of A875 and PC12 cell membranes have the properties predicted for the NGF receptor, which has been characterized extensively in intact cells, membranes, and octyl glucoside–soluble extracts. The molecular sizes of the purified receptor peptides are essentially identical to those expected from affinity labeling experiments using [^{125}I]NGF. In addition, the K_d value for [^{125}I]NGF binding is approximately the same for the purified receptor and the crude solubilized receptor. Thus, by two independent criteria, molecular size and equilibrium binding analysis, the affinity-purified peptides correlate directly with the NGF receptor–binding components.

Massague *et al.* (1981) first reported a significant difference in mobility on SDS gels in the presence and absence of dithiothreitol of the [^{125}I]NGF cross-linked receptor from rabbit superior cervical ganglia. Similar differences in mobility were observed under reducing and nonreducing conditions with the purified iodinated NGF-receptor proteins (Buxser *et al.*, 1984). The mobility shift results in a change in M_r from 65 kd to 85 kd for the smaller NGF-receptor protein and a similar degree of change in M_r for the larger NGF-receptor protein. These results suggest a significant internal disulfide structure for both NGF-receptor proteins. No evidence for interchain disulfides between NGF-receptor proteins was found.

When the iodinated purified NGF-receptor peptides were resolved on SDS gels and the bands were eluted and run a second time on SDS gels, the 85-kd peptide migrated exactly as it had on the first gel. However, when the 200-kd peptide was rerun, a significant fraction of the peptide ran with $M_r = 85$ kd. This indicates that the smaller, 85-kd NGF-binding peptide could be derived from the larger NGF-binding peptide. Initially, it was thought that the relationship between the 85-kd and the 200-kd NGF-binding proteins might be either as precursor–product or as closely related proteins, both capable of binding NGF. The similar shift on SDS gels after reduction with dithiothreitol, which indicated similar internal disulfide bonds, supported this notion. Peptide mapping of the iodinated purified NGF-binding proteins gave a striking result; the use of three different proteases resulted in identical maps from both proteins. If the two proteins were related as precursor–product, or if they were similar but nonidentical proteins, different iodinated peptide maps would be expected. The generation of the 85-kd peptide from the 200-kd peptide and the identity of proteolytic peptide maps suggest that the larger-molecular-weight receptor protein may be an aggregate, possibly a dimer, of the smaller NGF-binding protein. Generation of the 200-kd binding protein is not simply an artifact of the purification, because it can be detected by hydroxysuccinimydyl-azidobenzoate (HSAB) cross-linking of [^{125}I]NGF to intact A875 and PC12 cells.

IV. STATES OF THE NGF RECEPTOR

Two NGF-receptor affinity states have been described by several laboratories for NGF receptor in PC12 cells and neural ganglia. As discussed previously, the high-affinity state of NGF receptor is characterized by the slow rate of dissociation of bound [^{125}I]NGF and by trypsin resistance of the receptor complex. Similarly, high-affinity states of receptors for other hormones have been described, including thyrotropin-releasing hormone (Hinkle and Kinsella, 1982), insulin (Corin and Donner, 1982), and human growth hormone (HGH) (Donner *et al.*, 1980). In each case, the high-affinity state is apparently the result of receptor conversion from a lower-affinity state. The mechanisms for these conversions have not been ascertained. In other systems, changes in receptor affinity are associated with changes in activity of hormone-receptor complexes. For example, cholinergic agonists induce a receptor transition from a low- to a high-affinity state (Weiland and Taylor, 1979; Maelicke *et al.*, 1977; Sine and Taylor, 1979). The high-affinity form of cholinergic receptor is inactive, and, thus, the agonist-induced receptor transition is important in the regulation of neuromuscular function. Steroid receptors, in contrast, are converted from a low-affinity, inactive form to a high-affinity, active form (Weichman and Notides, 1977; Murakami *et al.*, 1979). Since the early events in NGF stimulation have not been well characterized, the importance of NGF-receptor conversions in early stimulation events is unclear. However, the biochemical basis for receptor conversion between affinity states and the relationship of receptor affinity state modulation to biological activity have been determined for the β-adrenergic receptor (Ross and Gilman, 1980). The affinity of the β-adrenergic receptor–agonist complex is regulated by interaction with the guanine nucleotide regulatory protein of adenylate cyclase (N_S). The interaction of the β-adrenergic receptor with specific agonist is high affinity when complexed with N_S in the absence of GTP. When GTP associates with N_S, adenylate cyclase is activated and the β-adrenergic–agonist complex dissociates from N_S. In this form the β-adrenergic–agonist binding is low affinity. Thus, alterations in receptor-binding affinity can be mediated by the interaction of the hormone–receptor complex with a nonreceptor protein and may be involved in initiation of the biological response to the hormone. Similar receptor–nonreceptor protein interactions may account for the affinity changes observed in NGF-, insulin-, TRH-, or HGH-receptor systems and may provide important information in explaining hormone-initiated signaling events. For this reason, we examined the properties of NGF-receptor conversions.

During the purification of NGF receptors from octyl glucoside extracts of A875 membranes, we observed that the receptor bound to WGA–sepharose but not to Concanavalin A (ConA)–sepharose. Reports in the literature indicated that plant lectins altered the binding properties of NGF receptor on PC12 cells (Vale and Shooter, 1982) and neural ganglia (Costrini and Kogan, 1981b). We confirmed these observations for receptor in PC12 and A875 cells (Buxser *et al.*, 1983a) and additionally determined that WGA, but not ConA, treatment resulted in conversion of NGF receptor to a high-affinity, trypsin-resistant state in microsomal membranes and in detergent-solubilized and reconstituted receptor preparations (Buxser *et al.*, 1983b). N-acetyl-D-glucosamine, which specifically inhibits binding of WGA, could inhibit or reverse NGF-receptor conversion. The change in NGF-receptor properties was not simply due to aggregation of NGF-receptor induced by WGA, since NGF-receptor preparations incubated with WGA in the absence of NGF were not trypsin resistant. Both NGF and WGA were simultaneously required to induce the trypsin-resistant, high-affinity NGF-receptor state. Additionally, substantial aggregation of receptor would be expected to affect the rate of [^{125}I]NGF association, but association rates for [^{125}I]NGF were not significantly different in the presence or absence of WGA. Finally, WGA was equally active on detergent-soluble NGF-receptor and on receptor reconstituted into PC vesicles. The reconstituted vesicles contained a large excess of PC, and the distribution of receptor among the vesicles should minimize the receptor–receptor association that would be required if WGA were active merely by causing receptor aggregation. Several lines of evidence support the hypothesis that receptor conversion results from a conformational change in the receptor molecule (Buxser *et al.*, 1983b). First, all soluble NGF receptor as well as NGF receptor in microsomal membrane or in reconstituted vesicle preparations was sensitive to trypsin digestion in the absence of WGA. Within minutes after addition of WGA, [^{125}I]NGF binding became resistant to trypsin degradation. This induction of trypsin resistance in the [^{125}I]NGF–receptor complex can be explained if the complex undergoes a conformational change that shields previously exposed trypsin-sensitive sites within the complex after binding of WGA and NGF to the receptor. Additionally, formation of the high-affinity complex is time dependent. Binding of both WGA and NGF was complete within 2 minutes, but the amount of high-affinity receptor complex increased for an additional 5–8 minutes. The amount of high-affinity binding was also directly dependent on the incubation temperature. Thus, the time- and temperature-dependent increase in high-affinity, trypsin-resistant NGF receptor is consistent with the induction of a conformational change in the NGF–receptor–WGA complex initiated by the binding of NGF and WGA. The order of addition of NGF and WGA did not affect receptor conversion. Conversion to the high-affinity, trypsin-resistant state began only after both NGF and WGA were present, indicating that both NGF and WGA are required for receptor conversion to take place.

This apparent conformational change in NGF receptor is similar to the change in β-adrenergic receptor properties induced by its interaction with the N_S protein. In the case of NGF receptor, an experimental system has been developed which modifies NGF-receptor properties by direct interaction with a nonreceptor protein (e.g., WGA). The resulting high-affinity, trypsin-resistant state of NGF receptor is indistinguishable from the high-affinity, trypsin-resistant state of NGF receptor that is present on intact PC12 cells, even in the absence of WGA. The factor in intact PC12 cells that is responsible for NGF-receptor conversion has not been unequivocally determined, but recent evidence indicates that the NGF receptor interacts with cytoskeletal elements and results in a high-affinity, trypsin-resistant NGF receptor (Vale and Shooter, 1982; Schechter and Bothwell, 1981).

The data summarized above demonstrate that the state of NGF receptor can be converted from a low-affinity, trypsin-sensitive state to a high-affinity, trypsin-resistant state by addition of WGA (Vale and Shooter, 1982; Buxser *et al.*, 1983b) or by fusion of NGF receptor–containing membranes with 3T3 cells (Block and Bothwell, 1983). Scatchard analysis and trypsin sensitivity data indicate that NGF receptors found in A875 cells or in membranes derived from A875 or PC12 cells are all sensitive to trypsin and have uniform, low-affinity binding in the absence of WGA. Additionally, detergent-solubilized NGF receptor from A875 or PC12 cells or membranes is in a trypsin-sensitive, low-affinity state. However, NGF receptor purified by affinity chromatography is not structurally homogeneous, but consists of two glycoproteins with $M_r = 85$ kd and $M_r = 200$ kd (Puma *et al.*, 1983). Two binding proteins with similar M_r to purified NGF receptor are also observed on A875 and PC12 cells by means of photoaffinity cross-linking of [125I]NGF to cell-surface proteins (Buxser *et al.*, 1983a). These results indicate receptor heterogeneity, but the equilibrium binding analysis detects a single species of NGF receptor.

A clue to understanding this discrepancy is suggested by the binding and structural properties of NGF receptors reconstituted into PC vesicles. Binding of [125I]NGF to detergent-soluble NGF receptor purified by one passage through NGF–sepharose generated a linear Scatchard plot. Scatchard analysis after reconstitution of NGF receptors into PC vesicles resulted in a nonlinear Scatchard plot and indicated nonhomogeneity of the NGF receptor after reconstitution. SDS–PAGE of radiolabeled NGF receptor before and after reconstitution revealed that the proportion of 200-kd material was greater in reconstituted vesicles than in the soluble starting material. Two possible explanations for the increase are (1) preferential reconstitution of the 200-kd in contrast to the 85-kd receptor protein into PC vesicles, or (2) formation of 200-kd protein as a result of the reconstitution procedure. Regardless of the reason for the increase in 200-kd protein, it appeared to correlate with an increase in high-affinity binding as determined by Scatchard analysis. The NGF receptor in soluble and reconstituted preparations remained highly sensitive to trypsin digestion. Consequently, the change in binding properties for the NGF receptor after reconstitution was not the result of conversion to the high-affinity, trypsin-resistant state. These results provoke the question of whether the high-affinity, trypsin-sensitive form of NGF receptor corresponds to a population of NCF receptor present on intact cells or membranes.

Since both the 200-kd and the 85-kd proteins of NGF receptor were detected in A875 membranes by photoaffinity cross-linking analysis (Buxser et al., 1983a), we carefully analyzed the kinetics of [^{125}I]NGF binding to A875 membranes. Receptor characterization in membranes is not complicated by the presence of the high-affinity, trypsin-resistant NGF-receptor state. Additionally, potential interactions of receptor with the cytoskeleton or receptor internalization are eliminated. Rates of [^{125}I]NGF dissociation were chosen since these assays provide kinetic rather than equilibrium binding parameters for receptor. Initial experiments also differed from most previous analyses in that dissociation of bound [^{125}I]NGF was initiated by dilution of the [^{125}I]NGF–membrane mixture, not by addition of unlabeled NGF. These experiments clearly indicated that dissociation from A875 and PC12 membranes was not monophasic. This supports the notion that NGF receptors on membranes are not homogeneous. More striking, however, was the observation that the ratio of apparent high-affinity to low-affinity binding was constant over a wide range of NGF concentrations. This indicates that the amount of apparent high-affinity binding was directly proportional to the amount of NGF bound. Thus, a high-affinity, trypsin-sensitive subpopulation of NGF receptors is apparently formed in direct proportion to the amount of NGF bound.

Previous dissociation experiments used addition of unlabeled NGF to induce dissociation (Landreth and Shooter, 1980; Olender and Stach, 1980; Sutter et al., 1979; Schechter and Bothwell, 1981; Riopelle et al., 1980). Analysis of these experiments is complicated by the presence of the conformationally altered high-affinity, trypsin-resistant state of the NGF receptor as well as the problem of receptor internalization. In such a population of receptors biphasic dissociation would be expected. In order to avoid these problems we repeated the dissociation experiments, in which bound [125I]NGF was dissociated by addition of unlabeled NGF, but used membranes that lack the high-affinity, trypsin-resistant NGF receptor. In the presence of a high concentration of unlabeled NGF, dissociation of bound [125I]NGF from NGF receptor was very rapid and monophasic. This is in sharp contrast to experiments in which dissociation was initiated by dilution and suggests that binding of NGF is more complicated than simple interaction of a single ligand with a single receptor.

In order to reconcile the data obtained from structural, kinetic, and equilibrium binding analyses, we have formulated a working hypothesis which also takes into account the structural properties of βNGF.

The hypothesis considers several observations: (1) Linear Scatchard plots are observed in experiments where other evidence, e.g., photoaffinity cross-linking, indicates that the NGF-receptor population is heterogeneous; (2) nonlinear Scatchard plots are observed in experiments using NGF receptor reconstituted into PC vesicles in which the ratio of 200-kd to 85-kd protein is increased; (3) the 200-kd purified receptor protein is indistinguishable from the 85-kd protein by analysis of peptide maps; (4) kinetic analysis of [125I]-NGF dissociation produces different results depending on whether dissociation is initiated by dilution or by addition of a high concentration of unlabeled NGF; and (5) the amount of high-affinity, trypsin-sensitive receptor is dependent on the concentration of NGF bound, but the ratio of high-affinity to low-affinity binding is maintained over a wide range of NGF concentrations.

β-NGF consists of a dimer of identical 13-kd peptides. Two monomeric β-NGF molecules are tightly associated in a noncovalent manner. The dimeric structure appears to be important functionally, since attempts to produce biologically active monomeric β-NGF have not been successful. The dimeric structure of β-NGF suggests that each monomer may bind to one 85-kd receptor protein. This assumption predicts several properties for binding of [125I]NGF to its specific receptor and provides an explanation for the identity of the 200-kd and 85-kd peptide maps of purified receptor. That is, the 200-kd protein is a dimer of the 85-kd protein, whose formation increases during binding of the receptor to affinity columns. This is apparent when the eluates from the first and second affinity columns are compared (see Fig. 2). The binding analysis that resulted in nonlinear Scatchard plots for data from reconstituted receptor indicates that the 200-kd binding protein has a higher affinity than the 85-kd protein. The stability of the 200-kd protein after affinity purification or reconstitution is not clearly understood. However, both procedures involve a step that may induce a localized, transient high density of receptor, i.e., binding of receptor to NGF on affinity columns and precipitation of receptor during reconstitution. This may enhance receptor–receptor associations to produce the stable 200-kd form of receptor.

The data, which characterize the binding of [125I]NGF to NGF–receptor reconstituted into PC vesicles, imply that the 200-kd form of receptor has higher affinity than 85-kd receptor. Our hypothesis, in which 200-kd receptor is a dimer consisting of two 85-kd receptors, provides an explanation for this increase in apparent affinity. Dissociation of β-NGF bound to two 85-kd receptors in a 200-kd complex requires dissociation from both 85-kd receptors simultaneously. This should be significantly less probable than dissociation of β-NGF from a single 85-kd receptor molecule. The correspondingly slower rate of dissociation for β-NGF bound to a 200-kd complex can explain the increased apparent affinity for that portion of binding. There is precedent for this predicted increase in apparent affinity since dimeric intact antibody or (Fab)$_2$ antibody fragments have higher apparent affinity than monomeric Fab antibody fragments. Linear Scatchard plots in the presence of nonhomogeneous receptor proteins are observed for membranes or A875 cells. The 200-kd form of receptor is probably not a stable dimer until covalently cross-linked with HSAB. Thus, the amount of high-affinity receptor may increase as the concentration of NGF increases, but the ratio of high-affinity to low-affinity receptor remains constant. Therefore, at any particular concentration of NGF, bound [125I]NGF is distributed with a constant proportion between high and low affinities. Over the usual range of NGF concentrations used, only the average or apparent affinity is detected by Scatchard analysis. As long as the ratio of high-affinity to low-affinity binding is constant, only the average of the two affinities is detected. The apparent affinity observed is therefore a weighted average of the high- and low-affinity binding complexes. This hypothesis is further supported by the observation that initiation of dissociation by dilution or by addition of unlabeled NGF produces different results. Dissociation initiated by dilution accurately demonstrated the presence of receptor with two different binding affinities. However, in the presence of a high (saturating) concentration of NGF, all binding sites should be associated with a single, dimeric β-NGF molecule. The receptor–β-NGF–receptor complex would be saturated to form two receptor–βNGF complexes that each contain monomeric binding sites (85 kd) and therefore exhibit lower affinity. This would result in rapid, monophasic dissociation of the [125I]NGF, as was observed. This is a simpler model than negative cooperativity, since it requires no change in intrinsic receptor binding properties but is the result of receptor dimerization induced by the structure of β-NGF itself.

The hypothesis proposed previously may have even broader application. In particular, comparison of the binding properties of insulin and NGF may be valuable. Insulin and insulin receptor have several properties in common with NGF and NGF receptor. For example, insulin and NGF have a significant degree of amino acid sequence homology (Bradshaw and Niall, 1978). Additionally, a portion of insulin receptors is converted to a higher-affinity state in a time-dependent manner after binding of insulin (Donner and Corin, 1980). This conversion to higher affinity was accompanied by an apparent conformational change in the insulin receptor (Donner and Yonkers, 1983). [^{125}I]Insulin dissociated from membranes in a biphasic manner when dissociation was initiated by dilution into a large volume of medium (Corin and Donner, 1982). This is very similar to the biphasic dissociation observed for [^{125}I]NGF dissociation from A875 membranes described previously. Dissociation of either insulin or NGF was enhanced by addition of unlabeled hormone to the dissociation medium. This enhancement of dissociation did not appear to be due to receptor site–site interactions (i.e., negative cooperativity) in either case. Other recent results indicate that an "affinity regulator" for insulin receptor exists, which interacts noncovalently with insulin receptor and can be separated from receptor chromatographically (Harmon *et al.*, 1983). The presence of the high-affinity, trypsin-resistant state of NGF receptor observed on intact PC12 cells or induced by WGA suggests that a similar affinity regulator may exist for NGF receptor. These results indicate striking similarities between binding of insulin and NGF to their respective receptors.

Analysis of the structure of insulin receptor also indicates similarities to NGF receptor, particularly if the 200-kd form of NGF receptor is a dimer of the 85-kd form. Results from affinity cross-linking analysis of [^{125}I]insulin bound to insulin receptor indicate that insulin receptor consists of α subunits and β subunits covalently linked by disulfide bonds (see Czech *et al.*, 1981, for review). The intact insulin receptor consists of a heterodimer as (β-s-s-α)-s-s-(α-s-s-β). The importance of maintaining the apparent dimeric receptor structure for biological activity is not clear.

In view of the results obtained from analysis of NGF receptor, which indicate an apparent NGF-induced receptor dimerization, a new interpretation of insulin binding to its specific receptor may be indicated. Specifically, the concept of negative cooperativity may require reevaluation. It has previously been suggested that the negative cooperativity exhibited by insulin receptor may be due to dimerization of insulin rather than to site–site interaction of insulin receptor (Cuatrecasas and Hollenberg, 1975). The observation that the "cooperative" site on the insulin molecular is also the site involved in insulin dimerization (DeMeyts *et al.*, 1978) is very interesting. It seems likely that insulin dimerization, which occurs at high concentrations of insulin, may also occur if two insulin molecules bind to a single dimeric insulin receptor and, thus, are brought into close proximity to produce a localized high insulin concentration. Additionally, the apparent conformational change in the insulin–insulin receptor complex could be either the cause or the result of insulin dimerization on the receptor. As evidenced by the studies of NGF binding to NGF receptor, analysis of negative cooperativity, primarily on the basis of experiments in which dissociation is initiated by the addition of unlabeled ligand, is subject to equivocal interpretation. Reevaluation of such a model in light of recent structural data is indicated.

In general, comparison of the NGF and insulin receptor systems suggests that a similar mechanism may govern multivalent hormone and/or multivalent receptor systems, especially by mediation of alterations in binding affinity. This model may be further expanded to include other hormone or growth factor systems where multivalent receptor is present or can be induced. The relationship between receptor structure and biological activity has not been established in most cases. Clearly, this is an area worthy of considerable further effort.

V. CONCLUSIONS AND PERSPECTIVES

The major goal of these studies is to define how the interaction of β-NGF with its receptor triggers the many cellular responses observed with PC12 cells and with other responsive cells derived form the neural crest. We have avoided this topic purposely, because we do not yet have an answer. Our NGF-receptor preparations do not appear to have a detectable tyrosine kinase activity, similar to that associated with insulin, EGF, and probably PDGF receptors. NGF receptors also do not appear to interact with GTP-binding proteins associated with hormone-responsive adenylate cyclase systems, nor have we succeeded in showing that NGF affects cAMP levels in PC12 cells. However, our data do indicate that NGF and cAMP effects are additive or greater than additive with several responses, such as neurite outgrowth and Na^+,K^+-ATPase activation. We have also failed to demonstrate an effect of NGF on arachidonic acid metabolism, suggesting that prostaglandin synthesis may not be involved. These frustrations are not new and have been experienced by everyone in the NGF field.

Several different approaches in different laboratories certainly will define NGF action in the future. Our ability to purify NGF receptors allows definition of receptor properties and the molecular basis for multiple kinetic states. Reconstitution procedures will probably lend themselves to defining the interaction of NGF receptors with other cell components. Several PC12 mutants that have altered responses to NGF have been isolated, which may prove useful in delineating specific cell components involved in NGF action, much like what has been done with the S49 mouse lymphoma system and hormone-sensitive adenylate cyclase (Ross and Gilman, 1980). Finally, recombinant DNA techniques are now being applied to the NGF-receptor system, and genes involved in NGF action will most certainly complement and accelerate our understanding of NGF action.

ACKNOWLEDGMENTS

This work has been supported by NIH Grant NS18779 and an award from the Juvenile Diabetes Foundation. P. Puma is a postdoctoral fellow of the Muscular Dystrophy Association. G. L. Johnson is an Established Investigator of the American Heart Association. S. Buxser was a postdoctoral fellow of the Juvenile Diabetes Foundation during much of the work described.

REFERENCES

Andres, R. Y., Jeng, I., and Bradshaw, R. A. (1977). *Proc. Natl. Acad. Sci. U.S.A.* **74**, 2785–2789.
Banerjee, S. P., Snyder, S. H., Cuatrecasas, P., and Greene, L. A. (1973). *Proc. Natl. Acad. Sci. U.S.A.* **70**, 2519–2523.
Banerjee, S. P., Cuatrecasas, P., and Snyder, S. H. (1976). *J. Biol. Chem.* **251**, 5680–5686.
Bernd, P., and Greene, L. A. (1983). *J. Neurosci.* **3**, 631–643.
Block, T., and Bothwell, M. (1983). *J. Neurochem.* **40**, 1654–1663.
Bradshaw, R. A., and Niall, H. D. (1978). *Trends Biochem. Sci.* **3**, 274–278.
Buxser, S. E., Watson, L., and Johnson, G. L. (1983a). *J. Cell Biochem.* **22**, 219–233.
Buxser, S. E., Kelleher, D. J., Watson, L., Puma, P., and Johnson, G. L. (1983b). *J. Biol. Chem.* **258**, 3741–3749.
Buxser, S. E., Puma, P., and Johnson, G. L. (1984). *J. Biol. Chem.* (in press).
Claude, P., Hawrot, E., Dunis, D., and Campenot, R. B. (1982). *J. Neurosci.* **2**, 431–442.
Corin, R. E., and Donner, D. B. (1982). *J. Biol. Chem.* **257**, 104–110.
Costrini, N. V., and Kogan, M. (1981a). *J. Neurochem.* **36**, 710–717.
Costrini, N. V., and Kogan, M. (1981b). *J. Neurochem.* **36**, 1175–1180.
Cuatrecasas, P., and Hollenberg, M. D. (1975). *Biochem. Biophys. Res. Commun.* **62**, 31–41.
Czech, M. P., Massague, J., and Pilch, P. F. (1981). *Trends Biochem. Sci.* **6**, 222–225.
DeMeyts, P., VanObberghen, E., Roth, J., Wollmer, A., and Brandenburg, D. (1978). *Nature (London)* **273**, 504–509.
Donner, D. B., and Corin, R. E. (1980). *J. Biol. Chem.* **255**, 9005–9008.
Donner, D. B., and Yonkers, K. (1983). *J. Biol. Chem.* **258**, 9413–9418.
Donner, D. B., Casadei, J., Hartstein, L., Martin, D., and Sonenberg, M. (1980). *Biochemistry* **19**, 3293–3300.
Fabricant, R. N., DeLarco, J. E., and Todaro, G. J. (1977). *Proc. Natl. Acad. Sci. U.S.A.* **74**, 565–569.
Frazier, W. A., Boyd, L. F., and Bradshaw, R. A. (1974a). *J. Biol. Chem.* **249**, 5513–5519.
Frazier, W. A., Boyd, L. F., Pulliam, M. W., Szutowitz, A., and Bradshaw, R. A. (1974b). *J. Biol. Chem.* **249**, 5918–5923.
Greene, L. A. (1978). *J. Cell Biol.* **78**, 747–755.
Greene, L. A., and Tischler, A. S. (1976). *Proc. Natl. Acad. Sci. U.S.A.* **73**, 2424–2428.

Greene, L. A., and Tischler, A. S. (1982). *Adv. Cell. Neurobiol.* **3**, 373–414.

Harmon, J. T., Hedo, J. A., and Kahn, C. R. (1983). *J. Biol. Chem.* **258**, 6875–6881.

Herrup, K., and Shooter, E. M. (1973). *Proc. Natl. Acad. Sci. U.S.A.* **70**, 3884–3888.

Herrup, K., and Thoenen, H. (1979). *Exp. Cell Res.* **121**, 71–78.

Hinkle, P. M., and Kinsella, P. A. (1982). *J. Biol. Chem.* **257**, 5462–5470.

Hogue-Angeletti, R., Stieber, A., and Ganatas, N. K. (1982). *Brain Res.* **241**, 145–156.

Landreth, G. E., and Shooter, E. M. (1980). *Proc. Natl. Acad. Sci. U.S.A.* **77**, 4751–4755.

Levi, A., Shechter, Y., Neufeld, E., and Schlessinger, J. (1980). *Proc. Natl. Acad. Sci. U.S.A.* **77**, 3469–3473.

Maelicke, A., Fulpius, B. W., Klett, R. P., and Reich, E. (1977). *J. Biol. Chem.* **252**, 4811–4830.

Massague, J., Guillette, B. J., Czech, M. P., Morgan, C. J., and Bradshaw, R. A. (1981). *J. Biol. Chem.* **256**, 9419–9424.

Murakami, T., Brandon, D., Rodbard, P., Loriaux, D. L., and Lipsett, M. B. (1979). *Endocrinology* **104**, 500–505.

Olender, E. J., and Stach, R. W. (1980). *J. Biol. Chem.* **255**, 9338–9343.

Puma, P., and Johnson, G. L. (1984). Submitted for publication.

Puma, P., Buxser, S. E., Watson, L., Kelleher, D. J., and Johnson, G. L. (1983). *J. Biol. Chem.* **258**, 3370–3375.

Riopelle, R. J., Klearman, M., and Sutter, A. (1980). *Brain Res.* **199**, 63–77.

Rohrer, H., Schafer, T., Korsching, S., and Thoenen, H. (1982). *J. Neurosci.* **2**, 687–697.

Ross, E. M., and Gilman, A. G. (1980). *Annu. Rev. Biochem.* **49**, 533–564.

Schechter, A. L., and Bothwell, M. A. (1981). *Cell* **24**, 867–874.

Seeley, P. J., Keith, C. H., Shelanski, M. L., and Greene, L. A. (1983). *J. Neurosci.* **3**, 1488–1494.

Sherwin, S. A., Sliski, A. H., and Todaro, G. J. (1979). *Proc. Natl. Acad. Sci. U.S.A.* **76**, 1288–1292.

Sine, S., and Taylor, P. (1979). *J. Biol. Chem.* **254**, 3315–3325.

Sutter, A., Riopelle, R. J., Harris-Warwick, R. M., and Shooter, E. M. (1979). *J. Biol. Chem.* **254**, 5972–5982.

Tait, J. F., Weinman, S. A., and Bradshaw, R. A. (1981). *J. Biol. Chem.* **256**, 11086–11092.

Vale, R. D., and Shooter, E. M. (1982). *J. Cell Biol.* **94**, 710–717.

Weichman, B. M., and Notides, A. C. (1977). *J. Biol. Chem.* **252**, 8856–8862.

Weiland, G., and Taylor, P. (1979). *Mol. Pharmacol.* **15**, 197–212.

Yankner, B. A., and Shooter, E. M. (1979). *Proc. Natl. Acad. Sci. U.S.A.* **76**, 1269–1273.

Yankner, B. A., and Shooter, E. M. (1982). *Annu. Rev. Biochem.* **51**, 845–868.

CHAPTER 14

The Thyrotropin Receptor*

Leonard D. Kohn, Salvatore M. Aloj, Donatella Tombaccini,
Carlo M. Rotella, Roberto Toccafondi, Claudio Marcocci,†
Daniela Corda, and Evelyn F. Grollman

Section on the Biochemistry of Cell Regulation
Laboratory of Biochemical Pharmacology
National Institute of Arthritis, Diabetes, Digestive and Kidney Diseases
National Institutes of Health
Bethesda, Maryland

*Abbreviations: TSH, thyrotropin; ConA, Concanavalin A; hCG, human chorionic gonadotropin; LATS, long-acting thyroid stimulator; LH, luteinizing hormone; FRTL-5 cells, functioning rat thryoid cells derived from normal Fisher rat thyroid glands; G_{M1}, galactosyl-N-acetylgalactosaminyl-[N-acetylneuraminyl]-galactosylglucosylceramide; G_{M2}, galactosyl-galactosyl-N-acetylgalactosaminyl-galactosylglucosylceramide; G_{D1a}, N-acetylneuraminylgalactosyl-N-acetyl-galactosaminyl-[N-acetylneuraminyl]-galactosylglucosylceramide; G_{D1b}, galactosyl-N-acetylgalactosaminyl-[N-acetyl-neuraminyl-N-acetylneuraminyl]-galactosylglucosylceramide; G_{T1}, N-acetylneuraminylgalactosyl-N-acetyl-galactosaminyl-[N-acetylneuraminyl-N-acetylneuraminyl]-galactosylglucosylceramide; T_3, triiodothyronine; T_4, thyroxine; CBA, cytochemical bioassay; TSAb, thyroid-stimulating autoantibody; TPI, tripolyphosphatidylinositol; DPI, dipolyphosphatidylinositol; PI, phosphatidylinositol; $TPMP^+$, triphenylmethylphosphonium$^+$; DPH, 1,6-diphenyl-1,3,5-hexatriene.

†Present address: Cattedra di Endocrinologia e Medicina Costituzionale, Universitá di Pisa, Via Roma 67, 56100 Pisa, Italy.

BIOCHEMICAL ACTIONS OF HORMONES, VOL. XII

I. INTRODUCTION

Thyrotropin (TSH) is a pituitary glycoprotein hormone whose primary role is to regulate the differentiated function of thyroid cells (see Dumont, 1971; Dumont *et al.*, 1978; Field, 1978; Robbins *et al.*, 1980). Thus, the interaction of TSH with a specific receptor on the thyroid cell surface induces changes in adenylate cyclase activity that result in the following tissue responses: enhanced iodide uptake, thyroglobulin biosynthesis, iodination of thyroglobulin, degradation of iodinated thyroglobulin to form thyroid hormone (T_3 and T_4), and the release of thyroid hormone into the bloodstream (Fig. 1).

Recent studies indicate that another important action of TSH is to stimulate the growth of thyroid cells. Initially this role was suggested by observations that TSH caused increases in the mitotic index of thyroid glands *in vivo* (Wollman and Breitman, 1970) and could induce thymidine uptake in primary cultures of thyroid cells (Winand and Kohn, 1975b) or thyroid follicles (Nitsch and Wollman, 1980). This role of TSH is now unequivocally established by the observations that (i) the growth of a clonal, continuous culture of functional thyroid cells is TSH dependent (Ambesi-Impiombato *et al.*, 1980; Valente *et al.*, 1983a), and (ii) antibodies that stimulate growth and are related to TSH receptor structure are present in the sera of Graves' patients (Valente *et al.*,

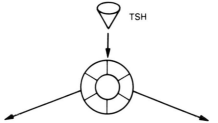

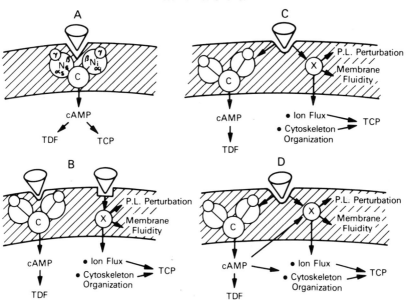

Fig. 1. Modification of the classical view of TSH receptor wherein TSH interaction with specific recognition site results in growth as well as adenylate cyclase stimulation and a sequence of second message–induced responses yielding thyroid hormone via the cAMP kinase cascade system. The β-subunit of TSH is depicted as carrying the primary evidence for recognition determinants; however, evidence for α-subunit involvement, direct and indirect, exists. Three possibilities are depicted that could account for TSH receptor–mediated growth activity: a single receptor and another cAMP-directed response; independent message and response systems coupled to a single recognition site; and independent message and response systems, each with its own recognition site. The data summarized in this report will suggest the last possibility depicted: a single recognition site with two major signal systems, cAMP- and phospholipid-based, each coded to different differentiated functions, operating together in a coregulated manner to achieve growth. Abbreviations: TH, thyroid hormone; TG, thyroglobulin.

1983b). TSH regulation of growth must also involve a specific cell-surface receptor, one that is either the same as that for regulating differentiated function or one that is an entirely different molecular entity (Fig. 1). In a similar vein, TSH regulation of growth may use the cAMP messenger system, one or more different signal systems, or combinations of signals (Fig. 1).

Initial studies presumed that the TSH receptor and the adenylate cyclase enzyme existed as a single molecular entity. It is now evident that the thyroid cell has both a membrane glycoprotein and a ganglioside, which mimic TSH receptor recognition phenomenon in reconstituted liposome systems (see below, as well as Kohn, 1978; Kohn and Shifrin, 1982; Kohn *et al.*, 1981, 1982a,b, 1983a,b, 1984a,b). Further, it is clear that the receptor is coupled to a series of separate molecular species necessary to generate second messenger signals. Thus, for example, in terms of receptor coupling to the classically defined adenylate cyclase messenger response, it is evident that the adenylate cyclase system is composed of at least four components: a catalytic unit, a stimulatory regulating subunit (N_S), an inhibiting regulatory subunit (N_I), and a low-molecular-weight γ chain whose function is unknown (Fig. 1). It is also evident that these can be linked to several receptors within the same cell (Rodbell, 1980; Ross and Gilman, 1980; Katada and Ui, 1982; Manning and Gilman, 1983; Hildebrandt *et al.*, 1984).

Thus, any current view of the TSH receptor must take into account the possibility that the TSH receptor as a recognition site may well involve more than one receptor, or several molecular components with different roles, and coupling mechanisms wherein more than one signal system is perturbed in a coregulated manner.

The present chapter will offer a molecular synthesis of the TSH receptor with respect to recognition, signal coupling, and signal transmission based on a sum of current data; this synthesis is in the nature of a current working hypothesis. The chapter will also discuss data concerning autoimmune antibodies in the sera of patients with Graves' disease, since these have been characterized as antibodies to the TSH receptor that can induce pathologic responses of hyperthyroidism as well as goiters or enlarged glands. Finally, TSH receptors will be discussed with respect to their existence and functional expression on nonthyroidal tissues and with respect to the structure and function of receptors for cholera toxin, tetanus toxin, and interferon.

II. AUTOIMMUNE THYROID DISEASE AND THE THYROTROPIN RECEPTOR

Graves' disease is an organ-specific autoimmune disorder of the thyroid characterized by (1) a diffusely enlarged thyroid gland (goiter), (2) symptoms of hyperthyroidism resultant from the overproduction of thyroid hormones, and (3) episodically associated connective tissue complications, for example, exophthalmos and pretibial myxedema.

The weight of evidence suggests that Graves' disease is a disturbance of the immune system that results in the entrance into the sera of autoantibodies that stimulate the thyroid and induce the hyperthyroid state (Adams, 1981). This concept derives from the discovery of the long-acting thyroid stimulator (LATS), an antibody in the sera of these patients that can stimulate thyroid function in mice. Today the concept of LATS as the stimulatory agent has evolved to the idea that there are a host of thyroid-stimulating autoantibodies (TSAbs) in the sera of patients with Graves' disease, which can perturb the thyroid; that some are species-specific in that they stimulate only humans and not mice; that they are readily measurable *in vitro*, using thyroid cells, slices, or membranes, by their ability to stimulate adenylate cyclase activity; and that they are related to or directed against the TSH receptor.

That TSAbs were related to the TSH receptor was suggested by their ability to influence many aspects of thyroid cell metabolism in a manner similar to that of TSH and by the fact that many patients with Graves' had antibodies in their sera that could inhibit TSH binding. Proof of the relationship was, however, clouded by conflicting experiments involving IgG preparations from the sera of Graves' patients. Thus, it was not clear whether stimulation of adenylate cyclase by TSAb might be due to a change in membrane configuration rather than to binding to a specific receptor site (Yamashita and Field, 1973). Further, despite numerous studies (Macchia *et al.*, 1981; Sugenoya *et al.*, 1979; Ozawa *et al.*, 1979a; Zakarija and McKenzie, 1980, 1981; Pinchera *et al.*, 1980), no clear correlation between TSAb stimulatory activity and the ability of the same immunoglobulin preparations to inhibit TSH binding to thyroid membranes could be found, nor were the antibodies that inhibited TSH binding shown to exhibit true competitive kinetics with respect to TSH. The problem of, and the relationship between, TSAbs and TSH receptors was rendered more complex by reports (Doniach *et al.*, 1981; Drexhage *et al.*, 1980, 1981) that antibodies promoting thyroid growth but unable to stimulate adenylate cyclase activity were also present in thyrotoxic patients with large goiters. At least some of these antibodies are argued to be directed against the TSH receptor, since these were like TSH in their effects on cell growth (Valente *et al.*, 1982a, 1983b).

In summary, clinical data led to a belief that antibodies to thyroid membranes existed in the sera of Graves' patients and were important in the pathogenesis of the hyperthyroid state. It was less clear that these antibodies were directed against the TSH receptor, whether there were multiple antibodies to this structure, or even whether there was more than one TSAb "receptor"—one involved in binding, one for adenylate cyclase activation, and one for goiter production (growth). Resolution of the apparent discrepancies in different clinical studies required a greater understanding of TSH-receptor structure and function as well as the characteristics of individual antibodies within the spectra present in a single patient's serum.

III. THE THYROTROPIN RECEPTOR: A FUNCTIONAL COMPLEX OF MORE THAN ONE MEMBRANE COMPONENT

A. Binding Studies: More Than One Membrane-Binding Component with TSH Recognition Properties

Although the TSH receptor was originally defined in terms of its adenylate cyclase or bioactivity response, it is now a well-accepted concept, as noted previously, that components of the adenylate cyclase complex are molecules without receptor recognition properties and that solubilized molecules with TSH recognition or binding properties do not cofractionate with hormone- or fluoride-stimulated adenylate cyclase activity. These results meant that membrane molecules important in the cell surface hormonal recognition process would have to be defined in binding studies rather than by functional response assays.

Numerous laboratories measured radiolabeled TSH binding to membrane preparations (Amir *et al.*, 1972; Lissitzky *et al.*, 1973; Moore and Wolff, 1974; Manley *et al.*, 1974; Tate *et al.*, 1975a; Verrier *et al.*, 1977; Azukizawa *et al.*, 1977; Powell-Jones *et al.*, 1979; Pekonen and Weintraub, 1980, etc.) with significant differences in results depending on the conditions chosen. Thus, studies using "more physiologic conditions," i.e., 50- to 100-mM salt concentrations, 37°, and a pH of ~7.4 (see Pekonen and Weintraub, 1980, for example) measured a single class of sites that exhibited high-affinity properties, a high degree of specificity, ready displacement with unlabeled TSH, but a low level of binding, usually <1% of radioactivity added. In contrast, studies that extended results over a broader range of salt concentrations and pH conditions (for example see Amir *et al.*, 1972; Tate *et al.*, 1975a), i.e., to "nonphysiologic conditions," measured much higher levels of binding, 40 to 80% of radioactive ligand added, but detected nonlinear binding curves, a lesser degree of specificity with respect to luteinizing hormone (LH) and human chorionic gonadotropin (hCG), and less sensitive displacement curves using unlabeled TSH. Although some argued that the "nonphysiologic" *in vitro* binding conditions were not measuring a high-affinity physiologically relevant TSH binding site (Pekonen and Weintraub, 1980), others argued that these conditions were in fact measuring both a high- as well as a low-affinity, salt-sensitive binding site (Kohn, 1978; Kohn and Shifrin, 1982; Kohn *et al.*, 1980, 1981, 1982a,b, 1983a,b, 1984a,b). This latter group pointed out that the displacement data could merely reflect the operational involvement of these low-affinity sites as higher concentrations of TSH were added to the assay, a phenomenon some interpreted as negative cooperativity.

The sum of the studies thus left the possibility that there might be more than one "specific" TSH binding site. Further, the studies suggested that the physiologic relevance of each might be a difficult problem to resolve once solubilization and purification studies were initiated to define them as molecular entities. Later we will note that this issue was finally resolved with receptor monoclonal antibodies and reconstitution experiments. However, it was the continued use of binding assays that first suggested that the TSH receptor might be composed of two components, a membrane glycoprotein and a ganglioside, which is a membrane glycolipid containing sialic acid (Kohn, 1978; Kohn and Shifrin, 1982; Kohn *et al.*, 1980, 1981, 1982a,b, 1983a,b, 1984a,b).

B. Evidence for a Glycoprotein Component of the Thyrotropin Receptor

Studies assaying TSH binding showed that limited tryptic digestion of thyroid cells resulted in a coincident loss and return of TSH binding and cell function; TSH stimulated adenylate cyclase activity (Winand and Kohn, 1975b) and TSH stimulated changes in membrane potential (Grollman *et al.*, 1978a). Tryptic digestion did not, however, destroy the receptor but rather released the TSH binding component into the media; the binding component also could be radiolabeled by pulsing cultures with [^{14}C]glucosamine (Winand and Kohn, 1975b). This component and a tryptic fragment were purified by applying affinity chromatographic procedures to tryptic digests of bovine thyroid membranes solubilized with lithium diiodosalicylate; they could also be adsorbed by Concanavalin A (ConA)–sepharose (Tate *et al.*, 1975a,b). Antisera prepared against the purified receptor fragment were able to precipitate the TSH binding activity in crude solubilized receptor preparations and reacted with the receptor fragment that was lost from the plasma membrane after trypsinization of the thyroid cells (Winand and Kohn, 1975b; Tate *et al.*, 1975a,b, 1976). There was no evidence for a change in the ganglioside composition of cells or membranes exposed to trypsin (Kohn and Shifrin, 1982; Kohn *et al.*, 1981, 1982a).

The solubilized glycoprotein membrane component with TSH binding activity was reconstituted in liposomes and shown to exhibit many of the characteristics of TSH binding exhibited by plasma membranes (Grollman *et al.*, 1978b; Kohn and Shifrin, 1982; Kohn *et al.*, 1981, 1982a). Moreover, using liposomes containing a self-quenched fluorescent dye, 6-carboxy-fluorescein, TSH could cause a dose-dependent release of 6-carboxyfluorescein that was not duplicated by hCG (Kohn and Shifrin, 1982; Kohn *et al.*, 1982a). This last result was obtained despite the observation that hCG could bind better to the liposomes reconstituted with the solubilized membrane glycoprotein component of the TSH receptor than to the intact thyroid cell or membrane. This observation indicated that the glycoprotein membrane component did exhibit a TSH interaction that resulted in a specific perturbation of the membrane bilayer structure and exhibited properties that could not be duplicated even by a structurally similar hormone, hCG, able to bind to the receptor when it was placed in a less restrictive *in vitro* environment.

In sum, the binding data supported the view that one TSH binding site was a membrane glycoprotein and that this glycoprotein exhibited properties of high-affinity and salt-insensitive TSH binding, that it exhibited properties of appropriate specificity in reconstituted liposomes, that it was a component of the physiologic TSH receptor since function was lost when its TSH binding properties were lost, but that it did not itself have biologic function with respect to catalytic adenylate cyclase activity.

C. Evidence for a Ganglioside Component of the Thyrotropin Receptor

As noted previously, studies of TSH binding to thyroid membranes in low-salt buffers identified a possible low-affinity membrane binding component. Studies of the properties of the glycoprotein component of the TSH receptor indicated that sialic acid might be a receptor determinant (Tate *et al.*, 1975a,b, 1976; Winand and Kohn, 1975b), i.e., the binding activity of the solubilized fragment was found to be sensitive to neuraminidase. With this result in mind and the evidence that the ganglioside G_{M1} was the receptor for cholera toxin (Bennett and Cuatrecasas, 1977; Holmgren, 1978), the idea that a ganglioside could also be a TSH receptor component was considered (Kohn, 1978). Accordingly, a variety of these gangliosides were evaluated for their effects on TSH binding to bovine thyroid receptors.

The gangliosides G_{D1b} and G_{T1} were found to be inhibitors of TSH binding to its specific membrane receptor by comparison to G_{M1} and G_{D1a}. This inhibition was caused by an interaction of these gangliosides with the hormone rather than the membrane, and the inhibition was hormone specific (Mullin *et al.*, 1976a,b; Kohn, 1978). Gangliosides could be reconstituted in liposomes and could both bind TSH and respond to TSH with the release of 6-carboxyfluorescein in a manner not significantly different from liposomes containing the glycoprotein component of the TSH receptor (Kohn, 1978; Kohn and Shifrin, 1982; Kohn *et al.*, 1981, 1982a). Thyroid plasma membranes contained gangliosides with the chromatographic characteristics of G_{D1b} and G_{T1}, but also had a higher order ganglioside which (1) was an even more potent inhibitor of TSH binding, and (2) did not appear to be present in the brain (Mullin *et al.*, 1978; Kohn, 1978). A TSH receptor defect in a rat thyroid tumor was correlated with an alteration in ganglioside biosynthesis and, as a result, in the loss of higher order gangliosides in the membrane (Meldolesi *et al.*, 1976; Kohn, 1978). Resynthesis or reconstitution of gangliosides in membranes from this rat tumor caused a return in both TSH binding and an effect on adenylate cyclase stimulation (Laccetti *et al.*, 1983, 1984) (see Table IV and associated text for further details).

D. A RECEPTOR MODEL

In sum, the binding studies identified a membrane ganglioside as well as a membrane glycoprotein as potentially important components in the cell surface recognition event (Fig. 2). Studies of the *in vitro* properties of [125I]TSH binding to each led to the following ideas concerning the process of recognition and the mechanism by which the hormone–receptor interaction induced a functional response in the cell (Kohn, 1978; Kohn and Shifrin, 1982; Kohn *et al.*, 1981, 1982a,b, 1983a,b, 1984a,b).

TSH binding to the glycoprotein component of the membrane was proposed to be the initial high-affinity recognition event on the cell surface, i.e., the necessary first step in receptor recognition; however, a full functional response was postulated to require the ganglioside.

The ganglioside was suggested to contribute to the following receptor functions. It completed specificity by helping to distinguish among glycoprotein hormones and related ligands such as tetanus toxin, cholera toxin, and interferon (see Section IV,A). It modulated the apparent affinity and capacity of the glycoprotein receptor component and induced a conformational change in the hormone believed necessary for subsequent message transmission. It allowed the ligand to perturb the phospholipid bilayer through alterations in lipid order and contributed to the ability of TSH to alter the ion flux across the membrane. Finally, the model proposed that, after the glycoprotein receptor component trapped the TSH, much as a sperm on the

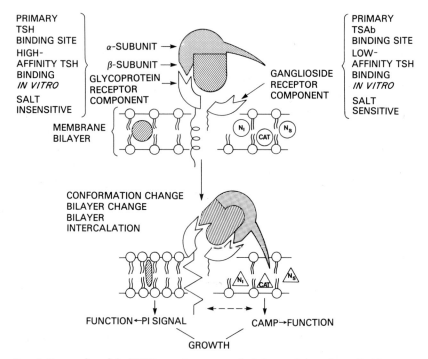

FIG. 2. Proposed model of TSH receptor composed of glycoprotein and ganglioside component. After the TSH β subunit interacts with the receptor, the hormone changes its conformation and the α subunit is brought into the bilayer where it interacts with other membrane components. The β subunit of TSH is presumed to carry the primary determinants recognized by the glycoprotein receptor component, but in no way does the model exclude an α subunit contribution, either direct or by conformational perturbations of β. The end result includes changes in the organization of the membrane bilayer, changes in transmembrane electrochemical ion gradients, changes in lipid turnover and cAMP levels, the expression of other receptors, the initiation of growth, and the expression of differentiated functions. The data to be summarized will suggest that the TSH and TSAb signal to the adenylate cyclase complex (N_S, N_I, Cat) is via the ganglioside; the glycoprotein component appears more directly linked to the phospholipid signal system.

surface of the ovum, the ganglioside acted as an emulsifying agent to allow the hormone to interact with other membrane components within the hydrophobic environment of the lipid bilayer and thereby to initiate the signal processes. The physical basis of the emulsification process was the formation of the anhydrous complex between the hormone and the oligosaccharide moiety of the ganglioside. By excluding water from the interface of the ligand–receptor complex, membrane penetration was facilitated, and interactions involving membrane components of the adenylate cyclase ensued.

IV. TSH RECEPTOR STRUCTURE

A. Monoclonal Antibodies Confirm the Two-Component Model and Relate Components to Autoantibodies in the Sera of Graves' Patients

In order to see whether these hypotheses derived from *in vitro* experiments were true for an *in vivo* system, a monoclonal antibody approach was evolved (Yavin *et al.*, 1981b,c; Valente *et al.*, 1982a,b; Kohn *et al.*, 1983a,b, 1984a,b), i.e., the aims were to identify monoclonal antibodies to the TSH receptor by assays of TSH receptor function, to relate these to specific membrane molecules, i.e., the ganglioside or glycoprotein receptor components, and then to further define their functional roles. The first step avoided a preconceived model wherein purified receptor components were injected, but rather involved the injection of crude solubilized thyroid membrane preparations into mice followed by spleen cell fusion with non-IgG-producing mouse myeloma cells, production of hybridomas secreting antibodies to the intact mouse preparation, functional identification of antibodies related to the TSH receptor structure, and, finally, characterization of the antigenic determinants of the antibodies with particular respect to the already identified TSH binding components.

The second step encompassed attempts to directly relate TSH receptor structure to the autoantibodies in Graves' sera since, as noted previously, this autoimmune disease had been linked to the possible presence in sera of antibodies directed against the TSH receptor. Since each antibody could be presumed to be the product of a specific clone of B-cells present in these patients, this approach involved the following steps: fusion of lymphocytes from patients with active Graves' disease with a non-IgG-secreting mouse myeloma cell line, identification of heterohybridomas that secreted antibodies capable of stimulating thyroid function or blocking TSH binding, and characterization of the antigenic determinants of these antibodies with respect to the structural or functional components of the TSH receptor identified by the monoclonal antibodies derived from the first approach or postulated in the receptor model.

A two-stage screening procedure with thyroid membranes was utilized. In the first stage, hybridomas producing antibodies reactive with thyroid membranes were identified by using ^{125}I-labeled staphylococcal protein A or a ^{125}I-labeled rabbit anti-mouse or anti-human IgG $(Fab')_2$ fragment-specific antibody. In the second stage, the assay was repeated as a competition assay by adding 1 μm TSH during the initial incubation of membranes and hybridoma medium. Hybridoma antibodies reactive with thyroid membranes in the first screening assay but blocked by unlabeled TSH in the second were chosen as potential TSH receptor antibodies.

Having identified potential anti-TSH receptor-producing clones, they were appropriately subcloned to ensure their monoclonal nature and were identified as monoclonal antibodies to the TSH receptor by the following criteria. (1) The antibody had to inhibit TSH binding to thyroid membranes or, conversely, be itself prevented from binding to thyroid membranes by TSH. (2) Inhibition had to be reasonably *specific* and had to be *competitive* as opposed to noncompetitive or uncompetitive. (3) The antibody had to competitively inhibit TSH-stimulated thyroid functions, i.e., adenylate cyclase activity, iodide uptake, or thyroid hormone release, or, conversely, had to mimic TSH activity and exhibit properties of competitive agonism.

Thus far, after over 15 fusions using both approaches and with the identification of over 30 antibodies satisfying the criteria above, all antibodies can be broadly grouped into three classes. The first group, originally termed "inhibitor" antibodies because their properties resembled autoantibodies in Graves' sera, which could inhibit TSH binding, exhibited the following properties: competitive inhibition of [^{125}I]TSH binding, competitive inhibition of TSH-stimulated adenylate cyclase activity, inhibition of TSH-stimulable thyroidal iodine release or uptake, and no direct stimulation of thyroid adenylate cyclase activity, T_3/T_4 release, or iodide uptake. No antibody could be reactive with TSH, i.e., they were not simply anti-TSH antibodies.

The second group was termed "stimulators" since they mimicked the activity of stimulating TSABs in Graves' patients by exhibiting the following characteristics: direct, TSH-like, stimulatory action with respect to adenylate cyclase activity as well as iodide uptake and T_3/T_4 release by the thyroid; competitive agonism when included with low concentrations of TSH in assays measuring adenylate cyclase activity; and significantly weaker inhibition of [^{125}I]TSH binding than the first group, despite equally potent competitive inhibition of TSH-stimulable adenylate cyclase activity. A third group, termed "mixed" antibodies, had all of the stimulatory properties of a stimulatory antibody (TSAb) but also had the ability to inhibit [^{125}I]TSH binding to a significant degree. The significance of the existence of antibodies with "mixed" properties will be discussed with respect to the organization of receptor components, their active site determinants, and signal transmission phenomena. Representative antibodies of each group, which are discussed in this report, and their categorization, as above, are summarized in Table I.

The antibodies in the "inhibitory" group mentioned previously were able to significantly block TSH binding to human, bovine, or rat thyroid membranes or cells (Yavin et al., 1981c; Valente et al., 1982a,b; Kohn et al., 1983a,b, 1984a,b) and to liposomes embedded with the glycoprotein component of the thyroid membranes with TSH binding activity (Table II). Inhibi-

TABLE I
REPRESENTATIVE MONOCLONAL ANTIBODIES TO THE TSH RECEPTOR

Clone number	TSH receptor source	"Activity" pattern
13D11	Bovine	Inhibitor
11E8	Bovine	Inhibitor
59C9	Human	Inhibitor
60F5	Human	Inhibitor
129H8[a]	Human	Inhibitor
122G3[a]	Human	Inhibitor
22A6	Bovine	Stimulator
206H3[a]	Human	Stimulator
307H6[a]	Human	Stimulator
52A8	Human	Mixed
208F7[a]	Human	Mixed

[a] Heterohybridomas.

tion was evident whether tested in preincubation, competition, or displacement assays, i.e., independent of the order of addition of TSH or antibody. Inhibition was competitive with respect to TSH whether measured using [^{125}I]TSH and unlabeled antibody or unlabeled TSH and unlabeled antibody, binding of antibody being measured with ^{125}I-labeled protein A. Since inhibition could be detected under all the *in vitro* conditions used to measure TSH binding, it seemed evident that arguments concerning the condition-dependent measurement of this receptor component were, in retrospect, misplaced.

Using cultured thyroid cells, the antibodies noted as inhibitors in Table I were all unable to mimic TSH as direct stimulators of adenylate cyclase activity, iodide uptake, or thyroid hormone release in a mouse bioassay (Table III, Fig. 3). They were, however, able to inhibit TSH-stimulated adenylate cyclase activity (Table III, Fig. 3), and inhibition in each case was competitive (Fig. 3). The antibodies also inhibited TSH-stimulated radioiodine uptake in thyroid cells (Table III) and TSH-stimulated T_3/T_4 release in a mouse bioassay used to measure *in vivo* TSH activity (Table III).

Stimulating monoclonals were able to enhance either human or rat thyroid cell adenylate cyclase activity (Table III, Fig. 3). They could also be potent inhibitors of TSH-stimulated adenylate cyclase activity (Table III) despite the fact that they were weak inhibitors of TSH binding. This apparent contradiction was resolved with the observation that their inhibitory action with respect to TSH was dependent on the TSH concentration (Fig. 3). Thus, at low TSH levels, 22A6, 206H3, and 307H6 were more than additive competitive agonists, and at high TSH concentrations they were competitive

TABLE II

Ability of Antibodies to Prevent [125I]TSH Binding to Liposomes Containing the Glycoprotein Component of TSH Receptor[a] or to React with Various Ganglioside Preparations[b]

| Antibody | [125I]TSH bound (cpm) Glycoprotein component | | | Ganglioside reactivity measured as [125I]protein A or [125I]antihuman (Fab)$_2$ binding to antibody ganglioside complexes in a solid phase assay (cpm) | | | |
	Bovine	Human	Rat	No added lipid	Human thyroid ganglioside	Rat thyroid ganglioside	Mixed brain ganglioside
Controls							
Monoclonal control	18,200	14,800	29,200	150	160	155	155
N1 mouse IgG	17,940	14,700	29,500	128	185	125	135
N1 human IgG	18,400	14,800	31,200	149	144	160	145
Inhibitors							
13D11	4,100	3,800	5,400	141	235	175	215
11E8	2,100	400	2,050	156	206	210	204
59C9	6,200	1,200	5,900	121	195	195	198
60F5	4,100	1,050	4,200	110	210	210	200
129H8	1,400	980	2,800	101	285	256	170
122G3	6,400	4,200	9,200	146	268	235	155
Stimulators							
22A6	14,800	13,600	26,800	137	870	982	410
206H3	15,500	12,200	24,500	156	2889	1210	128
307H6	16,200	12,800	26,400	129	4210	2450	240
Mixed							
52A8	9,800	5,400	15,300	135	1480	1210	205
208F7	12,400	6,100	14,400	136	920	1140	180

[a] Dipalmitoylphosphatidylcholine/cholesterol liposomes containing the glycoprotein portion of the TSH receptor were prepared as described (Aloj *et al.*, 1979b). Liposomes were mixed with [125I]TSH (50,000 cpm/50 μl) in Tris-acetate, 20 mM, pH 7.0. Liposomes were incubated at the noted temperatures for 1 hour. The reaction mixture was then filtered through EHWP-02500 Millipore filters, and liposome-bound [125I]TSH (that trapped on the filter after washing with the incubation buffer) was counted. Control IgG or monoclonal IgG was added concomitantly with the [125I]TSH. Values are ±5% and are the average result of triplicate incubations. Analogous data were obtained in 20 mM Tris-chloride, pH 7.4, containing 50 mM NaCl (Kohn *et al.*, 1984a,b) except that total binding values were lower. The monoclonal antibody control is one that interacted with thyroid membranes equally well in the presence or absence of TSH and was known not to perturb TSH binding to membranes.

[b] See Laccetti *et al.* (1983, 1984) for assay details.

antagonists. The antibodies were active in the mouse bioassay measuring thyroid hormone release and were able to enhance iodide uptake by thyroid cells in a manner similar to TSH (Table III), i.e., under conditions where cAMP-dependent iodide uptake was the measured response.

In a solid phase assay, the stimulating antibodies were all able to interact with ganglioside preparations of thyroid membranes (Table II) but only interacted minimally with bovine brain ganglioside preparations. It was notable that 22A6, an antibody made using bovine thyroid membranes as the antigen, was both a stimulator of bovine thyroid adenylate cyclase activity and reactive with bovine thyroid gangliosides. In contrast, 307H6, a heterohybridoma human stimulator, exhibited human specificity in both reactions. This would suggest that the phenomenon of TSAb species specificity defined in the concept of LATS vs. LATS protector (Adams, 1981) rests in structural differences in gangliosides from species to species.

The evidence that inhibitor and stimulator monoclonal antibodies were directed at distinct biochemical determinants of the membrane, which, nevertheless, functionally acted together, was supported by observations involving reconstitution experiments and mixing experiments.

As noted previously, an important study implicating that higher order gangliosides were a potential component of the thyrotropin receptor involved the recognition that membrane preparations from the 1-8 rat thyroid tumor with a TSH receptor defect were coincidentally devoid of higher order gangliosides (Meldolesi *et al.*, 1976). The TSH receptor defect was expressed as low TSH binding and no TSH-stimulated adenylate cyclase activity despite normal thyroid functional responses to prostaglandins or dibutyryl cAMP (Meldolesi *et al.*, 1976). The original 1-8 tumor also had no cholera toxin–stimulated adenylate cyclase response despite the ability of forskolin to activate adenylate cyclase activity (Table IV). Incubation of cultured cells from the 1-8 thyroid tumor with a ganglioside extract derived either from a line of functioning rat FRTL-5 thyroid cells or from human membrane preparations resulted in return to TSH, TSAb, and cholera toxin–stimulated adenylate cyclase activity (Table IV). No reconstitution of TSH receptor function occurred in control incubations containing no ganglioside extract, a ganglioside extract from the original 1-8 tumor (G_{M3}), mixed brain gangliosides, or the human or FRTL-5 ganglioside extracts treated with a mixture of neuraminidases capable of converting 85 to 94% of the sialic acid residues from a lipid-bound to free form. Incorporation of the gangliosides from the human or from FRTL-5 thyroid cell preparations into the 1-8 original tumor cells was monitored by reactivity with the 22A6 or 307H6 stimulating monoclonal antireceptor antibodies. Thus, for example, as measured by [125I]protein A, 22A6-binding to the no addition cells, to cells incubated with neuraminidase-treated FRTL-5 gangliosides, or to cells

TABLE III

Ability of Monoclonal Antibodies to Stimulate Adenylate[c] Cyclase Activity in Human Thyroid Cells, to Increase cAMP-Mediated Iodide Uptake in Rat FRTL-5 Thyroid Cells, or Release T_3T_4 into the Bloodstream as Measured by a Mouse Bioassay

Antibody added (0.1 mg/ml)	Adenylate cyclase activity[a] (cAMP level, pmoles/μg DNA)		Iodide uptake in rat FRTL-5 thyroid cells[b] (^{125}I cpm)		Mouse blood ^{125}I[c] (% of control)	
	Direct effect on human thyroid cells	Effect on 2.5×10^{-10} M TSH activity	Alone	+TSH 2.5×10^{-10} M	Alone	+TSH
Controls						
No addition	1.2 ± 0.2	8.8	680	7700	130	480
Normal human IgG	0.8 ± 0.2	8.8	700	8100	120	480
Normal mouse IgG	0.8 ± 0.2	8.8	820	7900	118	520
Monoclonal control	0.8 ± 0.2	7.4	540	8100	121	450
Inhibitors						
13D11	0.8 ± 0.2	3.8	700	2450	112	170
11E8	0.8 ± 0.2	3.3	650	1410	124	180
59C9	0.8 ± 0.2	4.1	730	2200	110	200
60F5	0.8 ± 0.2	3.4	810	1100	104	188
129H8	0.8 ± 0.2	3.9	740	1500	123	210
122G3	0.8 ± 0.2	2.5	920	2980	110	230

Stimulators					
22A6	3.0 ± 0.2	3.1	6840	600	—
206H3	1.5 ± 0.2	2.9	8200	440	—
307H6	3.4 ± 0.2	2.8	7400	510	—
Mixed					
52A8	2.8 ± 0.2	4.2	7800	340	—
208F7	1.8 ± 0.2	2.7	9400	520	—

[a] Human thyroid cell primary cultures were tested for the ability of bovine TSH and monoclonal antibodies to affect adenylate cyclase activity in 0.2 ml of Krebs Ringer Bicarbonate (KRB) buffer, pH 7.4, containing glucose (1.0 g/liter), bovine serum albumin (3.0 g/liter), and 3-isobutyl-1-methylxanthine (IMX) (0.6 mM). Direct stimulatory activity was measured at 37°C in a 10% CO_2 environment for 120 minutes. Ability of monoclonal antibodies to inhibit TSH responsiveness was tested by incubating cells for 30 minutes with TSH, in the same conditions as previously, but after a 120-minute preincubation in KRB buffer with the different monoclonal antibodies. Incubations were stopped by adding 0.2 ml of cold absolute ethanol and the plate was stored at −20°C overnight. Thawed broken cells were detached by means of a rubber policeman, the suspension was centrifuged at 2000 × g at 4°C, and aliquots were tested in cAMP radioimmunoassay.

[b] FRTL-5 rat cells are normally grown in medium containing TSH; cells are viable when TSH is removed for as long as 10 days, although cell growth stops. Five-day TSH-depleted FRTL-5 cells were given TSH or antibody at the noted concentration for 60 hours, after which 75,000 cpm ^{125}I-labeled sodium iodide was added. After 40 minutes, cells were washed, recovered, and the cell-associated iodide was measured in the presence or absence of an ionophore (FCCP) that releases free but not bound or organified iodide. The difference is the free iodide uptake values presented previously. Assays are in duplicate; standard errors are < ±5%.

[c] The mice were prepared with radioiodine by a standard procedure. In all experiments, 0.1 ml of material was injected into each of six mice. The means are reported; SEM was ±16%. Stimulatory activity is measured at 2 hours after injection. Antibody (0.2 mg/ml) and TSH (1 milliunit/ml) were mixed and injected together; assays were at 2 hours. Assays at different protein concentrations did reveal a dose–response for inhibition (+ inhibitors) in all cases (over the range 0.01 through 0.3 mg/ml). Similarly, stimulators also exhibited dose-related stimulation over the same range. Inhibitors were not stimulators when tested over the range 0.01 to 0.3 mg/ml.

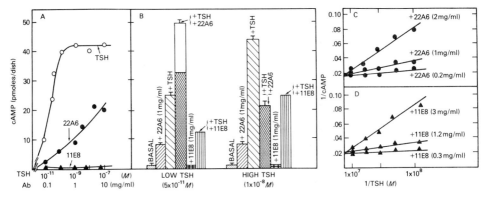

FIG. 3. (A) Effect of monoclonal antibodies on cAMP levels of FRTL-5 functioning rat thyroid cells in continuous culture. Inhibitor antibodies (60F5, 59C9, 13D11, 129H8, or 122G3) had no direct stimulatory action over the concentration range noted as represented by data for the 11E8 antibody (▲). Over the same concentration range, stimulating or mixed antibodies (307H6, 52A8, 208F7, and 206H3) increase adenylate cyclase activity in a concentration-dependent fashion as noted for 22A6 (●). The effect of the ligands on cAMP was measured using a technique similar to that in Valente *et al.* (1983b). Antibody molarity was calculated in this experiment using the total IgG protein content. (B) Effect on cAMP levels of FRTL-5 cells of mixing low or high TSH concentrations with either a stimulatory (22A6) or inhibitory (11E8) antibody. In the case of 11E8, TSH activity is decreased in each case. In the case of 22A6 there is more than additive agonism at low TSH values and an "inhibitory" agonism at high concentrations. Double reciprocal plot of the cAMP stimulatory activity of mixtures of 22A6 and TSH (C) and of 11E8 and TSH (D) at the noted concentrations. In both cases competitive inhibition is evident; the same results were evident for all stimulatory, inhibitory, or mixed monoclonals.

incubated with intact FRTL-5 gangliosides measured 170 ± 50, 180 ± 50 and 610 ± 40 cpm, respectively. A key observation relevant to the existence of distinct biochemical components within the TSH receptor complex evolved when the ganglioside reconstituted cells were treated with trypsin. Thus, 1-8 cells reconstituted with FRTL-5 gangliosides and then exposed to trypsin lost their ability to respond to TSH. It was notable, however, that the TSAb and cholera toxin stimulation activity were significantly less altered by the trypsin treatment (Table IV), i.e., the TSH receptor required both protein and ganglioside components, whereas the TSAb behaved as an autoimmune equivalent of cholera toxin.

Mixing experiments were equally revealing with respect to the existence of separate determinants within the functional TSH receptor complex (Ealey *et al.*, 1984). Thus, in a cytochemical bioassay (CBA), 22A6 and 307H6 were stimulators (Fig. 4) whose dose–response curves paralleled those of a LATS-B standard, a Graves' serum thyroid–stimulating autoantibody (TSAb). The CBA for thyroid stimulators is based upon quantification of changes in the staining of sections of guinea pig thyroids utilizing leucine-2 naphtylamide as a chromogenic substrate to meausre a lysosomel enzyme activity. In contrast to 22A6 or 307H6, 11E8 was inactive as a stimulator in the CBA over a wide dose range. Most important, however, was the observation that, whereas 11E8 inhibited TSH stimulation in the CBA, 11E8 was ineffective when inhibiting the stimulation activity of the thyroid-stimulating antibodies 22A6, 307H6, or LATS-B (Fig. 4). 11E8 had no affect on these TSAbs even at 10,000 fold higher dosage than that used to completely inhibit concentrations. It is intuitive that differences in the effect of 11E8 on TSH as opposed

TABLE IV

RECONSTITUTION OF TSH RECEPTOR EXPRESSION IN 1-8 RAT THYROID TUMORS

Thyroid membrane or cell preparation	Adenylate cyclase activity[a] (pmoles cAMP/μg DNA)			
	Basal	Cholera toxin $1 \times 10^{-9}\ M$	TSH $1 \times 10^{-9}\ M$	307H6 20 μg/ml
FRTL-5 thyroid cell	0.5	6.4	18	5.4
1-8 tumor (original)	0.8	0.4	0.8	0.7
+ FRTL-5 thyroid cell gangliosides	0.7	3.8	5.2	2.6
+ FRTL-5 thyroid cell disialoganglioside[b]	0.6	1.2	9.8	4.6
+ human thyroid gangliosides	0.5	3.9	4.7	3.5
+ NDase-treated FRTL-5 gangliosides	0.7	0.9	0.9	0.8
+ NDase-treated FRTL-5 disialoganglioside	0.8	0.7	1.4	0.9
+ NDase-treated human thyroid gangliosides	0.5	0.7	1.1	0.8
+ mixed brain gangliosides	0.8	3.1	1.1	0.8
+ 1-8 tumor gangliosides	0.5	0.7	0.5	—
+ G_{M3}	0.8	0.7	0.7	0.8
+ FRTL-5 thyroid cell gangliosides followed by trypsin treatment[c]	0.5	4.1	0.9	2.4
+ FRTL-5 thyroid cell disialoganglioside followed by trypsin treatment	0.6	1.1	0.6	3.8

[a] Assays were performed in triplicate; results are the average of at least three separate experiments. In no case did the standard deviation of any value exceed ±10%. Reconstitution procedures were as described by Laccetti *et al.* (1983).

[b] Purified by DEAE chromatography; added at 1/100 the concentration of total FRTL-5 ganglioside pool based on lipid bound sialic acid.

[c] Trypsin treatment of cell preparations used the procedures referred to Tate *et al.* (1975a,b) or Winand and Kohn (1975a).

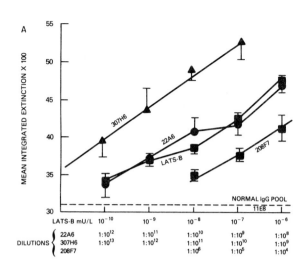

A

MEAN INTEGRATED EXTINCTION X 100

55

50

45

40

35

30

307H6

22A6

LATS-B

208F7

NORMAL IgG POOL

11E8

LATS-B mU/L	10^{-10}	10^{-9}	10^{-8}	10^{-7}	10^{-6}
DILUTIONS 22A6	$1:10^{12}$	$1:10^{11}$	$1:10^{10}$	$1:10^{9}$	$1:10^{8}$
307H6	$1:10^{13}$	$1:10^{12}$	$1:10^{11}$	$1:10^{10}$	$1:10^{9}$
208F7			$1:10^{6}$	$1:10^{5}$	$1:10^{4}$

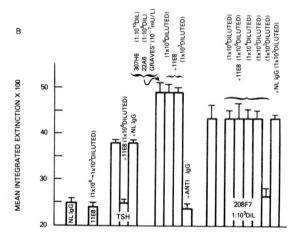

B

MEAN INTEGRATED EXTINCTION X 100

50

40

30

20

307H6 (1:10^{10}DIL)
22A6 (1:10^{8}DIL)
GRAVES' (10^{-7}mU/L)
(1x10^{6}DILUTED)
+11E8 (1x10^{2}DILUTED)

(1x10^{8}DILUTED)
+11E8 (1x10^{6}DILUTED)
(1x10^{4}DILUTED)
(1x10^{3}DILUTED)
(1x10^{2}DILUTED)
+NL IgG (1x10^{2}DILUTED)

NL IgG

11E8 (1x10^{6}→1x10^{2}DILUTED)

+11E8 (1x10^{6}DILUTED)
+NL IgG
TSH

+ANTI IgG

208F7
1:10^{3}DIL

C

TSH receptor

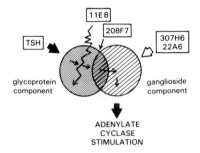

11E8

208F7

307H6
22A6

TSH

glycoprotein
component

ganglioside
component

ADENYLATE
CYCLASE
STIMULATION

to 22A6, 307H6, or LATS-B were not the result of a 10,000-fold difference in binding constants; thus, 307H6 was bioactive in the CBA at protein concentrations greater than tenfold lower than used to measure 11E8 inhibition of TSH binding. This was confirmed directly in binding experiments.

The ability of 11E8 and 22A6, 307H6, or 208F7 to block or stimulate selectively in mixing experiments clearly indicates that these two monoclonals are antibodies to different determinants on the TSH receptor. Since the separate experiments described indicate that the 11E8 monoclonal antibody interacts predominantly with a membrane glycoprotein, whereas the 22A6 and 307H6 monoclonal antibodies interact with a ganglioside (see previous discussion), the simplest way of reconciling the sum of observations is to apply the two-component receptor model suggested in receptor binding studies (Fig. 4). Thus, TSH can be envisaged to interact first with the glycoprotein component of the TSH receptor, which exhibits high-affinity binding properties. Its biological action, however, requires an additional or subsequent interaction with a ganglioside. In contrast, TSAbs represented by 307H6, LATS-B, and 22A6 can be envisaged to bypass the glycoprotein receptor component and interact with the ganglioside to initiate the hormone-like signal. This model would be consistent with the observations that TSH action can be blocked by 11E8, an antibody binding to the glycoprotein receptor component. The three TSAbs, 307H6, LATS-B, and 22A6, are, in contrast, minimally affected by 11E8 since they are directed at the next sequential step, the ganglioside, which is vital in ligand message transmission.

The existence of "mixed" antibodies, 208F7 and 52A8 for example, are revealing in their dual properties, that is, in their ability to be both a potent inhibitor of TSH binding and a potent stimulator of adenylate cyclase activity. These antibodies react with both the glycoprotein receptor compo-

---

FIG. 4. (A) Responses to increasing doses of monoclonal 22A6, 307H6, 208F7, and LATS-B reference preparation in the cytochemical bioassay for thyroid stimulators by comparison to 11E8 and normal IgG. The 12-μm sections of guinea pig thyroid tissue were exposed to the stimulators and to the controls, normal IgG or 11E8, for 3 minutes. The results are the mean values of mean integrated extinction obtained from triplicate sections, $\pm$SD. (B) 11E8 at a 10^6 dilution inhibits a maximal TSH response but even at 10^2 dilutions does not inhibit 22A6, 307H6, or LATS-B and just does inhibit 208F7. Increasing concentrations of 11E8 were added ($1:10^6$ dilution to $1:10^2$ dilution) together with optimal amounts of 22A6, 307H6, LATS-B, or 208F7. NIIgG (negative control IgG from euthyroid pooler sera) was added at 0.1 mg/ml. Mean integrated extinction was determined for duplicate sections. (C) Hypothetical model of TSH receptor as suggested by studies with monoclonal antibodies to the TSH receptor. TSH interacts with glycoprotein component but requires ganglioside to function. TSAb (307H6, 22A6) bypasses glycoprotein component to interact with ganglioside directly. The mixed antibody reacts with determinants common to both receptor components.

nent and the ganglioside (Table II), yet, like 307H6, 22A6, or LATS-B, are relatively insensitive to 11E8 in CBA mixing experiments (Fig. 4), requiring 10,000 fold higher 11E8 concentrations to inhibit by comparison to TSH. These results suggest that mixed antibodies are directed against a unique set of receptor determinants different from 11E8 or 307H6 yet common to both (see later for further evidence). The best explanation is that these are common carbohydrate determinants on the glycoprotein and ganglioside or that the true "physiologic TSH receptor" exists as a functional complex of ganglioside and glycoprotein.

If the TSH receptor does exist as a complex of the two glycoconjugates, a model of a receptor complex of both components in equilibrium with free ganglioside or glycoprotein is an intuitive extrapolation since each has different biosynthetic and biodegradation pathways (Fig. 5). Further, the gangliosides can be viewed as a group or series of similar structures with greater or lesser affinities for a particular ligand, but each with the potential for interacting with a glycoprotein—including the TSH receptor glycoprotein. The implications of such a model are far reaching.

The TSH receptor has been related to receptor structures for cholera toxin, tetanus toxin, and interferon (Kohn, 1978). Thus, each of these ligands has been associated with a receptor structure involving gangliosides, albeit structures with different ganglioside specificities. Cholera toxin interacts with G_{M1}, and, like the TSAb, bypasses any functional need for the glycoprotein receptor component despite the existence of glycoproteins capable of binding the cholera toxin (Grollman *et al.*, 1978b). Similarly, interferon appears to interact with a glycoprotein and ganglioside receptor structure. All three, TSH, cholera, and interferon, can influence the binding and bioactivity of the others (Kohn, 1978; Grollman *et al.*, 1978b). Thus, cholera can first enhance TSH binding, then inhibit it. Similarly, interferon can enhance and then inhibit cholera toxin binding and inhibit TSH binding. That these phenomena result in interactions involving the molecular components of the different receptors is illustrated by the fact that the cholera toxin interaction with its receptor, G_{M1}, resulted in enhanced surface exposure of higher order gangliosides between the G_{M1} and G_{D1b} areas (Mullin *et al.*, 1976b; Kohn, 1978). This same region of the chromatogram contains a unique thyroidal ganglioside with the highest affinity to TSH, as measured in binding as well as functional studies (see the following).

A possible simple explanation for these phenomena resides in the equilibrium model of Fig. 5, top. Thus, cholera toxin at low concentrations (Fig. 5, bottom) interacts with G_{M1} and favors the interaction of the more relevant TSH receptor ganglioside with the TSH receptor glycoprotein, since the competing free ganglioside pool is smaller and its affinity is best. The result is enhanced TSH bioactivity. At high concentrations, cholera toxin would

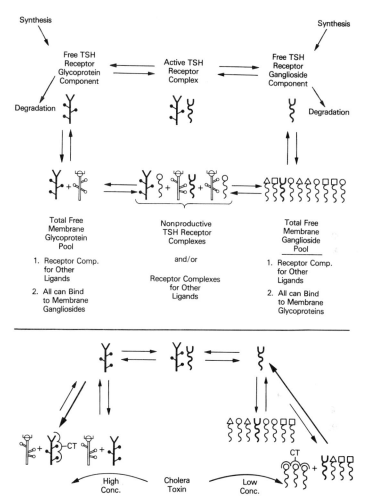

FIG. 5. (Top) Hypothetical model of active TSH receptor complex in equilibrium with its free component parts, which are in turn in equilibrium with other glycoproteins and gangliosides of the membrane. It is presumed that the complex of both units exists since mixed antibodies exist, i.e., these are presumed to be directed against the complex of both components. The possibility that TSH induces the complex to form, is not, however, excluded. (Bottom) The presumptive action of cholera toxin in this equilibrium system. These interactions could account for data concerned with the effect of cholera toxin on TSH binding and function (in the absence of exogenous NAD) when cholera toxin (CT) is added to membrane systems. This is not a unique model, but is based on reasonable presumptions from the current available data.

also interact with the TSH receptor glycoprotein and decrease its availability for forming the active TSH receptor complex, thereby inhibiting TSH bioactivity. This model could, in part, account for the complex of binding and stimulatory phenomena in experiments where TSH and cholera toxin are mixed (Mullin *et al.*, 1976b; Field *et al.*, 1979; Zakarija *et al.*, 1980).

In sum, the monoclonal data would appear to confirm the two-component receptor model envisaged from *in vitro* binding experiments and to show that the autoantibodies in Graves' sera are related to different components of the TSH receptor. An important clinical implication of the data is as follows. If a Graves' patient has both an "inhibiting" and stimulating antibody present in his or her serum, the phenotypic expression will be a hyperthyroid state. This is evident since the inhibitor antibody will not inhibit TSAb activity, but only TSH activity (Ealey *et al.*, 1984).

B. STRUCTURE OF THE GLYCOPROTEIN RECEPTOR COMPONENT

Immune precipitation of detergent-solubilized thyroid membrane preparations by monoclonal antibodies 11E8 or 13D11 indicate that there are two subunits involved in the TSH receptor, one of ~18–25K and one of ~50–60K (Fig. 6A).

Cross-linking studies to cells and membranes (Kohn *et al.*, 1983a) suggest

---

FIG. 6. Structure of glycoprotein component of TSH receptor. (A) Immunoprecipitation of detergent-solubilized radiolabeled bovine thyroid membrane preparation by 11E8 antibody is blocked by simultaneous presence of TSH (1×10^{-7} M), but not by similar concentration of albumin, insulin, glucagon, ACTH, normal IgG, hCG, LH, or FSH (not shown). Two major proteins are precipitated. The minor protein between 26 and 43K may be the 23K protein plus bound phospholipid since it disappears from phospholipase C–treated membranes. (B, C) Cross-linking of TSH to membranes in more physiologic conditions results in three major components plus material on top of gel. Cross-linking is specifically blocked by 11E8, 13D11, or TSH. See Kohn *et al.* (1983a) for procedural details. Cross-linking at pH 6.0 and low sites yields only one major band, which is again not present if TSH or 11E8 is present in the incubation. (Bottom) A model taking into account the above observations and data from earlier solubilization studies (Tate *et al.*, 1975a,b, 1976). This receptor component is proposed to have two subunits of approximately 20–25K and approximately 50–60K. At 37°, pH 7.4, and 50mM NaCl, the two receptor subunits exist cross-linked to one (~80K) or two TSH subunits (~95K) or exist as multimers in the image of the IgG heavy and light chain molecule cross-linked to one or more TSH subunits (~200K). Trypsin is suggested to split off a TSH binding fragment from the glycoprotein receptor component (Winand and Kohn, 1975b), which at this time is suggested to come only from the ~20–25K unit. The possibility that such a fragment comes from both subunits is not excluded nor is the idea that the binding site requires determinants from both subunits.

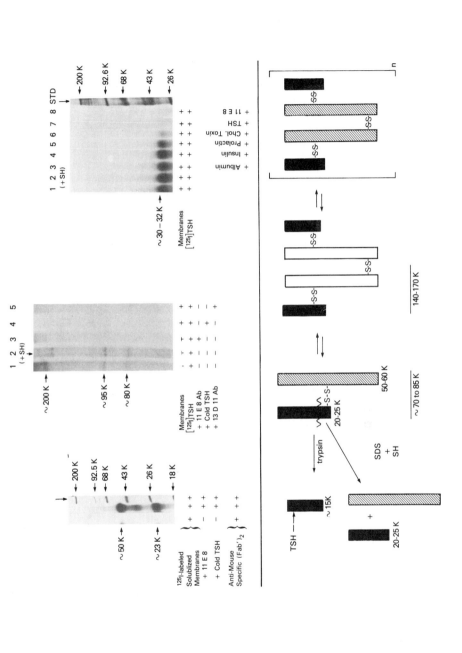

A. IMMUNOPRECIPITATION

B. CROSS-LINK pH 7.4 + SALT

C. CROSS-LINK pH 6.0, low SALT

that, at pH 7.4 at 37°C and in 50 mM or isotonic salt concentrations, the receptor exists as a complex of the two subunits with an approximate molecular weight of 80–90K or as a tetrameric structure of ~160–180K (Fig. 6B). The variability in specific numbers derives from the different receptor preparations used (i.e., membranes or cells from human, rat, porcine, etc.), from possible different levels of proteolysis in the preparations, from questions as to the number of TSH subunits cross-linked, and from the accuracy of numbers derived from gel electrophoresis data alone. Solubilization studies using nonreducing detergent systems or lithium diiodosalicylate indicate that the receptor can exist as a 300K, an ~175–200K, and an ~90K complex (Tate *et al.*, 1975a,b, 1976; Islam *et al.*, 1983) with disulfide bonding between the subunits (Tate *et al.*, 1975a,b, 1976; Ozawa *et al.*, 1979a; Ginsberg *et al.*, 1982; Islam *et al.*, 1983). The sum of these data would therefore indicate that the glycoprotein component of the TSH receptor is in the image of an immunoglobulin with heavy and light chains (Fig. 6, bottom), which can exist in a tetrameric (4-subunit) form or even as a higher multimer (8-subunit octamer) as well as in component monomers.

It is notable that, at pH 6.0 and 0–4°C in a low-salt milieu, where binding is very high with respect to capacity or percent (see previous discussion of added [^{125}I]TSH bound per milligram of protein, the predominant TSH receptor complex present in cross-linking studies (Kohn *et al.*, 1983a) is ~30–35K (Fig. 6C). This complex is believed to represent the ~18–25K receptor subunit plus one subunit of the TSH molecule. Consistent with this view is the observation that TSH binding under these conditions is associated with the disappearance of an ~18–25K protein present in [^{35}S]methionine-labeled solubilized thyroid membrane preparations. This 18–25K subunit appears to be related to the ~15K fragment of the TSH receptor purified after tryptic digestion of solubilized membrane preparations (Tate *et al.*, 1975a,b, 1976). Thus, the trypsin-produced fragment is also reactive with TSH and 11E8 on affinity columns in studies using [^{35}S]methioine-labeled membrane preparations. These results would indicate that the predominant TSH binding determinants may reside in the lower-molecular-weight subunit and that there is a trypsin-sensitive site in this subunit that can release the ~15K fragment without need for disulfide reduction (Fig. 6, bottom). The possibility that trypsin also releases a fragment with TSH binding properties from the ~50–60K subunit is, however, not unequivocally excluded.

In early studies, immobilized ConA was shown to remove TSH binding activity from soluble thyroid membrane preparations (Tate *et al.*, 1975a,b). Subsequent studies have shown that ConA can interact with thyroid membranes to increase the affinity of the glycoprotein receptor component for TSH (Kohn and Shifrin, 1982; Yavin *et al.*, 1981b,c). The probability thus exists that there is a ConA binding site on the glycoprotein component of the

TSH receptor as it exists *in situ* and that it is not involved in the TSH binding site. The possibility that this site is on the ~18–25K receptor subunit has been raised in the cross-linking studies (Kohn *et al.*, 1983a).

The glycoprotein receptor component may contain a site that recognizes immunoglobulin-reactive agents. Thus, protein A, which reacts with Fc sites on IgG molecules, can precipitate the receptor and can inhibit TSH binding. Given the structural analogy of the receptor to the heavy–light chain model of an IgG and the concept that IgGs themselves are "receptors" on lymphocytes, these data could have evolutionary as well as functional significance.

Finally, there is probably an acidic phospholipid attachment site to the glycoprotein receptor component. Thus phosphatidylinositol can prevent reconstitution of TSH receptor into liposomes by perturbing the activity of the glycoprotein component (Aloj *et al.*, 1979b). The effect on the latter is exerted in two ways: (1) by decreasing its incorporation into the lipid matrix, and (2) by inhibiting the binding activity of that fraction of glycoprotein that is incorporated. Phosphatidylinositol has no effect on the incorporation and the expression of receptor properties of gangliosides into liposomes as measured by TSH binding activity using reconstituted ganglioside–liposomes.

C. Structure of the Ganglioside Receptor Component

As noted previously, the reactivity with the ganglioside preparations is relatively thyroid-specific when using total ganglioside extracts, i.e., when comparing brain and thyroid ganglioside preparations (Table II). This is confirmed in experiments wherein thyroid gangliosides are shown to be better (>100 fold) than mixed brain gangliosides as inhibitors of the adenylate cyclase stimulatory activity of a monoclonal TSAb (307H6) or of a Graves' serum autoantibody TSAb preparation.

The ability of the monoclonal stimulating receptor antibodies to react with ganglioside preparations (Table II) is lost if the glycolipid preparation is pretreated with neuraminidase (Table V) and is highest in disialoganglioside fractions obtained by column chromatographic techniques (Laccetti *et al.*, 1984). The highest reactivity is, however, evident with a single minor component of the disialoganglioside preparation whether eluted from thin layer plates and tested in solid phase assays (Fig. 7) or evaluated by direct autoradiography (Fig. 7).

These observations are consistent with an earlier study showing that the ganglioside with the greatest ability to inhibit TSH binding to thyroid membranes was 0.015% of the total thyroid ganglioside pool and was not evident in brain ganglioside preparations (Mullin *et al.*, 1978). In that study, cholera vibrio neuraminidase treatment of the thyroidal ganglioside eliminated only

TABLE V

ABILITY OF MONOCLONAL TSH RECEPTOR–STIMULATING ANTIBODIES TO REACT
WITH MODIFIED OR PARTIALLY PURIFIED THYROID GANGLIOSIDE PREPARATIONS

Ganglioside preparation	Ganglioside reactivity (cpm)[a]			
	22A6	307H6	52A8	Graves' IgG[b]
Control human thyroid gangliosides	930	3,955	1,525	2,810
+ neuraminidase treatment	210	410	310	195
Control rat thyroid gangliosides	884	2,290	1,190	3,100
+ neuraminidase treatment	195	290	206	301
Human neutral glycolipid[c]	—	800	—	1,100
Monosialogangliosides[c]	—	2,000	—	2,100
Disialogangliosides[c]	—	10,700	—	14,000

[a] Assayed per Laccetti *et al.* (1983, 1984) using a solid phase technique.

[b] Graves' IgG from a patient with high stimulating activity obtained from A. Pinchera, University of Pisa. This is a total IgG preparation with many potential individual antibodies including some that can inhibit TSH binding.

[c] Prepared by DEAE chromatography as described by Mullin *et al.* (1978).

a portion of the sialic acid from this ganglioside, suggesting that the disialoganglioside had one neuraminidase-sensitive and one insensitive sialic moiety. If the original inhibition studies (Mullin *et al.*, 1976a; Kohn, 1978) involving TSH and gangliosides have meaning as evidence of cross reactivity at very high brain ganglioside concentrations, it can be presumed that the sialic residues have a G_{D1b} configuration rather than a G_{D1a} configuration, i.e., both residues on the internal galactose moiety.

FIG. 7. (Left) Thin layer chromatograph of purified fractions, i.e., neutral glycolipids, monosialoglycolipids, and disialoglycolipids, by comparison to the total human ganglioside starting preparation. Standards are in the first column; chromatography and purification was per Mullin *et al.* (1978). (Center) Reactivity of 307H6 with individual gangliosides scraped from the thin layer chromatograph eluted in methanol, and tested after drying and resolubilization in buffer. A solid phase assay was used wherein ganglioside is attached to the plate, incubated with the antibody preparation, and then, after washing, reacted with ^{125}I-labeled protein A (Laccetti *et al.*, 1984). As noted, the reactivity appears to coincide with a minor ganglioside component barely visible in the total human ganglioside extract but more apparent in the disialoganglioside fraction. (Right) Autoradiography of thin layer chromatograms of total human thyroid gangliosides (lanes 1–4) or disialoganglioside fraction (lanes 5–7). Plates were washed and sequentially treated with the noted antibodies, followed by normal mouse or human serum and ^{125}I-labeled anti-human IgG (for 307H6 or Graves IgG), ^{125}I-labeled anti-mouse IgG (for 22A6, 52A8, or 11E8), or ^{125}I-labeled cholera toxin (CT). In lane 4, the ganglioside preparation was pretreated with neuraminidase before chromatography.

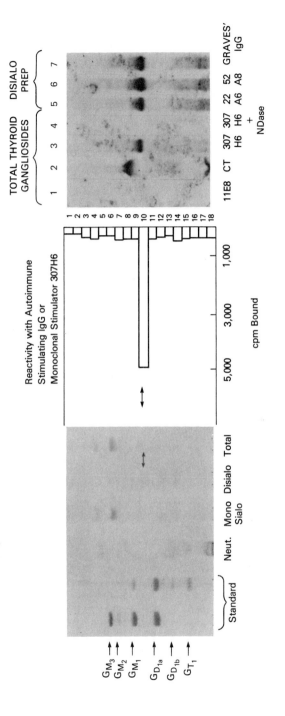

TOTAL THYROID GANGLIOSIDES   DISIALO PREP

1   2   3   4   5   6   7

11E8   CT   307   307   22   52   GRAVES'
             H6   H6   A6   A8   IgG
                  +
                 NDase

Reactivity with Autoimmune
Stimulating IgG or
Monoclonal Stimulator 307H6

cpm Bound

1,000   3,000   5,000

1 2 3 4 5 6 7 8 9 10 11 12 13 14 15 16 17 18

Standard   Neut.   Mono   Disialo   Total
                   Sialo

G_{M_3}
G_{M_2}
G_{M_1}
$G_{D_{1a}}$
$G_{D_{1b}}$
G_{T_1}

V. TSH RECEPTOR STRUCTURE AND TSH-RELATED
GROWTH ACTIVITY

As noted in the introduction, TSH is an important stimulator of thyroid cell growth. It would appear from monoclonal antibody data that the receptor structure defined previously is also used to signal growth activity and that maximal growth expression requires both receptor components because they can perturb independent signal mechanisms. Evidence for these conclusions is as follows.

All "stimulators" of adenylate cyclase activity also stimulate the growth activity of FRTL-5 rat thyroid cells measured either as cell number or as [³H]thymidine uptake (Table VI). All "mixed" antibodies also stimulate growth activity but have three- to tenfold higher ratios of growth to adenylate cyclase stimulatory activity when normalized to equivalence with respect to adenylate cyclase activity, i.e., when each is set to give comparable cAMP stimulatory activity over a linear dose–response region. "Inhibitor" antibodies can be, surprisingly, either inhibitors of TSH-stimulated growth as well as adenylate cyclase activity (122G3, 59C9) or stimulators of growth despite their ability to inhibit TSH-stimulated adenylate cyclase activity (129H8). Though these data clearly state that the same structural TSH receptor is used to signal growth as well as adenylate cyclase activity, differences in signal coupling seemed an intuitive likelihood.

The following observations suggested that this is true. TSH growth activity can be partially inhibited by indomethacin (Table VI); indomethacin is a cyclooxygenase inhibitor that limits arachidonic acid processing to form derivatives such as prostaglandins. Indomethacin also partially inhibits the mixed antibodies 208F7 and 52A8 (Table VI). It has, however, no affect on stimulator antibodies such as 307H6, yet it completely inhibits 129H8 activity. In short, it would appear that the TSH-modulated growth activity of the thyroid cell involves both adenylate cyclase and phospholipid modulation signals (see later for further details). Further, phospholipid signaling seems to be linked more to the glycoprotein receptor component; adenylate cyclase action, to the ganglioside component.

Before turning from this point, the clinical implications of this phemonemon are already becoming evident. Thus, growth-promoting TSAbs as well as cyclase stimulatory TSAbs exist in patients and can be present at different levels. Patients can have high levels of a growth-promoting TSAb but low levels of cyclase stimulatory activity, equal levels of each, or, conversely, high cyclase stimulatory TSAb activity and low-growth TSAb activity (Valente *et al.*, 1983b). Success of medical therapy may be better correlated with the disappearance of both; growth TSAbs may be more persistent; and goiter may be a reflection of the growth TSAb.

TABLE VI

EFFECT OF MONOCLONAL ANTIBODIES TO THE TSH RECEPTOR ON THE GROWTH OF
FRTL-5 THYROID CELLS AS MEASURED BY RADIOLABELED THYMIDINE UPTAKE INTO DNA

Monoclonal antibody	Alone	[³H]thymidine uptake[a] (cpm/μg DNA)	
		+TSH 1×10^{-10} M	+Indomethacin
None	1,600	6,700	1,400
N1 IgG	1,450	5,900	1,510
TSH 1×10^{-10} M	6,800	—	3,500
1×10^{-9} M	31,000	—	14,800
"Stimulating" antibodies			
22A6	6,800	11,200	6,900
307H6	8,700	13,200	9,200
"Mixed" antibodies			
52A8	18,500	25,100	7,400
208F7	17,200	23,800	6,500
"Inhibiting" antibodies			
122G3	1,350	2,300	1,460
59C9	1,410	1,900	1,390
129H8	5,600	14,200	1,480

[a] 72-Hour thymidine uptake measured as detailed by Valente *et al.* (1983b).

It seems possible, based on the monoclonal antibody studies, that thyroid stimulation in Graves' disease may, therefore, result from a small goiter potently stimulated by a 307H6-type antibody to actively release thyroid hormones; from a larger goiter, caused by a 129H8 antibody, whose release of excess thyroid hormone reflects the existence of an excess of responsive tissue; or from a combination of both types of antibodies. It is also possible that the presence of (1) a mixed antibody, or (2) a mixture of an autoantibody with the characteristics of 129H8, (i.e., an antibody to the glycoprotein component of the TSH receptor that is a growth stimulator and an antibody that is a cAMP stimulator such as 307H6) would result in two independent and potent stimulators being present simultaneously and, most likely, the most severe cases of thyroid stimulation. In the last mixture, it must be remembered (see previous discussion) that the 129H8 autoantibody capable of inhibiting TSH binding and function would have no inhibitory.action on cAMP stimulatory activity since inhibition of TSAb activity requires a <10,000-fold higher activity coefficient than inhibition of TSH (Fig. 4); the fundamental basis for this is the interaction of the different autoantibodies with distinct sites of the TSH receptor.

VI. TSH RECEPTOR REGULATION OF THE
ADENYLATE CYCLASE SIGNAL

A. REGULATION OF ADENYLATE CYCLASE ACTIVITY VIA ADP
RIBOSYLATION

Current evidence (Rodbell, 1980; Ross and Gilman, 1980; Katada and Ui, 1982; Manning and Gilman, 1983; Hildebrandt *et al.*, 1984) in nonthyroidal systems indicates that the adenylate cyclase complex includes a catalytic unit, two regulatory units of which one is stimulatory (N_S) and one is inhibitory (N_I), and a γ subunit (Fig. 1). Each regulatory subunit is believed to have a GTP binding site and GTPase activity that is important in its expression, and each is composed of two different-sized subunits making up a complex of ~75–80K. It is presumed that GTP binding to the regulatory subunits, regulated by GTP hydrolysis and a GTP–GDP exchange reaction, is important in regulatory subunit activation of the adenylate cyclase catalytic unit. The N_S subunit that binds GTP is ~40–42K, although subunits of ~45, 48, and 52K have been noted to be associated with N_S identification; it is ADP ribosylated by cholera toxin. The N_I subunit that binds GTP is presumed to be 39–41K; it is ADP ribosylated by pertussis toxin. The further presumption is that ADP ribosylation modulates the GTP binding, GTPase activity, or GTP–GDP exchange as its means of modulating adenylate cyclase activity. Both N_S and N_I are argued to have a similar, and possibly identical, 35K subunit.

In general, a two-subunit regulatory system such as this could achieve activation or inhibition of adenylate cyclase activity by several mechanisms. Thus, increased adenylate cyclase activity can result from an increase in stimulatory subunit (N_S) expression or a decrease in inhibitory subunit (N_I) activity. Conversely, decreased adenylate cyclase activity can result from a decrease in N_S expression or an increase in N_I activity. Mechanistically, each regulatory subunit could influence the catalytic subunit directly, or, alternatively, the inhibitory subunit can modulate the activity of the stimulatory subunit to transmit its effect on catalytic cAMP conversion.

The thyroid adenylate cyclase complex is stimulated by GTP and fluoride (Wolf and Cook, 1973; Asbury *et al.*, 1978). The complex has an N_S subunit as evidenced by cholera toxin ADP ribosylation (Goldhammer *et al.*, 1980; DeWolf *et al.*, 1980, 1981a,b,c; Vitti *et al.*, 1982), an N_I subunit as evidenced by pertussis toxin ADP ribosylation (see later), and two separate GTP binding sites that are on different ~40K units (Goldhammer and Wolff, 1982).

As noted earlier in the monoclonal antibody data, the ganglioside component of the TSH receptor has been linked most directly with adenylate cyclase stimulation. The ganglioside, G_{M1}, has been similarly involved in the cholera toxin receptor. Thus it is argued that, after interacting with the B subunit of cholera toxin, G_{M1} allows the cholera toxin A subunit to enter the membrane bilayer where its ADP ribosyltransferase activity catalyzes the ADP ribosylation of the N_S protein using NAD as a substrate (Bennett and Cuatrecasas, 1977; Holmgren, 1978; Ross and Gilman, 1980; Gill, 1977; Moss and Vaughan, 1979).

Since it is clear that mutant cells without the ganglioside G_{M1} are insensitive to cholera toxin, whereas the A subunit is still able to increase adenylate cyclase activity in membranes from these cells, the minimal ganglioside role must be to allow the A subunit to enter the bilayer to interact with the N_S regulatory protein. If one presumes that a major role of the ganglioside component of the cholera toxin receptor is to internalize the A subunit of the toxin to effect the ADP ribosylation reaction, a major presumptive role for the ganglioside in the TSH receptor emerges. It is important to note, however, that internalization does not mean into the cytoplasm, but rather into the hydrophobic plane of the membrane bilayer. Internalization also does not necessarily require subunit separation.

Studies that have compared the mechanism of action of TSH with cholera toxin have shown that TSH has no ADP ribosylation activity (Moss *et al.*, 1978). However, other studies (DeWolf *et al.*, 1981a,b,c; Filetti *et al.*, 1981; Filetti and Rapoport, 1981; Vitti *et al.*, 1982) have shown that TSH can perturb a membrane-associated ADP ribosyltransferase that carries out this same reaction or, in the absence of a receptor, the conversion of NAD to free ADP ribose and nicotinamide. In short, TSH, like cholera toxin, can alter ADP ribosylation activity. Since this appears to be linked to regulation of adenylate cyclase activity as will be shown later, the role of the ganglioside becomes, in the case of TSH and cholera toxin, similar, i.e., to bring a portion of the TSH molecule into the bilayer where it can perturb membrane enzymes (Kohn 1978; DeWolf *et al.*, 1981a,b,c; Kohn *et al.*, 1981, 1982a,b, 1983a,b, 1984a,b). The physical basis for this process is presumed to be the formation of the anhydrous complex between the hormone or toxin and the oligosaccharide moiety of the ganglioside. By excluding water from the interface of the ligand–receptor complex (Aloj *et al.*, 1979a) membrane penetration is facilitated, and interactions involving an ADP-ribosylation activity and membrane components of the adenylate system ensue.

Evidence that the TSH-modulated ADP ribosylation reaction is important in regulating thyroidal adenylate cyclase activity is several fold (DeWolf *et al.*, 1981a,b,c; Vitti *et al.*, 1982; Kohn *et al.*, 1982b). First, the TSH-modulated ADP ribosylation reaction is cAMP independent and is rapid, preceding in time the ability of TSH to stimulate adenylate cyclase activity. Second, the β subunit of TSH can coordinately inhibit the TSH-stimulated adenylate cyclase and ADP ribosylation activities. Third, conditions can be uncovered in normal membrane preparations wherein NAD increases basal and TSH-stimulated adenylate cyclase activity. Fourth, a thyroid tumor 1-5G, which has a high basal adenylate cyclase activity and limited stimulatory activity by TSH or cholera toxin, has a very high basal NAD hydrolysis activity, an activity presumably reflecting the ADP ribosylation half-reaction. The addition of high NAD concentrations to 1-5G membrane preparations resensitizes the membranes to TSH and cholera toxin regulation of adenylate cyclase activity. Fifth, thyroid cells whose adenylate cyclase response has been desensitized by chronic TSH treatment (i.e., cells which no longer exhibited increased levels of cAMP with further additions of TSH) could be resensitized if incubated with nicotinamide or arginine-L-methyl ester (Filetti *et al.*, 1981). Since these are, respectively, an end product and an artificial substrate of the ADP ribosylation reaction and are known to be effective inhibitors of the ADP riboxylation activity in thyroid membranes, the importance of the system in regulating adenylate cyclase activity was implied. Finally, and most important in this circumstantial array, is the nature of TSH-dependent ADP-ribosylated proteins in the thyroid membrane preparations.

Using bovine thyroid membranes and high (1 mM) NAD concentrations (Vitti *et al.*, 1982), it was noted that TSH increased the incorporation of [^{32}P]ADP ribose into several membrane components, including approximately 40,000 molecular weight components that appeared to be ADP ribosylated by cholera toxin and were believed to be related to the regulatory subunit of the adenylate cyclase complex. Though this suggested, initially, that TSH-modulated ADP ribosylation might, like cholera toxin, act via N_S, several problems suggested that this hypothesis was not necessarily correct. First, the identification of N_I with a 40K unit required resolution of this issue, i.e., was control through N_S or N_I? Second, in human thyroid membranes, TSH and cholera toxin exhibit additive adenylate cyclase action, a phenomenon which suggested different mechanisms rather than a common one (Field *et al.*, 1979; Zakarija *et al.*, 1980).

In studies of human membranes under conditions wherein there was additive cholera toxin and TSH stimulation of adenylate cyclase activity, it was indeed evident that there was also additive stimulation of ADP ribosylation activity (Fig. 8A). Further, when specific ADP-ribosylated proteins were evaluated, under conditions where both TSH and cholera toxin were cyclase stimulating, a different primary action of cholera toxin and TSH was evident. Thus, the data showed that in the human thyroid system, a ~140K GTP binding component was the major protein initially ADP ribosylated by cholera toxin (Fig. 8A). Appropriate *in vitro* conditions, i.e., changing to phosphate buffers, or *in vivo* treatment, did generate small amounts of an ADP-ribosylated 40–42K protein, but the 140K component dominated. In contrast to cholera toxin, and despite evidence that the 140K component may be ADP ribosylated in the first seconds and after prolonged (>30 minutes) exposure to TSH, the major TSH effect appeared to be to initially decrease (Fig. 8) the basal ADP ribosylation of the 140K component and increase the ADP ribosylation of smaller 35K, 40–42K, 48K, and 52K membrane proteins. The major 35K ADP-ribosylated product also seemed linked to a GTP site since GTP affinity chromatography of ADP-ribosylated preparations saw its recovery in Gpp(NH)p eluates (Table VII).

These data raised many new questions. It appeared that not only would there have to be different modulation of regulatory subunit activity, but also different processing activity (i.e., of the 140K GTP binding component) as well as different sites of ADP ribosylation. Fortunately, the answers appear to be emerging in studies of FRTL-5 thyroid cells. Thus, it was noted that TSH was a superagonist of adenylate cyclase activity when present with forskolin (Fig. 9A). This phenomenon had been noted as a characteristic feature of receptors wherein the ligand was an active modulator not of N_S, but of N_I (Seamon and Daly, 1982). The idea emerged, therefore, that TSH modulated not N_S, but N_I subunit action. Support for this view is as follows. First, pertussis toxin stimulates adenylate cyclase activity in FRTL-5 cells (Fig. 9B) and, like TSH in these cells, is a "super-agonist" in the presence of forskokin. Second, TSH and pertussis adenylate cyclase stimulation are not additive, but rather can be inhibitory (Fig. 9C). Thus, pertussis pretreatment prevents TSH stimulation of FRTL-5 cell cyclase activity, and, conversely, TSH pretreatment prevents pertussis action. Third, pertussis ADP ribosylates a ~40K thyroid membrane protein *in vitro* and *in vivo* (Fig. 8B); treatment *in vivo* or *in vitro* with TSH in these cells ADP ribosylates a ~120K protein. *In vivo* pertusis prevents *in vitro* ADP ribosylation of the ~120K protein by TSH, and, conversely, *in vivo* TSH prevents *in vitro* ADP ribosylation of the ~40K pertussis-modulated N_I unit (Fig. 8C).

In sum, then, it appears that TSH-stimulated adenylate cyclase and ADP ribosylation activities appear linked to pertussis- stimulated adenylate cyclase and ADP ribosylation activities as similarly active and as mutual inhibitors, whereas the respective TSH and cholera toxin actions are additive. This would indicate that the current best hypothesis is that TSH modulation of adenylate cyclase activity by ADP ribosylation involves modulation of N_I activity. The current best hypothesis would equally predict that the action of all the ligands will require a more complex model wherein a 120–140K, GTP binding protein may be a precursor ADP-ribosylated substrate common in each case and wherein different sites of ADP ribosylation as well as different processing or deribosylation reactions occur. Obviously,

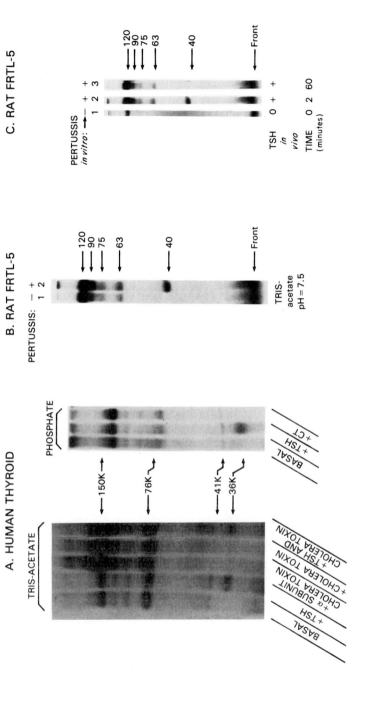

A. HUMAN THYROID

PHOSPHATE

TRIS-ACETATE

150K
76K
41K
36K

BASAL
+TSH
+CT

BASAL
+TSH
+α SUBUNIT
CHOLERA TOXIN
+TSH AND
CHOLERA TOXIN
CHOLERA TOXIN

B. RAT FRTL-5

PERTUSSIS: − +
1 2

120
90
75
63
40
Front

TRIS-
acetate
pH = 7.5

C. RAT FRTL-5

PERTUSSIS:
in vitro: − + +
1 2 3

120
90
75
63
40
Front

TSH
in
vivo
0 + +

TIME 0 2 60
(minutes)

the mechanisms by which these events occur will require much additional work, but, as a first approximation, they predict that the model wherein N_I regulates N_S to perturb the cyclase catalytic unit is a more likely possibility than that of independent interactions with the catalytic unit.

As suggested earlier, ADP ribosylation has been related to the ability of TSH to desensitize the adenylate cyclase response. Membranes from functioning thyroid cells have been shown to have *low* ADP ribosyltransferase but *high* NAD glycohydrolase activities (DeWolf *et al.*, 1981a,b,c; Vitti *et al.*, 1982); NAD glycohydrolase activity can be viewed as the half-reaction of ADP ribosyltransferase wherein water is substituted for an acceptor protein. In contrast to these results, membranes from nonfunctioning thyroid cells have a *high* ADP ribosyltransferase but a *low* NAD glycohydrolase activity. Both membrane preparations have an enzyme activity analogous to snake venom phosphodiesterase capable of removing AMP from monoADP-ribosylated acceptor molecules (DeWolf *et al.*, 1981a,b,c; Vitti *et al.*, 1982). Evidence also exists which shows that the different ADP ribosyltransferase activities in membranes from functioning and nonfunctioning thyroid cells really reflect a low level of available membrane acceptor in the functioning

---

FIG. 8. (A) Fluorographic analysis of ADP-ribosylated proteins in human thyroid membranes exposed for 30 minutes to no exogenous ligand (basal), to TSH, or to cholera toxin (or the α subunit of cholera toxin). 60 μg of membrane were incubated in the presence of 10 μM NAD containing 2×10^6 cpm [adenylate-^{32}P]NAD, 4 mM GTP, and 10 mM thymidine. The buffer was either 0.1 M Tris-acetate, pH 7.5, or 20 mM potassium phosphate, pH 7.2, as noted. When present, TSH and cholera toxin (or its α subunit) were 1 to 4×10^{-7} M concentrations. After 30 minutes of incubation in Tris-acetate buffer as noted, the reaction was arrested by the addition of 10% trichloroacetic acid. The trichloroacetic acid pellets were applied to a 10% acrylamide gel. The total counts applied to the gel were: basal, 2200; TSH, 3400; cholera toxin, 3500. Fluorographs were developed for 7 days. In the phosphate buffer incubations, a similar procedure was used. The counts in the TSH and cholera toxin samples were substantially the same, whereas the basal sample had 2600 cpm. Data were the same if the assay mixtures included 6 mM Mg^{2+} acetate, 0.2 mM cAMP, 2 mM dithiothreitol, 0.3 mM ATP, and ATP-regenerating system. (B) Fluorographic analysis of ADP-ribosylated proteins in rat FRTL-5 cell membranes from cells treated with TSH for 2 minutes *in vivo*. The assay mixture (~50 μl) included 50 μg of membrane protein, 0.1 M Tris-acetate, pH 7.5, 1 mM ATP, 20 mM dithiothreitol, and 12 pmoles of [adenylate-^{32}P]NAD (2.5×10^6 cpm). The incubation was carried out at 37°C for 15 minutes, and it was stopped by addition of cold phosphate buffered saline (PBS) (1 ml). Sample number 2 was incubated in the presence of 1×10^{-7} M pertussis toxin. The pellets, obtained after washing the samples twice in cold PBS, were resuspended in Laemmli buffer, incubated overnight at room temperature, and applied to a 10% acrylamide gel. Fluorographs were developed for 7–8 days. The ~40K protein ADP ribosylated in the pertussis sample is N_I. (C) Fluorographic analysis of FRTL-5 membranes from cells not treated with TSH (lane 1) and cells treated with TSH for 2 minutes (lane 2) and 1 hour (lane 3). Samples in lanes 2 and 3 were treated with pertussis *in vitro* as previously. The long-term TSH treatment *in vivo* prevents pertussis labeling of N_I (40K band) *in vitro*.

TABLE VII

GTP-Agarose Adsorption of [32P]ADP Ribosylated Human Membrane Components Formed in the "Basal" State or in 5-Minute Incubations with TSH ($\sim 1 \times 10^{-7}$ M), Cholera Toxin ($\sim 2 \times 10^{-7}$ M), or Pertussis Toxin ($\sim 1 \times 10^{-7}$ M) Using Tris-Acetate Buffer and Conditions that Are Optimal for Adenylate Cyclase Stimulation

Incubation components	Total counts applied[a] (cpm)	Counts bound GTP-agarose beads		Net GTP-related binding (cpm)	Counts eluted by Gpp(NH)p (cpm)	Molecular weight of labeled membrane protein[c] (cpm)
		Cts bound (cpm)	Cts bound in the presence of of Gpp(NH)p[b] (cpm)			
Basal	60,000	11,000	5,000	6,000	4,000	140K
+TSH	60,000	37,500	8,000	29,500	19,400	140K, 35K[d]
+Pertussis	60,000	29,000	7,000	22,000	15,600	40K
+Cholera toxin	60,000	27,000	6,000	21,000	15,800	140

[a] Equal number of counts were applied by pooling up to 20–30 membrane pellets from individual incubations. Radiolabeled components were solubilized by Lubrol.

[b] Radiolabeled counts that could bind were evaluated for specific GTP binding by examining the number of counts bound in duplicate experiments when samples were incubated with beads in the presence of 0.2 mM Gpp(NH)p.

[c] Molecular weights in Laemli SDS gels.

[d] Minor and major components, respectively.

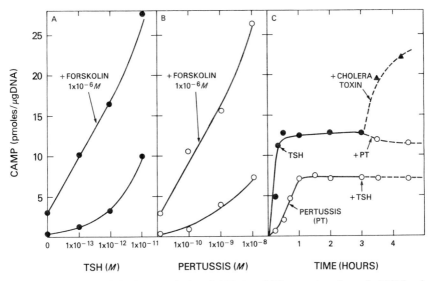

FIG. 9. Effect of forskolin $(1 \times 10^{-6} M)$ on (A) TSH- and (B) pertussis-enhanced cAMP levels in FRTL-5 thyroid cells. Effect (C) of pertussis addition on cAMP levels of TSH-stimulated FRTL-5 thyroid cells (●———●) and, conversely, effect of TSH on pertussis-stimulated FRTL-5 thyroid cells (○———○). The mixture period in both cases (○- - -○) shows no increase, whereas cholera toxin $(1 \times 10^{-9} M)$ can cause an increase when added to TSH-treated cells (▲- - -▲). Assays were performed in FRTL-5 cells without TSH for 7 days, as detailed by Valente *et al.* (1983b).

cell preparation and a high level of acceptor in the nonfunctioning cell preparation (DeWolf *et al.*, 1981a,b,c). In short, the difference is not in the enzyme, but in the acceptor and the "deribosylation" reaction. It is suggested that the "desensitized" state of functioning thyroid cells could thus be accounted for by correlating the following: a high level of ADP-ribosylated N_I acceptor, a high cAMP level, a stable functioning state, and a lack of responsiveness to additional amounts of TSH because of nonavailable free N_I acceptor, a requirement to synthesize new N_I before sensitization returns. This scheme is readily integrated into the speculative model of receptor regulation of adenylate cyclase activity via ADP ribosylation as the end sequence of the activation process.

B. REGULATION OF TSH RECEPTOR–MODULATED ADENYLATE CYCLASE ACTIVITY VIA MEMBRANE LIPID MODULATION

As will be noted in detail as follows, TSH can perturb membrane polyphosphoinositide metabolism as well as phosphatidylinositol synthesis and turnover by a non-cAMP mechanism (Aloj, 1982; Fains, 1982; Michell,

1975). Other ligands, norepinephrine and forskolin, can also do this even at concentrations or under conditions where each has no intrinsic ability to elevate cAMP levels in cells (Totsuka *et al.*, 1983; Weiss *et al.*, 1984c). This phenomenon may be important in regulating TSH-stimulated cyclase activity by affected receptor coupling mechanisms or in altering the "set point" sensitivity of the system to ADP ribosylation. Thus, as noted earlier, forskolin is a potentiator of TSH activity under conditions where it effects lipid and cyclic GMP but not cAMP changes (C. M. Rotella and R. Toccafondi, manuscript submitted). In an opposite regulatory mode, phentolamine can inhibit the TSH-stimulated cyclase response in FRTL-5 cells. Since norepinephrine perturbs polyphosphoinositide metabolism in these cells (Kohn *et al.*, 1984a), the phentolamine action may occur via the modulation of membrane lipids. This area is only now being explored in biochemical terms.

C. Coupling of TSH Receptor–Mediated Regulation of the Adenylate Cyclase System to a Functional Cell Response

TSH modulation of iodide transport is a well-recognized cAMP-mediated, receptor-mediated process (Wilson *et al.*, 1968; Tong, 1975; Halmi *et al.*, 1960; Williams and Malayan, 1975; Weiss *et al.*, 1984a,b,c). In FRTL-5 thyroid cells, the TSH-stimulated cAMP response is maximal in 15 minutes; however, TSH-induced iodide transport, which can be equally induced by cAMP, requires 60 hours to reach maximal levels (Weiss *et al.*, 1984a,b,c) (Fig. 10). The iodide transport response requires TSH to be present only for several hours and is blocked by cycloheximide; i.e., cAMP-dependent protein synthesis is important to achieve the cell response. No simple correlation of iodide transport exists with other overall protein synthesis or overall protein phosphorylation (Weiss *et al.*, 1984a,b,c) (Fig. 10).

Recently (Marcocci *et al.*, 1984), the sequence of TSH-induced protein

---

Fig. 10. (A) Iodide uptake stimulated by TSH (and mimicked by dibutyryl cAMP) in FRTL-5 thyroid cells (i) can be blocked by cyclohexamide; (ii) is not simply related to TSH-stimulated increases in cAMP levels, total protein synthesis, or total protein phosphorylation; and (iii) requires TSH to be present only for the first 2–4 hours to achieve a maximal response at 60 hours (Weiss *et al.*, 1984b). (B) TSH-stimulated protein synthesis studies in FRTL-5 thyroid cells can separate individual proteins into two general pools, those whose maximal synthetic rate is at 8 hours and those with a maximal rate at ~24 hours. Proteins #1 and #2 in this figure are representative of the two groups. Data are taken from SDS gels of cells equilibrium labeled with [³H]leucine and pulsed (30 minutes) with [³⁵S]methionine at different times after TSH addition. Data are presented as a ratio of the two radiolabels and cannot be accounted for by altered degradation or pool sizes. Data are from Cohen *et al.* (1983) American Thyroid Association. (C) Effect of actinomycin D on iodide efflux when added at different times after TSH. (D) Theoretic schema to account for results using a translation model.

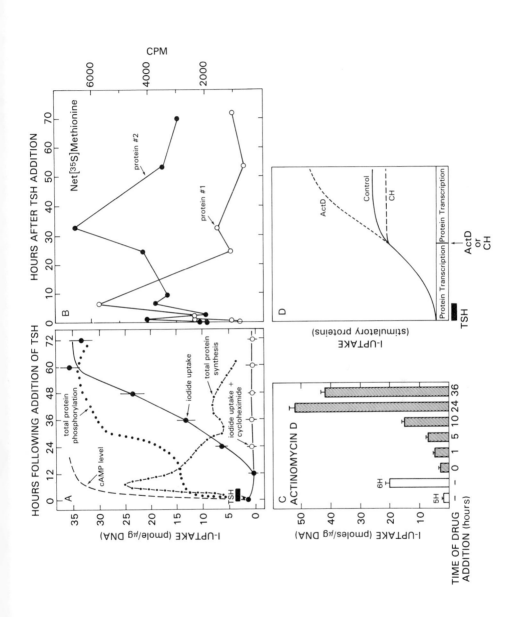

synthesis was evaluated in FRTL-5 thyroid cells in terms of specific proteins. To ensure that true protein synthesis was measured, cells were equilibrium labeled with [^{3}H]leucine and pulsed at different times after TSH addition by a 30 minute exposure to [^{35}S]methionine. It was evident on polyacrylamide gels that TSH induced the synthesis of a whole variety of proteins, thyroglobulin-induced biosynthesis, for example, being only one part of the overall response, not a unique synthetic product. On further analysis, however, it was recognized that there were two waves of protein synthesis (Fig. 10B). Thus, a group of proteins was synthesized with a rate that was maximal at ~8 hours; a second and different group of proteins was synthesized with a rate that was maximal at ~24 hours. Cyclohexamide or actinomycin D at early times, wherein the synthesis of the first wave of proteins was blocked, also blocked the induction of the transport system (Fig. 10B). In contrast, actinomycin D at 24 hours increased the uptake of iodide two-to fivefold over normal TSH-stimulated controls (Fig. 10C). This phenomenon is blocked by cyclohexamide, indicating that "super induction" requires protein synthesis and is not simply an activation process. The properties of iodide transport are normal; hence, this is not a new system coming into play. It is an effect on influx, not efflux (Marcocci *et al.*, 1984).

These data indicate that normally TSH must regulate at a messenger RNA (mRNA) level (Fig. 10D). As one possibility, there must be a unique stabilization of the mRNA for the iodide porter or another key component of the transport system. Alternatively, there is a sequential induction of messages. The second mRNA results in the formation of an inhibitor able to prevent the reading of the mRNA first component, able to cause mRNA degradation, or able to cause the degradation of the iodide porter. The key point with respect to the TSH receptor–cAMP coupling mechanism is that there must be a means to regulate at the transcription or translation level of one of the most important functional expressions of TSH activity, iodide transport. The mechanism of this coupling process at the level of transcription or translation should provide an area of intense research in the near future.

VII. THYROTROPIN RECEPTOR–MEDIATED SIGNAL PROCESSES INVOLVING PHOSPHOLIPID MODULATION

A. The Phosphatidylinositol Turnover Phenomenon

TSH is well known to increase the turnover of phosphatidylinositol in the thyroid (Michell, 1975; Aloj, 1982; Fains, 1982). The phospholipid effect is unrelated to the ability of TSH to elevate cAMP, but rather appears to be linked to a separate effect of TSH on cytosol Ca^{2+} since it is mimicked by muscarinic cholinergic agonists (Boeynaems *et al.*, 1979); and the ionophore A-23187. A schematic view (Michell, 1975; Putney, 1978; Berridge, 1984) of polyphosphoinositide and phosphatidylinositol turnover would suggest that Ca^{2+} released by the breakdown of tripolyphoinositol (TPI) to di-polyphosphoinositol (DPI) is an activator of phosphatidylinositol breakdown to yield arachidonic acid. The process results in the formation of products that can activate growth either directly or via a phorbol ester–sensitive kinase implicated in the regulation of growth (Fig. 11). In the thyroid, as in other tissues, arachidonic acid is the source of prostaglandins via a cyclooxygenase pathway or of leukotrienes via a lipoxygenase pathway (Boeynaems *et al.*, 1979; Dumont *et al.*, 1978; Igarashi and Kondo, 1981).

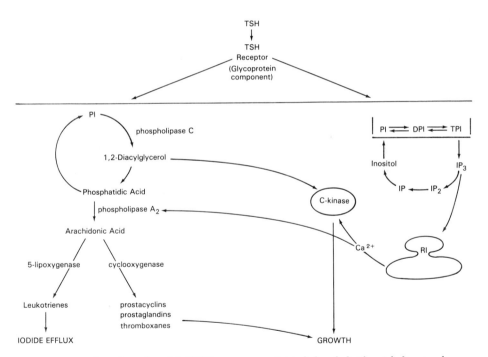

Fig. 11. A hypothetical model of TSH receptor–modulated phospholipid metabolism involving currently known complexities of the polyphosphoinositide (DPI and TPI) and PI turnover schemes. The release of inositol triphosphate (IP_3) as a signal to release Ca^{2+} from a pool in an endoplasmc RI pool is a currently proposed path in other systems; this phenomenon has not yet been seen in the thyroid. Similarly, the C-kinase role in growth is not clear in the thyroid.

B. TSH Receptor–Mediated Changes in Ion Flux and the Phospholipid Signal System

Electrochemical ion gradients play a role in receptor-mediated ligand signaling and the functional response of target cells (Grollman, 1982). One effect of TSH stimulation of thyroid tissue is an alteration in membrane potential as measured directly using microelectrodes or using a biochemical probe for membrane potential, the lipophilic cation triphenylmethylphosphonium$^+$ (TPMP$^+$) (Grollman, 1982; Grollman *et al.*, 1978a). Thyroid cells grown in culture accumulate TPMP$^+$. TSH stimulates the uptake of the cation three-fold, but this stimulatory effect of TSH on TPMP$^+$ accumulation is abolished if the TSH receptor activity of the cells is destroyed by treatment with trypsin. Analogous effects are observed with thyroid plasma membrane vesicles wherein the adenylate cyclase pathway is not operative (Grollman *et al.*, 1978a). The sum of these two observations links the TSH-ion flux signal to the glycoprotein component of the receptor and to a possible phospholipid perturbation. TPMP$^+$ uptake and stimulation of TSH occurs when NaCl, KCL or Tris-HCl concentration gradients are artifically imposed across the vesicle membrane, which is consistent with TSH either increasing the permeability of the membrane to anions or decreasing its permeability to cations. One cation which accumulates is H$^+$; this accumulation may contribute to the cAMP-dependent iodide uptake process.

A second important action of TSH on ion flux in thyroid tissue or cells, one mimicked by norepinephrine or A23187, is the efflux of iodide from inside to outside the cell. This process is linked to the efflux of iodide through the apical membrane into the follicular lumen since it is associated with the organification process, i.e., the iodination of thyroglobulin stored within the follicular lumen (Maayan *et al.*, 1981).

The TSH effect, like that of norepinephrin and A23187, is Ca^{2+} dependent (Table VIII). It is not mimicked by cAMP (Table VIII); instead, it is associated with TPI breakdown and can be duplicated by arachidonic acid; i.e., a phospholipid metabolic path is the signal mechanism. The iodide efflux by TSH is inhibited by quinicrine, suggesting that a Ca^{2+}-activated phospholipase activity is involved. It is minimally affected by indomethacin, suggesting that arachidonate metabolism via the cyclooxygenase pathway is not involved but is inhibited by agents that would block arachidonate metabolism by lipoxygenases to form leukotrienes. In sum, a TSH receptor–mediated signal for iodide efflux is linked to phosphatidylinositol (PI) turnover and lipoxygenase-dependent metabolism of arachidonic acid to form leukotrienes.

The effect is not seen with the 307H6 monoclonal, but is seen with 52A8 and 129H8, i.e., the glycoprotein receptor component seems to be more

TABLE VIII

PROPERTIES OF TSH EFFECT ON IODIDE EFFLUX^a IN FRTL-5 RAT THYROID CELLS

Ligand	Causes iodide efflux	Ca^{2+} dependent	Stimulates adenylate cyclase	TPI DPI breakdown	Quiniqrine (1×10^{-3} M) inhibition	Indomethacin^b (1×10^{-4} M) inhibition	Eicosatetraynoic^b acid (1×10^{-5} M) inhibition
TSH	+	+	+	+	+	0	+
Norepinephrin	+	+	0	+	+	0	+
A23187	+	+	0	+	+	0	+
8-Bromo cAMP	0	0	−	0	0	0	0
307H6	0	0	+	0	0	0	0
207H8	+	+	+	+	+	0	+
129H8	+	+	0	+	+	0	+

^{a} Measured as described in Weiss et al. (1984c).

^{b} Indomethacin inhibits only the cyclooxygenase pathway; eicosatetraynoic acid inhibits the cyclooxygenase and lipoxygenase pathway.

directly coupled via a phospholipid signal iodide efflux response (Table VIII) as it is in the case of the membrane potential–anion flux response.

VIII. TSH RECEPTOR–MEDIATED GROWTH RELATED TO MULTIPLE SIGNAL COUPLING MECHANISMS

Indomethacin, an inhibitor of arachidonic acid metabolism and prostaglandin biosynthesis, can partially block TSH-stimulated growth (Sluszkiewicz and Pawlikowski, 1980; Rotella *et al.*, 1984) as measured by thymidine uptake in thyroid cells (Table VI); the PI path must thus also be involved in the growth response.

Another agent inhibiting growth is amelioride, an inhibitor of sodium proton exchange (Aloj *et al.*, 1984). This inhibition is associated with a decrease in internal pH of the FRTL-5 thyroid cells; a high internal pH is a phenomenon associated with growth. However, when a series of amelioride analogs are studied, the growth inhibition potency correlates best with another activity of these drugs, inhibition of sodium–Ca^{2+} exchange.

A third parameter that has been linked to thyroid cell growth is the fluidity of the plasma membrane, which is related to lipid composition of the bilayer and which is particularly sensitive to changes in the relative proportions of phospholipids and cholesterol (Beguinot *et al.*, 1983). A widely used technique to measure membrane fluidity involves the use of the hydrophobic fluorescent dye 1,6-diphenyl-1,3,5-hexatriene (DPH), which readily penetrates the lipid region of plasma membranes. The polarization of fluorescence of the dye incorporated into the membranes is inversely related to their fluidity. DPH polarization is low in a growing thyroid cell, i.e., cell growth is associated with high membrane fluidity. After TSH withdrawal, the DPH polarization rapidly increases, i.e., membrane fluidity decreases, with cessation of growth. When TSH is returned to the cell, there is an initial, 2–3-hour duration further increase in polarization (or decrease in membrane fluidity) followed by a decrease in polarization (or increase in fluidity) over the next 24 hours. The second phase can be duplicated by dibutyryl cAMP, yet dibutyryl cAMP, under these conditions, i.e., after cells are deplete of TSH for 10 days, cannot itself initiate cell growth. Since, however, cAMP can eliminate a prolonged 48–72 hour lag phase in TSH-stimulated growth when TSH is returned to hormone-depleted cells after 10 days (Rotella *et al.*, 1984), it is presumed that the cAMP effect and membrane fluidity change is permissive, i.e., it is a necessary, although not sufficient, membrane alteration for growth to occur. Other non-cAMP-mediated, TSH-dependent signals are necessary.

One can address the question of the basis for these changes. Studies using experimental conditions identical to those mentioned previously show that the initial 2–3-hour TSH-induced decrease in fluidity is associated with a decrease in phosphatidylethanolamine (PE) and an increase in phosphatidylcholine (PC) membrane concentrations. Altered lipid methylation has been linked to this phenomenon already by others (Hirata and Axelrod, 1978). The decrease in membrane fluidity that follows TSH depletion is associated with PI changes in the membrane and an increase in cholesterol. TSH-induced membrane lipid changes are thus linked to both TSH-modulated cAMP and phospholipid alterations; they appear necessary but permissive in their linkage to TSH-modulated growth, and they are consistent with alterations in membrane fluidity measurable with DPH fluorescence.

In sum, it is evident (Figs. 1, 2, and 11) that TSH-modulated growth involves a concerted and coregulated modulation of multiple cellular processes involving both cAMP and the phospholipid signal system.

In a previous section of this chapter, data were summarized showing that monoclonal antibodies to the ganglioside and glycoprotein receptor components of the TSH receptor could both stimulate growth in FRTL-5 thyroid cells. When comparing antibodies, it was noted that indomethacin completely inhibited the growth effect of 129H8, partially inhibited that of 208F7 or 52A8, and minimally inhibited that of 307H6 (Table VI). In short, the explanation for the larger spectrum of growth activity associated with the antireceptor monoclonals may best be explained as resulting from linkages of the different receptor components to different signal systems. An interaction with the glycoprotein component (129H8) signals through a pure phospholipid route; an interaction with the ganglioside (307H6) signals through a pure ganglioside route; and an interaction with both receptor components (TSH, 208F7, 52A8) gives a dual, coregulated signal. As anticipated, the growth rate effected by TSH or the mixed antibodies, 208F7 and 52A8, is significantly better than those effected by either 208F7 or 52A8 (Table VI).

In the context of the mechanism of TSH-stimulated growth and a TSH-stimulated adenylate cyclase response, it should be recalled that ADP ribosylation seemed to be involved in regulating the cyclase signal. Since TSH-stimulated growth is a property of cells desensitized to TSH with respect to adenylate cyclase activation, the question of a link between ADP ribosylation and growth can be raised. Thyroid tumors can be formed by chronic stimulation of TSH. These tumors effectively lose their TSH-regulated growth function. Examination of two such tumors (1-5G and 1-8) have demonstrated that they also lose their TSH-regulated ADP ribosyltransferase activity and have instead a tenfold elevated "basal" ADP-ribosylating activity (Kohn et al., 1983a,b, 1984a,b; Aloj et al., 1984). The possibility thus exists that deregulated ADP ribosylation can result in increased growth, i.e., that this reaction is interposed between some or all of the TSH-modulated signal processes involved in growth.

In sum, TSH receptor–mediated growth appears to involve multiple coregulated signals and initial evidence suggests that the individual signals are coupled more directly to one receptor component than to another (Figs. 1 and 2).

IX. TSH RECEPTORS ON NONTHYROID TISSUE

Target tissue specificity as a criterion for identifying a receptor evolved in early studies defining a receptor by its response. Thus, TSH-stimulated adenylate cyclase activity and cAMP increases were measured in the thyroid and in thyroid membrane preparations, but not in liver, brain, muscle, adrenal gland, pancreas, or even target sites for LH and hCG. When binding was the assay of receptor recognition and when receptor solubilization and purification became the issue, this rule was immediately violated.

When TSH binding was used to directly measure the recognition function of the receptor particularly using nonphysiologic conditions, binding to fat cells, lymphocytes, mouse L-cells, neural membranes, and even thyroid fibroblasts could be measured (Kohn, 1978). Since this binding was usually lower than that to the thyroid measured per milligram of membrane protein, it was considered by many to be nonspecific and irrelevant. In fact, however, functional responses to TSH could be measured in several of the nonthyroid tissues mentioned. Thus, fat cells did have a TSH-responsive adenylate cyclase system. In mouse L-cells, the TSH interaction resulted in inhibition of the antiviral effect of interferon (Friedman and Kohn, 1976; Kohn et al., 1976; Friedman et al., 1982). Even in neural tissue, TSH could be shown to undergo retrograde transport as did tetanus toxin (Lee et al., 1979; Habig et al., 1981; Yavin et al., 1981a). In sum, the binding has defined a TSH "receptor" site on nontarget tissues which may be coupled to very different responses in these tissues than the functional response we have historically associated with thyroid action.

Nonthyroidal "receptors" have been argued to be important in the pahtogenesis of exophthalmos and the connective tissue complications of Graves' disease. Thus, in the 1970s, studies of experimental exopthalmos in experimental animal models suggested that there was a TSH receptor response in retroorbital tissues and that the response required both TSH or a derivative of the TSH molecule and an abnormal serum γ-globulin found in exophthalmos patients (Winand and Kohn, 1970, 1972, 1973, 1975a; Kohn and Winand, 1971, 1974, 1975). It was postulated that TSH, or its exophthalmogenic derivative, was the direct effector mediating changes through cAMP elevations and that the γ-globulin was an antibody that enhanced binding of the derivative to retroorbital tissue but decreased binding to the thyroid.

The evidence for this idea was based on the studies that showed the following. TSH was exophthalmogenic in experimental animals. The exophthalmogenic activity of the TSH molecule was associated with a portion of the molecule separate from that responsible for thyroid-stimulating activity. Both the exophthalmogenic derivative of the TSH molecule and/or γ-globulin from the sera of patients could induce experimental exophthalmos. *In vitro* binding studies showed that TSH or its exophthalmogenic derivative were able to bind to retroorbital tissue membranes, and the γ-globulin increased this binding to retroorbital but not to thyroid membranes. TSH or its exophthalmogenic derivative induced adenylate cyclase elevations in retroorbital tissue membranes, and the adenylate cyclase activation occurred at lower hormone concentrations in the presence of the γ-globulin from exophthalmos patients.

The argument that this was a phenomenon relevant only to the animal models, for example to the Harderian glands of the guinea pig or to guinea pig adipose tissue, appeared to be negated by experiments confirming these effects in human retroorbital tissue adipocyte membranes (Mullin *et al.*, 1976c). The major difficulties with this hypothesis were the *in vitro* conditions necessary to demonstrate TSH receptors in human adipocyte membrane preparations, the absence of a TSH derivative in Graves' sera analogous to that created by partial pepsin digestion of bovine TSH *in vitro*, and the absence of any information concerning the "exophthalmogenic" γ-globulin that was present in Graves' sera. Further, until the use of the monoclonal antibody approach cited as follows, there was no simple approach that could be reasonably anticipated to resolve these questions.

The adaption of the monoclonal approach to the mechanism of exophthalmos involved a simple extension of the monoclonal approach to define the TSH receptor in the thyroid and relate it to autoantibodies causative of thyroid hyperfunction. In the first approach, monoclonal antibodies derived from the lymphocytes of patients with Graves' disease without exophthalmos were compared with those of patients with Graves' disease plus exophthalmos. Thymidine uptake in fibroblasts as well as in thyroid cells was the screening tool. One stimulating antibody (307H6) derived from the exophthalmos group was found to stimulate thymidine uptake in fibroblasts (Kohn, 1984) as well or better than in thyroid cells and to also stimulate collagen biosynthesis in these fibroblasts (Fig. 12).

This antibody had all the characteristics of a stimulator antibody to the TSH receptor defined above; its existence as only one of over a dozen TSAb monoclonals and as originating from a patient with exophthalmos clearly established that a unique stimulator TSAb could exist that also stimulated fibroblasts.

A second important observation evolved during the testing of a range of

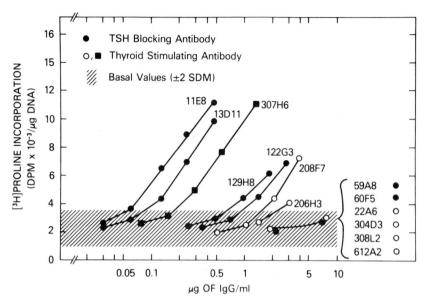

Fig. 12. Effect of different anti–TSH receptor monoclonal antibodies on collagen synthesis in human fibroblasts. Inhibiting antibodies (●) are either mouse IgGs (11E8, 13D11, 59A8) or human IgGs (129H8, 122G3). Stimulating mouse and human antibodies with no activity (○) are compared with 307H6 (■), the one stimulatory TSAb with fibroblast activity. Only 307H6 also has growth stimulatory activity in fibroblasts (Kohn, 1984). The assay measures collagen biosynthesis as incorporation of [^{3}H]proline into collagen over a 24-hour period.

monoclonal antibodies to the TSH receptor that were in the "inhibitory" group. None of the antibodies had growth activity with respect to fibroblasts even if they exhibited growth activity with respect to thyroid cells (129H8). None stimulated cAMP activity in fibroblasts. Surprisingly, however, several had potent activities as stimulators of collagen biosynthesis in fibroblasts (Fig. 12). These data also, therefore, indicated that a select group of TSH receptor antibodies might perturb fibroblast but not thyroid function.

A fundamental question was whether the fibroblast collagen biosynthesis assay is relevant to exophthalmos. In this respect, the following experimental observation suggests an affirmative response. In studies using the same collagen biosynthesis assay involving measurement of [^{3}H[proline incorporation into fibroblasts, IgG preparations from 17 of 20 patients with Graves' ophthalmopathy were shown to stimulate collagen (Kohn, 1984). This activity, correlated with the severity of the ophthalmopathy, was not associated with TSAb activity in a thyroid cell cAMP assay in 50% of cases; it disappeared in remission; and it was not evident in IgGs from 12 normals of 7 of 8 Graves' with no exophthalmos, 4 Hashimoto's, 7 nontoxic goiters, or 4 thyroid atrophy patients. The activity of the "exophthalmogenic" IgGs was comparable to the positive monoclonals discussed previously. Thus, in the same assay, 11E8 and 13D11, the two mouse monoclonal antibodies to the bovine TSH receptor, and 307H6, the human monoclonal to the TSH receptor from a Graves' patient with exophthalmos, were as active in stimulating collagen incorporation of [³H]proline as the most potent IgG preparations from exophthalmos patients, but were active at >1000- to 10,000-fold lower IgG concentrations (0.1–0.5 μg/ml as opposed to >1 mg/ml). In sum, it seemed possible to conclude that (1) the fibroblast collagen biosynthesis assay was a valid means of measuring exophthalmogenic autoantibodies, whether TSAb positive or not, and (2) selected populations of autoantibodies to the TSH receptor could interact with fibroblasts to account for the activity *in vitro*.

These observations have implications with respect to the original hypotheses involving TSH receptor structure on nonthyroidal tissues as well as providing strong support for a TSH receptor involvement in human as well as experimental exophthalmos. First, the TSH receptor on nonthyroid tissues may require non-TSH-related determinants on the antibody molecules since the activity of the 11E8, 13D11, and 307H6 antibodies in the collagen biosynthesis assay cannot be duplicated by TSH alone. In addition, the activity is clearly linked to an antigen common to fibroblast and thyroid membranes since the fibroblast activity of each of these antibodies is lost if the antibody is preadsorbed on thyroid but not on liver or kidney membranes.

It is evident that continued studies in this area should afford a new approach to understanding not only exophthalmos but also the structure, function, and expression of TSH receptors on nonthyroid tissue.

X. SUMMARY

The purpose of this chapter is not to present the final or ultimate model of TSH receptor structure and function. Any model or concept propagated here is simply a current hypothesis for designing further experimental attacks. It is striking that several diverse lines of clinical and biochemical evidence are beginning to be reconciled and are compatible with a complex receptor structure with multiple transmission modes or signals. It is equally interesting that current views of TSH receptor structure have begun to evolve at the molecular level despite problems associated with limited hormone availability, which would allow a coordinate ligand modification approach to resolve the detailed molecular events. This last issue may be resolved by studies of antiidiotypes, i.e., antibodies directed against the "active sites" of the TSH receptor monoclonals. This approach already has reached a promising level of development in several laboratories.

REFERENCES

Adams, D. D. (1981). *Vitam. Horm. (N.Y.)* **38**, 119–203.

Aloj, S. M. (1982). *Horiz. Biochem. Biophys.* **6**, 83–100.

Aloj, S. M., Lee, G., Consiglio, E., Formisano, S., Minton, A. P., and Kohn, L. D. (1979a). *J. Biol. Chem.* **254**, 9030–9039.

Aloj, S. M., Lee, G., Grollman, E. F., Beguinot, F., Consiglio, E., and Kohn, L. D. (1979b). *J. Biol. Chem.* **254**, 9040–9049.

Aloj, S. M., Marcocci, C., De Luca, M. L., Shifrin, S., Grollman, E. F., Valente, W. A., and Kohn, L. D. (1984). *In* "Proceedings of the International Meeting on Peptide Hormones, Biomembranes, and Cell Growth." Plenum, New York (in press).

Ambesi-Impiombato F. S., Parks, L. A. M., and Coon, H. G. (1980). *Proc. Natl. Acad. Sci. U.S.A.* **77**, 3455–3459.

Amir, S. M., Carraway, T. F., Kohn, L. D., and Winand, R. J. (1972). *J. Biol. Chem.* **248**, 4092–4100.

Asbury, R. F., Cook, G. H., and Wolff, J. (1978). *J. Biol. Chem.* **253**, 5286–5292.

Azukizawa, M., Kurtzman, G., Pekary, E., and Hershman, J. M. (1977). *Endocrinology* **101**, 1880–1889.

Beguinot, F., Formisano, S., Rotella, C. M., Kohn, L. D., and Aloj, S. M. (1983). *Biochem. Biophys. Res. Commun.* **110**, 48–54.

Bennett, V., and Cuatrecasas, P. (1977). *In* "The Specificity and Action of Animal, Bacterial, and Plant Toxins" (P. Cuatrecasas and M. F. Greaves, eds.), pp. 3–66. Chapman & Hall, London.

Berridge, M. J. (1984). *Biochem. J.* **220**, 345–360.

Boeynaems, J. M., Waelbroeck, M., and Dumont, J. E. (1979). *Endocrinology* **105**, 988–995.

Cohen, J., Marcocci, C., Philp, N., and Grollman, E. (1985). *Endocrinology* (in press).

DeWolf, M. J. S., Yavin, E., Yavin, Z., Consiglio, E., Vitti, P., Shifrin, S., Epstein, M., Gill, D. L., Grollman, E. F., Lee, G., and Kohn, L. D. (1980). *In* "Radioimmunoassay of Hormones, Proteins, and Enzymes" (E. Albertini, ed.), pp. 3–12. Elsevier/North-Holland, Amsterdam.

DeWolf, M. J. S., Fridkin, M., Epstein, M., and Kohn, L. D. (1981a). *J. Biol. Chem.* **256**, 5481–5488.

DeWolf, M. J. S., Fridkin, M., and Kohn, L. D. (1981b). *J. Biol. Chem.* **256**, 5489–5496.

DeWolf, M. J. S., Vitti, P., Ambesi-Impiombato, F. S., and Kohn, L. D. (1981c). *J. Biol. Chem.* **256**, 12287–12296.

Doniach, D., Bottazzo, G. F., and Khoury, E. L. (1981). *In* "Autoimmune Aspects of Endocrine Disorders" (A. Pinchera, D. Doniach, G. F. Fenzi, and L. Baschieri, eds.), pp. 25–55. Academic Press, London.

Drexhage, H. A., Bottazzo, G. F., and Doniach, D. (1980). *Lancet* **2**, 287–291.

Drexhage, H. A., Bottazzo, G. F., Bitensky, L., Chayen, J., and Doniach, D. (1981). *Nature (London)* **289**, 594–596.

Dumont, J. E. (1971). *Vitam. Horm. (N.Y.)* **29**, 287–412.

Dumont, J. E., Boeynaems, J. M., Decoster, C., Erneux, C., Lamy, F., Lecocq, R., Mockel, J., Unger, J., and Van Sande, J. (1978). *Adv. Cyclic Nucleotide Res.* **9**, 723–734.

Ealey, P. A., Kohn, L. D., Ekins, R. P., and Marshall, N. J. (1984). *J. Clin. Endocrinol. Metab.* **58**, 909–915.

Fains, J. N. (1982). *Horiz. Biochem. Biophys.* **6**, 237–276.

Field, J. B. (1978). *In* "The Thyroid" (S. C. Werner and S. H. Ingbar, eds.), 4th ed., pp. 185–195. Harper & Row, Hagerstown, Maryland.

Field, J. B., Dekker, A., Titus, G., Kerins, M. E., Worden, W., and Frumess, R. (1979). *J. Clin. Invest.* **64**, 265–271.

Filetti, S., and Rapoport, B. (1981). *J. Clin. Invest.* **68**, 461–467.

Filetti, S., Takai, N. A., and Rapoport, B. (1981). *J. Biol. Chem.* **256**, 1072–1075.

Friedman, R. M., and Kohn, L. D. (1976). *Biochem. Biophys. Res. Commun.* **70**, 1078–1084.

Friedman, R. M., Lee, G., Shifrin, S., Ambesi-Impiombato, F. S., Epstein, D., Jacobsen, H., and Kohn, L. D. (1982). *J. Interferon Res.* **2**, 387–400.

Gill, D. M. (1977). *Adv. Cyclic Nucleotide Res.* **8**, 85–118.

Ginsberg, J., Rees Smith, B., and Hall, R. (1982). *Mol. Cell. Endocrinol.* **26**, 95–98.

Goldhammer, A., and Wolff, J. (1982). *Biochim. Biophys. Acta* **701**, 192–199.

Goldhammer, A., Cook, G. H., and Wolff, J. (1980). *J. Biol. Chem.* **255**, 6918–6922.

Grollman, E. F. (1982). *Horiz. Biochem. Biophys.* **6**, 157–174.

Grollman, E. F., Lee, G., Ambesi-Impiombato, F. D., Meldolesi, M. F., Aloj, S. M., Coon, H. G., Kaback, H. R., and Kohn, L. D. (1978a). *Proc. Natl. Acad. Sci. U.S.A.* **74**, 2352–2356.

Grollman, E. F., Lee, G., Ramos, S., Lazo, P. S., Kaback, H. R., Friedman, R. M., and Kohn, L. D. (1978b). *Cancer Res.* **38**, 4172–4185.

Habig, W. H., Kohn, L. D., and Hardegree, M. C. (1981). *In* "Bacterial Vaccines (Seminars on Infectious Diseases Series)" (J. B. Robbins, J. C. Hill, and G. Sadoff, eds.), Vol. 4, pp. 48–53. Thieme-Stratton, New York.

Halmi, N. S., Granner, D. K., Doughman, D. J., Peters, B. H., and Muller, G. (1960). *Endocrinology* **67**, 70–81.

Hildebrandt, J. D., Codina, J., Risinger, R., and Birnbaumer, L. (1984). *J. Biol. Chem.* **259**, 2039–2042.

Hirata, F., and Axelrod, J. (1978). *Nature (London)* **275**, 219–220.

Holmgren, J. (1978). *In* "Bacterial Toxins and Cell Membranes" (J. Jeljaszewicz and T. Waldstrom, eds.), pp. 333–366. Academic Press, New York.

Igarashi, Y., and Kondo, Y. (1981). *Biochem. Biophys. Res. Commun.* **99**, 1045–1052.

Islam, M. N., Briones-Urbana R., Bako, G., and Farid, N. R. (1983). *Endocrinology* **113**, 436–438.

Katada, T., and Ui, M. (1982). *J. Biol. Chem.* **257**, 7210–7216.

Kohn, L. D. (1978). *Recept. Recognition, Ser. A* **5**, 133–212.

Kohn, L. D. (1984). *In* "The Thyroid" (S. Werner, S. Ingbar, and L. Braverman, eds.), 5th ed. Harper & Row, Hagerstown, Maryland (in press).

Kohn, L. D., and Shifrin, S. (1982). *Horiz. Biochem. Biophys.* **6**, 1–42.

Kohn, L. D., and Winand, R. J. (1971). *J. Biol. Chem.* **246**, 6570–6575.

Kohn, L. D., and Winand, R. J. (1974). *Isr. J. Med. Sci.* **10**, 1348–1363.

Kohn, L. D., and Winand, R. J. (1975). *J. Biol. Chem.* **250**, 6503–6508.

Kohn, L. D., Friedman, R. M., Holmes, J. M., and Lee, G. (1976). *Proc. Natl. Acad. Sci. U.S.A.* **73**, 3695–3699.

Kohn, L. D., Consiglio, E., De Wolf, M. J. S., Grollman, E. F., Ledley, F. D., Lee, G., and Morris, N. P. (1980). *In* "Structure and Function of Gangliosides" (L. Svennerholm, P. Mandel, H. Dreyfus, and P. F. Urban, eds.), pp. 487–504. Plenum, New York.

Kohn, L. D., Consiglio, E., Aloj, S. M., Beguinot, F., DeWolf, M. J. S., Yavin, E., Yavin, Z., Meldolesi, M. F., Shifrin, S., Gill, D. L., Vitti, P., Lee, G., Valente, W. A., and Grollman, E. F. (1981). *In* "International Cell Biology 1980–1981" (A. G. Schweiger, ed.), pp. 696–706. Springer-Verlag, Berlin and New York.

Kohn, L. D., Aloj, S. M., Beguinot, F., Vitti, P., Yavin, E., Yavin, Z., Laccetti, P., Grollman, E. F., and Valente, W. A. (1982a). *In* "Membranes and Genetic Diseases" (J. Shepard, ed.), Vol. 97, pp. 55–83. Alan R. Liss, Inc., New York.

Kohn, L. D., Beguinot, F., Vitti, P., Laccetti, P., Valente, W. A., Grollman, E. F., Rotella, C. M., and Aloj, S. M. (1982b). *In* "Membranes in Tumor Growth" (T. Galeotti, A. Cittadini, G. Neri, and S. Papa, eds.), Vol. 7, pp. 389–395. Elsevier Biomedical Press, Amsterdam.

Kohn, L. D., Valente, W. A., Laccetti, P., Cohen, J. L., Aloj, S. M., and Grollman, E. F. (1983a). *Life Sci.* **32**, 15–30.

Kohn, L. D., Yavin, E., Yavin, Z., Laccetti, P., Vitti, P., Grollman, E. F., and Valente, W. A. (1983b). *In* "Monoclonal Antibodies: Probes for the Study of Autoimmunity and Immunodeficiency" (B. I. Haynes and G. S. Eisenbarth, eds.), pp. 221–258. Academic Press, New York.

Kohn, L. D., Tombaccini, D., DeLuca, M. L., Bifulco, M. Grollman, E. F., and Valente, W. A. (1984a). *In* "Receptors and Recognition: Antibodies to Receptors" (M. F. Greaves, ed.), pp. 201–234. Chapman & Hall, London.

Kohn, L. D., Valente, W. A., Laccetti, P., Marcocci, C., DeLuca, M., Ealey, P. A., Marshall, N. J., and Grollman, E. F. (1984b). *In* "Receptor Biochemistry and Methodology—Monoclonal and Antiidiotypic Antibodies: Probes for Receptor Structure and Function" (J. C. Venter, C. M. Fraser, and J. M. Lindström, eds.), pp. 85–116. Alan R. Liss, Inc., New York.

Laccetti, P., Grollman, E. F., Aloj, S. M., and Kohn, L. D. (1983). *Biochem. Biophys. Res. Commun.* **110**, 772–778.

Laccetti, P., Tombaccini, D., Aloj, S. M., Grollman, E. F., and Kohn, L. D. (1984). *In* "Ganglioside Structure Function and Biomedical Potential" (R. Leadeen, R. Yu, M. Rapport, and K. Suzuki, eds.), pp. 355–367. Plenum, New York.

Lee, G., Grollman, E. F., Dyer, S., Beguinot, F., Kohn, L. D., Habig, W. H., and Hardegree, M. C. (1979). *J. Biol. Chem.* **254**, 3826–3832.

Lissitzky, S., Fayet, G., Verrier, B., Hennen, G., and Jacquet, P. (1973). *FEBS Lett.* **29**, 20–24.

Maayan, M. L., Volpert, E. M., and From, A. (1981). *Endocrinology* **109**, 930–934.

Macchia, E., Fenzi, G. F., Monzani, F., Lippi, F., Vitti, P., Grasso, L., Bartalena, L., Baschieri, L., and Pinchera, A. (1981). *Clin. Endocrinol. (Oxford)* **15**, 175–183.

Manley, S. W., Rourke, J. R., and Hawker, R. (1974). *J. Endocrinol.* **63**, 437–448.

Manning, D. R., and Gilman, A. G. (1983). *J. Biol. Chem.* **258**, 7059–7063.

Marcocci, C., Cohen, J., and Grollman, E. F. (1984). *Endocrinology* **115**, 2123–2132.

Meldolesi, M. F., Fishman, P. H., Aloj, S. M., Kohn, L. D., and Brady, R. O. (1976). *Proc. Natl. Acad. Sci. U.S.A.* **73**, 4060–4064.

Michell, R. H. (1975). *Biochim. Biophys. Acta* **415**, 81–147.

Moore, W. V., and Wolff, J. (1974). *J. Biol. Chem.* **249**, 6255–6263.

Moss, J., and Vaughan, M. (1979). *Annu. Rev. Biochem.* **48**, 581–600.

Moss, J., Ross, P. S., Agosto, G., Birken, S., Canfield, R. E., and Vaughan, M. (1978). *Endocrinology* **102**, 415–419.

Mullin, B. R., Fishman, P. H., Lee, G., Aloj, S. M., Ledley, F. D., Winand, R. J., Kohn, L. D., and Brady, R. O. (1976a). *Proc. Natl. Acad. Sci. U.S.A.* **73**, 842–846.

Mullin, B. R., Aloj, S. M., Fishman, P. H., Lee, G., Kohn, L. D., and Brady, R. O. (1976b). *Proc. Natl. Acad. Sci. U.S.A.* **73**, 1679–1683.

Mullin, B. R., Lee, G., Ledley, F. D., Winand, R. J., and Kohn, L. D. (1976c). *Biochem. Biophys. Res. Commun.* **69**, 55–62.

Mullin, B. R., Pacuscka, T., Lee, G., Kohn, L. D., Brady, R. O., and Fishman, P. H. (1978). *Science* **199**, 77–79.

Nitsch, L., and Wollman, S. H. (1980). *Proc. Natl. Acad. Sci. U.S.A.* **77**, 2743–2747.

Ozawa, Y., Chopra, I. J., Solomon, D. H., and Smith, F. (1979a). *Endocrinology* **105**, 1221–1226.

Ozawa, Y., Maciel, R. M. B., Chopra, I. J., Solomon, D. H., and Beall, G. N. (1979b). *J. Clin. Endocrinol. Metab.* **48**, 381–388.

Pekonen, F., and Weintraub, B. D. (1980). *J. Biol. Chem.* **255**, 8121–8127.

Pinchera, A., Fenzi, G., Bertalena, L., Chiovato, L., Marcocci, C., Toccafondi, R., Rotella, C., Aterini, S., and Zonefrati, R. (1980). *In* "Thyroid Research VIII" (J. R. Stockit and S. Nagataki, eds.), pp. 707–710. Australian Academy of Science, Canberra.

Powell-Jones, C. H. J., Thomas, C. G., Jr., and Nayfeh, S. N. (1979). *Proc. Natl. Acad. Sci. U.S.A.* **76**, 705–709.

Putney, J. W., Jr. (1978). *Pharmacol Rev.* **30**, 209–245.

Robbins, J., Rall, J. E., and Gorden, P. (1980). *In* "Metabolic Control and Disease" (P. K. Bondy and L. E. Rosenberg, eds.), pp. 1325–1426. Saunders, Philadelphia, Pennsylvania.

Rodbell, M. (1980). *Nature (London)* **284**, 17–22.

Ross, E. M., and Gilman, A. G. (1980). *Annu. Rev. Biochem.* **49**, 533–564.

Rotella, C. M., Tramontano, D., Kohn, L. D., Aloj, S. M., Ambesi-Impiombato, F. S., and Toccafondi, R. (1985). *Endocrinology* (in press).

Seamon, K. B., and Daly, J. W. (1982). *J. Biol. Chem.* **257**, 11591–11596.

Sluszkiewicz, E., and Pawlikowski, M. (1980). *Endocrinol. Exp.* **14**, 227–235.

Sugenoya, S. A., Kidd, A., Row, V. V., and Volpe, R. (1979). *J. Clin. Endocrinol. Metab.* **48**, 398–402.

Tate, R. L., Schwartz, H. I., Holmes, J. M., Winand, R. J., and Kohn, L. D. (1975a). *J. Biol. Chem.* **250**, 6509–6515.

Tate, R. L., Holmes, J. M., Kohn, L. D., and Winand, R. J. (1975b). *J. Biol. Chem.* **250**, 6527–6533.

Tate, R. L., Winand, R. J., and Kohn, L. D. (1976). *In* "Thyroid Research" (J. Robbins and L. E. Braverman, eds.), pp. 57–60. Exerpta Medica, Amsterdam.

Tong, W. (1975). *In* "Methods in Enzymology" (B. W. O'Malley and J. G. Hardman, eds.), Vol. 37, pp. 256–279. Academic Press, New York.

Totsuka, Y., Ferdows, M. S., Nielsen, T. B., and Field, J. B. (1983). *Biochim. Biophys. Acta* **756**, 319–327.

Valente, W. A., Vitti, P., Yavin, Z., Yavin, E., Rotella, C. M., Grollman, E. F., Toccafondi, R. S., and Kohn, L. D. (1982a). *Proc. Natl. Acad. Sci. U.S.A.* **79**, 6680–6684.

Valente, W. A., Yavin, Z., Yavin, E., Grollman, E. F., Schneider, M. D., Rotella, C., Zonefrati, R., Toccafondi, R. S., and Kohn, L. D. (1982b). *J. Endocrinol. Invest.* **5**, 293–301.

Valente, W. A., Vitti, P., Kohn, L. D., Brandi, M. L., Rotella, C. M., Toccafondi, R., Tramontano, D., Aloj, S. M., and Ambesi-Impiombato, F. S. (1983a). *Endocrinology* **112**, 71–79.

Valente, W. A., Vitti, P., Rotella, C. M., Aloj, S. M., Ambesi-Impiombato, F. S., and Kohn, L. D. (1983b). *N. Engl. J. Med.* **309**, 1028–1034.

Verrier, B., Planells, R., and Lissitzky, S. (1977). *Eur. J. Biochem.* **74**, 243–252.

Vitti, P., De Wolf, M. J. S., Acquaviva, A. M., Epstein, M., and Kohn, L. D. (1982). *Proc. Natl. Acad. Sci. U.S.A.* **79**, 1525–1529.

Weiss, S. J., Philp, N. J., and Grollman, E. F. (1984a). *Endocrinology* **114**, 1090–1099.

Weiss, S. J., Philp, N. J., Ambesi-Impiombato, F. S., and Grollman, E. F. (1984b). *Endocrinology* **114**, 1099–1107.

Weiss, S. J., Philp, N. J., and Grollman, E. F. (1984c). *Endocrinology* **114**, 1108–1113.

Williams, J. A., and Malayan, S. A. (1975). *Endocrinology* **97**, 163–168.

Wilson, B., Raghupathy, E., Tonoue, T., and Tong, W. (1968). *Endocrinology* **83**, 877–884.
Winand, R. J., and Kohn, L. D. (1970). *J. Biol. Chem.* **245**, 967–975.
Winand, R. J., and Kohn, L. D. (1972). *Proc. Natl. Acad. Sci. U.S.A.* **69**, 1711–1715.
Winand, R. J., and Kohn, L. D. (1973). *Endocrinology* **93**, 670–680.
Winand, R. J., and Kohn, L. D. (1975a). *J. Biol. Chem.* **250**, 6522–6526.
Winand, R. J., and Kohn, L. D. (1975b). *J. Biol. Chem.* **250**, 6534–6540.
Wolff, J., and Cook, G. H. (1973). *J. Biol. Chem.* **248**, 350–355.
Wollman, S. H., and Breitman, T. R. (1970). *Endocrinology* **86**, 322–327.
Yamashita, K., and Field, J. B. (1973). *Biochim. Biophys. Acta* **304**, 686–692.
Yavin, E., Yavin, Z., Habig, W. H., Hardegree, M. C., and Kohn, L. D. (1981a). *J. Biol. Chem.* **256**, 7014–7022.
Yavin, E., Yavin, Z., Schneider, M. D., and Kohn, L. D. (1981b). *In* "Monoclonal Antibodies in Endocrine Research" (R. E. Fellows and G. Eisenbarth, eds.), pp. 53–67. Raven Press, New York.
Yavin, E., Yavin, Z., Schneider, M. D., and Kohn, L. D. (1981c). *Proc. Natl. Acad. Sci. U.S.A.* **78**, 3180–3184.
Zakarija, M., and McKenzie, J. M. (1980). *Endocrinology* **107**, 2051–2054.
Zakarija, M., and McKenzie, J. M. (1981). *In* "Autoimmune Aspects of Endocrine Disorders" (A. Pinchera, G. F. Fenzi, L. Baschieri, and D. Doniach, eds.), pp. 83–90. Acadmeic Press, New York.
Zakarija, M., Witte, A., and McKenzie, J. M. (1980). *Endocrinology* **107**, 2045–2050.

Index

Contents of Previous Volumes